Progress in Ambulatory Assessment

Computer-assisted psychological and psychophysiological methods in monitoring and field studies

J. Fahrenberg & M. Myrtek (Editors)

Progress in Ambulatory Assessment

Computer-assisted psychological and psychophysiological methods in monitoring and field studies

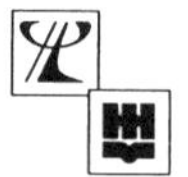

Hogrefe & Huber Publishers
Seattle · Toronto · Bern · Göttingen

Library of Congress Cataloging-in-Publication Data

is available via the Library of Congress Marc Database under the
LC Control Number 2001093610

National Library of Canada Cataloguing in Publication Data

Main entry under title:

Progress in ambulatory assessment : computer-assisted psychological and psychophysiological methods in monitoring and field studies

Includes bibliographical references and index.
ISBN 0-88937-225-X

1. Medicine, Psychosomatic—Research—Methodology. 2. Psychophysiology—Methodology. 3. Ambulatory medical care. 4. Diagnosis—Data processing.
I. Fahrenberg, Jochen II. Myrtek, Michael

BF176.5.P76 2001 616.08 C2001-901983-1

Hogrefe & Huber Publishers

USA:	P.O. Box 2487, Kirkland, WA, 98083-2487 Phone (425) 820-1500, Fax (425) 823-8324
CANADA:	12 Bruce Park Avenue, Toronto, Ontario M4P 2S3 Phone (416) 482-6339
SWITZERLAND:	Länggass-Strasse 76, CH-3000 Bern 9 Phone (031) 300-4500, Fax (031) 300-4590
GERMANY:	Rohnsweg 25, D-37085 Göttingen Phone (0551) 496090, Fax (0551) 4960988

Printed and bound in Germany
ISBN 0-88937-225-X

Preface

Ambulatory Assessment involves the acquisition of psychological data and/or physiological measures in everyday life, that is, in natural settings. Field studies are not solely concerned with the ambulatory monitoring of patient blood pressure or ECG, but rather include a wide spectrum of objectives and applications. Our *first* volume, *Ambulatory Assessment*, published in 1996, was the first edited work to examine—in 24 chapters—the real-time measurement of both behavioral and physiological data, with a particular emphasis upon how interrelationships between self-report, behavioral and physiological events may be illumined by concurrent, naturalistic recordings. The *present* volume, *Progress in Ambulatory Assessment*, is not a second edition. The 35 new chapters explore the use of computer-assisted methods as assessment tools in research and applied settings. Common features covered are recordings in everyday life, state-of-the-art computer-assisted methodology, maintenance of ecological validity, and practical utility.

Previous research has focussed upon the novelty of certain applications, the limited equivalence of computer-assisted *vs.* traditional paper-and-pencil measures of self-report, and issues relating to laboratory-field generalizability. Some of these topics were covered in depth in the first volume. As indicated in the last volume, portable computers have, so far, predominantly been used for collecting psychological and physiological data. The current volume examines more innovative approaches, applying new strategies in controlled or interactive assessment supported by on-line analysis and feedback: Electronic diaries and ambulatory physiological and behavioral measures can now be supplemented by real-time information processing and event-contingent applications. Ambulatory assessment appears to be entering a phase of transition, in which the challenge is how to best make use of advanced information technology and internet-based systems. Health care and telemedicine, orienting toward self-management of the chronically ill, may provide major fields for applications of computer-assisted strategies in daily life. Ergonomic and occupational psychophysiology are evolving into disciplines in which ecologically valid assessments require ambulatory methodologies.

The present book originated from a workshop on ambulatory assessment, hosted at the University of Freiburg in 1999, and was, once again, supported by the Deutsche Forschungsgemeinschaft. This English language publication was prepared to reach the English speaking audience. Translation may have affected the stylistic elegance of some chapters but, hopefully, not the meaning. Contributions were received from Austria, Germany, the Netherlands, Switzerland, the United Kingdom, and the United States. We appreciate the assistance of Ulla Probst and Thomas Hammelmann in the preparation, editing and lay-out of manuscripts. Marcus Cheetham significantly improved the English of several manuscripts. We also wish to thank Dr. Michael Vogtmeier and Mr. Robert Dimbleby from Hogrefe & Huber Publishers, who made this publication possible.

That most authors from the first volume were prepared again to contribute summaries of recent findings is evidence of the continuing confidence in this approach, the rewards of this line of research, and, indeed, the fact that there is *Progress in Ambulatory Assessment.*

Jochen Fahrenberg Michael Myrtek

Contents

Part I
Psychological Assessment

Chapter 1
Computer-Assisted Ambulatory Performance Tests in Everyday Situations: Construction, Evaluation, and Psychometric Properties of a Test Battery Measuring Mental Activation

Lothar Buse and Kurt Pawlik
Department of Psychology, University of Hamburg, Germany

Introduction

Ambulatory assessment refers to the systematic collection of psychological and/or physiological data in everyday situations, outside the laboratory. Two different kinds of data collection can be distinguished. In an *event controlled* mode data collection is triggered by the occurrence of a particular event, whereas in a *time controlled* mode records are made according to a time sampling schedule. This latter approach has been followed in a large number of research studies, also known as experience sampling method (Buse & Pawlik, 1984, 1996; Csikszentmihalyi & Larson, 1987; deVries, 1992; Diener & Larsen, 1984; Fahrenberg & Myrtek, 1996; Hormuth, 1986; Larson & Csikszentmihalyi, 1983; Pawlik & Buse, 1982, 1992; Tennen, Suls & Affleck, 1991).

Numerous possibilities for improvement of ambulatory assessment haven risen from progress in the design of portable devices that electronically collect and save data. On this point, the device can be either a special product (behavior data recorder) or standard equipment (electronic notebook) with varying memory capacities. Next to data collection, some types of equipment also allow for additional functions, such as to serve as an alarm for the implementation of a time sampling schedule, a display screen for the presentation of text or tests, or a register, or recording device for the collection of physiological data.

Such devices allow ambulatory performance tests to be employed in the daily life course of a person. Actually, this equipment allows the self-administration of tests in everyday situations for the first time. An important and absolutely necessary function is the control of the test administration, so that time requirements can be exactly met. The on-line presentation of the items on the screen ensures that the items cannot be inspected before actual testing begins. Also, the electronic memory prevents a given answer from being corrected at a later time. In addition, such devices can also serve as a precision clock to measure reaction times at high levels of precision.

Numerous applications are to be considered in the scope of psychodiagnostics, with regard to the assessment of individual differences in cognitive (information-processing) and/or intellectual abilities. In a representative sample of everyday situations external ("ecological") validity is likely to arise. This means that the data are more easily generalizable to real-life situations as compared to when they came from a laboratory setting.

The present test battery was developed with two goals in mind: (1) the measurement of cognitive performance within subjects at various times to evaluate the effects of environmental stressors on current performance level, and (2) the measurement of differences in ability level between subjects as for personnel selection or neuropsychologial assessment.

To collect data in a large number of everyday situations, ambulatory assessment is a necessary prerequisite. Repeated measurement is required in studies following multiple-baseline experimental design where the subjects serve as their own controls. Besides, test aggregates derived from repeated measures will be more reliable and can be more easily generalized than single test data. Further, repeated serial assessment is indispensable to the study of seasonal or cyclic variations as conducted in time series analysis.

Areas requiring such serial assessment may include: (1) evaluating the effects of environmental stress, for example, sleep deprivation, fatigue, monotony, boredom, shift-work, temperature, altitude, or noise; (2) assessing the effects of toxic substances, for example, nickel, lead, or cadmium; or (3) assessing the effects of psychoactive drugs, for example, alcohol, nicotine, amphetamines, benzodiazepines, or antidepressants.

From a neuropsychological point of view, Kane and Kay (1992) add some other areas requiring serial assessment. In fact, they include (1) monitoring disease progression and recovery from injury, (2) assessing the effects of medication on performance, (3) assessing the effects of medical and surgical intervention, and (4) evaluating training effects and the effects of cognitive rehabilitation.

Tests used in this line of research are required to be responsive to variations in the state of cognitive performance. In this way, test scores must increase or decline, respectively, depending on whether someone is, for example, alert or sleepy at the time of testing. In addition, it is required that changes caused by measurement errors be small. Tests fulfilling these requirements will be described as reliably sensitive to change.

A problem with ambulatory assessment is caused by the fact that test situations are often poorly standardized. Actually, bad lighting, noise or disruptions by other people can negatively affect test performance, so it may be difficult to compare test scores obtained at different times. For this reason, the external circumstances of a test session must be specified as precisely as possible.

Though not in fact developed for ambulatory assessment, the *Battery of Standardized Tests for Research with Environmental Stressors* (Santucci, 1989), abbreviated *STRES,* comes close to our needs. Test examples are Grammatical Reasoning, Spatial Processing, Visual-Motor Tracking, and Memory Search. Test administration requires a stationary computer, however, self-administration of the tests outside the laboratory, but indoors, for example at home or in the workplace, is possible, though for the majority of subjects, examiner assistance will be required. The maximum time for each test is three minutes. With respect to sensitivity to change, there is a lot of experimental evidence that test performance is negatively affected by environmental stressors. For example, subjects have been tested in a shuttle during a space mission (Manzey, Lorenz, Schiewe, Finell& Thiele, 1995). Before introducing experimental treatment, the tests are practiced over multiple test sessions to establish an asymptotic level of performance.

Some other suggestions came from the *Performance Tests for Environmental Research (PETER)* (Bittner, Carter & Kennedy, 1986). The goal of the *PETER* program was "to identify a set of measures of human cognitive, perceptual, and motor capabilities for a use in the study of environmental and other time course effects" (p. 684). The tests were required "to be sensitive to subtle changes in performance and for other repeated measures applications" (p. 684). To meet these as goals, random samples of people were tested over 14 days, each day at the same time with the same test. The tests "were drawn from environmental, informational processing, and microcomputer task batteries" (p. 684). Only for some of the tests was administration computer-assisted. Tests yielding a linear slope on the practice curve were recommended, provided that their reliability coefficients were sufficiently high. For reasons of comparison, the coefficients were converted for each test by taking a constant test time of three minutes as a common time basis. Above all and as expected, derived test measures (for example, differences, ratios, and angle degrees) proved less reliable. Statements on the tests' sensitivity to change are missing. The test collection was not checked on conditions of ambulatory assessment.

A result of the *PETER* program is the *Automated Portable Test System*, which was originally designed to run a lightweight, battery-operated notebook computer. Tasks included are, for example, Simple and Complex Reaction Time, Continuous Performance, Spatial Visualization, Serial Addition, Code Substitution, Memory Search, etc.

The *Testbatterie zur Aufmerksamskeitsprüfung [Battery of Alertness Tests]* , abbreviated *TAP*, (Becker, Sturm, Willmes & Zimmerman 1996; Zimmerman & Fimm, 1993) provided further suggestions. The test battery was developed for neuropsychological assessment. It consists of 12 task groups. Examples are Alertness, Working Memory, Interference, Selective Attention, and Vigilance. The test administration requires a stationary computer. Statements on the sensitivity to change are missing.

The goals of the current research were development, evaluation, and psychometric analysis of a computer-assisted test battery for ambulatory assessment of performance functions of alertness, attention and information processing in everyday situations. This required the following steps: (1) Hardware development, in cooperation with a production company for psychological testing equipment. (2) Construction of a test battery of potentially change-sensitive performance tests. (3) Software development for the online administration of the tests. (4) Empirical examination of the tests and the machine. (5) State-trait analysis to evaluate sensitivity to change. (6) Analysis of within-subject correlations among the tests.

Method

The Testing Device

The portable recording apparatus (behavior data recorder AMBU: Ambulatory Monitoring and Behavior-Test Unit, Pawlik & Buse, 2001) has to meet a number of requirements essential for ambulatory assessment. It has to serve as a signaling device to call upon the subject at a given observation point ("occasion") according to a time sampling schedule. It has to contain a display for presenting instructions as well as checklist items and test items. It has to serve as a data storage. And it has to be freely programmable to implement a time sampling or event sampling plan for data acquisition and details of test-selection, testware, etc..

Our own development of a computer-based behavior data recorder for ambulatory psychological assessment goes back to 1980 (Buse & Pawlik, 1984; Pawlik & Buse, 1982). An improved second-generation version was developed in 1984 (Buse & Pawlik, 1996; Pawlik & Buse, 1992) and a totally redesigned third-generation recorder (*AMBU*) in 1995, and, with minor changes, in 1998.

AMBU testing device. Size: 17.5 x 8.3 x 3 cm. Weight: 435g. Processor: Intel 801188 EB 13. Storage capacity: 1 MB RAM. Display: 6 x 4 cm active LCD surface, 128 x 64 pixel with full graphics. Keyboard: 0-9; 4 arrow keys (for cursor movement and special responses), specially marked home key. Additional response module: endless turn knob (opto-electronic encoder) for continuous circular motor response. (In the 1998 version, functions executed via the knob have been re-programmed via the arrow keys.) Power supply: rechargeable battery 900 mAh (with separate unit for overnight recharging). Programming languages: Turbo Pascal, C.

The Test Battery

In the development of the test battery, several conditions had to be met: 1) The tests should measure cognitive performance with particular reference to attention, working memory, perception, and motor performance. In addition, some ability tests should serve as trait markers. 2) The tests should be psychometrically reliable. 3) The tests must allow computer-assisted self-administration in everyday situations. 4) Total test times should not exceed 1 or 2 minutes per test. 5) The computer should generate items automatically, wherever possible. 6) Each test should have infinite parallel forms, if possible. 7) The measurement errors should be as small as possible. 8) Test performance should change as little as possible due to practice. 9) The tests should be language-independent. The eleven tests explained below, seemed well-suited to fulfill these requirements.

Alertness Test

When holding the home key down, a vertical cross appears on the display. The "0" key should be pressed as quickly as possible after the cross appears. Half of the time, a warning tone precedes the appearance of the cross; this tone must not be reacted to. Subjects are instructed to use the same finger for holding the home-key and for pressing the reaction key. The test consists of 28 trials. In the middle 14 trials the warning tone is offered. In the test for reliability, the first 14 trials were compared with the second 14 trials.

Anagram Test

Five letters are displayed next to one another, from which a noun must be built by rearranging the letters. The letters are numbered 1, 2, 3, 4, 5 from left to right. The first letter of the unscrambled word must be marked by entering its number. Each test administration consists of 12 items. The response time is limited to 15 seconds per item and displayed on a small clock shown on the display. The test is to serve as a trait marker of word fluency. Odd/even reliabilities across items serve as reliability estimates.

Continuous Performance Test

When pressing the home key, 60 times a number between 1 and 8 is shown, one after another in a seemingly random order. When three odd or three even numbers appear in direct succession, this constitutes a target and the "0" key should be pressed as quickly as possible. Subjects are again instructed to use the same finger to hold down the home key and to press the reaction key. The test consists of two blocks, each comprising 30 numbers and 6 targets. To examine reliability, the two blocks were compared. The test can serve as a measure of sustained attention.

Corsi Block Tapping
On the display screen several squares (fields) are seen, some of which, one after another, randomly blacken. The subject must retain the sequence in which this occurs. Afterwards the fields will be numbered. By entering the respective numbers, the sequence are to be repeated. Mistakes can be corrected by moving backwards (pressing the left arrow key (¬) and subsequently typing over the mistake). Pressing the star key enters the repeated number sequence. Nine fields are always shown; of these nine fields, six darken. The selection of these six fields and their sequence is random as well as the numbering of the fields. The test should measure visuospatial short-term memory. To test for reliability, the test was divided odd/even.

d2- Cancellation Test
A series of letters are shown simultaneously, in which "d" and "p" switch randomly. The letters are presented with one or two vertical short lines (strokes) above and/or below. Target stimulus is a "d" with two strokes – be it both above, both below, or above and below. At the start a cursor flashes under the letter at the far left of the screen. This shows which letter is being considered. If the letter is a "d" with two lines, then the star key is to be pressed, causing a slash to appear across the letter (the letter is "crossed out"). The cursor then moves one letter to the right. The decision process begins again. By repeatedly pressing the star key, one can move back to incorrect entries. When the letter is not a "d" with two lines, the cursor is moved one letter to the right by pressing the right arrow (®). Then the decision process begins again. When a target is overseen, one can move back by pressing the left arrow (¬). Subjects are instructed to work as quickly and exactly as possible. The test can serve as a measure of selective attention. To evaluate reliability, the test was divided into two halves, at every thirty seconds.

Grammatical Reasoning Test
Each item consists of a pair of sentences accompanied by three symbols in a particular order. Each sentence either correctly or incorrectly describes the order (before / after) of an adjacent pair of symbols within the set of three. The subjects are required to compare the truth of the sentences. If both sentences are true or if both are false, the "1" key is to be pressed. If one sentence is true and the other one false, the "0" key is to be pressed. The test consists of 12 items. To examine reliability, the items are distributed odd/even.

Go/NoGo Test
After pressing the home key, either an "X" or a vertical cross appears. Both symbols are graphically composed of 17 small diamond-shaped patterns. Inserting an approximately equal number of patterns in the free spaces between the axes makes

distinguishing the "X" and the cross more difficult. The "0" key is to be pressed as quickly as possible after presentation of the "X" (Go), whereas the home key must be kept pressed when the cross appears (No Go). Subjects are instructed to use the same finger in holding the home key down and in pressing the reaction key. The test consists of 40 trials, presented in four ten-trial blocks. A block consists of 7 targets (Go's) and 3 non-targets (No Go's) or, in the reverse, of 7 non-targets and 3 targets. Blocks 1 and 3 are of the first, and blocks 2 and 4 of the second type. The sequence of targets and non-targets within a block is random. The test serves as a measure of selective attention. To test for reliability, the first two blocks were compared with the last two blocks.

Mental Rotations Test

In each item 2 figures are shown, which can be seen as three-dimensional shapes built of several small cubes. In some items the figures are the same but are rotated against one another, so that they can be merged by rotating them back. In the remaining items the shapes are different, so they can not be merged. Subjects must decide as quickly as possible between "same" and "different" block configurations. Each test consists of 12 items; in six items the two figures are identical, in the remaining six they are different. Rotation angles of 45°, 90°, and 135° were employed. The task was adopted from the *Mental Rotations Test* of Vandenberg and Kuse (1978), the figures originating from research by Shepard and Metzler (1971). The test should serve as a trait marker of spatial visualization. To examine reliability, the items were distributed odd/even.

Rota Test

In two rows a total of fourteen clocks are shown on the display screen, each consisting of a circle and a hand (pointer). In each clock the hand moves clockwise at the same speed. Thirteen clocks show the same time, while one clock is fast. The subject must identify this clock and mark it with the cursor. The right and left arrow keys are pressed until the cursor shows the "wrong" clock. Pressing the star key enters the clock chosen. Immediately afterwards another clock pattern is presented. Subjects are instructed to work as quickly and accurately as possible. The test was developed by the authors (Buse & Pawlik, 1996). To evaluate reliability, the test was divided into two test halves of thirty seconds each.

Sternberg Memory Search

Upon pressing the home key, several capital letters (*memory set*) are shown simultaneously for a few seconds. Several lower case letters (*probe letters*), shown successively, follow. The subject must decide which of these lower case letters were among the upper case letters. When so, the "0" must be pressed as quickly as possible and when no, the "9". The subjects are instructed to use the same finger to hold down the home key and to press the reaction key. Each test consists of four sets, of which the first and fourth contain three letters and the second and third contain six. The exposition time for each set is 5 seconds. Afterwards the probe letters are shown. The test should measure processing speed in short-term memory. To evaluate reliability, the first two sets were compared with the last two sets.

Unstable Tracking Task

On the display screen appears a vertical center line, from which a horizontal band stretches left or right with increasing speed, that is develops from a stroke into a more or less long strip. By turning the reaction knob against the direction of the strip (or using the proper arrow keys), further movement to this side is prevented. Contact with a sideline (edge) of the display results in a short interruption (termed below *control loss*). In such a case the strip is set back automatically to the center line. Subjects are instructed to keep the band as close to the center line and as long as possible. The test time is 30 seconds. Every 50 msec the band's position is recorded in the number of pixels of deviation from the center line. Following a control loss, the time between contacting the side line and the moment when the band is reset was not counted; in this way, the real test time always amounts to exactly thirty seconds, independent of the number of control losses. The test is an adaptation of the Critical Tracking Task by Jex, McDonnell, and Photak (1966). The instability of the test line is brought about by a positive feedback loop, the speed of the band changing proportionally to the distance from the center line. The greater the distance, the harder movement will be to control. As a consequence, the subject has to respond both to the velocity and the length of the band. A subject's performance in a single trial can be presented graphically on a scale of 600 points (x-axis), with the distance from the center line in pixels on the y-axis. The length of the resulting curve ("string") serves as measure of performance. In addition, the number of control losses is counted. To examine reliability, the first fifteen seconds are compared with the second fifteen.

The Inventory

In addition to the performance tests, several checklists had to be completed at each test occasion to assess variations in the subject's physical and psychological state as well as exogenous circumstances, under which a test session took place. They are: a position list (6 items on body position previous to testing); a setting list (46 items on current surroundings.); a mood list (28 items on current mood); a complaint list (15 items on physical complaints); a behavior list (43 items on behaviors occurring previous to testing); a person list (5 items on the presence or absence of people); a work list (15 items on the external circumstances while taking the tests).

Study 1

Procedure. Subjects were recruited by advertisements in two Hamburg daily newspapers. Addressees were people who thought they "could interrupt their activities for 8-10 minutes for a psychological experiment" several times during any part of the day, over three weeks. Interested people who replied either in writing or by telephone, were mailed a brochure explaining details of the planned experiment. Subjects who gave informed consent to participate were invited to a two and one-half hour preliminary inquiry, where several standard performance tests and a multidimensional personality questionnaire were completed. In addition, they were asked about time preferences in regard to the study. Several weeks later they were informed about the planned assessment period and invited to a second, one and one-half hour conference. At this occasion they received detailed instructions on operating the recording device. In addition, test proceedings were explained and several practice tests administered. The *AMBU*-testing device was distributed with a DIN-A5 booklet, that served as a manual and a reference book for the three week test period and contained important user information (description of the testing device and instructions on use; potential problems; precautionary measures; the energy supply; description of the tests along with instructions; function of the keys; finding the online help function; description of the inventories and lists). In addition, a hotline was established during the day to respond to subjects' queries. Each week the subject had to return, so the data could be retrieved. Upon returning the device at the end of the third week, the subjects took part in a debriefing interview. They were asked, for example, what they enjoyed most or did not enjoy at all. In order to maintain test motivation, the subjects were promised feedback information on their individual performance at the end of the test period. Moreover, subjects received information on their current performance online after each test (in the form of number correct, mistakes, and/or time). Subjects received a modest financial remuneration for participation. The data collection was carried out between September 1995 and February 1997.

Subjects. Recruitment took place in several waves. Altogether, 244 individuals answered the ads. Of those, 45 were excluded because their age and/or gender were already over-represented. An additional 69 respondents declined to participate, after they had been informed about the time needed to complete the tests and to comply with the demands of the study. Further, 15 individuals remained unconsidered because of age (over 60 years) or because they suffered from chronic diseases. In all, fifty-two men and sixty-three women participated. Three age groups were formed: 30 to 39, 40 to 49, and 50 to 59, occupied with almost equal numbers of men and women (between 16 and 23) per age group. One third (36.5 %) of the subjects were employed fulltime, 19.5% part-time, 15% were homeworkers, unemployed, or retired; 29.5% did not answer this question. With respect to education, 13% reported they had earned at least a college degree. An additional 38.3% had high school graduation (13 years of schooling); 37.4% had passed first examination in secondary school (10 years), and 11.3% had completed junior high school (9 years).

Time Schedule. Each subject was tested for three successive weeks. Eight test sessions per day were pre-set, with an average inter-session interval of about 90 minutes. The time schedule was decided individually with the subjects, for example, roughly beginning at 8 a.m. In all, 168 test occasions were offered for each subject.

Administration Scheme. A selection of five tests was presented at each occasion. The tests differed from week to week, however remained constant within the same week. The Alertness Test was given in each week. Three tests (Corsi, Tracking, and d2) were administered only for two weeks and the other six tests only one week.

Compliance. Of the 168 test occasions, an average of 133 were fully completed; this results in an average response rate of 79.4%. Test administrations took place at home (59%), in the workplace (19%), at another person's home (6%), while shopping (2%), at other places (8%).

Study 2

Subjects. The study was carried out in cooperation with the Psychological Services of the *Bundeswehr* [German Armed Forces]. Subjects were 130 conscripts (aged 18 to 26) completing their basic training (that is, in their first three months of military service) in two garrison towns in the Federal State of Schleswig-Holstein. A total of 12 training groups from 3 different training units were tested, each consisting of about 12 conscripts.

Time Schedule. Data collection took place between April and November 1999. Each subject was tested for three successive weeks, with test sessions scheduled on working days only. From Monday to Thursday eight test sessions were arranged from about 6 a.m. to 5 p.m. and on Friday from about 6 a.m. to 12 a.m. A total of 108 test sessions was programmed per subject. An event-controlled mode of data collection was employed. (A time-controlled mode as used in the previous study was unsuitable because the soldiers should never have to interrupt ongoing training activities.) Instead, the soldiers were called upon at suitable points of time chosen so as to sample the range of test situations typical for this phase of military training. The signal to initiate a test occasion was given by a project co-worker, who stayed with the soldiers throughout their working time (inside the barracks, during practical or theoretical instruction, on the shooting range, during physical education, during a cross-country march, in the ground, etc). The signal was set in consultation with the group's instructor. Care was taken that a representative sample of working-day situations was thus collected.

Administration Scheme. A selection of 5 tests was presented at each test occasion.

The selection differed from one week to the other, but remained constant within a week. Only the Alertness Test was given in each week. Three tests (Rota, Tracking, and d2) were administered over two weeks each, the other six tests one week only.

Pilot Study. Prior to the main study, a pilot study was conducted with 25 conscripts. The objective was to bring checklist item content in line so that the coverage of settings, activities, and physical complaints would be typical of the military environment studied.

Compliance. A total of 12.628 test sessions was fully completed. Thus, the average response rate amounts to about 90 %. Note that in the previous study the response rate was lower. The higher response rate in the Study 2 may be due to the fact that the examiner was present during all data collection (and could watch whether or not the subjects complied with the request). Following data collection, subjects were again interviewed about their evaluation of the testing program. About 50 % said they would be willing to participate once more. In the previous study about 57% had expressed their readiness. The higher percentage may be due to the fact that subjects in Study 1 have been paid for participation.

The State-Trait Model

To examine the degree of sensitivity to change, a state-trait model of analysis was employed (Buse & Pawlik, 1991). The model assumes that the test score of any given person at any given point in time is comprised of three components: a time-stable and situation-invariant performance level of the person (trait), a temporary deviation from this level caused, for example, by varying degrees of mental activation (state), and an unsystematic error component that varies randomly within a situation (error).

From repeated administrations of a test with different people at different times (in different situations) one can analyze how much of the total variance can be accounted for by each of the three components. Depending on the variance amount of the state component, a test can serve either as a change-sensitive state marker or as a trait marker (if state-variations are small to negligible).

The state-trait model refers to typical variations in behavior and mood in everyday situations. The approach differs from measuring experimentally induced changes in the laboratory, where conditions are often atypical of everyday life.

To measure sensitivity to change, the between-subjects and within-subject variances of the test scores are needed. The between-subjects variance is calculated for each occasion across subjects, and the within-subject variance for each subject across occasions, respectively. The between-subjects variance can be used to estimate the size of the trait variance. (With a large number of occasions, the variance of the individual means will approximate the trait variance.)

In an extension of this state-trait model we wished to analyze the within-subject variance into variance due to practice, due to state, and error of measurement. In this we differentiated between monotonic and non-monotonic variations. Monotonic components refer to systematic intraindividual variations which follow an inflection-free trend over successive occasions of assessment. Psychologically, they may be due to practice and/or training. Here we distinguished between two kinds of non-monotonic components: 1) systematic (true score) fluctuations over time, occasions, and settings/situations reflecting changes in the internal make-up of a person (mood state, level of activation, etc.) and/or varying extraneous demands, and 2) unsystematic errors of assessment, observation, and recording.

To separate the three components, a best-fitting practice curve was calculated individually for each subject and test. The deviation of raw test scores from this practice curve was computed to serve as a trend-free estimate of test performance at any one test occasion (termed *residual* below). This residual variance was then separated into two components: a systematic non-monotonic variation (state variation s.s.) and variation due to unsystematic measurement error. To evaluate the within-subject reliability of these residuals, which is necessary for this variance decomposition, the split-half method was used. As a consequence, the curve-fitting had to be performed separately for each of the two test halves. To ensure reliability of the full test, the split-half-correlation was upgraded to full test length according to the Spearman-Brown formula. These coefficients serve as trend-free measures of test sensitivity to change. Multiplied by 100 they give the percentage of within-subject variance between occasions due to true-score state variations.

Results and Discussion

Within-Subject Reliability

To break down within-subject variance into state, practice, and error components, the following calculations were carried out for each person and test separately:

Reliability coefficients of test raw scores. To assess within-subject reliability, the correlation between test halves was calculated across occasions (over 1, 2 or 3 weeks, depending on the test). In Study 1 these reliability estimates are based on an average of 42, 88, and 131 occasions, in Study 2 of 30, 63, and 97 occasions, respectively. The coefficients, averaged across subjects using Fisher's z'-transformation, can serve as a measure of within-subject reliability. As practice takes place in both test halves, thereby acting as a common source of variance, these coefficients may be increased for tests showing a substantial practice component.

Curve fitting. To remove a monotonic practice trend, exponential functions were fitted to the individual test data. The data were processed in chronological order.

Incomplete or omitted occasions were ignored. The curve fitting was performed for each test half separately and also for both halves together. The difference between raw and estimated scores (termed *residuals* below) is an indicator of test performance free of monotonic practice effects.

Elimination of outliers. The term outlier refers to test scores substantially below the individual performance level of a person. Most likely, outliers can reflect external disturbances during testing. They are easily noticeable in graphic data representations. Numerically, the problem was solved by calculating the amount by which a test score departs from the monotonic trend curve. To this end, the residuals were z-transformed in each of the two test halves. Occasions with a score equal to $z \leq -2.4$ in at least one of the two test halves were eliminated for that person in that test. Approximately 3.5 % of test scores available for analysis were thus eliminated.

Reliability coefficients of residuals. Correlations between test halves across occasions were then calculated for the residuals, again employing the Spearman-Brown formula. These correlations can serve as a measure of within-subject reliability corrected for spurious effects due to practice and outliers. The coefficients were averaged across subjects using again the Fisher z'-transformation. Table 1 shows the results for Study 1 and Study 2.

Depending on the test, within-subject reliabilities of residuals range from .14 to .80 in Study 1 and from .31 to .73 in Study 2, respectively. In all, there are only small differences between the studies. In each study the median amounts to about .60. The coefficients clearly show that the within-subject variance is not largely due

Table 1. AMBU-Tests of cognitive performance: Within-subjects reliabilities corrected for outliers and practice effects

Tests	Study 1	Study 2
Alertness (T)	.80	.73
Continuous Performance (T)	.73	.59
Go/NoGo (T)	.65	.66
Sternberg (T)	.64	.56
Mental Rotations (T)	.52	.43
Anagrams (T)	.20	a
Grammatical Reasoning (T)	a	.43
Rota (C)	.36	.56
d2-Cancellation (C)	.37	.55
Corsi (C)	.17	.31
Tracking	.59	.92

Note. T = time, C = number correct.
Study 1: averaged across n=115 subjects; Study 2: averaged across n=130 subjects. [a] not used.

to measurement error, as one might have expected. Several tests yield indeed a considerable true state score variance. Furthermore, true score variance within subjects is not exhausted even after the removal of the monotonic practice component. However, considerable differences between tests warrant further comment.

Calculation of variance proportions. According to the model, the within-subject variance of the raw scores is composed of three components (state, practice, and error), whereas the within-subject variance of residuals consists only of two (state and error). The variance components are calculated as follows:

$$s^2_P = s^2_t - s^2_r \quad (1)$$
$$s^2_S = s^2_r \, r_{tt(r)} \quad (2)$$
$$s^2_E = s^2_r \, (1 - r_{tt(r)}) \quad (3)$$

with: s^2_P = practice variance; s^2_S = state variance; s^2_E = error variance; s^2_t = test raw score variance; s^2_r = residual variance; $r_{tt(r)}$ = reliability of the residuals.

For each subject the proportions of variance due to state, practice, and error components were calculated and subsequently averaged across subjects. In Table 2 mean values are shown for Study 1 and Study 2.

A test's sensitivity to change depends heavily on the proportion of state variance. Here highest values were obtained for decision times: Alertness: Study 1: 70% /

Table 2. AMBU-Tests of cognitive performance: Proportions of variance due to state, practice, and error components

Tests	Study 1			Study 2		
	State	Practice	Error	State	Practice	Error
Alertness	.70	.13	.17	.68	.10	.21
Continuous Performance	.66	.10	.24	.53	.06	.41
Go/NoGoNo	.56	.14	.30	.60	.08	.32
Sternberg	.48	.25	.27	.36	.39	.25
Mental Rotations	.28	.34	.27	.42	.31	.38
Anagrams	.21	.06	.73		not used	
Grammatical Reasoning		not used		.32	.10	.58
Rota	.24	.38	.38	.33	.37	.30
d2-Cancellation	.20	.52	.28	.18	.66	.16
Corsi	.15	.12	.73	.31	.06	.63
Tracking	.41	.31	.28	.61	.34	.05

Note. Study 1: averaged across n=115 subjects. Study 2: averaged across n=130 subjects.

Study 2: 68%; Continuous Performance: 66% / 53%; Go/NoGo: 56% / 60%; Sternberg: 48% / 36%. Likewise, the proportions for Tracking were high: 41% / 61%. For other measures the values were substantially lower: Mental Rotations: 38% / 27%; Rota: 23% / 33%; d2: 20% / 18%; Corsi: 15% / 31%; Anagrams: 18%; Grammatical Reasoning: 32 %.

Time measures also stand out in that they have the lowest error terms. This again holds true especially for decision times: Alertness: 17% / 21 %; Continuous Performance: 24% / 41%; Go/NoGo: 30% / 32%; Sternberg: 27% / 25%. Smaller error variances were obtained for some other variables as well (Rota: 40% / 30%; d2: 28% / 16%; Tracking: 28% / 5%). For power tests, the proportion of error variance was, by comparison, small in one test (Mental Rotations: 34% / 31%) and large in some others (Anagrams: 73%; Grammatical Reasoning: 58%; Corsi: 73% / 63%).

In some tests the percent practice variance is strikingly high (d2: 52% / 66%; Rota: 35% / 37 %; Tracking: 34% / 34 %). Likewise, higher values were obtained for Mental Rotations (28% / 42%) and Sternberg (25% / 39%).

Why do the time measures result in larger state variances? One possible explanation is that the reaction time on a simple decision task is better measure of a person's state (for example, alertness) than the completion of a test with higher demands on word fluency, reasoning or spatial visualization. Furthermore, in less demanding tests larger numbers of items can be responded to because of the little time required per item. With larger numbers of items, however, the error variance is to decrease. In addition, time measures meet interval scale properties to a higher degree. While psychometric items differentiate only between "false" and "correct", chronometric measurements are carried out at a much finer level (here: in milliseconds).

Why do certain tests show larger practice effects? It is assumed that the obtained practice effects are largely due to improvement of motor response. In fact, for the two tests with the strongest practice effects (d2 and Rota), each response requires an ordered sequence of finger movements. Likewise, a strong practice effect was obtained for the tracking task, where finely graded motor responses are required. So it seems reasonable to infer that the practice effects were mainly due to improved dexterity in complex motor responses.

Within-Subject Correlations Between Tests

To what extent do the tests measure different aspects of mental activation? To address this question, the residual scores were correlated within subjects across occasions. As only five of the ten tests could be administered at a time and the selection of tests differed between weeks, Alertness was chosen to serve as reference test in all weeks. Three tests were limited to two weeks (Corsi, Tracking, and d2, in Study 1, Rota, Tracking, and d2, in Study 2) and the rest to one week. Tests with similar demands were assigned to different weeks (Rota and d2, Sternberg and Corsi, Continuous Performance and Go/NoGo). Table 3 shows the matrix of correlations for Study 1, averaged across subjects, after use of Fisher's z'-transformation. The matrix is incomplete; missing values indicate that there is no common time basis. Given the high numbers of test sessions, even the lowest coefficients already prove to be significant (coefficients above .03 at the 5% level, above .04 at the 1% level, and above .05 at the .01% level).

Consistent with expectation, the correlations among time measures were positive. Correlations among number correct measures were positive as well, whereas correlations between time and number correct measures were negative. Correlations between time measures and Tracking were positive, while correlations between number correct measures and Tracking were negative. Alertness, Go/NoGo, Continuous Performance, and Sternberg correlate on average between .44 and .56. Thus, decision time measures have a substantial part of variances in common, irrespective of the particular task requirement. With within-subject reliabilities between .65 and .80, the coefficients for these tests are remarkably high.

Alertness, Go/NoGo, Continuous Performance and Sternberg correlate with Rota and d2 between -.18 and -.26 on average. This suggests that there is a common source of variance also between reaction tests and speed tests. Presumably, the low values are due to the low degree of sensitivity of the two speed tests (around .35).

Moreover, Tracking correlates with Alertness, Continuous Performance, Sternberg, and d2 at .23, .21, .12, and -.15, respectively. The lowest correlations were found for Mental Rotations, Corsi, and Anagrams. Altogether, the results suggest

Table 3. AMBU-Tests of cognitive performance: Within-subjects correlations among selected measures[a]. Study 1

	AS	CP	GN	ST	d2	RO	TR	CO	MR	AN
AS		.56	.50	.44	-.26	-.25	.23	-.09	-.03	-.05
CP			b	.44	-.18	b	.21	b	b	b
GN				b	b	-.25	b	-.02	-.05	b
ST					-.26	b	.12	b	b	b
d2						b	-.15	.10	b	.04
RO							b	.08	.04	b
TR								-.05	b	-.06
CO									.04	.02
MR										b
AN										

Note. AS = Alertness; CP = Continuous Performance; GN = Go/Nogo; ST = Sternberg Memory Search; d2 = Cancellation; RO = Rota; TR = Tracking; CO = Corsi Block Tapping; MR = Mental Rotations; AN = Anagrams. [a] averaged across n=115 subjects. [b] no common time basis.

that there is a correlations cluster, albeit low, among seven of the tests.

For Study 2 the correlation matrix is shown in Table 4. Though coefficients are generally lower, the pattern was essentially confirmed. Again, correlations among time measures are positive, correlations among number correct measures are positive as well, whereas correlations between time and number correct measures are negative. Besides, correlations between Tracking and time measures are negative, while correlations between Tracking and number correct measures are positive. The lowest values were found for Mental Rotations, Corsi, and Grammatical Reasoning.

The fact that most of the tests have true state variance in common, seems to lend new support to the old hypothesis of a unitary activation system. Yet, each test also includes a significant specific component; so it will be necessary to distinguish between multiple activation states, like effort and arousal, which are tapped by the tests differentially. As a consequence, in relating activation to performance it will be necessary to employ a properly balanced battery of tests measuring distinct dimensions of activation.

Between-Subjects Reliability

The between-subject reliability indicates how much of the test score variance can be accounted for by time-stable true score variations between subjects. Empirically, this value can be determined by correlating the test scores at different occasions across subjects. Our expanded state-trait model assumes that the test score variance at any occasion is composed of four components (trait, state, practice, and error). Moreover, the trait component is the only one our model does not allow to

Table 4. AMBU-Tests of cognitive performance: Within-subjects correlations among selected measures[a]. Study 2

	AS	CP	GN	ST	d2	RO	TR	CO	MR	GR
AS		.33	.39	.15	-.26	-.35	-.24	-.11	.07	.05
CP			b	b	b	-.18	-.23	b	.16	b
GN				b	-.21	b	-.17	-.06	b	b
ST					-.19	-.17	b	b	b	.10
d2						.30	.17	.15	b	-.10
RO							.17	b	-.07	-.06
TR								.09	-.04	b
CO									b	b
MR										b
GR										

Note: AS = Alertness; CP = Continuous Performance; GN = Go/Nogo; ST = Sternberg Memory Search; d2 = Cancellation; RO = Rota; TR = Tracking; CO = Corsi Block Tapping; MR = Mental Rotations; AN = Anagrams.

[a] averaged across n=130 subjects. [b] no common time basis.

Table 5. AMBU-Tests of cognitive performance: Between-subjects reliabilities

Tests	Study 1		Study 2	
	with[a]	without[b]	with[a]	without[b]
Rota	.75	.83	.50	.63
Tracking	.74	.82	.68	.73
d2	.64	.80	.46	.72
Sternberg	.62	.71	.48	.57
Alertness	.58	.62	.45	.47
Corsi	.56	.60	.50	.51
Mental Rotations	.51	.59	.48	.61
GO/NoGo	.52	.56	.54	.54
Continuous Performance	.44	.47	.53	.55
Anagrams	.30	.32	not used	
Grammatical Reasoning	not used		.47	.52

Note. [a] with practice variance [b] without practice variance

vary within subjects. Thus, the correspondence of the test scores at any two occasions must depend exclusively on the trait component. It follows that the correlation can be estimated from the trait variance in proportion to the test variance. However, if performance improves with practice, the test score variance will be inflated by the practice component. So for reasons of comparison two analyses have been performed: in one analysis the practice component was removed while it was retained in the other. The coefficients are shown in Table 5.

Results. (1) Without exception, coefficients are higher after practice variance has been removed. This holds true especially for tests in which the practice variance is high (d2, Tracking, Rota, Sternberg and Mental Rotations). (2) In Study 1 the coefficients are generally higher. Most likely, this is because the sample was more heterogeneous with respect to age, gender, and education, thereby increasing the variances of the tests. (3) In Study 1 the values are highest for Rota, d2, and Tracking. At the same time, the sensitivities (within-subject reliabilities) for these tests are strikingly low. Conversely, for tests that have revealed the highest sensitivities, the between-subjects reliabilities are moderately high. Though a high degree of sensitivity does not preclude a stable rank order between subjects, tests combining both properties are obviously rare. A necessary prerequisite is that measurement errors be small. (4) In Study 2 the highest values were obtained for Tracking and d2. Although the relationship is less pronounced, the order of good versus poor trait markers is similar to Study 1.

Conclusions

Ambulatory performance measurement in everyday situations is feasible. With a response rate averaging approximately 80 % in Study 1 and 90 % in Study 2, respectively, the compliance is sufficiently high. Likewise, by common standards the psychometric properties of the tests can be regarded as satisfactorily high. Nevertheless, application of such tests in research and practice is rare. Many reasons come into light. For one, ambulatory assessment places more demands on time, cost, and personnel, compared with questionnaires or paper-and-pencil tests under laboratory-like conditions. Second, ambulatory performance measurement is not feasible without portable microcomputers. Thirdly, the development of the software implies programming with special hardware-software experience.

The psychometric properties of the tests differ. Decision times in four simple attention and memory tests yielded within-subject reliabilities that can be regarded as sufficiently high. In contrast, the values were rather low for speed and power tests. With regard to the between-subjects reliability, the coefficients were highest for speed tests. The coefficients were lower for tests whose sensitivities were high.

The tests show shortcomings in test construction. 1) Some of the tests are too short. This holds true especially for the power tests, where the number of items is small. This can partially explain why the reliabilities for these measures are low. By adding further items, reliability can be expected to rise according to the Spearman-Brown rule. 2) Performance in some of these tests drastically improved with practice, a fact that makes within-subject comparisons between different occasions at raw score level more difficult to evaluate. In this study all monotonic practice variance was statistically removed. This procedure can be criticized on the grounds that different mental processes may be involved in a state of low or high practice.

To our knowledge the research reported here constitutes the first systematic large-scale study of the computer assisted ambulatory assessment of cognitive performance measures in everyday situations. Not surprisingly, the test battery is still far from perfect and will need to be improved further.

Acknowledgement

We would like to thank Johannes Drepper, Wilfried Kunde and Hilmar Böhm for programming the behavior data recorder. We also wish to thank Ute Kopp, Inken Prytulla, Christina Reitz, Stefan Rustenbach, Frank Spohn and Grit Weiland for their assistance in collecting and analyzing the data.

References

Becker, M., Sturm, W., Willmes, K. & Zimmermann, P. (1996). Normierungsstudie zur Aufmerksamkeitstestbatterie (TAP) von Zimmermann und Flimm [Standardization of a computer-assisted battery of attention tests]. *Zeitschrift für Neuropsychologie,* 7, 3–15.

Bittner, A.C., Carter, R.C., Kennedy, R.S., Harbeson, M.M. & Krause, M. (1986). Performance evaluation tests for environmental research *(PETER)*: Evaluation of 114 measures. *Perceptual and Motor Skills, 63,* 683–708.

Buse, L. & Pawlik, K. (1984). Inter-Setting-Korrelationen und Setting-Persönlichkeit-Wechselwirkungen: Ergebnisse einer Felduntersuchung zur Konsistenz von Verhalten und Erleben [Transsetting correlations and setting-personality interactions: Results of a field investigation into the consistency of behavior and mood]. *Zeitschrift für Sozialpsychologie, 15,* 44–59.

Buse, L. & Pawlik, K. (1991). Zur State-Trait-Charakteristik verschiedener Meßvariablen der psychophysiologischen Aktivierung, der kognitiven Leistung und der Stimmung in Alltagssituationen [On the state-trait characteristic of various measurement variables of psychophysiological activation, cognitive performance, and mood in daily life situations]. *Zeitschrift für experimentelle und angewandte Psychologie, 38,* 521–538.

Buse, L. & Pawlik, K. (1994). Differenzierung zwischen Tages-, Setting- und Situationskonsistenz ausgewählter Verhaltensmerkmale, Maßen der Aktivierung, des Befindens und der Stimmung im Alltagssituationen [Distinction between temporal, transsetting, and transsituational consistency of selected behavior items, measures of activation, health, and mood in daily life situations]. *Diagnostica, 40,* 2–26.

Buse, L. & Pawlik, K. (1996). Ambulatory behavioral assessment and in-field performance testing. In J. Fahrenberg & M. Myrtek (Eds.), *Ambulatory Assessment. Computer-assisted psychological and psychophysiological methods in monitoring and field studies* (pp. 29–50). Seattle, Toronto, Bern, Göttingen: Hogrefe.

Csikszentmihalyi, M. & Larson, R. (1987). Validity and reliability of the experience sampling method. *Journal of Nervous and Mental Disease, 175,* 526–536.

Diener, E. & Larsen, R. J. (1984). Temporal stability and cross-situational consistency of affective, behavioral, and cognitive responses. *Journal of Personality and Social Psychology, 47,* 871–883.

Fahrenberg, J. & Myrtek, M. (Eds.), *Ambulatory Assessment. Computer-assisted psychological and psychophysiological methods in monitoring and field studies.* Seattle, Toronto, Bern,Göttingen: Hogrefe.

de Vries, M.W. (Ed.) (1992). *The experience of psychopathology. Investigating mental disorders in their natural settings.* Cambridge: Cambridge University Press.

Hormuth, S.E. (1986). The sampling of experiences in situ. *Journal of Personality, 54,* 262–293.

Jex, H.R., McDonnell, J.D. & Phatak, A.V. (1966). A "critical" tracking task for manual control research. *IEEE Transactions of Human Factors in Electronics, HFE-7,* 138–145.

Kane, R.L. & Kay, G.G. (1992). Computerized assessment in neuropsychology: A review of tests and test batteries. *Neuropsychology Review, 3,* 1–117.

Larson, R. & Csikszentmihalyi, M. (1983). The experience sampling method. In H. Reis. (Ed.), *New Directions for Naturalistic Methods in the Behavioral Sciences.* San Francisco: Jossey-Bass.

Manzey, D., Lorenz, B., Schiewe, A., Finell, G. & Thiele, G. (1995). Dual-task performance in space: Results from a single-case study during a short-term space mission. *Human Factors, 37,* 667–681.

Pawlik, K. (1996). Contributions to differential psychology from ambulatory assessment: A researcher's plaidoyer. In J. Fahrenberg & M. Myrtek (Eds.), *Ambulatory Assessment. Computer-assisted psychological and psychophysiological methods in monitoring and field studies* (pp. 21–25). Seattle, Toronto, Bern, Göttingen: Hogrefe.

Pawlik, K. & Buse, L. (1982). Rechnergestützte Verhaltensregistrierung im Feld: Beschreibung und erste psychometrische Überprüfung einer neuen Erhebungsmethode [Computer-assisted behavior assessment *in situ:* Description and first psychometric examination of a new assessment technique*]. Zeitschrift für Differentielle und Diagnostische Psychologie, 3,* 101–118.

Pawlik, K. & Buse, L. (1992). Felduntersuchungen zur transsituativen Konsistenz individueller Unterschiede im Erleben und Verhalten [Field investigations into the transsituational consistency of individual differences in mood and behavior]. In K. Pawlik & K.H..Stapf (Eds.). *Umwelt und Verhalten [Environment and behavior]*. Bern: Huber.

Pawlik, K. & Buse, L. (2001). *Ambulatory Monitoring and Behavior-Test Unit. Handbuch für den AMBU.* Göttingen: Hogrefe (in press).

Santucci, G., Farmer, E., Grisett, J.D., Wetherall, A., Boer, L., Goeters, K.M., Schwartz, E. & Wilson, G., (1989). Battery of Standardized Tests for Research with Environmental Stressors. *Human Performance Assessment Methods No. 308*. Neuly Sur Seine: AGARD (Advisory Group for Aerospace Research & Development).

Shepard, R.N., Metzler, J. (1971). Mental rotation of three-dimensional objects. *Science, 171,* 701–703.

Vandenberg, S.G. & Kuse, A.R. (1978). Mental Rotations, a group test of three-dimensional spatial visualization. *Perceptual and Motor Skills, 47,* 599–604.

Tennen, H., Suls, J. & Affleck, G. (1991). Personality and daily experience. *Journal of Personality, 59*, No 3.

Zimmermann, P. & Fimm, B. (1993). *Testbatterie zur Aufmerksamkeitsprüfung (TAP) Version 1.02. Handbuch [Battery of computer-assisted alertness tests. Manual]*. o.O.: Psytest.

Chapter 2
Simultaneous Computer-Assisted Assessment of Causal Attribution and Social Coping in Families

Meinrad Perrez, Peter Wilhelm, Dominik Schoebi, and Monique Horner
Psychology Department, University of Fribourg, Switzerland

Introduction

Most computer-aided self-monitoring procedures were devised for the assessment of individual emotional or somatic states or ongoing cognitive conscious processes relevant for dysfunctional behavior (cf. de Vries, 1992; Fahrenberg & Myrtek, 1996, 2001; Wilhelm & Perrez, in press). For dyadic or family processes, ambulatory assessment methods have only recently been developed. However, an impressive volume of work has been done with a booklet-approach – without the advantages of micro-computers – by Larson and Richards (1994). They studied fifty-five families with adolescents using the experience sampling method. The main emphasis of the authors was a representative sample of the experiences in families with adolescents for studying the common and divergent realities they encounter. An electronic pager carried by all members of the family simultaneously beeps at eight random times per day over a week. At these moments the subjects had to complete a page in the booklet in order to observe their daily family experience. We have proposed a conceptual basis (Perrez, Berger & Wilhelm, 1998) to assess social regulation of emotions in couples and families in natural settings. An initial aim focuses on the emotional states in daily life of parents and adolescents. How do they evolve throughout the day and over the week for parents and adolescents ? How do parents perceive their own emotional states and those of the partner? A second aim refers to stress emotions. The framework distinguishes between the experienced stressful events in couples and families according to the different possible disturbances of equilibria, namely the equilibrium of individual family members (individual stress), the equilibrium of a subsystem of the family, or of the entire family system (see Table 1). Another aspect consists of how an individual, a subsystem or indeed the whole family react to stress emotions of an individual, a subsystem or to the family as a whole.

We assume that essential components of the social regulation of emotions are characteristics of appraisal and perception processes (or tendencies) of the actors. As variables, important for stress experience and coping ,involving appraisal and interpersonal perception, we focus on valence (positive and negative), controllability, causal attribution, and the accuracy of decoding the partners' emotions. One

Table 1. Matrix of equilibria and coping disturbances

<table>
<tr><th>Adaptive reactions
(dysfunctional or functional)
disturbance of equilibrium</th><th>❶
Father</th><th>❷
Mother</th><th>❸
Child</th><th>❹
Sub-system from 1 to 3</th><th>❺
Family</th></tr>
<tr><td>❶ Father</td><td>intra-individual</td><td>dyadic</td><td>dyadic</td><td rowspan="4">Sub-system involved episode</td><td rowspan="5">Family involved episode</td></tr>
<tr><td>❷ Mother</td><td>dyadic</td><td>intra-individual</td><td>dyadic</td></tr>
<tr><td>❸ Child</td><td>dyadic</td><td>dyadic</td><td>intra-individual</td></tr>
<tr><td>❹ Subsystem from 1 to 3</td><td colspan="3">Subsystem involved episode</td></tr>
<tr><td>❺ Family</td><td colspan="4">Family involved episode</td></tr>
</table>

ty, causal attribution, and the accuracy of decoding the partners' emotions. One aspect of interest is if tendencies in these variables can be identified, which are typical for specific situations, for specific activities with respect to gender and generation. A second aspect concerns emotional and somatic states (positive and negative). They are assumed to be related to cognitive and appraisal process in a theoretically predictable way (Lazarus, 1991; Scherer, 1988). A third question consists of the social effects of causal attributions, if they are ascribed to other members of the family (for couples see Fincham, Harold & Gano-Phillips, 2000). A fourth aspect consists of the adaptive coping responses (individual or social). We assume that functional and dysfunctional individual and social coping reactions can be distinguished from each other. For the *individual* forms we built on the idea, that the functionality or the adequacy of coping responses depend on the fitting of the response with the demands of the coping-task (Reicherts & Perrez, 1992; Reicherts, 1999). For the *social* forms we refer to a taxonomy, that essentially covers the criteria of self-esteem and the system-internal (adaptation to the stressor) versus system-external adaptation (reaction is intended to alter the stressor).

We formulated hypotheses about the relationship of specific attributions patterns with emotional states, as well as for the social effects of specific attributions. For the social coping we expect that the interaction patterns considered to be functional are related in the *short term* to better emotional and social well being (state) of the actor and the actor's partner, and in the *mean term* lead to better individual well being (trait), at the subsystem level to greater partner satisfaction and at the family level to greater cohesion and family satisfaction.

The behavioral analysis of social regulation of emotions should record such processes and identify how far the emotional states can be explained by attribution and social coping tendencies. Such knowledge is of theoretical interest for basic research as well as for the dyadic behavior analysis being a first step in therapy to prepare intervention programs.

In the following paragraphs we describe and summarize the work of the Fribourg research group over the last years, in which several Ph.D. and undergraduate students were involved.

How to assess such intra-individual and interaction patterns under natural conditions?

The microanalysis of the social regulation of emotions needs four types of psychological information corresponding to the temporal structure of the events involved. These are (i) information on antecedents of emotions (such as causal attributions, controllability and interpersonal perception features, co-occurring features such as setting, activity), (ii) information on emotional and somatic states, (iii) on individual and social (adaptive and maladaptive) responses, and (iv) on the individual and social short term effects.

The usual access to such information consists in the use of questionnaires which focus on the variables of interest. Typical, and especially retrospective self-report data, mirror the subjects' cognitive representation of their behavior, emotion and cognition and not how they behaved, felt and thought in particular situations; the same is valid for the estimation of frequencies of behaviors, emotions and cognitions. This assessment approach may be useful and valid for the observation and measurement of the cognitive representation of the subjects' experiences. However if it is not cognitive representations of behavior, of emotional experiences and cognitive activities, but behavioral, emotional and cognitive activities that are our object of study, we need other methods than traditional questionnaires (Wilhelm & Perrez, in press). In order to avoid the impairing effects on validity of usual self-report data, we need assessment strategies which meet the three following criteria: (i) The procedure should allow assessing the above mentioned information in daily life under the social and environmental conditions in which these states and events occur. (ii) The time lag between the experienced states and behavior and their recording should be as short as possible, to minimize memory distortions. Information should be recorded when the subjects are still in the state of emotional arousal for storing "hot emotions" and "hot cognition". (iii) The method should assess psychological relevant data, not using a diary style free text self description, but structured according to the theoretical framework.

To accomplish this aim we have in recent years developed a systematic self observation method based on the use of pocket computers. Our assessment procedure has its root in the experience of the COMRES (COMputer Recording System), that

Table 2. FASEM-C information types and item formats

Information type	Item types
1. Duration and quality of sleep (1st observation of the day)	5 Items (6- and 7-point scales)
2. Emotional and somatic state	11 (6-point scales)
3. Causal attribution	
• internal or external attribution	9 Items (3-point scales)
• other persons	9 Items (3-point scales)
4. Control expectation	(triggered by 2.)
• by myself or by other persons	10 Items (3-point scales)
• which other persons	
5. Somatic complaints / pain	10 Items (3-point scales)
• Attribution	13 Items (categories)
6. Place	6 Categories
7. Setting	14 Items (categories)
• presence of other persons	9 Items (categories)
• evaluation of pleasantness	1 Item (4-point scale)
8. Evaluation of partner's affective state (only for parents)	8 Items (categories and 6-point scales)
9. actual activity	16 Items (categories)
• valence of activity	2 Items (6-point scales)
• consumption of drugs	7 Items (categories)
10. Conflicts with others	Yes/No, triggers:
Social coping	3 Items (3-point scales)
• description of own behavior	12 Items (3-point scales)
• description of other's behavior	12 Items (3-point scales)
11. Individual stress	2 Items (category and 3-point scale)
12. Individual coping	(triggered by 11.)
	12 Items (3-point scales)
13. Social support	Yes/No, triggers:
• by whom?	4 Items (categories)
	triggered by 13.
14. Evaluation of own and other's behavior	2 Items (6-point scales)

Perrez and Reicherts (1996) developed and evaluated in earlier projects on recording individual stress experiences and coping with them. The pocket computer is used as an external memory for stress, that is applied directly in daily stressful situations. This allows minimizing problems of memory and the consequent subjective retrospective distortion.

The purpose is to have access to the emotional life of families, including positive emotional and somatic states as well as negatives. The new approach had not only to integrate a broader range of emotional states; it had in addition to involve the social contingencies of an individual's emotional state in the form of the behavior of other family actors present. With this aim in mind the event-sampling method, for the assessment of individual stress experiencc and coping, was adapted to a time-sampling instrument to assess positive or negative emotional states, related cognitive activities and the social regulative activities of emotions from all members of the family simultaneously.

What is self-recorded?

The method is devised for couples and families with adolescents. Tablc 2 summarizes the different information types and item formats assessed by the family-self-monitoring system (FASEM-C).

Experience and behavior sampling

The social interconnection of the behavior experience assessed, to the behavior of other family members plays a major role for the analysis of the social regulation of emotions. A time sampling strategy is therefore indispensable. The system works with such a method with one exception: In order to avoid waking up the subjects for the first self-observation of the day, the user of FASEM-C start their first recording after getting up in the morning. For the other five measurement points the computer alerts the subject acoustically according to a random time point inside a time window of roughly three hours, five times per day for a weekly period. At these measurement points all subjects had to record their current emotional and somatic state and the other information mentioned above including information on stressful individual or social events and coping with respect to the period between the previous recording and the present moment. The question-program is in some ways adaptive. The presentation of several questions depend on previous answers; for example, if the question "Do you feel any pain or physical complaints?" is answered with "yes", one has to answer supplementary menus. The signal contingent assessment assures the simultaneous recording of all members of the family or couple (older than 13 years). In the same way social support and coping reactions are assessed. Coping responses are only asked if an individual or a social stressful situation has been previously noted. Questions on social coping depend on the involvement of other people in the situation (for example, conflicts). For situations, requiring adaptation without social involvement, individual coping items are presented. Furthermore the program only presents questions concerning control expectations, if a negative emotional state has been recorded.

Technical aspects

The palmtop computer chosen for our studies was the HP 360 LX based on the windows CE operating system. It has a pencil pointing device, a complete Qwerty and touch screen with a resolution of 640 * 240. Data entry was done almost exclusively using the pointing device with the keyboard being only of marginal utility. These characteristics make it possible to carry it during everyday activities and allow the immediate entry of information in a structured format.

Use of a computer has several advantages: it allows the questionnaire to be personalized for each family, using the individual first names of the family members. It also allow a control of user input making it impossible that a user misses completely or incorrectly fills in a question as sometimes occurred in the booklet versions. It also hides some of the questionnaire's complexity from a user as questions that do not apply are not asked and it minimizes reactivity in that once the question displayed is answered no backtracking to a previous question is possible.

Our program separates the questionnaire interpreter from the questionnaire specification. This allows preparation of the questionnaire without any knowledge of computer programming. It also allows easy adaptation to different languages, which is important in Switzerland, with several official languages. Versions in French, German and Portuguese have been tested.

Method

Description of the sample

The data reported here, was gathered in the context of an interdisciplinary project supported by the Swiss National Foundation (see Perrez, Schoebi & Wilhelm, 2000).

For the selection of the families we used the following criteria: Each family should consist of both parents and at least one adolescent between 14 and 17 years, living together in the same household. We also made sure that the self-observation took place during a normal family week and not during holidays or when the family is travelling.

We recruited families with the help of the German and French-speaking school secondary school administrations of canton Fribourg and by using the town population census, (information freely available to the public). A letter was written to each family (about 5200), informing about the purpose of our study and inviting the family to participate.

Interested families sent back a coupon, signed by each participating family member. 101 two-parent-families were willing to participate. Two families cancelled their participation before starting. One stopped the participation because of computer problems. One family was from the Balkans and was dropped from data analysis because the mother had language problems.

The following results are based on 96 families with 314 persons (96 mothers, 96 fathers, 56 female and 66 male adolescents). 40 families were French-speaking the other 56 were German speaking. The average parent was 46.13 years old (SD =

5.86), and the adolescents/young adults 15.45 years (SD = 1.12). Most families belong to the middle class with a comparably high educational level.

Additional questionnaires

In addition, the subjects answered several questionnaires:

Relationship Assessment Scale (Hendrick, 1988; Sander & Böcker, 1993), Family Life Satisfaction Scale (cohesion, adaptation, communication and family satisfaction) (Schneewind & Weiss, 1999), Frankfurter Selbstkonzeptskalen (Deusinger, 1986), Socio-demographic variables and further scales not relevant for the current paper were given. All scales were translated to French and back translated into the original version.

Procedure

Data acquisition took place from November 1998 to April 2000. The interviewer visited the family at home. The participants were given a first introductory training in self-observation with the help of the pocket computer. In addition, the subjects answered the questionnaires. For motivational reasons, the adolescent participants received a coupon for a CD with a value of about 30.- SFr at the end of their self-monitoring task. All families took part on a raffle for a holiday prize with a value of about 3500.- SFr, and they could ask for feedback on their results.

Results with respect to methodological criteria

Acceptance, Accuracy and Duration of recording

All subjects were questioned after the self-observation week about their experience with the assessment method. For most of the participants the duration of the recording task was acceptable (76 %), and nearly all participants (94 %) judged the work with the pocket computer as positive. These results are in accordance with the experience of the first study and belies the expectation, that ambulatory computer-aided self-monitoring disturb participants as suggested by Asendorpf and Wilpers (1999).

The palmtop computer automatically stores the real recording time and the duration of every assessment. This allows strong control on the subject's accuracy and commitment. More than 60 percent of the subjects have been started within five minutes after the signal. 75–80 % of the subjects completed their self-monitoring task within a 30 minutes time-limit.

Concerning the duration, the time is depending on the question, whether more detailed information was asked or not in function of the previous answers. For the shortest version the mean needed time for the protocol was 4.65 min (SD = 2.89) and for the complete version 7.28 minutes per protocol (S.D = 3.82).

Reliability

In the context of self-observation methods there are different possibilities of estimating the reliability of measures (Buse & Pawlik, 1996, Wilhelm & Perrez, in press): The local reliability, the total aggregate reliability and situation-specific-reliability and for simultaneous observations the inter rater reliability. Table 3 summarizes some results on psychometric properties, and we refer to Perrez, Schoebi and Wilhelm (2000) for more detailed results.

Table 3. Reliability coefficients

Local reliability (Cronbach's alpha for the state-items) computed for each of the 42 observations	
Emotional state	.92 to .95 (Mdn = .935)
Somatic state	.46 to .81 (Mdn = .708)
Total-aggregate reliability (odd-even over the 42 observations)	
Emotional state	r= .98
Somatic state	r= .98
Variability (split half)	
Emotional state	r= .85
Somatic state	r= .86

To compute the total-aggregate-reliability the 42 observations were divided into two samples according to the odd-even-method. To calculate the average split-half-reliability for the items belonging to a question, the coefficients were subjected to a Fischer's-z-transformation. The odd-even reliability coefficients for other self-observation categories vary between .34 and .98 with a mean of .69. If the values of strongly situation-dependent items, which are triggered by previous answers (and have therefore a low frequency) are eliminated, the mean is .80. This average total-aggregate-reliability is quite high. For the average emotional state as well as for the average somatic state the total aggregate reliability was r = .98, for bodily complaints (answering the question "Do you feel any pain or do you have any physical complaints in the moment?" with yes or no) it was r = .97, for feeling hungry it was r =.91 and for the evaluation of the activity as pleasant or unpleasant it was r = . 89.

Reactivity

On one hand the reactivity question can be considered as the core question for a self-monitoring procedure – comparable to the memory problem for retrospective assessment methods – , on the other hand it should not be forgotten as Fahrenberg (1994) emphasized, that methodologically conditioned reactivity is a feature of (nearly) all psychological measurement methods. In any case we should know the extent of the influence. We have some objective and some subjective indicators for the question how far FASEM-C has itself an influence on the observed phenomena. If the same questions are asked six times a day over the course of a week, it is probable that the procedure will have learning, fatigue or sensitivity effects. For these analyses we refer to Perrez, Schoebi and Wilhelm (2000). Their results show that over the course of the observation people learn how to use the observational system in a more economic way: They tend to avoid answering questions that are followed by more detailed questions. They also tend to protocol their emotional state in a more stereotype way. This results in a slight increase of the emotional state score. However, even if the effects are statistically significant, the effects are rather small.

Another indicator for reactivity is the subjective estimation of the persons concerning the experienced influence of the assessment procedure. The participants were asked after their self-observation period to what extent the self-monitoring influenced family life, professional activity and their affective states. 57 % answered that the self-observation had no impact on family life, respect. 74 % on professional activity; 36 % estimated a little influence.

With respect to the effects on their affective state, 62 % could not observe any effect, and 33 % a little effect, and for the remainder it was experienced as stronger.

The role of causal attributions for the individual and social regulation of emotion in the family

The self-monitoring study tries to identify cognitive regulation mechanisms, which influence the individual and social regulation of emotion within the family. Causal attributions are supposed to be prominent antecedents and consequences of emotions. Their dimensions (for example, causal locus, controllability) should influence the quality of the emotions (cf. Weiner, 1986; Scherer, 1988), and the quality of emotions may influence the type of attribution. Many studies have been done on the relationship of appraisal components as defined by Lazarus (1991) with specific emotions; less attention has been paid to the role of causal attribution. Lazarus and Smith (1988) and Smith, Haynes, Lazarus and Pope (1993) distinguished two types of cognitive implications: knowledge and appraisal; the latter evaluates the significance of stressors for one's personal wellbeing. The present study focuses on *causal attribution as antecedent and consequence* of emotional states, which is considered as an element of appraisal processes (deviating from the distinction of Lazarus and Smith, 1988). We analyze particularly the self-protective function of internal vs. external causal attributions in positive and negative states and the multi-causality in negative states. A second goal concerns the *social effects of attributions*. How are the attributions toward the family members, and what are the effects? Karney and Bradbury (2000) observed the effects of attributions on marital satisfaction in a longitudinal study. Studies dealing with the connection of children's attribution with features of the relationship in the family can be located in the same context (for example, Fincham, Beach, Arias & Brody, 1998). Our objective is to observe causal attributions and their social consequences in the natural family setting.

For the *assessment* of causal attributions FASEM-C asks family members in every situation, why they feel the way they feel. As causes could be selected oneself, other family members, other persons, and impersonal external circumstances. Answers are rated on a 3-point scale indicating their importance. The specification of the variables "internal attribution", "external attribution", "external attribution addressed to a member of the family", or "external attributions addressed to a person outside the family" was determined by the selection of the answer with the most intensive value, if more than one answer was given. If the subject select more than one cause, then a multi-causal, more complex explanation for the current state is present.

Causal attributions are analysed *(1)* as emotion-consequences by comparing the attributions with respect to positive and negative emotional states, emotional states will be *(2)* examined as antecedents of consecutive emotional states, and *(3)* the social aspects and effects of causal attributions in dyadic situations will be observed.

"Emotional state" consists of a score based on eight bipolar items that create a consistent factor and show high reliability (Perrez, Schoebi & Wilhelm, 2000). Because negative emotional states were rather rare and a large part of the sample only reported one or two negative emotional states, we preferred to take the first positive resp. negative situation reported instead of an aggregation of the data.

Results on causal attributions

The *self-protective function* of causal attributions is suggested by the fact that the subjects explained their *negative* emotional states more intensively by external causes (M=2.27, SD=.99) than by internal (M=1.23, SD=1.20), and they attribute more intensively internal causes for *positive* emotional states (ANOVA: causal attribution x emotional state: $F_{(1,167)}$=33.39, p=.000, eta^2=.17, n=168). In the previous study the percentage of mono-causal internal explanation was significantly higher for good mood states than for bad ones; and mono-causal external explanations were inversely more frequent for bad mood than for good mood (Perrez & Wilhelm, 2000).

The role of *multi-causality of causal explanations:* For every explanation of an emotional state the subject can use one or several causes for explaining his or her state. The variable "multi-causality" is defined by the number of causes used to explain the state. We can observe that negative emotional states are followed by more complex explanations compared with positive emotional states (M_{neg} = 2.70, SD = 2.21 vs M_{pos} = 2.20, SD = 2.14, $t_{(166)}$ = 3.93, p = .000, d = .30). Human beings seem to have a stronger need to explore the possible causes for negative states than for positive. Weiner (1986) noticed that the subjects produce spontaneously attributions when the events are unexpected or the goal non-attained. Positive emotional states and moods are experienced as a matter of course, whereas negative states demand explanation, and the explanation may have an self-reassuring and calming effect.

This need to explore causes seems to be influenced by traits: multi-causality is correlated with indicators of "neuroticism", in particular with lower self-esteem (r = -.24, p =. 002, n = 172), more psychosomatic symptoms (r =. 17, p = .02, n =

172) and higher depressive scores (r = . 15, p = .04, n = 172). These are rather small effects, that reach significance only when we treat family members as independent individuals.

Emotional states tend to be followed by different causal attributions according to the valence of the emotion, if subjects are asked for explanation, and according to personality traits.

This self-protecting phenomenon is in some way confirmed by the short term effects; the causal attributions are here taken into account as *antecedents of emotions*: Because external attributions with respect to negative emotional state are more likely to maintain the self-esteem, they should be more prone to change the mood in a positive direction than internal attributions. We predicted as a short term-effect that positive mood swing between the previous observation t_0 and the following observation t_1 will be larger, if the person attributes external attributions at observation t_0, and it will be lower, if it reports an internal attribution. The intra-personal comparison showed in the previous study (Perrez & Wilhelm, 2000), and in the present, that after external attributions the positive emotional state is significantly larger than after internal (M_{ext}= 3.93, SD= .81 *vs* M_{int} = 3.63, SD = 1.13, $t_{(30)}$= 1.69, p = .05 (one tailed) d= .30). This difference is not due to differences in the emotional state at observation t_0.

Social aspects of attributions: To what extent do family members attribute their positive and their negative emotional states to other members of the family? We compared the intensity of the causal attributions during positive and negative emotional states (Wilcoxon, two-tailed). Family members report other members of the family more intensively as the cause for *negative* states than for positive emotional states (Z = 5.46, p< .001, n = 168). These findings confirm the results of the previous study (Horner, Perrez, Berger, Wilhelm & Schoebi, 2000).

The adolescents tend to explain *positive* emotional states as in the previous project more with causes attributed to persons outside the family than inside (Z = 5.91, p< .001, n = 119), which underlines the important role of peers for adolescents. They spent significantly more time with persons not belonging to the family than their parents. The adolescents met friends in settings outside the school and home in 61 % of the observations; parents record meeting friends in 30 % of their observations outside work place and home.

Interpersonal effects of causal attributions: We assumed that an external attribution should have an influence on the addressee, especially if negative emotions are at stake. Therefore, we compared the emotional state of B, if subject A attributes the causes for his or her negative emotional state to B (t test with dependent samples), with his or her state in the cases when A *does not* attribute the causes for his or her negative emotional state to B. The within-comparison of the emotional states (as addressee or as non-addressee of the causal attribution for the negative state of the partner) is based on situations in which both persons are present.

The analysis confirmed our expectations. If the father attributes his negative emotional state to the mother, her emotional state is significantly worse than if he doesn't make her responsible for his negative state. The same tendency can be observed if sons and daughters are the targets of the father's attributions (see table 4). The observed effect sizes are comparable, but do not reach significance due to the small sample sizes.

If we have a look to the mothers' attribution, similar effects can be observed. None of the adolescents' attributions had a significant effect on their parents' emotional state, but at least for the mother, they follow the same general trend. Larger samples would be required to confirm the rather small effects.

In the previous study the effects were strongest for fathers, according to the power location in the family, then for mothers, and finally for the female adolescents. The latter's attribution were associated with the mother's emotional state (Horner, Perrez, Berger, Wilhelm & Schoebi, 2000; and Horner, in preparation).

The results confirm findings of the previous study (Horner, Perrez, Berger, Wilhelm & Schoebi, 2000; Perrez & Wilhelm, 2000; Wilhelm, Horner & Perrez, 2000).

Table 4. Matrix of the differences of emotional states in association of father's and mother's attributions

	Father	Mother	Son	Daughter
Father		d=.25, p=.06, n=37	d=.22, p=ns, n=12	d=.22, p=ns, n=12
Mother	d=.29, p=.03 n=44		d=.29, p=.08 n=24	d=.12, p=ns n=28

Social coping in families

In the German speaking area, social coping in families was discussed by Laux and Schütz (1996) and by the Fribourg group (Perrez, Berger & Wilhelm, 1998). Bodenmann's (1995, 2000) contributions deal with the dyadic coping as a special case of social coping.

We define *social coping* as social behavior of a person A which intends to reduce stress-emotions. The stress-emotions can affect the person A itself, and A tries for example, to reduce stress by asking person B for help. They can also affect actor B, and A tries to help B to solve his or her emotional distress; or both actors are involved in a same stressful encounter, for example, in a conflict or in the common loss of a loved person.

We define a social coping response as *functional*, if it is favorable to one's self-esteem or, at least, does not impair the self-esteem of the persons who are involved in the stressful encounter. Impairing responses are qualified as *dysfunctional*. We consider for example, the category "give way against the own will" as dysfunctional accommodation. Examples for functional social coping are: "Negotiating", "convincing" (assimilative social coping), "accepting the opinion of the other" (accommodative social coping).

The *assessment of the social coping* with FASEM-C consists first of the question if the subject was involved in a problem with somebody else since the last observation point (about 3 hours). In the affirmative the person has to record first the behavior of the conflict partner and then his or her own social coping behavior using 12 three-point scales (the items correspond to the responses, listed in table 5). This procedure enables assessing information on the self-perception and the interpersonal perception of the social coping.

Table 5: Functional and dysfunctional social coping responses

Functional social coping responses	Dysfunctional social coping responses
Negotiating	Reproaching
Support/trying to understand	Obeying against the own will
Accepting the other's intention	Devaluing others/not taking the other seriously
Taking in good humor	Concealing his feelings
Convincing	Avoiding contact/fleeing the partner
Declaring oneself	Covering negative feelings*

Note: * This category has not been recorded.

Dependency of social coping from situations

The question which type of social coping responses is favored by persons presumably does not only depend on personal styles, but depends also on features of the situation. In the field of emotion research, Ekman knew already in the sixties that emotions are impressively influenced by social situations. He called the phenomenon "display rules of emotions" (Ekman, 1972). Analogous influences can be suspected for social coping. We expect more dysfunctional social coping responses, if they are addressed to family members than if they focus on persons outside the family. The family facilitates not only the expression of negative emotions, but also of dysfunctional social behavior as a comparably tolerant environment for deviation. We expect this difference in both the recording of own and other's behavior.

The following results based on a subsample of the initial 96 families. 213 subjects of a total of 314 persons reported more than two conflict situations within the observation period and were therefore included. Subjects with less than three conflict reports were excluded for reasons of feasibility of the intended analyses. This sample of 213 persons (out of 67 families) reported a total of 853 conflicts. In 10 of these situations family members as well as persons from outside the family were involved in the stressful encounter. They were excluded from the comparison. The

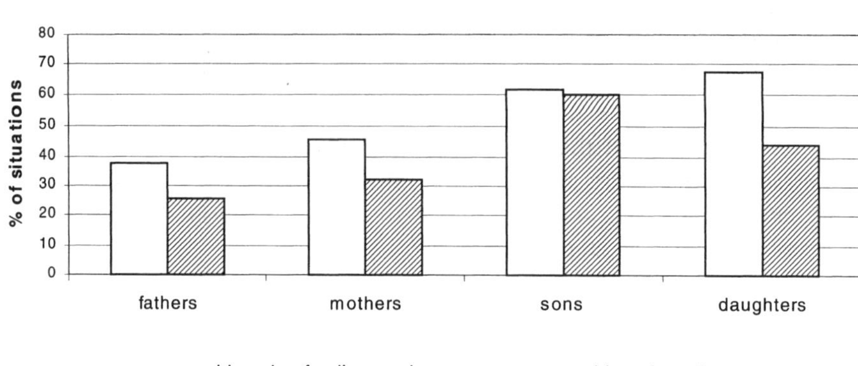

Figure 1. Dysfunctional social coping towards family members and others

database for the analysis finally included data of 58 fathers (157 conflict situations with family members and 51 with others), 63 mothers (255 vs. 31), 45 sons (106 vs. 55) and 47 daughters (138 vs. 50). The percentage of situations with predominantly dysfunctional social coping has been calculated for each individual separately for conflicts with family members and conflicts with others. Figure 1 illustrates the means of the individual percentages according to the addressees:

The results concerning the perceived coping behavior of the conflict partner show congruent patterns, as illustrated in Table 6.

Table 6. Distribution of predominantly dysfunctional coping responses of the conflict partners

Recorded by	Predominantly dysfunctional social coping by	
	Family members	others
Fathers	46.5%	37.3%
Mothers	54.5%	45.2%
Sons	61.3%	76.4%
Daughters	68.1%	56,0%

To test the descriptive results, reported above, within subject comparison would be most appropriate. Therefore, the sample described above was further restricted to persons who reported at least one conflict situation with family members *and* another with others.

98 persons out of 67 families (26 fathers, 21 mothers, 24 sons and 27 daughters) remained for the analysis. The within-comparison (Wilcoxon-test) shows a significant difference (p=.021) as expected. This is in accordance with an alternative analysis of the same data (Perrez & Schoebi, in press) and with the results of a previous study (Wilhelm, Horner & Perrez, 2000), where subjects recorded significantly more dysfunctional coping responses with family members. The within-

comparison for the subsamples (fathers, mothers, sons and daughters) indicate tendencies (p ranges between .052 and .081) in the same direction, except for the sons.

For the reported social coping responses observed by conflict partners, the differences do not reach the level of significance if analyzed over the whole sample, but show a comparable pattern. The sons differ from the general pattern found for the other family members. They record a rather equal distribution of their own functional and dysfunctional behavior and their reports on the other's behavior even contradict the general tendency.

Discussion

The above described computer-aided self-monitoring system for couples and families with adolescents has proven it's *applicability* in normal families and in selected cases of families with patients (anorexia) (Rach, 1998). In all cases it requires motivated couples or families. With this prerequisite the drop out rates are surprisingly low. Families who decide to participate showed, in general, a reliable commitment. Most of the participants accepted the self-monitoring task with the help of the pocket computer, even if there were sometimes technical problems to solve, especially with the energy supply of the computers. The results on *reliability* are satisfactory. For some predominantly situations-specific variables we found, as we expected, lower aggregate reliability coefficients. The *reactivity* of this assessment procedure is significant, but small. For our method, we assume a strong *ecological validity*, because in contrast to laboratory or questionnaire methods, behavioral and mood data are gathered in the context and under the conditions under which behavior and emotional states usually occur.

The advantages of this assessment procedure are evident for the purpose of data collection on psychological and social processes, on "hot cognition" and "hot emotions" in daily life. The traditional questionnaire methods usually assess rather the subject's cognitive representation of his or her emotions, cognitions and behaviors than properties of theses psychological phenomena. The described method requires that the phenomena assessed are conscious to the subject. Some developments can be observed in the context of psychotherapeutic intervention (cf. Wilhelm & Perrez, in press) for individual therapies. FASEM-C is opening new ways for the behavior and cognition analyzes of couples and families. This new procedure of analyzing the individual and social regulation of emotion may be helpful in the future for the planing of therapeutic intervention for couples and families. The *clinical importance* consists – compared with traditional methods – of a more appropriate assessment of psychological phenomena. The direct observation of actual behavior, emotional states, and cognition fits better the theoretical assumptions on functional relationships between cognitive or other antecedents and their behavioral consequences. The advantage of reliable self-monitoring consists in information on behavior, recorded in daily life close to the events. Using FASEM-C, dysfunctional social patterns and their intra-personal cognitive antecedents can be discovered. The utility is not restricted to the functional analysis; it also concerns the assessment of base-line and follow-up data for treatment evaluation.

The results show with regard to the connection of causal attributions with emotional states promising relationships. The importance of causal attributions as antecedents of emotional states is confirmed on a correlation-level; and on the other hand emotional states are revealed as predictors of causal attributions. The self-protecting function of external causal attributions and the social effects by the addressees inside the family have been replicated in the new data. They also confirm the self-serving biases, as has been observed by Laux and Schütz (1996) and Schütz (1999) with respect to the attributions for one's own and spouse's behavior in conflicts. The results do not contribute to the distinction of attributions and appraisals, as Smith, Haynes, Lazarus and Pope (1993) proposed.

The confirmation of the results of the previous FASEM-study is furthermore true for the analyses of the social regulation of emotions. It seems to exist what could be termed "display rules for social coping" by analogy to the display rules for emotions (Ekman, 1972). Functional social modalities of emotion regulation happen easier during exchange with persons not belonging to the family than with family members, and for dysfunctional modalities the inverse is true.

With respect to the limits of conventional statistic computing of serial data as they are generated by FASEM-C, we emphasize that they can be helpful for clarifying very specific and limited questions such as, if dysfunctional coping is more often addressed to family members than to others, or if one type of causal attribution to explain a stressor is more associated with some specific emotional states than with others. However, these analyses are confronted with the problem of the multiple dependency of the data. The data can be referenced to different levels: to subjects, to families, to time points, etc. Conventional methods focus on *one* level (cf. Schallberger, 2000). In this chapter we reported results, that are based on standard statistical methods (mostly paired sample t-test or Wilcoxon-test). These tests are well known and the results are easy to communicate. For most of the analyses we collapsed the data over the repeated observations a person reported in two (or more) different types of situations, and then we computed within subject comparisons on the base of such aggregated scores. One problem of that strategy is that the persons who did not report self-observations data in every situation, which is going to be analyzed, had to be dropped. This leads to a reduction of statistical power to detect effects and complicates the generalization of the results.

In family data a second source of dependence is between subjects, because family members are more similar to each other than random sampled individuals. To take care of a second source of dependence is quite complicated in standard statistical analysis (for example, Wilhelm, Horner & Perrez, 2000). In this chapter some of the analyses ignore family membership and treat subjects as independent units. These significance tests are in danger of being to liberal. One way to protect against such an inflation of the alpha error is to check if the results are still significant if one corrects degrees of freedom. The right correction has to take the amount of similarity between family members into account, that can be measured as an intra-class correlation (Kenny, Kashy & Bolger, 1998). A crude and conservative, but easy way to check whether the significance test holds, is to look if a result is still significant after the degrees of freedom have been reduced from the number of individuals to the number of families involved into the analysis (minus the corrective for number of parameters estimated). Applying this check to the results reported here, reveals that significance holds even under that condition.

Wilhelm gives in a separate chapter an example of how the problems discussed here can be solved alternatively by applying multilevel analysis to the family self observation data.

Acknowledgements

The authors express their thanks to Ian Law for his excellent programming work, Regula Berger, Karin Kronenberg, Nicola Jacobshagen for their continuous cooperation, and Marie-Hélène Marra, François Gremaud, Marlène Wicky, Alexandra Lebrun, Michael Schmidhauser, Cornelia Gut, Sandra König and Marcel Fankhauser for their help with the data collection. We thank the Swiss National Science Foundation for its financial support (Proj. Nr. SNF 1114–041935.94/1).

References

Asendorpf, J.B. & Wilpers, S. (1999). Kontrolliertes Interaktions-Tagebuch zur Erfassung sozialer Interaktionen, Beziehungen und Persoenlichkeitseigenschaften. *Diagnostica, 45*, 82–94.

Bodenmann, G. (1995). *Bewältigung von Stress in Partnerschaften. Der Einfluss von Belastungen auf die Qualität und Stabilität von Paarbeziehungen.* Freiburger Beiträge zur Familienforschung. Bd. 2. Freiburg: Universitätsverlag / Bern: Hans Huber.

Bodenmann, G. (2000). *Stress und Coping bei Paaren.* Göttingen: Hogrefe.

Buse, L. & Pawlik, K. (1996). Ambulatory behavioral assessment and in-field performance testing. In J. Fahrenberg & M. Myrtek (Eds.), *Ambulatory assessment* (pp. 29–50). Seattle, WA: Hogrefe & Huber Publishers.

de Vries, M.W. (Ed.). (1992). *The experience of psychopathology. Investigating mental disorders in their natural settings.* Cambridge: Cambridge University Press.

Deusinger, I.-M. (1986). *Frankfurter Selbstkonzeptskalen (FSKN).* Göttingen: Hogrefe.

Ekman, P. (1972). Universals and cultural differences in facial expressions of emotion. In J.K. Cole (Ed.), *Nebraska Symposium on motivation* (pp. 207–285). Lincoln: University of Nebraska press.

Fahrenberg, J. (1994). Ambulantes Assessment. Computerunterstützte Datenerfassung unter Alltagsbedingungen. *Diagnostica, 40* (3), 195–216.

Fahrenberg, J. & Myrtek, M. (Eds.), (1996). *Ambulatory Assessment: Computer-assisted psychological and psychophysiological methods in monitoring and field studies.* Seattle, WA: Hogrefe & Huber Publishers.

Fahrenberg, J. & Myrtek, M. (2001). Ambulantes Monitoring und Assessment. In F. Rösler (Ed.), *Enzyklopädie der Psychologie, Bd. 4: Grundlagen und Methoden der Psychophysiologie* (pp. 657–798). Göttingen: Hogrefe.

Fincham, F.D., Beach, S.R.H., Arias, I. & Brody, G.H. (1998). Children's Attributions in the Family: The Children's Relationship Attribution Measure. *Journal of Family Psychology, 12* (4), 481–493).

Fincham, F.D., Harold, G.T. & Gano-Phillips, S. (2000). The longitudinal association between causal attributions and marital satisfaction: Direction of effects and role of efficacy expectations. *Journal of Family Psychology, 14* (2), 267–285.

Hendrick, S.S. (1988). A generic measure of relationship satisfaction. *Journal of Marriage and the Family, 50*, 93–98.

Horner, M. (in preparation). *Attributions causales comme antécédents d'émotions. Etude à la base d'autoobservation systématique dans le cadre naturel.* (Dissertation en préparation). Fribourg: Université, Département de Psychologie.

Horner, M., Perrez, M., Berger, R., Wilhelm, P. & Schoebi, D. (2000). *Austausch von Kausalattributionen innerhalb der Familie. Analyse auf der Basis computer-unterstützter Self-monitoring Daten* (Forschungsbericht Nr. 148). Fribourg: Universität, Departement für Psychologie.

Kenny, D.A., Kashy, D.A: & Bolger, N. (1998). Data analysis in social psychology. In D.T. Gilbert, S.T. Fiske & G. Lindzey (Eds.), *Handbook of social psychology, vol 1* (pp. 233–265). Boston: McGraw-Hill.

Karney, B.R. & Brodbury, T.N. (2000). Attributions in Marriage: State or Trait? A Growth Curve Analysis. *Journal of Personality and Social Psychology, 78* (2), 295–309.

Larson, R. & Richards, M. (1994). *Divergent realities. The emotional lives of mothers, fathers, and adolescents.* New York: BasicBooks.

Laux, L. & Schütz, A. (1996). Unter Mitarbeit von Burda-Viering, M., Limmer, R., Renner, K.-H. Trapp, W., Vogel, S. & Weiss, H. *Stressbewältigung und Gesundheit in der Familie.* (Schriftenreihe des Bundesministeriums für Familie, Senioren, Frauen und Jugend. Bd. 108.) Stuttgart: Kohlhammer.

Lazarus, R.S. (1991). *Emotion and Adaptation.* New York, Oxford: University Press.

Lazarus, R.S. & Smith, C.A. (1988). Knowledge and appraisal in the cognition-emotion relationship. *Cognition and Emotion, 2*, 281–300.

Perrez, M. & Reicherts, M. (1996). A computer-assisted self-monitoring procedure for assessing stress-related behavior under real life conditions. In J. Fahrenberg & M. Myrtek (Eds.), *Ambulatory Assessment. Computer-assisted psychological and psychophysiological methods in monitoring and field studies* (pp. 51–71). Seattle; Toronto; Bern; Göttingen: Hogrefe & Huber.

Perrez, M. & Wilhelm, P. (2000). Control psychology under the control of questionnaires? The search for an alternative assessment procedure. In W.J. Perrig & A. Grob (Eds.), *Control of Human Behavior, Mental Processes, and Consciousness* (pp. 245–261). Mahwah, N.J. and London: Lawrence Erlbaum.

Perrez, M., Berger, R. & Wilhelm, P. (1998). Die Erfassung von Belastungserleben und Belastungsverarbeitung in der Familie: Self-Monitoring als neuer Ansatz. *Psychologie in Erziehung und Unterricht, 45*, 19–35.

Perrez, M., Schoebi, D. & Wilhelm, P. (2000). How to Assess Social Regulation of Stress and Emotions in Daily Family Life? A Computer-assisted Family Self-monitoring System (FASEM-C). *Clinical Psychology and Psychotherapy, 7*, 326–339.

Perrez, M. & Schoebi, D. (in press). Soziales Coping in der Selbst- und in der Fremdperspektive. In S. Walper & R. Pekrun (Eds.), *Familie und Entwicklung: Perspektiven der Familienpsychologie.* Göttingen: Hogrefe.

Rach, N. (1998). *Belastungen und ihre Verarbeitung in Familien mit einer magersüchtigen Tochter* (Lizentiatsarbeit). Fribourg: Universität, Departement für Psychologie.

Reicherts, M. (1999). *Règles cognitivo-comportementales. Bases theoriques et méthodologiques* (Habilitationsschrift). Fribourg: Universitätsverlag.

Reicherts, M. & Perrez, M. (1992). Adequate coping behavior: The behavior rules approach. In M. Perrez & M. Reicherts (Eds.), *Stress, coping, and health: A situational- behavior approach. Theory, methods, applications* (pp. 161–182). Seattle; Toronto; Bern; Göttingen: Hogrefe & Huber.

Sander J. & Böcker, S. (1993). Die Deutsche Form der Relationship Assessment Scale (RAS): Eine kurze Skala zur Messung der Partnerschaftszufriedenheit. *Diagnostica, 39*, 55–62.

Schallberger, U. (2000). *Qualität des Erlebens in Arbeit und Freizeit. Untersuchungen mit der Experience Sampling Method* (Projektbericht). Zürich: Universität, Psychologisches Institut.

Scherer, K.R. (1988). Criteria for emotion-antecedent appraisal: A review. In V. Hamilton, G.H. Bower & N.H. Frijda (Eds.), *Cognitive perspective on Emotion and Motivation* (pp. 89–126). Dodrecht: Nijkoff.

Schneewind, K.A. & Weiss, J. (1999). *Gesundheit- und Stress-Fragebogen.* Bern: Hans Huber.

Schütz, A. (1999). It was your fault! Self-serving biases in autobiographical accounts of conflicts in married couples. *Journal of Social and Personal Relationships, 16* (2), 193–208.

Smith, C.A., Haynes, K.N., Lazarus, R.S. & Pope, L.K. (1993). In Search of the "Hot" Cognitions: Attributions, Appraisals, and Their Relation to Emotion. *Journal of Personality and Social Psychology, 65* (5), 916–929.

Weiner, B. (1986). *An attributional theory of motivation and emotion.* New York: Springer.

Wilhelm, P. & Perrez, M. (in press). Felddiagnostik. In R.-D. Stieglitz & U. Baumann (Eds.), *Psychodiagnostik psychischer Störungen.* Stuttgart: Enke.

Wilhelm, P., Horner, M. & Perrez, M. (2000). Humeur et gestion du stress dans les interactions familiales: Résultats à partir de la méthode FASEM. In J.-P. Pourtois & H. Desmet (Eds.), *Relation familiale et résilience* (pp. 255–274). Paris: L'Harmattan.

Chapter 3
Psychological Monitoring in Sociodiagnostics

Urs Baumann[1] , Ludwig Feichtinger[1], and Claudia Thiele[2]

[1] *Department of Psychology,* [2] *Department of Educational Studies*
both University of Salzburg, Austria

Core concepts in sociodiagnostics

The complex assessment of a person requires a multimodal diagnostic approach in which various levels of data are differentiated. This chapter focuses on the social data level, which assesses social interactions and social relationships among others (sociodiagnostics). The term *social interaction* (Hinde, 1992) refers to any situation, in which the behavior of two or more people relates to each other. Table 1 depicts those categories which proved important in the description of interactions and the interaction partners (Laireiter & Thiele, 1995).

The term interaction is limited by the term *social relation.* Hinde (1992) defines the existence of a social relation rather formally in terms of duration, which ascribes a temporal perspective to the interaction (including the past, present, and future). Moreover, social relations subsume relations which are low in contact frequency but still subjectively important (for example, having friends living in another country).

In characterising social relations the concepts of social network, social support, and social strain are of great importance (Laireiter, 1993a; Veiel & Baumann, 1992). In contrast to various other disciplines, the fields of psychology and psychiatry ascribe a very specific meaning to the term "network". In these fields the term *social network* refers to the system of social relations of a *single* person (compare to "personal social network", "egocentric network"). In the literature several dimensions have been developed to describe this individual system of personal relations (Pfingstmann & Baumann, 1987): structural (for example, size), interactional (for example, duration of the relation), functional (for example, support, strain), and evaluational (for example, satisfaction) parameters. Various criteria are used to define and operationalize this system of relations (for example, social roles, duration of contact).

Social support refers to meeting specific social needs for intimacy, security, information, practical help, relaxation, and comfort etc. (Veiel & Ihle, 1993). Thus, the

Table 1. Contact persons and social interactions: dimensions and examples (modified according to Laireiter & Thiele, 1995)

Dimensions	Contact partner	Interaction
	Examples for characteristics	
Structural aspects	Number Cluster (sub-groups)	Duration (min./hours) Number of interactions
Formal & content conditions	Age Gender Social role/s Homogeneity (e.g. same age)	Place Mode (directly, via phone, email, etc.)
Contents		Topics
Dynamics		Reciprocity Regulation Concern/rejection
Emotionality	Attractiveness Sympathy vs. Antipathy Familiarity	Emotional intensity Emotional quality (positive, indifferent, ambivalent, negative) Strain/conflict
Functional aspects		Help Support Care Sociability Relief Love Sexuality etc.
Evaluation		Satisfaction Importance

term describes a central functional aspect of social relations and relational networks. Research in the 1980s lead to further differentiations of the term with respect to assessment and evaluation (for example, construct components like perceived supp-port, enacted support; source of support (social role of the support person); the type of support (psychological vs. instrumental); Laireiter & Baumann, 1992).

Although the complex nature of social relations was pointed out by Rook (1984) in the 1980s, the positive aspects of social relations have dominated the area of sociodiagnostics for a much longer period, in particular those of social support. For example, any kind of social support creates a feeling of inferiority in the recipient and a decrease in self-esteem. An example is overprotection which is generally per-ceived negatively (by the recipient) but intended positively (by the person extending it) (compare also with the concept of expressed emotions). Therefore it seems useful to include, besides social support, another aspect which subsumes the negative aspects of social relations; this area can be referred to with the term *social strain* (similar constructs are for example, social conflict, social network-stressors, negative interactions). Taking a theoretical stance, Rook and colleagues posited three broad categories of social strain (Rook, 1984):

- ineffective social support (ineffective and excessive help);
- undesirable or aversive social contact (negative behavior/interactions such as criticism, disapproval);
- negative regulatory mechanisms (attempts at social control, which promote deviant or unhealthy behavior).

In sociodiagnostics the question is how these social constructs come into effect and how they are interrelated. Classical research focused on the interdependence of social support and well–being, as well as impairment of the latter. Studies have mainly been conducted in accordance with the buffer- and main-effect-hypothesis (Cohen & Wills, 1985; Schwarzer & Leppin, 1989). Building on these two central hypotheses and influenced by the stress concepts of Lazarus, later research has developed more complex concepts which cannot be discussed further in this chapter (Perrez, Laireiter & Baumann, 1998).

Research on the impact of social strain has been less systematic than research on social support. Most studies concentrated on the relationship to well-being (Rook, 1992). More recently there has been increased interest in the interrelationship between social support and social strain. For one thing, the frequencies of social support and social strain have been compared, and social support proved to be more prevalent than social strain (Müller & Baumann, 1999); moreover, the relative importance of each in terms of well-being has also been investigated.

From this research four deductions can be made (Lettner, Sölva & Baumann, 1996):

(1) Numerous studies suggest that the impact of social strain on well-being outweighs the impact of social support: a phenomenon referred to as the negativity effect.

(2) Only a few studies suggest a positivity effect, where the impact of social support is greater than the impact of social strain.

(3) Likewise, there is little evidence of a symmetrical effect, namely that social support and social strain have an equally strong impact on well-being.

(4) All three effects discussed above are usually found with respect to a single parameter. If several target criteria are used, domain specific effects are found which can be combined with variants (1) to (3).

Essential for this area of research is the complex assessment of subjective well-being (positive and negative affect; cognitive components; Sölva, Baumann & Lettner, 1995).

Measurement methods in sociodiagnostics with specific focus on diaries

Parameters in sociodiagnostics are mainly assessed by either oral (interviews, exploration) or written (questionnaires, rating procedures) inquiries (Baumann & Laireiter, 1995; Perrez, Laireiter & Baumann, 1998; Laireiter, 1993b). In a few cases behavior observation in real or laboratory settings or content analysis is used. For the most part, data are gathered cumulatively over several days or weeks (for example, "How often did you.... during the last week?"); diaries are used less often, although several diary procedures have been suggested in sociodiagnostics (for an overview see Laireiter & Thiele, 1995; Baumann, Thiele, Laireiter & Krebs, 1996). These diaries usually contain a self-observation report, where the subject rates his or her experiences and behaviors in social situations according to predetermined categories. In addition to these formal characteristics, diaries can be described by their principles of assessment (Laireiter & Thiele, 1995):

sampling procedure: event sampling, momentary time sampling or interval recording;

- mode of registration: paper-pencil or computer-assisted (for example, COMES-SOZU: Perkonigg, 1991; Perrez & Reicherts, 1996);
- data source: usually a single person in self-observation; more rarely subjects are two people (= double-diary).

According to Laireiter and Thiele (1995) diaries in sociodiagnostics can be subdivided into three groups (cf. Baumann et al., 1996):

- *Interval-contingent registration*: the subject observes his/her social interactions over a certain period of time (mostly 24 hours) which is subdivided into smaller time periods.
- *Event-contingent registration*: recording is triggered by an event (for example, contacts of a certain duration; supporting contact; straining contact).
- *Signal-contingent registration*: the subject assesses the relevant parameters (whether with or without a contact) whenever the signal occurs.

In addition to diaries in sociodiagnostics (for an overview see Baumann et al., 1996) a multitude of diaries – mostly non computer-aided – exist for different areas. In these other diaries the parameters of interaction diagnostics are also partly included, but are not the main purpose (overview: Thiele, Laireiter & Baumann, 2001; mood: Vittengl & Holt, 1998; elderly: Tesch-Römer, 1998; anxiety disorders: Margraf & Jacobi, 1997; pain: Feldman, Downey & Schaffer-Neitz, 1999).

In the clinical area two recent *computer-assisted* procedures which include interaction assessment are:

- *Computer-aided setting assessment* (CASA; Schick & Schmidt, 1997).

  Computer-aided behavior rating instrument for inpatient psychiatry with time sampling (a 5 seconds observation interval with consecutive coding every 10 minutes); the procedure assesses interactive and non-interactive behavior, aggress-sion, emotions/mood and movement/position through 89 items. Interrater reliability across all items is .87 (Cohen's kappa).

- *Interaction record* (Steiger, Gauvin, Jabalpurwala, Seguin & Stotland, 1999). The instrument has been developed in research on bulimia nervosa. Every social interaction longer than 10 minutes in duration is recorded. In addition to eating behavior, the areas of interaction tone, self-perception, and mood are assessed with several items each (alpha for each of the three areas >.89).

The following chapter presents the *SONET-CT-96*, a computer-aided instrument for interaction diagnostics. Given the multiple aspects of interaction diagnostics and in order to assess them in a reasonably complex manner, an extensive set of parameters is necessary, especially in describing social network, social support, and social strain. As these aspects include direct and indirect strain, the coping processes and subjective well-being as a demonstration of interaction dynamics are of great interest.

Our own approach has been empirically tested in a complex diary study, in an attempt to answer the following questions:
Description of daily structures pertaining to sociodiagnostics.
Formal accuracy of the procedure (reliability of results).
Relationship between social support, social strain, and subjective well-being.

In addition, the relationship between the interval-contingent registration of interaction assessment (the "classical" form of sociodiagnostics) and the diary data has been analysed, but is not reported here. Essential to our study is the *differential* question as to how well results correspond between the clinical and non-clinical population. For that reason, all research questions have been investigated separately for a clinical and a non-clinical sample. To date, computer-aided diary studies of sociodiagnostics have rarely been applied to patients, so in this respect the following study is an exploratory one.

Diary measurement SONET-CT-96

Description of the method

Our approach is based on SONET (Baumann & Laireiter, 1993; Laireiter, Baumann, Untner, Feichtinger & Reisenzein, 1997), which has been constructed as a complex measure of sociodiagnostics. The social network is assessed according to contact frequency and social roles. The period of observation is the previous six months. Reliability has proved to be very satisfactory (Schwarzenbacher & Baumann, 1990). Based on this concept various diary versions have been developed:

- *Computer-aided self registration system on stress and coping and social support* (COMES-SOZU; Perkonigg, 1991; Perkonigg, Baumann, Reicherts & Perrez, 1993).

This procedure represents an extension of Perrez' approach combining the stress-concept with the coping-approach (COMES: Perrez & Reicherts, 1996). The diary is event-contingent.

- *Interval-contingent diary* SONET-T (developed as paper-pencil method; observation interval is one day; Laireiter, Baumann, Reisenzein & Untner, 1997). Interval-contingent registration of contacts (contacts which are at least 10 minutes in duration and/or important ones) with social support or social strain.
- SONET-CT represents a *computer-assisted interaction diary on social network*, which assesses social support and social strain (Baumann, Laireiter & Thiele, 1994; Baumann et al., 1996; Thiele, 1994).

The original version SONET-CT has been extended to the current SONET-CT-96. With the latter, contact events (single contacts and group contacts) are being assessed (see Table 2 and Figure 1). Single contacts are differentiated into three forms:

- "pure" single contact;
- single contact within a group setting (for example, a person is in a group setting but mainly interacts with a single person);
- discontinous single contact (for example, co-operation of two team colleagues in the work place).

Every contact of 10 minutes or more, and important contacts of lesser duration are registered. Different kinds of contacts, as well as the support and strain questions, trigger jumps, so that normally all the questions do not have to be covered (see Figure 1). For instance, the very first question leads either to the section on single or group contacts. In case no support has been received (item 11; see Table 2 for the respective item description), the programme jumps to item 34 (strain). If there was neither direct nor indirect social strain (in conjunction with social support), the last section (item 56 to 71) is skipped.

In the new version SONET-CT-96 both sections – social support and social strain – are assessed in more detail:

- with social support: in addition to the appraisal of received support the aspect of strain is assessed as well;
- with social strain: this area is covered more comprehensively.

Along with increased assessment of social strain the question of how the strain is dealt with arises (coping). Therefore a detailed coping section (according to Lazarus) has been added. The computer technology has been substantially improved as well.

Technical Data of the Palmtop PC

The HP 1000CX Palmtop PC is a pocket-computer (16 x 8,64 x 2,54 cm) with a weight of 312 g (with batteries). This very small battery-powered palmtop has an operating system that should be completely MS-DOS (Ver. 5.0) compatible and has

Table 2. Structure of parameters (71 Items) of SONET-CT-96 with item examples (incl. response categories) (see also flow-chart - Figure 1)

Dimensions	Number of items	Item examples with item-number
Structural aspects *Item 1, 3, 5*	3	- 1: Are you about to describe a single or a group contact? (1) Single contact (2) Single contact in group setting (3) Discontinuing single contact (4) Group contact. *Enter corresponding number.* - Single: 5.1 How long was this contact altogether (in minutes)? *Enter duration in minutes.* - Group: 5.2 How long have you participated in this group contact (in minutes)? *Enter duration in minutes.*
Formal/content conditions *Item 2, 4, 6*	3	- 2: Please enter gender of contact partner (1) male (2) female. *Enter corresponding number.* - 4: Which form of relationship exists between you and the named person? Please check each applicable answer. (1) partner (2) child (3) household (4) relative/s......... (9) helping professions. .... other social role. *Enter corresponding number/s.*
Evaluation *Item 7, 8*	2	- Single 7.1 How important and significant was this contact with the named person altogether for you? (1) very important (2) important (3) neither important nor unimportant (4) less important (5) unimportant. *Enter corresponding number.* - Group: 7.2 How important and significant were these contacts in the group setting altogether for you? (1) very important (2) important (3) neither important nor unimportant (4) less important (5) unimportant. *Enter corresponding number.*
Well-being *Item 9, 10*	2	- 9: To which extent did you feel sad and depressed in this contact? (1) not at all (2) somewhat (3) quite much (4) very much. *Enter corresponding number.* - 10: To which extent did you feel happy in this contact? (1) not at all (2) somewhat (3) quite much (4) very much. *Enter corresponding number.*
Functional aspects (social support including associated distress) *Item 11-33*	23	- 11: In this contact, did you receive any kind of support (e.g. help, advice, affection, money, etc.)? (1) yes (2) no. *Enter corresponding number.* *If yes, various forms of support are presented (item 12, 15, 18, 21, 24, 27):* - 12: Did the named person relieve, comfort, encourage you in this contact? (1) yes (2) no. *Enter corresponding number.* *If yes, associated support and distress has to be rated:* - 13: How supportive was the contact for you? (1) very supportive (2) supportive (3) hardly supportive (4) not supportive. *Enter corresponding number.* - 14: How distressing was this for you? (1) very distressing (2) distressing (3) hardly distressing (4) not distressing. *Enter corresponding number.*
Emotionality (Social strain) *Item 34-55*	22	- 34: Did your contact partner/s distress you in any respect? (1) yes (2) no. *Enter corresponding number.* *If yes, different forms of distress are presented (Item 35, 37, 39, 41, 43, 45, 47, 49, 51):* - 35: Did the named person act capriciously in this contact? (1) yes (2) no. *Enter corresponding number.* *If yes, experienced distress has to be rated:* - 36: How distressing was this for you? (1) very distressing (2) distressing (3) hardly distressing (4) not distressing. *Enter corresponding number.*
Coping *Item 56-71*	16	- 56: How large would you rate the probability that the situation would change without any undertakings by yourself? Select any number between 0 and 100! *Enter number between 0 and 100.* *In case distress has been identified either in the domain of social support (item 11 – 33) or emotionality (item 34 – 55), various forms of coping are presented (item 59-68):* - 59: Did you distract yourself from the situation? (1) not at all (2) somewhat (3) quite much (4) very much. *Enter corresponding number.*

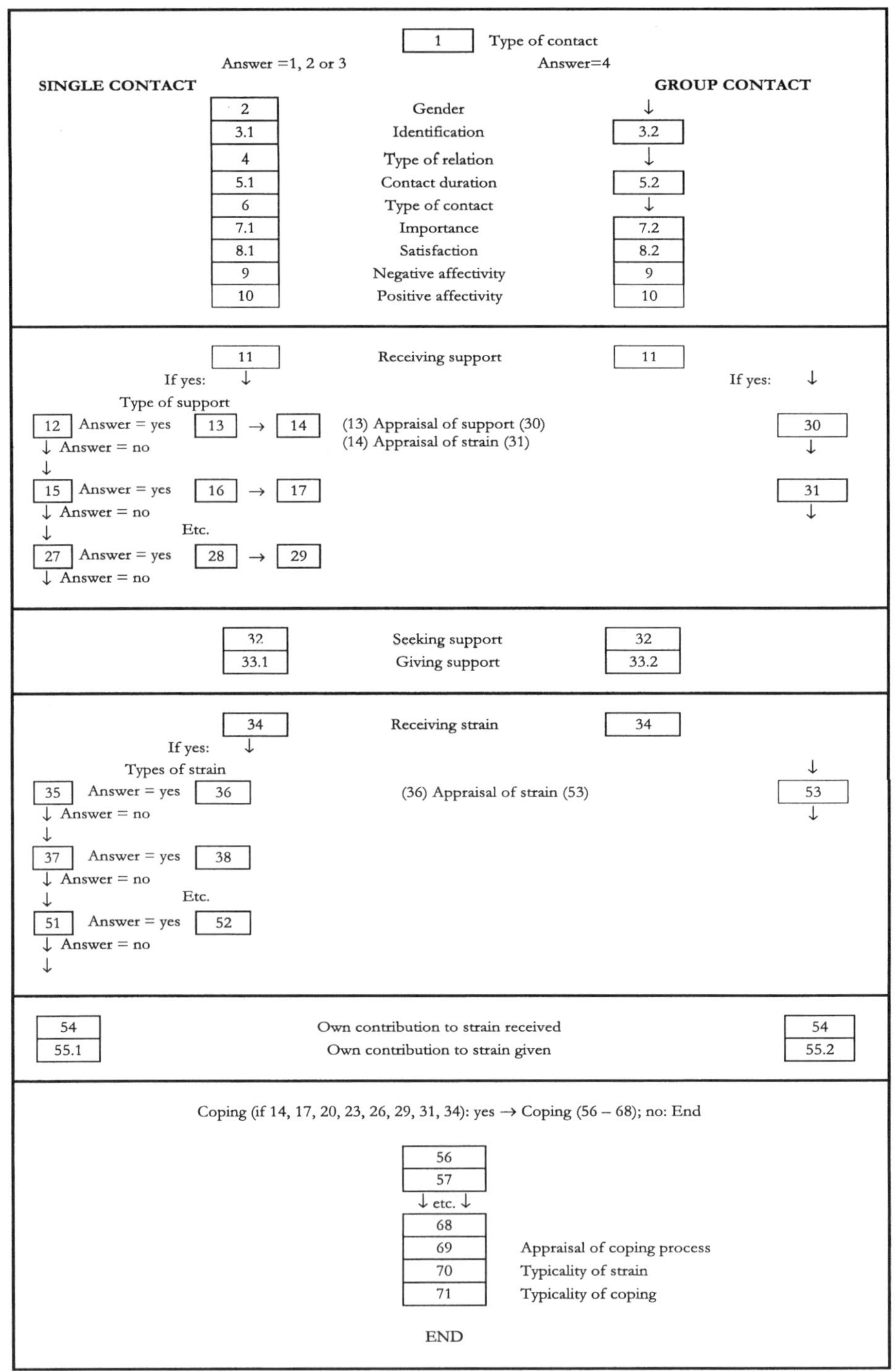

Figure 1. Overview over sequence of questions with single and group contacts(Numbers: Item Numbers; Examples of Items see Table 2)

a permanent memory of 1 MB RAM. It's possible to change the memory allocation between the RAM Disk (drive C, used for storage) and system RAM (application workspace), but the amount of RAM inside the palmtop is constant. The Palmtop is equipped with an Intel 80C186 CPU processor (7.91 MHz) and one serial optional port but without floppy drive. The FTN-display is compatible with CGA and a resolution of 640 x 200 pixels (80 columns by 25 rows) and a zoom fuction; it will automatically shut off to save power if the palmtop is not used for a period of 3 minutes. The HP 1000CX palmtop PC includes LapLink Remote, which facilitates migration of existing MS-DOS applications on a desktop or laptop computer to a palmtop PC. The diary program was written in Visual Basic. The user interface is very simple: once the program was started, the subjects answer multiple choice questions. This structure was used for all the questions in this interview. The equivalent number of the answer given was chosen on the display. To avoid data entry errors, the subjects could correct or confirm the answers. A particular problem was the limited storage space on the pocket computer; after each session the interview data had to be saved on a standard PC.

Methods of empirical investigation

As mentioned above, the SONET-CT-96 was empirically investigated by applying various research questions over a period of 2 weeks. This time period proved useful in a study by Baumann et al. (1996). It allows for a good insight into the daily experience of support and strain and is still reasonable for the subjects, especially patients, in terms of the amount of time necessary to complete it.

Samples. For this study two ad-hoc samples were used; the non-clinical sample was deemed sociodemographically representative of the average population in the age range of 20 to 60 years. The clinical sample was drawn from the outpatient sector of psychosocial care institutions; sociodemographic data were supposed to correspond to the non-clinical sample. Subjects diagnosed with a psychological disorder were selected. The disorder was not in its early stages, but was still affecting the patient. The clinical sample was very heterogenous. Considering the difficulties in implementing such a study (to date there have been no large computer-aided diary studies over a lengthy period of time that included a clinical sample) it was not possible to obtain a more homogenous sample. Because of the very time-consuming methods of measurement, sample sizes have been limited. As a means of motivation, every subject was paid a compensation of ATS 2000, which corresponds to approximately USD 130.

Both samples (see Table 3) have corresponding ages, genders, and occupations, however they differ with respect to education and marital status. Marital status is only associated with single parameters of social network (Laireiter, Ganitzer & Baumann, 1993), but not with overall network size. Married subjects for example, have more relatives within their network, but fewer friends, acquaintances, and also fewer supporters in single areas. With respect to education, the clinical sample probably corresponds more to a lower socio-economic status than the non-clinical sample, which may in turn influence subjective well-being. As this aspect is only mentioned in passing, it is not discussed further here.

Table 3. Description of samples

Characteristics	Non-clinical sample (N=35)	Clinical sample (N=20)	Comparison
Age	M= 34, Range 20-60	M = 35, Range 19-56	U-test, p>.05
Gender (F : M)	60 : 40	35 : 65	Chi squared, p>.05
Marital status - attached (married, long term relationship) - single (single, widowed, divorced)	 63% 37%	 15% 85%	Chi squared, p<.05
Educational status - no high school degree - high school degree	 46% 54%	 75% 25%	Chi squared, p<.05
Occupational status - employed - unemployed	 57% 43%	 55% 45%	Chi squared p>.05
Clinical notifications to the clinical sample - ICD-10-diagnoses F3: 8 Affective disorders (dysthymic disorder, out of which 3 include alcohol-, and/or drug abuse) F4: 8 Neurotic-, stress- and somatoform disorders (4 panic disorders with other disorders; 2 social phobias, 1 obsessive-compulsive disorder; 1 somatoform disorder) F1: 3 Addictive disorders F6: 1 Personality disorder (borderline) - Duration of morbidity: overall duration 4 years (median; range: ½ - 23 years); current episode 1.2 years (median; range: 0.3 – 10 years) - Psychotherapy/ treatment: currently 7 months (median; range: 0.3 – 13 years; including 3 cases with 6, 8, and 13 years, respectively)			

The non-clinical sample corresponds well to the sample used with the SONET-CT (Baumann et al., 1996); therefore the data from the prior study can be used for comparison with the current study:

- SONET-CT: N=20; Age M=35 years (20–59); 55% living in longterm relationships or married; 60% highschool degree.
- SONET-CT-96: N=35; Age M=34 years (20–60); 63% living in longterm relationships or married; 54% highschool degree.

Additional measures. At the beginning and the end of the data registration period, subjective well-being and a few social indicators (social network, social support, social strain) were assessed during an interview including standardized testing (results are not reported here):

- Subjective well-being: *Affect Balance Scale* ABS (Bradburn, 1969); 2 affectivity scales of the *Profil der Lebensqualität bei Chronisch-Kranken* PLC (English "profile of quality of life in chronically-ill patients" ; Siegrist, Broer & Junge, 1994); Life satisfaction assessed by *Satisfaction with Life Scale* SWLS (Pavot, Diener, Colvin & Sandvik, 1991).
- Social network, social support, and social strain: SONET-B, modified version of SONET (Baumann & Laireiter, 1993), assessing the actual behavior as opposed to resources per se.
- Life events: *Münchner Ereignisliste* MEL (english "Munich event checklist"; Maier-Diewald, Wittchen, Hecht & Eilert, 1983).

Essential to the application of more complex and lengthier diary studies – whether traditional or computerized – are specific accompanying and preventive actions for maintaining the quality of data and subject compliance (Foster, Laventry-Finch, Gizzo & Osantowski, 1999). In the literature, the following standards have been discussed (compare Foster et al., 1999; Korotitsch & Nelson-Gray, 1999): payment of subjects, limited interval of observation, personal supervision of subjects, method training, periodic submission of data, and control of data accuracy. In the study at hand, each of these actions have been taken and have lead to a high level of compliance.

Results of empirical testing

Comparison of results with other studies is difficult because similar studies are rare for both the non-clinical and the clinical sample, but especially for the latter. An exception is the study by Thiele (1994; Baumann et al., 1996), which can serve for comparison with the non-clinical sample.

When interpreting the data it is important to consider the self-reporting nature of the data. The question of how well these data correspond to behavior data still remains open. Studies (Laireiter, Reisenzein, Baumann, Untner & Feichtinger, 1997) have shown that correspondance is mostly good with non-clinical samples, but varies between sectors. Within a patient sample this question is even more important, because patients may not perceive support received as such (compare cognitive distortions in depressive patients); lower values may reflect deficiencies in perception rather than a real deficiency. Another possibility is a combination of both factors. These methodological limitations should be kept in mind when looking at the following interpretations.

Data analysis has been conducted based on absolute figures and also on relative values. Because the clinical sample had fewer overall contacts than the non-clinical sample, most of the other parameters differ significantly if absolute figures are used. Therefore, using relative values provides more information in this context, because it allows for detection of structural differences.

Description of contacts

Formal, interactional, and *evaluational* parameters are shown in Table 4. The recorded number of contacts (4.4 contacts/day) in the non-clinical sample corresponds more or less with results reported in the literature, with the biggest concordance being found with the study by Baumann et al. (1996) showing almost the same number of contacts per day (4.8 contacts/day). The number of contacts has been slightly higher in studies using different methods of measurement: 7 contacts/day (Wheeler & Nezlek, 1977); 6 contacts/day (Schumacher, 1991). The duration of contacts (60 minute – mean across all contacts; 65 minute – mean across all subjects) has been longer in the current study than in Baumann et al. (1996; 49 minute – mean of single contacts). There are no differences in the median (20 minute).

No comparison data are available for the clinical sample; in the literature patients have been often reported as showing a lower number of contacts, so that our findings concur with general clinical findings. The clinical sample is characterized by the following significant differences ($p<.05$): reduced number of contacts/day, consequently also a lower number of overall single and group contacts; group contacts generally occur in smaller groups, personal contacts are slightly less than phone contacts, group contacts are appraised as rather unimportant, they are less satisfied with contacts.

While *well-being* (see Table 4) is rather positively connotated within the non-clinical sample (positive values are clearly higher than negative ones), this is less obvious within the clinical sample; as expected, this can also be seen in the fact that the clinical sample shows increased negative well-being and reduced positive well-being compared to the non-clinical sample.

Results of *social support* are partly shown in Table 5; the following discussion also includes data not depicted in the table (the same holds true for social strain). The proportion of contacts including social support is much higher in this study (45%) compared to the study reported in Baumann et al. (1996; 13%). The reasons for the observed divergence cannot be completely explained, but the following aspect may play a role. The support domain was more complicated to record in the old version of the computerized diary in that each kind of support had to be gone through, which subjects may have found tiresome and eventually caused them to reduce the number of support contacts recorded.

Emotional support is the main focus in both samples, whereas financial support is relatively rare. Within the non-clinical sample of Baumann et al. (1996) as well as within the sample at hand, support through affection, comfort, and advice ranks high, whereas support via money ranks lowest. Within the non-clinical sample any kind of support is perceived as supportive and scarcely as a burden; this is also true for the clinical sample, yet one significant difference ($p<.05$) is that patients perceive support through comfort as being less supportive. The clinical sample felt more of a burden with most kinds of support (comfort, compliments, money, work; but not with advice and affection) than the non-clinical sample. Social support was clearly

Table 4. SONET-CT-96: Formal, interactional, evaluative parameters; well-being (14 days; means of both samples)

Characteristics	Non-clinical sample	Clinical sample	Clinical compared to non-clinical sample	p
Number of contacts/day	4.4	2.2	decreased	.00
Overall single contacts	46	25	decreased	.01
Overall group contacts	15	5	decreased	.00
Gender of contact partner (single contacts): men/women	42%/58 %	45%/55 %	-	n.s.
Group size of group contact	6.8	4.4	decreased	.01
Contact duration (min.)				
- single contact	65	68	-	n.s.
- group contact	157	130	decreased	.02
mode of contact				
- personal	78%	71%	decreased	.10
- via phone	22%	29%	increased	.03
Importance of contact *very important (1) – unimportant (5)*				
- single contact	2.0	2.2	-	n.s.
- group contact	2.2	2.7	less important	.06
Satisfaction with contact *very satisfied (1) – very dissatisfied (5)*				
- single contact	1.8	2.2	more dissatisfied	.01
- group contact	1.9	2.2	more dissatisfied	.01
Well-being during contact *not at all (1) – very much (4)*				
- negative affect	1.1	1.3	Negative well-being increased	.04
- positive affect	2.7	2.1	Positive well-being decreased	.00

Note. Statistical testing was executed using U-tests; n.s. $p>.05$.

less actively sought than received (non-clinical sample: received by 45%, sought by 21%); the difference between receiving and seeking social support is lower within the clinical sample (received by 33%, sought by 19%).

In summary, with respect to social support the clinical sample can be described as follows (differences according to p<.05): fewer supportive contacts absolutely (ties in with the overall lower number of contacts) as well as relatively; with the four

Table 5. SONET-CT-96: social support and social strain (selected parameters) (14 days; means of both samples)

Characteristics	Non-clinical sample	Clinical sample	Clinical compared to non-clinical sample	p
Supportive contacts (global support)				
- *absolute (all contacts)*	27.2	9.2	less contacts with support	.01
- *relative (to all contacts/person)*	45%	33%	less contacts with support	.03
Single contacts with specific types of support *(relative: to all single contacts/person)*				
- comfort				
- advice	26%	25%	-	n.s.
- praise	25%	24%	-	n.s.
- affection	20%	15%	-	n.s.
	39%	27%	fewer contacts with support	.02
- monetary			more contacts with support	
	3%	8%	-	.01
- work				
	16%	14%		n.s.
Active seeking of support				
- *absolute (all contacts)* yes	13	9	-	n.s.
no	49	22	with fewer persons	.00
- *relative (to all contacts/person)* yes	21%	28%	-	n.s.
Strain contacts (global strain)				
- *absolute (all contacts)*	5.4	5.8	-	n.s.
- *relative (to all contacts/person)*	10%	19%	more contacts with strain	.05
Single contacts with specific types of strain *(relative: to all single contacts/person)*				
- expressing caprice				
- control	5%	9%	more contacts with strain	.01
- hostility	5%	10%	more contacts with strain	.01
- causing worries	4%	10%	more contacts with strain	.01
- causing anger	7%	17%	more contacts with strain	.01
- insulting	6%	12%	more contacts with strain	.01
- conflicts	6%	9%	more contacts with strain	.01
- disappointment	5%	13%	more contacts with strain	.01
- lack of empathy	4%	11%	more contacts with strain	.01
	6%	14%	more contacts with strain	.01
Active contribution to strain *(relative: to all strain contacts/person)*				
- yes	35%	34%	-	n.s.

Note. Statistical testing was executed using U-tests; n.s. p>.05

kinds of support there are no relative differences, whereas with money there are relatively more supportive contacts and with affection there are relatively fewer supportive contacts. Receiving support is more of a burden to the patients than to the non-clinical sample, although absolute values do not suggest very high distress.

Results of *social strain* are partly depicted in Table 5. In absolute as well as relative figures, straining contacts are distinctly rarer than supportive contacts; this concurs with results in the literature saying that fewer straining network participants are mentioned as compared to supporting persons (Lettner, Sölva & Baumann, 1996). In the study of Baumann et al. (1996) 4% of contacts have been straining ones, in this study this is true for 10% of contacts of the non-clinical sample. This difference may also be due to the inconvenient recording procedure which may have reduced the recording of strain contacts in the earlier study (compare to supportive contacts as mentioned above).

The different types of social strain do not vary much between the two samples; the main kind of strain is "causing worries". All kinds of social strain are very distressing. In approximately one third of the strain contacts the subjects themselves contributed to the strain (no difference between samples). The clinical sample difffers from the non-clinical one in that patients have relatively more strain contacts ($p<.05$), which is reflected by each subdivision of strain. The two samples do not differ with respect to strain intensity.

As expected, the two samples do differ with respect to *coping* (see Table 6). The clinical sample perceives fewer possibilities of personal regulation. The more constructive coping-mechanisms (reflection, reappraisal, active influence) are less available within the clinical sample, while passive strategies (distraction, self-reproach, calming down/soothing) are more prevalent. Confidence in coping (quality of coping) is lower and the strain situation is less familiar.

In *summary*, the *non-clinical sample* can be characterized as follows: 4 to 5 important contacts are realized per day, the median duration of which is 20 minutes. Most contacts are single contacts (approximately two-thirds), which are carried out in person as opposed to over the phone. Contact situations are related to positive rather than negative affects. Almost half of the contacts (45%) include supportive elements, of which affection is the one most often received. Social support is more frequently received than sought after. Support is mostly perceived as supportive and rarely distressing. Strain contacts per se appear distinctly less often than support contacts. Distress related to contacts is resolved constructively (reflection, reappraisal, active influences).

For the *clinical sample* the domain of contacts is reduced altogether; the question as to whether the reduction in these patients reflects a personal optimum or an undesirable deficiency cannot be answered here. With most clinical groups – with the exception of schizophrenic patients – lower numbers of contacts represent defi-

Table 6. SONET-CT-96. coping in contacts (single, group) with strain (14 days; means of both samples)

Characteristics	Non-clinical sample	Clinical sample	Clinical compared to non-clinical sample	p
Appraisal of situation				
- possibility of change without active contribution (0-100%)	42%	30%	-	n.s.
- possibility of improvement by own person (0-100%)	55%	38%	not by own person	.03
- probability of reoccurence (0-100%)	53%	53%	-	n.s.
Coping *not at all (1) – very much (4)*				
- withdraw attention	1.5	1.8	increased	.03
- soothing	1.3	1.7	increased	.09
- reflecting	2.5	2.0	decreased	.05
- reproaches of others	1.8	1.9	-	n.s.
- reappraisal	2.1	1.6	decreased	.08
- self reproach	1.3	1.9	increased	.01
- evasion	1.3	1.5	-	n.s.
- passivity	1.9	1.7	-	n.s.
- active influence	2.3	1.8	decreased	.01
- getting support	1.3	1.1	-	n.s.
Appraisal				
- quality of coping *not at all (1) – very much (4)*	2.9	2.3	lower quality	.01
- familiarity *almost every day (1) – never (5)*	3.4	3.1	-	n.s.
- typicality *not at all (1) – very much (4)*	3.1	2.4	less typical	.01

Note. Statistical testing has been executed using U-tests. n.s. p>.05.

cits rather than an optimum. Although single contacts are still viewed as being as important as in the non-clinical sample, as satisfaction with contacts decreases, coupled with reduced well-being, contacts become increasingly distressing for these patients. Strain and reduced well-being are supposedly caused by deficiencies in social aptitude and these are frequently observed in clinical samples. But deficits in the domain of support are probably etiologically important conditions as well. In absolute and relative figures, patients have fewer contacts that include social support. In addition, social support is accompanied by distressing components within this group, whereas this does not hold true for the non-clinical sample. A further aspect contributing to reduced well-being are strain contacts, which clearly occur more often in the clinical sample as compared to the non-clinical sample (19% vs. 10%). Thus, we have a lower number of supportive contacts in conjunction with the increased distress associated with the support, as well as a higher number of strain contacts. This unfavorable condition is accompanied by coping deficits, so that the overall contact situation has to be viewed as an area of enormous difficulty for these patients.

Formal reliability of the procedure

Formal reliability was tested on 38 characteristics (the missing ones partly had no variance, were not appropriate for testing: for example, abbreviations of names, or have not been selected for testing for technical reasons: for example, intensity of support and strain, coping). Analyses included comparisons of means and computation of correlations with splitting of the data in two ways:

- Comparison of first vs. second half (split-half reliability): assessing stability over time and systematic change;
- Odd-even numbers of contact (random allocation): split-half reliability with avoidance of systematic tendencies;

Comparison of means (Wilcoxon-test for dependent samples) hardly yielded any significant differences (38 comparisons) in either variant of computation:

- first/second half: 0 comparisons (non-clinical sample), 1 comparison (clinical sample) with $p<.05$.
- odd/even: 4 comparisons (non-clinical sample), 1 comparison (clinical sample) with $p<.05$.

The level of non-significance (mostly $p>.2$) even suggests great similarity of values in both samples. Significant results of the odd/even-method in the non-clinical sample are mostly due to the rather low number of strain contacts.

Correlations (rank-correlations) are satisfactorily high and range (after revaluation according to Spearman-Brown) from .68 to .77 (see Table 7). Global values are especially high, as shown by the following examples (odd/even; revaluation according to split-half reliability); values are higher than those of the SONET-CT version (Baumann et al., 1996):

- number of contacts: .99 (non-clinical), .98 (clinical sample)
- number of supportive contacts: .97 (non-clinical), .86 (clinical sample)
- number of straining contacts: .69 (non-clinical), .73 (clinical sample)
- positive affectivity: .89 (non-clinical), 62 (clinical sample)
- negative affectivity: .82 (non-clinical), .70 (clinical sample)

It is interesting to note that positive affectivity is slightly higher in the non-clinical, and negative affectivity is higher in the clinical sample than the respective opposite affectivity.

Values of the non-clinical sample are slightly more stable than those of the clinical sample. Altogether these values are slightly lower (especially those of the split-half method) than those reported by Perrez and Reicherts (1996; odd/even: mean value of COMES-characteristics: $r=.85$). The difference is mainly due to the nine

Table 7. Stability (rank-correlations; percentage of all 38 coefficients)

Level of correlation	Non-clinical sample		Clinical sample	
	1./2. week	Odd/even contacts	1./2. week	Odd/even contacts
>.8	16%	34%	3%	13%
.6-.8	24%	18%	29%	26%
.4-.6	16%	32%	39%	37%
.0-.4	43%	16%	29%	24%
Median	.53	.62	.52	.55
Median revalued[1]	.69	.77	.68	.71
Number of r with p>.05	24%	26%	37%	29%

Note[1] Revaluation according to Spearman-Brown split-half reliability

relatively rarely occuring types of strain, which can be clearly observed in the first/second half method. Within the clinical sample, the low overall number of contacts further influences various characteristics in that these are as a consequence low in number as well. All in all, formal examination yielded very satisfactory results and confirms that diary data can be assessed with high accuracy in a relatively short period of time. Nevertheless, for clinical studies as well as in the case of rather infrequent events (for example, distressing relationships) longer periods of observation (3 to 4 weeks) should be considered.

Relationship between social support, social strain, and subjective well-being

To analyze the relationship between social support, social strain, and subjective well-being multiple correlations have been computed using absolute values as well as percentages (number with respect to network size) (see Table 8).

Analyses yielded the following results:

- In both cases (absolute and relative values) correlations were significant, with relations being higher with negative affectivity than with positive affectivity.
- Within the non-clinical sample, positive affectivity only relates to social support, whereas negative affectivity is mainly dependent on social strain. Using absolute values, social support has a slight influence on negative affectivity, but this relationship is distinctly weaker than the relationship between social strain and negative affectivity. Looking at percentages there is a very clear *domain specific effect* along with a *negativity effect* (impact on negative affectivity is larger than on positive affectivity). With absolute values this is less clear.

Table 8. Well-being as a function of social support and social strain: multiple correlations A = f (Su, St); A = f (Su%, St%)

	Positive affectivity A+		Negative affectivity A-	
	Non-clinical sample	Clinical sample	Non-clinical sample	Clinical sample
A = f(Su, St) Significant components	.49* Su**	.57* - St*	.57** - Su*, St***	.77** St**
max (r(A, Su); r(A, St))	.41	.61	.30	.74
A = f(Su%, St%) Significant components	.48* Su%**	.50* - St%*	.79** St%***	.83** St%***
max (r(A, Su%), r(A, St%))	.34	.62	.56	.72

Note. Rank-correlations positive/negative affectivity: -.28 (non-clinical); -.56** (clinical). * p<.05; ** p<.01; *** p<.001

- Within the clinical sample only social strain is meaningful, whereas social support does not relate significantly to affectivity. Thus, we have a *negativity effect.*

Positive and negative affectivity are not correlated within the non-clinical sample, but within the clinical sample there is a significant negative correlation. This indicates that within the clinical sample, affectivity only has one state at a time (either positive or negative); within the non-clinical sample both states can be applied independently of each other to describe situations, thus indicating a more differentiated affectivity. Yet, in both samples social strain proves more important than social support.

Clinical implications of these results are that it is important for patients to aim at a more differentiated affectivity, allowing for complex evaluations of individual situations. Having a less differentiated affectivity may also contribute to the fact that these patients experience more distress with individual situations, because positive affectivity is not an alleviating factor.

Concluding comments

The results of this study provide a differential insight into the contact structure of different groups. For both the clinical and the non-clinical sample an observation period of 14 days is sufficient for most parameters to yield formally satisfactory values. Results with respect to subjective well-being are particularly interesting as they are provided by field data for the first time. This study also supports the hypothesis that in the end the amount of stress experienced is more crucial to subjective well-being than social support. These results tie in with questions as to vulnerability and protective factors. As for interaction studies, one consequence of the findings is that it is important to assess the strain potential as well as the support potential, whereat both domains should display a similar degree of resolution.

Further analyses intend to look for particular trends, that is, analysis of non-agglutinated data to investigate micro-structural characteristics. Such data may prove especially useful for intervention studies, as they provide precise information about contact situations. Parameters such as support, strain, coping, and subjective well-being provide behavioral information on social situations, which cannot be assessed by common coping assessment procedures. Yet, for wider application the coping approach should be further developed, complementing the approach of Perrez and Reichert (1996). On the other hand, it may prove useful to reduce the number of categories of social strain (that is, provide fewer types of strain), because several of the single subtypes are relatively rarely used.

If the contact domain is to be assessed in combination with other areas (performance, psychophysiological parameters, etc.), the contact domain itself should be reduced substantially. One possibility is to refrain from differentiating various types of support and strain, and simply use the global questions (see item 11 and 34 in Table 2).

Thus, diary studies yield a precise insight into daily experience and in addition allow for validation of common procedures, which mostly use agglutinated data measures. Up to now, the question whether the agglutinated data approach and the diary data approach yield corresponding results has been neglected (see Epstein, 1979). Thus, future research should focus on validation upon daily experience, for which computer-aided procedures provide helpful support.

Acknowledgement

With the kind support of FWF-Austria Project P 10970 Soz. Thanks to A.R. Krebs for the technical production of the diary. We would like to thank Ms. Monika Brandstätter for translating this article.

References

Baumann, U. & Laireiter, A. (1993). SONET. Interview zum Sozialen Netzwerk und zur Sozialen Unterstützung. In G. Westhoff (Ed.), *Handbuch psychosozialer Meßinstrumente* (pp. 811–814). Göttingen: Hogrefe.

Baumann, U. & Laireiter, A. (1995). Individualdiagnostik interpersonaler Beziehungen. In K. Pawlik & M. Amelang (Eds.), *Enzyklopädie der Psychologie: Grundlagen und Methoden der Differentiellen Psychologie* (Band 1, pp. 609–643). Göttingen: Hogrefe.

Baumann, U., Laireiter, A. & Thiele, C. (1994). Erfassung interpersoneller Beziehungen mittels Tagebuch. In D. Bartussek & M. Amelang (Eds..), *Fortschritte der Differentiellen Psychologie und Psychologischen Diagnostik* (pp. 365–375). Göttingen: Hogrefe.

Baumann, U., Thiele, C. Laireiter, A.-R. & Krebs, A. (1996). Computer-assisted diary on social interactions, social relationships, social support and interpersonal strain. In J. Fahrenberg & M. Myrtek (Eds.), *Ambulatory Assessment: Computer-assisted psychological and psychophysiological methods in monitoring and field studies* (pp. 69–84). Seattle, Toronto: Hogrefe & Huber Publishers.

Bradburn, N.M. (1969). *The structure of psychological well-being.* Chicago: Aldine.

Cohen, S. & Wills, T.A. (1985). Stress, social support, and the buffering hypothesis. *Psychological Bulletin, 98*, 310–357.

Epstein, S. (1979). The stability of behavior: I. On predicting most of the people much of the time. *Journal of Personality and Social Psychology, 37, 1097–1126.*

Feldman, S.I., Downey, G.& Schaffer-Neitz, R.(1999). Pain, negative mood, and perceived supp-port in chronic pain patients: A daily diary study of people with reflex sympathetic dystrophy syndrome. *Journal of Consulting and Clinical Psychology, 67*, 776–785.

Foster, S.L., Laventry-Finch, C., Gizzo, D.P. & Osantowski, J. (1999). Practical issues in self-observation. *Psychological Assessment, 11*, 426–438.

Hinde, R.A. (1992). Auf dem Weg zu einer Wissenschaft zwischenmenschlicher Beziehungen. In A.E. Auhagen & M. von Salisch (Eds.), *Zwischenmenschliche Beziehungen* (pp. 7–36). Göttingen: Hogrefe.

Korotitsch, W.J. & Nelson-Gray, R.O. (1999). An Overview of Self-Monitoring Research in Assessment and Treatment. *Psychological Assessment, 11*, 415–425.

Laireiter, A. (Ed.). (1993a). *Soziales Netzwerk und Soziale Unterstützung: Konzepte, Methoden und Befunde.* Bern: Huber.

Laireiter, A.-R. (1993b). Begriffe und Methoden der Netzwerk- und Unterstützu ngsforschung. In A. Laireiter (Ed.), *Soziales Netzwerk und Soziale Unterstützung: Konzepte, Methoden und Befunde* (pp. 15–44). Bern: Huber.

Laireiter, A.-R. & Baumann, U. (1992). Network structures and support functions - Theoretical and empirical analyses. In H.O.F. Veiel & U. Baumann (Eds.), *The meaning and measurement of social support* (pp. 33–55). Washington DC: Hemisphere.

Laireiter, A.-R., Baumann, U., Reisenzein, E. & Untner, A. (1997). A diary method for the assessment of interactive social networks: the interval-contingent diary SONET-T. *Swiss Journal of Psychology, 56,* 217–238.

Laireiter, A.-R., Baumann, U., Untner, A., Feichtinger, L. & Reisenzein, E. (1997). Interview und Fragebogen zum Sozialen Netzwerk und zur Sozialen Unterstützung SONET. *Rehabilitation, 36*, 15–30.

Laireiter, A., Ganitzer, J. & Baumann, U. (1993). Soziale Netzwerk und Unterstützungsressourcen als differentielle Konstrukte – Bezüge zu sozialen und demographischen Variablen. In A. Laireiter (Ed.), *Soziales Netzwerk und soziale Unterstützung. Konzepte, Methoden und Befunde* (pp. 88–101). Bern: Huber.

Laireiter, A.-R., Reisenzein, E., Baumann, U., Untner, A. & Feichtinger, L. (1997). Zur Validität der Erfassung Sozialer Netzwerke und Sozialer Unterstützung: Vergleich von Selbst- und Fremdbeurteilung – Eine Pilotstudie. *Zeitschrift für Differentielle und Diagnostische Psychologie, 18*, 127–150.

Laireiter, A.-R. & Thiele, C. (1995). Psychologische Soziodiagnostik: Tagebuchverfahren zur Erfassung sozialer Beziehungen, sozialer Interaktionen und Sozialer Unterstützung. *Zeitschrift für Differentielle und Diagnostische Psychologie, 16,* 125–151.

Lettner, K., Sölva, M. & Baumann, U. (1996). Die Bedeutung positiver und negativer Aspekte sozialer Beziehungen für das Wohlbefinden. *Zeitschrift für Differentielle und Diagnostische Psychologie, 17,* 170–186.

Maier-Diewald, W., Wittchen, H.-U., Hecht, H. & Eilert, W. (1983). *Die Münchener Ereignisliste (MEL). Anwendungsmanual.* Max-Planck-Institut für Psychologie, München.

Margraf, J. & Jacobi, F. (1997). Marburger Angst- und Aktivitätstagebuch. In G. Wilz & E. Brähler (Eds..), *Tagebücher in der Therapie und Forschung. Ein anwendungsorientierter Leitfaden* (pp. 119–138). Göttingen: Hogrefe.

Müller, R. & Baumann, U. (1999). Das SASB-Modell: ein Konzept für Soziale Unterstützung und Soziale Belastung. *Zeitschrift für Differentielle und Diagnostische Psychologie, 20,* 272–289.

Pavot, W., Diener, E., Colvin, C.R. & Sandvik, E. (1991). Further validation of the satisfaction with life scale: Evidence for the cross-method convergence of well-being measures. *Journal of Personality Assessment, 57,* 149–161.

Perkonigg, A. (1991). *Die Bedeutung Sozialer Netzwerke und Sozialer Unterstützung bei der Verarbeitung von Belastungen.* Unveröff. Diss., Salzburg: Universität.

Perkonigg, A., Baumann, U., Reicherts, M. & Perrez, M. (1993). Soziale Unterstützung und Belastungsverarbeitung: Eine Untersuchung mit computergestützter Selbstbeobachtung. In A. Laireiter (Ed.), *Soziales Netzwerk und soziale Unterstützung. Konzepte, Methoden und Befunde* (pp. 128–141). Bern: Huber.

Perrez, M. , Laireiter, A.R. & Baumann, U. (1998). Stress und Coping als Einflussfaktoren. In U. Baumann & M. Perrez (Eds.), *Lehrbuch Klinische Psychologie – Psychotherapie* (2. Aufl., pp. 277–305). Bern: Huber.

Perrez, M. & Reicherts, M. (1996). A computer-assisted self-monitoring procedure for assessing stress-related behavior under real life conditions. In J. Fahrenberg & M. Myrtek (Eds.), *Ambulatory Assessment: Computer-assisted psychological and psychophysiological methods in monitoring and field studies* (pp. 51–67). Seattle, Toronto: Hogrefe & Huber Publishers.

Pfingstmann, G. & Baumann, U. (1987). Untersuchungsverfahren zum Sozialen Netzwerk und zur Sozialen Unterstützung. *Zeitschrift für Differentielle und Diagnostische Psychologie, 8,* 75–98.

Rook, K.S. (1984). The negative side of social interaction: Impact on psychological wellbeing. *Journal of Personality and Social Psychology, 46,* 1097–1108.

Rook, K.S. (1992). Detrimental aspects of social relationships: Tacking stock of an emerging literature. In H.O.F. Veiel & U. Baumann (Eds.), *The meaning and measurement of social support* (pp. 157–170). Washington DC: Hemisphere.

Schumacher, A. (1991). *Ein Tagebuchverfahren zur Erfassung sozialer Interaktionen.* (Mainzer Berichte zur Persönlichkeitsforschung, Nr. 38). Mainz: Psychologisches Institut der Universität.

Schwarzenbacher, K. & Baumann, U. (1990). Personennennungen versus Größenangaben: Zwei unterschiedliche Daten zur Reliabilitätsbestimmung Sozialer Netzwerke und Sozialer Unterstützung. *Zeitschrift für Differentielle und Diagnostische Psychologie, 11,* 27–36.

Schwarzer, R. & Leppin, A. (1989). *Sozialer Rückhalt und Gesundheit: Eine Meta-Analyse.* Göttingen: Hogrefe.

Schick, A. & Schmidt, L.R. (1997). Computer-aided Setting Assessment. Beschreibung einer Feldselbstbeobachtungsmethode (CASA). *Zeitschrift für Klinische Psychologie und Psychiatrie, 45,* 408–420.

Siegrist, J., Broer, M. & Junge, A. (1994). *PLC, Profil der Lebensqualität bei Chronischkranken.* Weinheim: Beltz.

Sölva, M., Baumann, U. & Lettner, K. (1995). Wohlbefinden: Definitionen, Operationalisierungen, empirische Befunde. *Zeitschrift für Gesundheitspsychologie, 4,* 292–309.

Steiger, H., Gauvin, L, Jabalpurwala, S., Séguin, J.R.& Stotland, S. (1999). Hypersensitivity to social interactions in bulimic syndromes: Relationship to binge eating. *Journal of Consulting and Clinical Psychology, 67,* 765–775.

Tesch-Römer, C. (1998). Alltagsaktivitäten und Tagesstimmungen im Alter. *Zeitschrift für Gerontologie und Geriatrie, 31,* 257–262.

Thiele, C. (1994). *Soziale Kontakte in Alltag: Eine Tagebuchstudie.* Unveröff. Diss., Salzburg: Universität.

Thiele, C., Laireiter, A.-R. & Baumann, U. (2001). Deutschsprachige Tagebuchverfahren in Klinischer Psychologie und Psychotherapie – Ein Überblick. *Zeitschrift für Klinische Psychologie, 30*, X–Y.

Veiel, H.O.F. & Baumann, U. (Eds.). (1992). *The meaning and measurement of social support.* New York: Hemisphere.

Veiel, H.O.F. & Ihle, M. (1993). Das Copingkonzept und das Unterstützungskonzept: Ein Strukturvergleich. In A. Laireiter (Ed.), *Soziales Netzwerk und Soziale Unterstützung: Konzepte, Methoden und Befunde* (pp. 55–65). Bern: Huber.

Vittengl, J.R.& Holt, C.S. (1998). A time-series diary study of mood and social interaction. *Motivation and Emotion, 22,* 255–275.

Wheeler, L. & Nezlek, J. (1977). Sex differences in social participation. *Journal of Personality and Social Psychology, 35,* 742–754.

Chapter 4
Ecological Momentary Assessment: Real-World, Real-Time Measurement of Patient Experience

Michael R. Hufford[1], Saul Shiffman[1, 2], Jean Paty[1, 2], and Arthur A. Stone[3]
[1]*invivodata, inc.*, [2]*University of Pittsburgh*, [3]*State University of New York at Stony Brook*

Introduction

Researchers have been attempting to collect real-time data from subjects in their natural environment for more than 50 years (Verbrugge, 1980). Recently, advances in both the technology and methodology of real-time data collection have enabled researchers to capture reliable and valid momentary data from subjects in the real world. This chapter first describes the rationale for moving away from retrospective measurement of clinical phenomena by reviewing the inaccuracies and biases associated with many types of retrospective reports. The use of diaries, experience sampling methods, and self-monitoring is reviewed as steps in the progression from retrospective to momentary data collection. Next, we describe a unifying framework for collection of real-time data in the real world, by a variety of methodologies, under the rubric of *Ecological Momentary Assessment* (Stone & Shiffman, 1994). Finally, the importance of subject compliance is reviewed as one critical component to the successful execution of real world data collection methods.

Patient Experience Data

Researchers frequently ask subjects to report on a variety of types of subjective experiences and objective events. We distinguish three types of data that are frequently collected from subjects: *self-observations*, *objective events*, and *quality of life* (QoL). We do not address here the collection of physiological data, which has itself been the subject of parallel methodological and technological developments, many detailed elsewhere in this volume. Many of the same methodological issues apply to both the self-report domain of patient experience and to ambulatory monitoring of physiological parameters, but there are also important differences.

Studies often rely on subjects to provide data based on *self-observations*; examples from the medical literature include coughing, urinary incontinence, and eating. These events are objective and could, in principle, be observed by others, but the subject is in a unique position to report on them as they occur in the real world. In these instances, the subject is acting as a proxy research observer, uniquely positioned to observe symptoms and events over time and across a spectrum of real-world environments and circumstances. In a second class of reporting targets, subjects are also often asked to report on important *subjective symptoms* that could not, even in principle, be observed by a third party; examples include pain, fatigue, anxiety, or drug withdrawal symptoms. Finally, researchers also ask subjects to report on their Quality of Life (QoL), which refers to a subject's evaluation of their mental and physical well-being. Conceptually, QoL data differ from symptom data largely in focusing on the impact of symptoms on a patient's life and incorporating an explicit evaluation (not just description) of that impact. A number of QoL domains have been proposed, including: symptom severity, social interaction, objective functioning, subjective well-being, mental health, physical health, and health-related QoL (Gill & Feinstein, 1994; Muldoon, et al., 1998; Schipper, Clinch & Powell, 1990). We term these classes of data collectively as *Patient Experience*. Collectively, they cover the range of assessment targets typically assessed by subject self-report.

From retrospective to real-time measures of patient experience

Reliance on recall

Traditionally, researchers have relied heavily on subjects' ability to retrospectively recall details regarding their experience. Many inquiries require subjects to summarize their behavior to yield estimates of past frequency ("How many headaches per week have you had in the past month?"), intensity ("How severe were the headaches, on average?"), or other – sometimes quite complex – characteristics ("Did you have more headaches in the evenings?" "Were the headaches related to stress?"). These types of questions require that subject not only recall the relevant data but also accurately summarize it and/or make a judgment about it. Other inquiries focus on specific, episodic personal memory to recall details of a specific episode without any requirement for summary (Brewer, 1994).

Cognitive scientists and survey researchers have been examining the limitations of retrospective data for several decades. We will not attempt to summarize this large literature (the interested reader is referred to Schwarz and Sudman's (1994) book on autobiographical memory), but will rather highlight some of the most pertinent findings as they relate to the recent shift toward momentary data collection methods. It is important to acknowledge that forgetting of past experiences is not simply the fading of memory traces over time. If they were, adjustments could be incorporated into recall assessments correcting for time expired since the experience. Instead, a number of much more complex processes affect the quality of retrospective data. Research on autobiographical memory demonstrates that recall is not a straightforward retrieval of events. Instead, memory relies on heuristic strategies to *reconstruct* past events (Bradburn, Rips & Shevell, 1987). Such retrieval or reconstruction is imperfect and subject to a range of biases resulting from the layers of processing that are necessary to answer the typical research inquiry. Each step or process has the potential to introduce significant inaccuracy and bias into recall data.

Encoding. In order for any content to be available for later recall, it must first be encoded into memory. Encoding is incomplete and imperfect and is influenced by a variety of processes. For example, whether something is encoded at all is influenced by its perceived salience at the time, which may be a function of the person's subjective state, distraction by other stimuli, etc., (Erickson & Jemison, 1991; Linton, 1991). How it is encoded (that is what is stored) is similarly influenced by the person's state and situation. This is particularly true for evaluative information (for example, Teasdale & Fogarty, 1979). Thus, autobiographical memory does not even start with an objective accurate record of events, but is error- and bias-prone from the start.

Retrieval. When people are asked to recall events, they do not always (or even most of the time) simply retrieve and 'replay' a detailed mental record of the event. Particularly when the recall task is challenging (as research inquiries typically are), we often rely on a retrospective reconstruction of what "must have" happened. This is not a function of sloppiness or non-cooperation; it is simply the way that autobiographical memory works. Several biases affect the retrieval of information. *Availability heuristics* can bias recall by ensuring that events that are more easily retrieved from memory – because they are more salient, more recent, more surprising, or more congruent with current mental state – will have an undue biasing effect on memory (Eisenhower, Mathiowetz & Morgenstein, 1991; Joffe, MacDonald & Kutcher, 1989). *Saliency* (that is, personal relevance) can also affect encoding, as salient events are more likely to be encoded initially and are more likely to be recalled later (Menon & Yorkston, 2000). *Recency* effects make more recent events more accessible to memory, and, as a result, exercise undue influence over recall (Schwarz & Sudman, 1994; Shiffman, Hufford, Hickcox, Paty, Gnys & Kassel, 1997). *State biases* can affect recall by virtue of making certain content more accessible. For example, people are more likely to retrieve negative information when they are in a negative mood, thus introducing substantial bias (Clark & Teasdale, 1982, 1985; Teasdale & Fogarty, 1979). Retrospective recall is notoriously poor for the *timing* of events (Friedman, 1993; Thompson, Skowronski & Betz, 1993). Research inquiries often ask about experience over a certain interval of time, requiring respondents not only to retrieve memory of experiences, but also to place them in time. A large body of research shows that autobiographical memory is particularly error-prone in making these temporal judgments, and the error is directional: We systematically recall events as having been more recent than they actually were (Bradburn, 2000). Finally, a most profound bias can be introduced by subjects' *effort after meaning* – that is, people's natural and unconscious tendency to re-construe events so as to make them consistent with subsequent events, or to make them amenable to the construction of a coherent and comfortable story of the past (Brown & Harris, 1978; Eich, Reeves, Jaeger & Graff-Radford, 1985; Means, Swan, Jobe & Esposito, 1994; Schwartz, Kowalski & McNally, 1993). This bias is particularly insidious because it tends to produce consistent and systematic results that often conform to the research hypothesis (for example, that stress precedes illness, based on post-diagnosis recall of prior stress), but only reflect the operation of the subjects' own 'theories' of their behavior.

Aggregation and summary. To answer the sort of questions commonly asked by researchers, subjects not only have to retrieve the relevant information, but to aggregate and summarize it over some period or sequence of events. This processing is necessary to respond to questions about the occurrence or frequency of events ("How many headaches did you have this week?") or their average or typical characteristics ("How much gastric discomfort did you have this week?"). Research on autobiographical memory makes clear that the human brain usually does not processes these requests by counting or averaging, but rather relies on a variety of heuristic strategies for estimating answers. These heuristic strategies potentially introduce substantial biases, similar to those that affect retrieval. For example, recent research shows that recall over 'average' pain using a pain episode is heavily influenced by the saliency (peak pain) and recency (pain intensity at the end of the episode) of the subject's pain experience (Eich, Reeves, Jaeger & Graff-Radford, 1985; Redelmeier & Kahneman, 1996; Stone et al., 2000). Recency also has profound effects on recall of frequency: people estimate frequency of events in part by noting the recency of the most recent occurrence (Bradburn, Rips & Shevell, 1987).

Instruction set. One often overlooked source of error in retrospective reports is subjects' misunderstanding of questionnaire instruction sets that require subjects to aggregate and summarize their experience in the recent past. For example, Bailey and Martin (2000) analyzed subjects' understanding of what time interval 'past month' referred to during completion of QoL questionnaires across 11 studies. If subjects were asked on the 15th of a month to recall the past month, only 64% of subjects correctly interpreted 'past month' to refer to the period from the 15th of the current month to the 15th of the previous month. In other words, 36% used an incorrect interval as the basis of their recall (for example, subjects used the past 2 weeks only, the entire month previous to the current month, or a 6-week period). Additional research is needed to better understand how frequently these sorts of errors occur in other types of retrospective patient experience measures. Furthermore, it is not evident that researchers are explicit in their instructions to participants regarding aggregation. For example, when asked to recall the level of pain over the last week, are researchers asking for the average level of pain or some other index of central tendency (the modal pain level, for instance)?

Summary. Cognitive science has documented a wide variety of inaccuracies and biases associated with retrospective recall. Even relatively banal inquiries aimed to collect patient experience data rely on the subject to engage in complex and fallible cognitive processes to recall the information. These processes render recall vulnerable to inaccuracy, thus undermining the quality of data on which the research enterprise depends. Worse, recall is also rife with systematic biases that can lead to incorrect scientific conclusions, thus undermining the process of scientific inference.

Avoiding Recall Biases

A number of methods have been developed to acquire patient experience data with less distortion than is found using recall methodologies. They accomplish this by trying to bring the assessment closer to real time.

Daily diaries. In the 1940s, written diaries were introduced as a way to collect health data from subjects in the field (Verbrugge, 1980). Initially, diary entries were meant to cue subjects' subsequent recall of health events, and were not seen as a primary source of data. Over time, diaries became a way to capture recall and summary data over a relatively brief interval, such as a day, to reduce bias sufficiently to be acceptable.

Many studies use diaries to collect once-daily data (for example, Lewis, Lewis & Cumming, 1994; Neugebauer, 1989). Given that retrospective questionnaires often ask for recall over intervals of weeks or months, daily summaries are seen as a substantial advance in bringing data collection closer to real time and minimizing recall. Indeed, for some types of events and recall tasks, daily summary recall may well be adequate. For example, it is likely that subjects can recall singular and prominent events, such whether or not they had a headache at any time during the day. However, although the shorter recall interval may reduce the demand on memory processes, even recall over the interval of a day is subject to the same cognitive processes that bias autobiographical memory over longer intervals. Thus, even over a day, it is less likely that subjects can accurately recall or summarize details or characteristics of events (for example, how intense the pain was), more frequent events (for example, how many cigarettes they smoked that day), or continuous quantities (for example, average intensity of pain in a chronic pain condition). For example, Stone et al. (1998) have shown that subjects' 24–48 hour recall of how they coped with difficulties is subject to substantial error (subjects forget a substantial proportion of their coping responses) and bias (cognitive strategies are especially likely to be omitted).

Moreover, the procedures typically used in daily diary studies are likely to introduce substantial bias. Subjects are typically directed to complete the diary at bedtime or at the end of the day (so that they can provide a complete overview). However, subjects' physical and mental state at bedtime is not at all representative of their state throughout the day (for example, more tired, etc.). Since state at the time of recall affects recall and summary, this introduces bias. Recall at the end of the day is also particularly likely to omit events that happened early in the day, simple because they are more distant. Finally, to the extent that subjects have discretion in when they choose to complete it, this can introduce further bias. Thus, a chronic pain patient in a pain study may be reminded and prompted to complete the diary by experiencing an episodic exacerbation of pain, and thus complete the diary when in particularly intense pain. Or the subject may avoid doing the diary when they are in pain, completing instead when they have a moment of respite from symptoms, thus completing the diary when experiencing uncharacteristically little pain. Since subject state at the time of recall influences the recall, these processes could profoundly bias the daily summaries.

Thus, while bringing reporting closer to experience, daily diaries still often require substantial recall and summary and may be subject to the same biases that infect retrospective questionnaires. Consideration of these biases may be especially important when targeting minor experiences or when measuring subjective qualities of daily experiences.

Momentary assessment. The realization of how profound recall bias can be led many researchers to focus on momentary assessment – that is, asking a person to report about how they feel or what they were doing at that moment – in order minimize or eliminate recall bias. These methods also circumvent biases due to summary processing, since respondents are not asked to summarize their experience over time or occasions, but simply to report current experience. In lieu of summaries made by subjects, these methods use aggregations of multiple momentary reports to capture and describe experience. For example, instead of asking subjects to recall how much pain they experienced over the last week, as is common in the practice of research and clinical care, momentary techniques might instead ask patients to complete pain reports several times a day for the entire week. Movement towards momentary assessment was also driven by the recognition that the respondent's current state and context may profoundly influence recall and reporting. Thus, momentary reports are ideally collected in the person's natural environment, so as to sample real-world experience, and avoid the bias potentially introduced by artificial reporting contexts. Finally, because momentary reporting is based on sampling real time experiences, it is critical that care be taken to design a sampling scheme that adequately represents the domain of experience studied. The real-time sampling of subject experience in real-world setting is the core of Ecological Momentary Assessment (Stone & Shiffman, 1994).

Collecting momentary patient experience data in real-world settings has several advantages over data collection gathered at the research site or during in-person interviews (Houpt, McMillan, Wein & Paget-Dellio, 1999; Norman, McFarlane, Streiner & Neale, 1982). First, the problems of autobiographical memory and recall biases are avoided if patients make their entries in real-time. Second, the repeated completion of assessments potentially adds to the reliability of the data, by allowing aggregation of multiple assessments over time. Aggregation of multiple measures reduces noise in data (that is, unreliability), making the measurement potentially more sensitive to changes in patient experience. Third, such data are more representative of subjects' everyday life, because subjects repeatedly provide data in real-world settings. Fourth, the richness of momentary data potentially allows for a more detailed analysis of a variety of experiences, particularly with regard to processes that exert their influence over time (for example, analyzing the onset and duration of medication effects or the sequelae of stressful occurrences). It is possible to examine trends in patient experience over time (for example, assessing speed of pain relief), the relationship between different aspects of subject behavior and response (for example, medication taking and daily peak pain intensity), or their relationship to other variables (for example, stress, diet, workload, etc.). Thus, compared to reports obtained periodically at the research site, momentary diaries have several potential advantages in terms of validity and efficiency.

Experience Sampling Method. As pagers and various types of programmable wrist-watches became widely available, researchers were able to actively prompt subjects to complete reports at specified times. The family of techniques that utilize these strategies is often referred to as the Experience Sampling Method (ESM; Csikszentmihalyi & Larson, 1987; DeVries, 1992). ESM was developed as a method for studying individuals' experiences in their natural environments by means of signaled random assessments. Each assessment would entail completion of a brief questionnaire. Assessments were typically completed several times a day for many days or even weeks. At the University of Chicago, landmark studies in adolescents (Csikszentmihalyi & Larson, 1984; Larson, 1989), and optimal experience or "flow" (Csikszentmihalyi, 1994), succeeded in establishing ESM as an ecologically valid way to collect data from subjects. ESM methods have been used to study a wide variety of populations and issues (see Csikszentmihalyi & Larson, 1987 for a review).

ESM researchers utilized new technology to investigate dynamic daily influences on health and behavior. They took the first steps in seeking a degree of ecological validity (Bronfenbrenner, 1979) in subjects' data. ESM provided a first step towards collecting empirical data on patient experience with a precision that had previously been only available in medicine.

Self-monitoring. There is also a large literature on the recording of event data (where events might be medication taking, symptom episodes, or some other definable discrete event), which is often referred to as self-monitoring (McFall, 1977). Self-monitoring refers to a two-stage process in which subjects first identify that a target event or behavior has occurred and then record their responses (Nelson, 1977). Researchers may ask subjects to report on antecedents, momentary experiences, or consequences of specific events. In this way, subjects are acting as a proxy for the researcher, recording details of specific events (for example, migraine headaches) or behaviors (for example, smoking).

Unlike ESM, which is focused on understanding the daily ebb and flow of subjects' daily lives, self-monitoring allows subjects to indicate when certain events occur. This is both a significant advantage and limitation of self-monitoring methods. Relatively infrequent events that could not be picked up via randomly-scheduled prompts asking about immediate experiences (for example, migraine headaches) can be picked up. However, the researcher is also reliant on the subject to faithfully record events of interest.

Self-monitoring data are often used to support a "naturalistic functional analysis" (Schlundt, Johnson & Jarrell, 1985) of the role of antecedent stimuli in prompting the target behavior (for example, do stressful events lead to increased symptoms?). However, self-monitoring data by themselves cannot logically support conclusions about the association between a target behavior and its antecedents. This method only provides information about the antecedents of the target behavior, which cannot be interpreted without comparison or control data (Epstein & Collins, 1977). For example, even if one observed that subjects frequently reported stress immediately preceding episodes of pain, it would be improper to conclude that pain was associated with – much less caused by – stress: the subjects might be equally likely to feel stressed when they were *not* experiencing pain. Establishing the association requires independent data on the base-rate of stress (or any other antecedent factor; Paty, Kassel & Shiffman, 1992). This is a general concern that applies to self-monitoring, ESM, and EMA methods.

Summary. The application of ESM and self-monitoring as methods to collect momentary data from subjects brought new advantages and challenges for researchers. For the first time, researchers were able to begin assessing the naturalistic variability of stimuli and responses. In other words, data could be collected from subjects that avoided the uniform context of research settings as well as the uniform processes of recall. These advantages were balanced against a new set of challenges. By definition, naturalistic field data lacks the stringent control over stimuli and responses present in the laboratory. Also, to reliably capture momentary data from subjects as they go about their daily lives, researchers began having to take into account issues of response burden (for example, how often is reasonable to prompt subjects each day) and compliance with the monitoring protocol (for example, how many assessments are missed during the study).

The importance of real-time data collection and the broad applicability of these methods has made self-monitoring and diary methods increasingly common for studying an impressive variety of health-relevant phenomena. A partial list includes mood (Marco & Suls, 1993), stress and coping (Jandorf, Deblinger, Neale & Stone, 1986; Eckenrode, 1984), pain (Follick, Ahearn & Laser-Wolston, 1984; Affleck, Urrows, Tennen & Higgins, 1992), sleep (Haythornthwaite, Hegel & Kerns, 1991), cigarette smoking (Shiffman & Prange, 1988), alcohol use and abuse (Samo, Tucker & Vuchinich, 1989), eating and eating disorders (Schlundt & Bell, 1987), and cardiovascular reactivity (Hedges et al. 1990). These methods have been used with children (Wolff & Wolff, 1991; Beidel et al. 1991), adolescents (Inderbitzen & Foster 1992; Larson, 1989), and the elderly (Spence, 1992; Samo, Tucker & Vuchinich, 1989) as well.

Ecological Momentary Assessment

The term *Ecological Momentary Assessment* (EMA; Stone & Shiffman 1994) refers to a conceptual strategy, including ESM and self-monitoring approaches, which can be used to collect real-time momentary data from subjects in the real world. First, the characteristics of EMA are described, including how different sampling schemes can be used to tailor the research protocol to match the study objectives. Next, the technology that can be used to implement EMA is presented, along with the pros and cons of each.

Characteristics of EMA

There are three characteristics that define EMA (Stone & Shiffman, 1994). First, subjects are studied in the environments they typically inhabit, to maximize ecological validity and real-world generalization. This requirement of EMA is in contrast to laboratory- or clinic-based studies where subjects respond to various tasks in circumstances considerably different from those they are usually in. The issue concerns the ecological validity of the measurements. In other words, environmental characteristics may affect responses of individuals, both behavioral and physiologic. A good example of the effect of artificial contexts on subjects is the well-documented phenomenon of 'white coat hypertension,' where blood pressures taken by 'white-coated' medical personnel in clinical settings are falsely elevated relative to actual real-world physiological parameters (Pickering, et al., 1999). In short, EMA maximizes ecological validity by allowing respondents to provide data in their normal environment.

Second, EMA depends on real-time data collection about momentary or near-immediate states to avoid retrospective distortion of data to maximize the validity of subjects' reports. This is a central element of EMA and one for which considerable evidence exists supporting the position. As reviewed above, a considerable empirical literature demonstrates that recall has a pernicious effect on the quality of the data.

Third, EMA typically involves a sampling strategy, usually of many momentary assessments per day, to ensure representative characterization of momentary experience. The idea of data collection as sampling is central to EMA. Unlike recall data where a single point is regarded as "the data," EMA methods recognize that subjective states and contexts vary, that data collection occasions are rooted in a particular state and context, and that patient experience is thus best characterized by a representative sampling of moments, states, and contexts. Broadly, EMA focuses attention on sampling of moments as an important component of design validity, much as research design focuses on respondent sampling as a component of valid inference to populations.

Collecting data at multiple time points also enables research to examine changes in patient experience over time. It ensures a reasonable characterization of phenomena and to enable the researcher to examine fluctuations of phenomena over time. This may be very important when the phenomenon has an important temporal component. For example, blood pressure, hormones, pain, and fatigue can all vary dramatically over the course of a day. Various methods of analyzing data may be employed to characterize EMA information (see, for example, Schwartz & Stone, 1998).

Recording paradigms

EMA typically uses a combination of recording paradigms to capture real-time data from subjects. Three basic types of sampling paradigms can be employed: interval contingent, event-contingent, and signal-contingent (Wheeler & Reis, 1991).

Event-contingent recording relies on the subject to self-monitor when events occurs and then complete an assessment (see Figure 1). Common uses for this type of assessment included tracking the details of specific events, such as asthma attacks or precipitants of pain exacerbations. This type of self-monitoring ensures that significant events to the subject are not missed, but they do require vigilance to constantly monitor for specific events and compliance with the recording paradigm on the part of the subject.

Interval-contingent recording requires subjects to complete an assessment at preselected times of the day (for example, 10am, 2pm, 8pm). The most common form is daily assessment, which typically is not meant to be momentary. These types of assessments can be used to ensure that specific times during the day are adequately

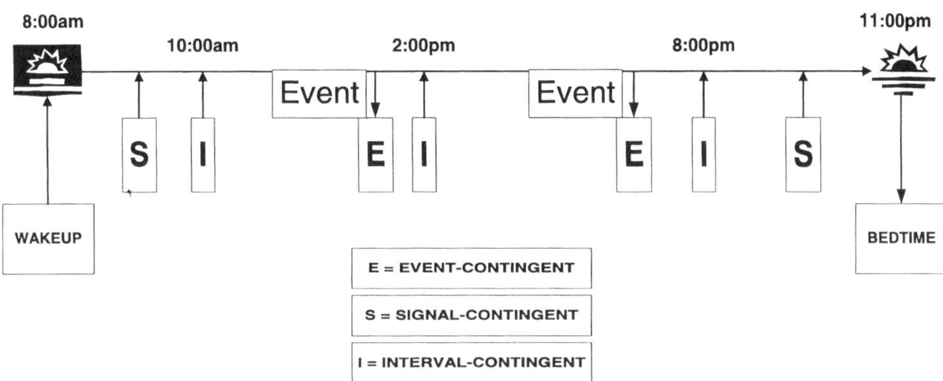

Figure 1. A sample subject's day using a combination of event-contingent (E), signal-contingent (S), and interval-contingent (I) assessments. For example, a subject could record significant pain exacerbations as events, be signaled randomly twice a day to complete an assessment of their well-being, and complete interval-based assessments every six hours of their baseline pain.

sampled, and can also be used to prompt or record certain behaviors from subjects, like medication taking. Drawbacks of interval-contingent assessments include that they may miss important, episodic events, they may be non-representative of the subject's day, the inflexible schedule may result in poor subject compliance if a scheduled assessment conflicts with another activity (for example, morning swim), and the timing of the assessment can be anticipated, which may lead to certain response biases. Generally speaking, the drawbacks of interval-contingent sampling schemes argue against their usage.

Signal-contingent recording uses some type of prompting device (for example, pager, handheld computer, see below) to signal the subject when to complete an assessment. The schedule can be determined by the needs of the research protocol. For example, signaled assessments may occur at random to collect representative data from subjects. Alternatively, stratified random sampling can be used to ensure a set number of assessments during different blocks of the day. More dynamic sampling can be employed to over-sample during critical periods of the day; for example, to detect a medication effect that is hypothesized to be greatest shortly after waking (for example, Shiffman, Elash, Paton, Gwaltney, Paty, et al., 2000). In other words, much as with sampling design for subjects, sampling of moments can be designed to address the particular research question. Drawbacks to signal-contingent recording are the reliance on subject compliance with prompting and, like interval-contingent recording, they may miss important episodes.

These recording paradigms each have a unique utility for researchers. The approaches can also be combined. For example, Shiffman et al. (1996) used event-contingent monitoring to capture data about particular and unique events (smoking relapse episodes and episodes of temptation). To help interpret the character of these events, they were compared with subjects' typical experience and state, as characterized via randomly-scheduled signal-contingent data. A variety of creative designs can be used to address particular research questions.

Implementing EMA

The execution of EMA protocols typically involves some type of technology to either prompt subjects for assessments and/or record their responses. Although it is possible to design a study that would rely solely on subjects to remember to make timed entries and record events as they occur, recent advances in EMA signaling devices make it possible to help subjects comply with the EMA protocol. A variety of methods have been used to signal subjects to complete real-time assessments. Radio-signaled pagers were frequently used in early ESM studies. "Smart" wristwatches have been used as the signaling device. They allow for individualized scheduling and have been frequently used in psychiatric studies in particular. Both pagers and "smart" wristwatches often have to limit their data collection to specific windows during the day, often between 8am and 8pm to avoid waking subjects with varying sleep habits. This is far from trivial, as studies have found that up to 26% of fell outside an 8am to 8pm time window and assessments outside of this window differed significantly from assessments within the window (Shiffman, 2000). A very substantial limitation of these signaling devices is that, although issuance of the signal can be controlled or confirmed, timely compliance with assessments cannot. A study by Litt et al. (1998) suggested that subjects often completed assessments long after they were beeped.

More recently, advances in handheld computing have allowed researchers to implement EMA designs. These handheld computers, which we have termed *Patient Experience Diaries* (PEDs), offer several unique advantages to researchers. PEDs can manage both prompting and data collection. As prompting devices, their programmability allows enormous flexibility to implement optimal research and sampling designs, including some where the prompting and sampling protocol changes dynamically (for example, prompting more frequently during an episodic increase in symptoms). The ability to turn prompting off dynamically for sleep or other 'time-out's is also valuable. PEDs can also prompt and track compliance with other aspects of the protocol, such as medication taking. Sophisticated solutions can also be designed that promote compliance, for example, by providing subjects feedback.

Handheld computers also offer enormous advantages as assessment platforms. Entries can be date and time-stamped so that compliance can be monitored. The user-interface can be developed and refined so that it is easy and fast to use, allowing subjects to complete assessments quickly and naturally. With modern interfaces (for example, point and touch) these devices can be used by a wide variety of subjects. Computerized data collection can ensure completion of obligatory fields, thus preventing missing data. It can also improve data quality, both by restricting entries to a valid range (for example, preventing entry of '6' on a 1–5 scale), and by implementing on-line real-time data checks to enforce even sophisticated validity rules. Furthermore, even complex branching within assessments can be administered using PEDs. Perhaps one of the most exciting prospects of applying handheld computers to the study of real world patient experience is that the possibility now exists to link PEDs with other types of ambulatory physiological data collection devices (for example, glucometers, instrumented inhalers, ambulatory blood pres sure cuffs) to collect parallel streams of both psychological and physiological data (for example, Fahrenberg, Foerster & Müller, 1996; Guyll & Contrada, 1998; Kamarck, Shiffman, Smithkline, Goodie, Paty, et al., 1998).

The considerable advantages of using handheld computers to implement EMA protocols also must be balanced against inevitable drawbacks. There is a considerable financial commitment that is required to conduct an EMA study that uses the highest level of technological innovation. Moreover, it is clear that a purely technical solution will not produce valid momentary data from subjects. Several studies that have failed to adequately address the user-interface and other programming issues have had high rates of failure and poor subject compliance (for example, Johannes, Crawford, Woods, Goldstein, Tran, et al., 2000; Litt, Cooney & Morse, 1998).

Challenges to using EMA

Despite its many advantages, EMA poses important challenges for researchers as well. One hypothesized challenge that faces all types of real-time patient experience data collection is the potential distortion of EMA data by reactivity. A reactive effect describes the degree to which the intensity, frequency, and/or quality of a target variable will change when being observed, monitored, or assessed (Nelson, 1977). Two studies have examined whether EMA engenders significant reactivity among subjects. Both studies, using pain patients, failed to find evidence that EMA produces significant reactivity (Cruise, Broderick, Porter, Kaell & Stone, 1996; Peters, Sorbi, Kruise, Kerssens, Verhaak, et al., 2000). Regardless, it is important that additional research examine the conditions under which reactive effects may emerge and how they can be controlled.

EMA methodologies involving frequent (especially random) prompting also pose reporting challenges for certain types of participants, such as those with occupations where it is difficult to respond to a signaled assessment (for example, airline pilot, surgeon, grocery checkout clerk, etc.). Likewise, certain activities are not conducive to momentary reporting and the inability to sample such times may pose a threat to the validity of EMA data. Fortunately, PED studies that have monitored compliance have generally shown very high compliance rates (many over 90%), suggesting that inability to respond may not be a serious threat.

Because EMA is based on samplings of daily life, there is a concern that infrequent events or extreme states (for example, intense pain, ecstatic mood, etc) may be missed with certain sampling schemes (interval and random). One solution to minimize this potential problem is to increase sampling density, thereby decreasing the probability of omitting important experiences. Consideration of the duration of the study and the sampling density are important, to avoid overburdening subjects.

More broadly, the type of data collected by EMA methods can pose data management and analysis challenges. First, a relatively simple EMA design prompting 100 subjects 5 times per day for a brief 10-item assessment, along with an average of 3 additional subject initiated reports per day, over a 3-week period will produce 168,000 data points. Some researchers may choose to create aggregates of patient experience by collapsing across multiple assessments each day, as these aggregates will now be free of the retrospective inaccuracies and biases associated with recall data. These aggregates lend themselves to traditional parametric analyses. More sophisticated analytic approaches have also appeared in the literature (for example, Schwartz & Stone, 1998; Tennen & Affleck, 1996) and are now available in commercial statistical packages.

Summary

EMA evolved as a collection of methods to collect real-time data on patient experience in the real world. Incorporating principles from both ESM and self-monitoring, EMA uses a combination of sampling schemes to characterize patient experience while allowing subjects to also enter important disease episodes or events. The technology used to implement EMA must allow subjects to easily enter the required data, and also must be rugged enough to survive field use for weeks at a time.

To date, EMA has been used to study a wide variety of phenomena, including psychiatric symptoms (Barge-Schaapveld, Nicolson, Berkhof, DeVries, 1999; DeVries, 1992), daily activities (Hank & Schwenkmezger, 1996), cognitive performance (Shiffman, Paty, Gnys, Kassel & Elash, 1995; Totterdell & Folkard, 1992), smoking (Shiffman, Paty, Gnys, Kassel & Hickcox, 1996), drinking (Collins, Morsheimer, Shiffman, Paty, Gnys & Papandonatos, 1998), pain (Affleck, Tennen, Urrows, Higgins, Abeles, et al., 1998), stress and coping (Stone, Neale, Schwartz, Shiffman, Marco, et al. 1998), changes in endocrine functioning (Okenfels, Porter, Smyth, Kirschbaum, Hellhammer & Stone, 1995, VanEck, Berkhof, Nicolson & Sulon, 1996), and cardiovascular reactivity (Guyll & Contrada, 1998; Kamarck et al., 1998).

Subject Compliance with Momentary Data Collection Methods

The promise of real-time, real world, momentary data collection depends on the methods used to capture patient experience data. Since subjects are directly reporting the data in the context of their natural environment, the methods used must facilitate subjects' adhering to the research protocol, that is, being compliant.

Compliance with paper diaries

Compliance with paper diaries, or methods that use an electronic device to prompt for a response but paper diaries to record the entry, is hard to assess. As nearly all researchers who have run paper diary trials can attest, many subjects correctly discern that researchers may be able to count diary entries, but cannot tell when they were filled out. Thus, many subjects complete their entries after the fact, often just before they are due to be returned to the research site. For example, a recent study by Litt and colleagues (1998) revealed that fully 70% of subjects falsified at least some of their diary entries every single day by writing the time they were prompted but then completing the entry at their convenience. This is more than a methodological curiosity, as faked diary entries rely on the very retrospective memory processes whose avoidance motivated the use of diaries in the first place. It is also likely that back-filled entries are of poor quality and validity, and not representative of the natural ebb and flow of patient experience, as subjects' use of heuristics to reconstruct the data may be more homogeneous than their actual real-time experience.

Diary compliance has been objectively, though indirectly, assessed in eight studies that used various instrumented devices (for example, inhalers, blood glucose monitors) to track the actual time and date of events recorded in the diary (Chmelik & Doughty, 1994; Jonasson et al., 1999; Mazze et al., 1984; Milgrom et al., 1996; Simmons et al., 2000; Spector et al., 1986; Straka et al., 1997; Verschelden et al., 1996). The correspondence between these data from the instrumented devices and the paper diary entries were then compared. A dramatic difference between subjects' reported versus actual compliance was observed. Whereas the paper diaries appeared to indicate high rates of compliance (88%), the objectively validated actual rates of compliance were significantly lower (54%). In other words, almost 40% of the paper diaries were false, due to a mix of subject data entry errors and outright back-filling and falsification of data.

Poor and faked compliance is the greatest limitation of paper diary methods. When 'momentary' diary data is actually entered retrospectively via subject noncompliance with the diary protocol, the validity of the data has been compromised. When subjects intermittently are noncompliant with the diary protocol, the remaining data are likely biased, as subjects do not miss assessments at random. Diary noncompliance can also threaten the statistical power of the study. Given the high rates of noncompliance reports above, many paper diary studies may be underpowered to test study hypotheses because of subject noncompliance. Moreover, invalid entries not only degrade reliability and thus statistical power, they have potential to introduce significant bias, since back-filled or incorrect entries are unlikely to represent the subject's actual experience during that moment.

Reasons for subject noncompliance

Why are subjects so noncompliant with paper diaries? First and foremost, it is not because they are bad people. In volunteering for research projects, most subjects are acting on a genuine desire to help researchers. But the hassles of everyday life and natural human forgetfulness serve to dramatically compromise compliance with paper diaries.

Who is noncompliant? The empirical literature on noncompliance has not found any consistent relationship between noncompliance and demographic characteristics or disease severity (Chmelik & Doughty, 1994; Jonasson et al., 1999; Mazze et al., 1984; Milgrom et al., 1996; Simmons et al., 2000; Spector et al., 1986; Straka et al., 1997; Verschelden et al., 1996). A number of general factors likely play a role in producing subject noncompliance with diary protocols.

A subject's desire to participate in clinical research and be a 'good subject' may also create motivation to retrospectively complete missed diary entries. Empirical evidence confirms that subjects' noncompliance is related to whether or not they are aware that the researcher is tracking their compliance (for example, Simmons et al., 2000). Second, subjects are sometimes asked to make entries at varying intervals (for example, each hour of the day), requiring them to faithfully remember when to make diary entries. For complex diary protocols, or those that require multiple entries per day, the demand on working memory escalates. Third, when diary entries are supposed to be cued by events, such as symptom flare-ups, the subject's diary burden is proportional to symptom severity or frequency. That is, an increasing rate of symptoms can overwhelm subjects as they try to complete an assessment for each occurrence. Increasing subject burden can introduce systematic bias in the data because subjects may systematically stop entering the specific types of events (for example, the most severe pain episodes). Finally, like the rest of us, subjects in clinical trials respond to incentives and cues. Most diaries make it difficult to comply and easy to be noncompliant. Without cues to structure subject behavior and incentives to establish, reward, and maintain it, compliance is difficult to achieve. In sum, while research has not fully identified the precise reasons for noncompliance, we can determine that subjects are, indeed, noncompliant with diaries. In addition, we can identify a number of factors likely promote both noncompliance and faked compliance.

Obtaining subject compliance with EMA studies

The problem of subject compliance is fundamentally one of guiding subjects' behavior. Researchers and clinicians are perhaps most aware of noncompliance issues from the extensive literature on subject noncompliance with medication regimens (for example, Boudes, 1998; Urquhart, 1996; Urquhart & DeKlerk, 1998). Indeed, this literature, in combination with principles from behavioral science, informs the key components of an EMA system that can be used to both achieve and maintain high rates of subject compliance with research protocols.

First, compliance considerations must be part of design, execution, and write-up of a study (Boudes, 1998; Stone & Shiffman, manuscript in preparation). In short, compliance must be given adequate attention throughout the development and implementation of an EMA study. Standard features need to be incorporated into the PEDs, so that subjects know their compliance is being tracked, receive feedback on their compliance, and are prompted to improve compliance.

Second, to be compliant with the protocol, subjects must be adequately trained (Verbrugge, 1980). The PED system should be extremely simple and intuitive, and therefore require little training regarding the system's basic functions. Protocol-specific features of the software must be adequately explained to allow the subject to comply with the procedures.

Third, the PEDs should be easy for subjects to use (Boudes, 1998). Ensuring that the user-interface is friendly and intuitive is essential to enhance compliance. User-interface issues that are not often considered when developing an electronic diary include how memory, attention span, habit formation, effortful cognitive processsing, and the graphical interface all combine to affect the subject (for example, Raskin, 2000). Subjects' tolerance for diaries that do not make intuitive sense is extremely limited, and it is of paramount importance that compliance with the protocol be a natural extension of following the prompts and reminders that are part of the PED system.

Fourth, programmed reminders have consistently been found to improve compliance rates in clinical studies (Boudes, 1998; Trick, 1993). Real-time compliance reminders should be built into PEDs to prompt subjects to complete diary entries. Moreover, by providing subjects with timely, real-time compliance reminders, electronic PEDs encourage the type of habit-forming interactions with the device that are characteristic of effective computer interfaces (Raskin, 2000).

Fifth, PEDs should easily handle complex branching within assessments. Rather than forcing the subject to decide whether or not they should complete certain assessment items depending on their answers to other items, PEDs should be programmed to administer the correct items in the correct logical sequence.

Sixth, collecting real-time, real world diary data requires that subjects incorporate the electronic PEDs into their daily lives. As a result, electronic PEDs should include a number of 'livability' functions that help subjects be compliant with the protocol. For example, functions allowing the subject to suspend any active beeping for sleeping at night, napping during the day, and when programmed reminders might be inappropriate (for example, at church), all help the subject remain compliant with the diary protocol. Empirically, it has been shown that the inclusion of these 'livability' functions does not result in subjects abusing them to avoid monitoring (Shiffman, et al., 2000).

Seventh, subjects are more compliant with research protocols if they feel a sense of accountability for the data (Urquhart, 1994). If subjects know that their compliance with the diary protocol is being tracked, and they receive real-time feedback regarding their compliance, they report feeling very engaged in the study protocol. In other words, if subjects know that they will be held accountable for their data, they tend to be more vigilant with the diary protocol (for example, Simmons et al., 2000).

Optimized, computer-supported EMA

Applications that apply EMA methods and designs, implemented on sophisticated modern palm-top hardware and software, with careful attention to compliance principles, can be used to successfully address a variety of research problems. These methods can achieve extraordinary compliance and data quality.

One example of the rates of subject compliance that can be achieved using the compliance features outlined above, implemented in a sophisticated PED, is a recent study of cardiovascular reactivity. In addition to carrying a PED for self-reports, subjects were also wearing devices that captured cardiovascular data in real time. In this intensive 6-day trial of 120 men and women, subjects were asked to complete a 27-item report of their affect, arousal, social situation, activity, and posture every 45 minutes during the waking day (a fixed-interval approach). Analyses of a subjects' compliance with the diary protocol revealed that subjects completed 99% of all scheduled assessments (Kamarck, et al., 1998). This study linked subjective and contextual data to cardiovascular parameters (systolic and diastolic blood pressure), helping to document psychological and contextual contributions to cardiovascular function and health.

Another study assessed the effects of nicotine patches on craving in 244 subjects in a smoking cessation trial. This study used a stratified random sampling plan to over-sample the first few hours of the day, in order to assess the effect of pharmacokinetic differences between nicotine patches, which are most evident in the first few hours after patch application. Subjects were prompted 8–12 times a day in a stratified random sampling plan. Excellent compliance was again achieved: Subjects responded to 93% of all assessment prompts within 2 minutes over a period of three weeks (Shiffman, et al., 2000). As a result of the sensitive measurement, the data were able to distinguish the clinical effects of two very similar medications.

In sum, electronic PEDs have been shown to achieve and maintain high rates of compliance with EMA protocols through an integration of recent advances in handheld technology and behavioral science.

Conclusions

Historically, researchers have heavily relied on recall data to understand subjects' experience. The pernicious inaccuracies and biases inherent in recall data have confronted researchers with the realization that the convenience of cross-sectional, retrospective data collection is paralleled by its limited validity and sensitivity to changes in patient experience. Fortunately, as our understanding of the limitations of recall data has grown, so too has our ability to apply recent advances in the technology and methodology of momentary measurement to the study of subjects in their natural environment. Ecological Momentary Assessment evolved as a way to allow researchers to collect real-time patient experience data in the real world. No study, no matter how well-designed, can collect valid momentary data if subjects are noncompliant with the research protocol. An application of behavioral science principles to the problem of noncompliance can allow researchers to successfully execute EMA studies while obtaining high rates of subject compliance.

References

Affleck, G., Tennen, H., Urrows, S., Higgins, P., Abeles, M., Hall, C., Karoly, P. & Newton, C. (1998). Fibromyalgia and women's pursuit of personal goals: A daily process analysis. *Health Psychology, 17*, 40–47.

Affleck, G., Urrows, S., Tennen, H. & Higgins, P. (1992). Daily coping with pain from rheumatoid arthritis: Patterns and correlates. *Pain, 51*, 221–229.

Bailey, A. S., Martin, M. L. (October, 2000). *In Quality of Life Questionnaires, What Do Patients Understand "Past Month" to Mean?* Poster presented at the International Society for Quality of Life Research conference, Vancouver, Canada.

Barge-Schaapveld, D. Q., Nicolson, N. A., Berkhof, J. & DeVries, M. W. (1999). Quality of life in depression: Daily life determinants and variability. *Psychiatry Research, 88*, 173–189.

Beidel, D. C., Neal, A. M. & Lederer, A. S. (1991). The feasibility and validity of a daily diary for the assessment of anxiety in children. *Behavior Therapy, 22*, 505–517.

Boudes, P. (1998). Drug compliance in therapeutic trials: a review. *Controlled Clinical Trials, 19*, 257–168.

Bradburn, N. M. (2000). Temporal Representation and Event Dating. In A. A. Stone, J. S. Turkkan, C. A. Bachrach, J. B. Jobe, H. S. Kurtzman & V. S. Cain (Eds.) *The Science of Self Report: Implications for Research and Practice* (pp.49–63). Mahwah, N.J.: Lawrence Erlbaum Associates, Publishers.

Bradburn, N. M., Rips, L. J. & Shevell, S. K. (1987). Answering Autobiographical Questions: The Impact of Memory and Inference on Surveys. *Science, 236*, 157–161.

Brewer, W. F. (1994). Autobiographical memory and survey research. In N. Schwarz & S. Sudman (Eds.) *Autobiographical memory and the validity of retrospective reports* (pp.11–20). New York: Springer-Verlag.

Bronfenbrenner, U. (1979). *The ecology of human development.* Cambridge, USA: Harvard University Press.

Brown, G. W. & Harris, T. (1978). *Social Origins of Depression.* London: Tavistock.

Chmelik, F. & Doughty, A. (1994). Objective measurements of compliance in asthma treatment. *Annals of Allergy, 73*, 527–532.

Clark, D. M. & Teasdale, J. D. (1982). Diurnal variation in clinical depression and accessibility of memories of positive and negative experiences. *Journal of Abnormal Psychology, 91*, 87–95.

Clark, D. M. & Teasdale, J. D. (1985). Constraints on effects of mood on memory. *Journal of Personality and Social Psychology, 48*, 1595–1608.

Collins, R. L., Morsheimer, E. T., Shiffman, S., Paty, J. A., Gnys, M. & Papandonatos, G. D. (1998). Ecological momentary assessment in behavioral drinking moderation training program. *Experimental and Clinical Psychopharmacology, 6,* 306–315.

Cruise, C. E., Broderick, J., Porter, L., Kaell, A. T., Stone, A. A. (1996). Reactive effects of diary self-assessment in chronic pain patients. *Pain, 67*, 253–258.

Csikszentmihalyi, M. & Larson, R. (1984). *Being adolescent: Conflict and growth in the teenage years.* New York: Basic.

Csikszentmihalyi, M. & Larson, R. (1987). Validity and reliability of the Experience Sampling Method. *Journal of Nervous and Mental Disease, 175*, 526–536.

Csikszentmihalyi, M. (1994). *Flow: The Psychology of Optimal Experience.* New York: HarperCollins.

DeVries, M. W. (Ed.) (1992). *The Experience of Psychopathology: Investigating mental disorders in their natural settings.* Cambridge, Cambridge University Press.

Eckenrode, J. (1984). Impact of chronic and acute stressors on daily reports of mood. *Journal of Social Psychology, 46*, 907–918.

Eich, E., Reeves, J. L., Jaeger, B. & Graff-Radford, S. B. (1985). Memory for Pain: Relation between Past and Present Pain Intensity. *Pain, 23*, 375–379.

Eisenhower, D., Mathiowetz, N. A. & Morganstein, D. (1991). Recall error: Sources and bias reduction techniques. In P. Beimer, R. Groves, L. Lyberg, N. Mathiowetz & S. Sudman (Eds.), *Measurement errors in surveys.* New York: Wiley.

Epstein, L. H. & Collins, F. L. (1977). The measurement of situational influences of smoking. *Addictive Behaviors, 2*, 47–50.

Erickson, J. R. & Jemison, C. R. (1991). Relations among measures of autobiographical memory. *Bulletin of the Psychonomic Society, 29*, 233–236.

Fahrenberg, J., Foerster, F. & Muller, W. (1996). Laboratory and field studies for improvement of ambulatory monitoring methodology. In J. Fahrenberg & M. Myrtek (Eds.) *Ambulatory Assessment: Computer-Assisted Psychological and Psychophysiological Methods in Monitoring and Field Studies* (pp.237–256). Seattle, WA: Hofgrefe & Huber Publishers.

Follick, M .J., Ahearn, D. K. & Laser-Wolston N. (1984). Evaluation of a daily activity diary for chronic pain patients. *Pain, 19*, 373–382.

Friedman, W. J. (1993). Memory for the Time of Past Events. *Psychological Bulletin, 113*, 44–66.

Gill, T. M. & Feinstein, A. R. (1994). A critical appraisal of the quality-of-life measurements. *Journal of the American Medical Association, 272*, 619–626.

Guyll, M. & Contrada, R. J. (1998). Trait hostility and ambulatory cardiovascular activity: responses to social interaction. *Health Psychology, 17*, 30–39.

Hank, P. & Schwenkmezger, P. (1996). Computer-assisted versus paper-and-pencil-based self-monitoring. In J. Fahrenberg & M. Myrtek (Eds.) *Ambulatory Assessment: Computer-Assisted*

Psychological and Psychophysiological Methods in Monitoring and Field Studies, pp.85–99. Seattle, WA: Hofgrefe & Huber Publishers.

Haythornthwaite, J. A., Hegel, M. T., Kerns, R. D. (1991). Development of a sleep diary for chronic pain patients. Journal of Pain Symptom Management, 6, *65–72.*

Hedges, S. M., Krantz, D.S., Contrada, R.J. & Rozanshi, A. R. (1990). Development of a diary for use with ambulatory monitoring of mood, activities, and physiological function. *Journal of Psychopathology Behavioral Assessment, 12*, 203–217.

Houpt, J. B., McMillan, R., Wein, C. & Paget-Dellio, S. D. (1999). Effect of Glucosamine Hydrochloride in the Treatment of Pain of Osteoarthritis of the Knee. *Journal of Rheumatology, 26,* 2423–2430.

Inderbitzen, H. M. & Foster, S. L. (1992). The Inventory of Social Skills: Development, reliability, and validity. *Psychological Assessment, 4*, 451–459.

Jandorf, L., Deblinger, E., Neale, J. M. & Stone, A. A. (1986). Daily versus major life events as predictors of symptom frequency: A replication study. *The Journal of General Psychology, 113,* 205–218.

Joffe, R. T., MacDonald, C. & Kutcher, S. P. (1989). Life events and mania: a case-controlled study. *Psychiatry Research, 30*, 213–216.

Johannes, C. B., Crawford, S. L., Woods, J., Goldstein, R. B., Tran, D., Mehrotra, S., Johnson, K. B. & Santoro, N. (2000). An electronic menstrual cycle calendar: comparison of data quality with a paper version. *Menopause, 7*, 200–208.

Jonasson, G., Carlsen, K., Sodal, A., Jonasson, C. & Mowinckel, P. (1999). Patient compliance in a clinical trial with inhaled budesonide in children with mild asthma. *European Respiratory Journal, 14,* 150–154.

Kamarck, T. W., Shiffman, S., Smithline, L., Goodie, J. L., Thompson, H., Ituarte, P., Jong, J. Y., Pro, V., Paty, J., Kassel, J., Gnys, M., Perz, W. (1998). The diary of ambulatory behavioral states: a new approach to the assessment of psychosocial influences on ambulatory cardiovascular activity. In D. Krantz & A. Baum (Eds.) *Perspectives in Behavioral Medicine: Technology and Methodology in Behavioral Medicine,* pp. 163–193. Mahwah, NJ: Lawrence Erlbaum Associates.

Larson, R. (1989). Beeping children and adolescents: A method for studying time use and daily experience. *Journal of Youth and Adolescence, 18*, 511–530.

Lewis, B., Lewis, D. & Cumming, G. (1994). The Comparative Analgesic Efficacy of Transcutaneous Electrical Nerve Stimulation and a Non-steroidal Anti-flammatory Drug for Painful Osteoarthritis. *British Journal of Rheumatology, 33*, 455–460.

Linton, S. J. (1991). Memory for chronic pain intensity: Correlates of accuracy. *Perceptual and Motor Skills, 72*, 1091–1095.

Litt, M. D., Cooney, N. L. & Morse, P. (1998). Ecological momentary assessment (EMA) with treated alcoholics: Methodological problems and potential solutions. *Health Psychology, 17,* 48–52.

Marco, C. A. & Suls, J. (1993). Daily stress and the trajectory of mood: spillover, response assimilation, contrast, and chronic negative affectivity. *Journal of Social Psychology, 64*, 1053–1063.

Mazze, R. S., Shamoon, H., Pasmantier, R., Lucido, D., Murphy, J., Hartmann, K., Kuykendall, V. & Lopatin, W. (1984). Reliability of blood glucose monitoring by patients with diabetes mellitus. *The American Journal of Medicine, 77*, 211–217.

McFall, R. M. (1977). Parameters of self-monitoring. In R. B. Stuart (Ed.), *Behavioral self-management: Strategies, techniques, and outcome.* New York: Brunner/Mazel.

Means, B., Swan, G. E., Jobe, J. B. & Esposito, J. L. (1994). The Effects of Estimation Strategies on the Accuracy of Respondents' Reports of Cigarette Smoking. In, N. Schwartz & S. Sudman

(Eds.) *Autobiographical Memory and the Validity of Retrospective Reports* (pp. 107–119). New York: Springer-Verlag.

Menon, G. & Yorkton, E. A. (2000). The Use of Memory and Contextual Cues in the Formation of Behavioral Frequency Judgments. In A.A. Stone, J. S. Turkkan, C. A. Bachrach, J. B. Jobe, H. S. Kurtzman & V. S. Cain (Eds.) *The Science of Self Report: Implications for Research and Practice* (pp. 63–80). Mahwah, N.J.: Lawrence Erlbaum Associates, Publishers.

Milgrom, H., Bender, B., Ackerson, L., Bowry, P., Smith, B. & Rand, C. (1996). Noncompliance and treatment failure in children with asthma. *Journal of Allergy and Clinical Immunology, 98*, 1051–1057.

Muldoon, M. F., Barger, S. D., Flory, J. D. & Manuck, S. B. (1998). What are the quality of life measurements measuring? *British Medical Journal, 316*, 542–545.

Nelson, R. O. (1977). Assessment and therapeutic functions of self-monitoring. In M. Hersen, R. M. Eisler & P. Miller (Eds.), *Progress in Behavioral Modification* (pp. 3–41). New York: Academic Press.

Neugebauer, R. (1989). Reliability of Seizure Diaries in Adult Epileptic Patients. *Neuroepidemiology, 8*, 228–233.

Norman, G. R., McFarlane, A. H., Streiner, D. L. & Neale, K. (1982). Health diaries: strategies for compliance and relation to other measures. *Medical Care, 20,* 623–629.

Okenfels, M. C., Porter, L., Smyth, J., Kirschbaum, C., Hellhammer, D. H. & Stone, A. A. (1995). The effect of chronic stress associated with unemployment on salivary cortisol: Overall cortisol levels, diurnal rhythm, and acute stress reactivity. *Psychosomatic Medicine, 57*, 460–467.

Paty, J., Kassel, J. & Shiffman, S. (1992). The importance of assessing base rates for clinical studies: An example of stimulus control of smoking. In M.W. DeVries (Ed.) *The Experience of Psychopathology: Investigating Mental Disorders in Their Natural Setting* (pp. 347–352). Cambridge: Cambridge University Press.

Peters, M. L., Sorbi, M. J., Kruise, D. A., Kerssens, J. J., Verhaak, P. F. & Bensing, J. M. (2000). Electronic diary assessment of pain, disability and psychological adaptation in patients differing in duration of pain. *Pain, 84*, 181–192.

Pickering, T. G., Coats, A., Mallion, J. M., Mancia, G. & Verdecchia, P. (1999). Blood pressure monitoring. Task force V: White-coat hypertension. *Blood Pressure Monitoring, 4*, 333–341.

Raskin, J., (2000). *The Humane Interface: New Directions for Designing Interactive Systems.* Reading, MA: Addison Wesley Longman, Inc.

Redelmeier, D. & Kahneman, D. (1996). Patients' memories of painful medical treatments: real-time and retrospective evaluations of two minimally invasive procedures. *Pain, 66*, 3–8.

Samo, J. A., Tucker, J. A. & Vuchinich, R. E. (1989). Agreement between self-monitoring, recall, and collateral observation measures of alcohol consumption in older adults. *Psychology of Addictive Behaviors, 11*, 391–409.

Schipper, H., Clinch, J. & Powell, V. (1990). Definitions and conceptual issues. In B. Spilker (Ed.), *Quality of Life Assessments in Clinical Trials* (pp.11–24). New York: Raven Press.

Schlundt, D. G. & Bell., C. (1987). Behavioral assessment of eating patterns and blood glucose in diabetes using the self-monitoring analysis system. *Behavior Research Methods, Instruments & Computers, 19*, 215–223.

Schlundt, D. G., Johnson, W. G. & Jarrell, M. P. (1985). A naturalistic functional analysis of eating behavior in bulimia and obesity. *Advances in Behavior Research and Therapy, 7*, 149–162.

Schwartz, E. D., Kowalski, J. M. & McNally, R. J. (1993). Malignant memories: Post-traumatic changes in memory in adults after a school shooting. *Journal of Traumatic Stress, 6*, 545–553.

Schwartz, J. E. & Stone, A. A. (1998). Strategies for analyzing ecological momentary assessment data. *Health Psychology, 17*, 6–16.

Schwarz, N. & Sudman, S. (1994). *Autobiographical memory and the validity of retrospective reports*. New York: Springer-Verlag.

Shiffman, S. (2000). Real-time self-report of momentary states in the natural environment: Computerized ecological momentary assessment. In A. A. Stone et al. (Eds.) *The Science of Self-Report: Implications for Research and Practice* (pp. 277–296). Mahwah, New Jersey: Lawrence Erlbaum Associates, Publishers.

Shiffman, S. & Prange, M. (1988). Self-reported and self-monitored smoking patterns. *Psychology of Addictive Behaviors, 13*, 201–204.

Shiffman, S., Elash, C. E., Paton, S. M., Gwaltney, C. J., Paty, J. A., Clark, D. B., Liu, K. S. & DiMarino, M. E. (2000). Comparative efficacy of 24-hour and 16-hour transdermal nicotine patches for relief of morning craving. *Addiction, 95*, 1185–1195.

Shiffman, S., Hufford, M., Hickox, M., Paty, J. A., Gnys, M. & Kassel, J. (1997). Remember that? A comparison of real-time versus retrospective recall of smoking lapses. *Journal of Consulting and Clinical Psychology, 65*, 292–300.

Shiffman, S., Paty, J. A., Gnys, M., Kassel. J. A. & Hickcox, M. (1996). First lapses to smoking: Within-subjects analysis of real-time reports. *Journal of Consulting and Clinical Psychology, 64*, 366–379.

Shiffman, S., Paty, J. A., Gnys, M., Kassel, J. D., Elash, C. (1995). Nicotine withdrawal in chippers and regular smokers: subjective and cognitive effects. *Health Psychology, 14*, 301–309.

Simmons, M. S., Nides, M. A., Rand, C. S., Wise, R. A. & Tashkin, D. P. (2000). Unpredictability of deception in compliance with physician prescribed bronchodilator inhaler use in a clinical trial. *Chest, 118*, 290–295.

Spector, S., Kinsman, R., Mawhinney, H., Siegel, S., Rachelefsky, G., Katz, R. & Rohr, A. (1986). Compliance of patients with asthma with an experimental aerosolized medication: Implications for controlled clinical trials. *Journal of Allergy and Clinical Immunology, 77*, 65–70.

Spence, S. H. (1992). Psychosexual dysfunction in the elderly. *Behavior Change, 9*, 55–64.

Stone, A. A. & Shiffman, S. (1994). Ecological Momentary Assessment: Measuring real world processes in behavioral medicine. *Annals of Behavioral Medicine, 16*, 199–202.

Stone, A. A. & Shiffman, S. (manuscript in preparation). *Capturing momentary, self-report data: A proposal for reporting guidelines.*

Stone, A. A., Broderick, J. B., Kaell, A. T., Delespaul, P. A. E. G. & Porter, L. (2000). Does the peak-end phenomenon observed in laboratory pain studies apply to real-world pain in rheumatoid arthritics? *Journal of Pain, Fall (1)*, 203–218.

Stone, A. A., Schwartz, J. E., Neale, J. M., Shiffman, S., Marco., C. A., Hickox, M., Paty, J., Porter, L. S. & Cruise, L. J. (1998). A comparison of coping assessed by ecological momentary assessment and retrospective recall. *Journal of Personality and Social Psychology, 74*, 1670–1680.

Stone, A. A., Schwartz, J. E., Neale, J. M., Shiffman, S., Marco., C. A., Hickox, M., Paty, J., Porter, L. S. & Cruise, L. J. (1998). A comparison of coping assessed by ecological momentary assessment and retrospective recall. *Journal of Personality and Social Psychology, 74*, 1670–1680.

Straka, R., Fish, J., Benson, S. & Suh, J. (1997). Patient self-reporting of compliance does not correspond with electronic monitoring: An evaluation using isosorbide dinitrate as a model drug. *Pharmacotherapy, 17*, 126–132.

Teasdale, J. D. & Fogarty, S. J. (1979). Differential effects of induced mood on retrieval of pleasant and unpleasant events from episodic memory. *Journal of Abnormal Psychology, 88*, 248–257.

Tennen, H. & Affleck, G. (1996). Daily Processes in Coping with Chronic Pain: Methods and Analytic Strategies. In M. Zeidner & N. S. Endler (Eds.) *Handbook of Coping: Theory, Research & Applications* (pp. 151–177). New York: John Wiley & Sons, Inc.

Thompson, C. P., Skowronski, J. J. & Betz, A. L. (1993). The use of partial temporal information in dating personal events. *Memory & Cognition, 21*, 352–360.

Totterdell, P. & Folkard, S. (1992). In situ repeated measures of affect and cognitive performance facilitated by use of a hand-held computer. *Behavior Research Methods, Instruments, and Computers, 24*, 545–553.

Trick, L. R. (1993). Patient compliance–don't count on it! *Journal of the American Optometric Association, 64*, 264–270.

Urquhart, J. (1996). Patient compliance with crucial drug regimens: implications for prostate cancer. *European Urology, 29*, 124–131.

Urquhart, J. (1994). Role of patient compliance in clinical pharmacokinetics: A review of recent research. *Clinical Pharmacokinetics, 27*, 202–215.

Urquhart, J. & De Klerk, E. (1998). Contending paradigms for the interpretation of data on patient compliance with therapeutic drug regimens. *Statistics in Medicine, 17*, 251–267.

VanEck, M., Berkhof, H., Nicolson, N. & Sulon, J. (1996). The effects of perceived stress, traits, mood states, and stressful events on salivary cortisol. *Psychosomatic Medicine, 58*, 447–58.

Verbrugge, L. M. (1980). Health diaries. *Medical Care, 18,* 73–95.

Verschelden, P., Cartier, A., L'Archeveque, A., Trudeau, C. & Malo, J. L. (1996). Compliance with and accuracy of daily assessment of peak expiratory flows (PEF) in asthmatic subjects over a three month period. *European Respiratory Journal, 9*, 880–885.

Wheeler, L. & Reis, H. T. (1991). Self–recording of everyday life events: Origins, types, and uses. *Journal of Personality, 59*, 339–354.

Wolff, R. P. & Wolff, L. S. (1991). Assessment and treatment of obsessive-compulsive disorder in children. Special Issue: Current perspectives in the diagnosis, assessment, and treatment of child and adolescent disorders. *Behavior Modification, 15*, 372–393.

Chapter 5
MONITOR: Acquisition of Psychological Data by a Hand-held PC

Jochen Fahrenberg, Paul Hüttner, and Rainer Leonhart
Forschungsgruppe Psychophysiologie, Department of Psychology, University of Freiburg, Germany

Introduction

Computer-assisted data acquisition

Methods of recording psychological data in everyday life have a long history in differential psychology and clinical psychology. Event recorders for the timed registration of stimuli and responses, "beeper" studies in which a programmable wristwatch prompts the subject to respond to a questionnaire, self-ratings on diary cards, and electronic data logger have all been used for this purpose. The arrival of pocket-sized (hand-held, palm-top) computers has eased the acquisition of data considerably. Many Book Chapters in this volume and in the previous volume refer to this methodology (for reviews, see Fahrenberg, 1996; Fahrenberg & Myrtek, 2001; Pawlik & Buse, 1996; Perrez, 1994; Stone & Shiffman, 1994; see also Hufford et al., this Volume). An overview on the origins and developments of psychological data acquisition was included here (Fahrenberg, this Volume).

Following the progress made in pocket-sized computers, software to facilitate the use of hand-held PCs in field studies has been developed in many institutions, more or less geared to the needs of certain studies. More flexible software systems suited to the requirements of a variety of applications are still an exception (see also, the Behavior Observation System, Noldus Information Technology, AG Wageningen, NL; AMBU for in-field performance testing, cf. Buse & Pawlik, 1996, Hogrefe Verlag, Göttingen, Germany; see also their Chapter in this Volume). At Freiburg University, the course of development progressed from the use of an analog cassette recorder (Fahrenberg, Foerster, Schneider, Müller & Myrtek, 1984) to hand-held PCs (Heger, 1990, Käppler, 1994, Myrtek et al., 1988, Myrtek, Brügner & Müller, 1996) during which time the MONITOR software emerged (Brügner, 1998).

Advantages and Limitations

The application of programmable pocket-PCs in ambulatory assessment has many advantages:

- alarm functions for prompting the subject at predefined intervals and a built-in reminder signal;
- reliable timing of input, delay of input, and duration of input;
- flexible layout of questions and response categories;
- branching of questions and tailor-made sequential or hierarchical strategies;
- concealment of previously recorded responses from the subjects;
- convenience and ease of transfer of data to a stationary PC for statistical analysis.

One can generally assume a higher reliability in the timing and saving of responses and a higher ecological validity of such assessments. Self-reports in the form of paper-and-pencil questionnaires and diaries cannot be designed in such a way that they can be applied flexibly and provide the exactness needed when timing responses. In psychology the hand-held PC so far has been predominantly used for recording self-reports on mood and other aspects of subjective state, including physical complaints and symptoms, that is, as an "electronic diary". There are other kinds of data, which can be obtained in field studies: objective features of a behavior setting, behavior observations, behavior and performance measures (in-field psychometric testing, see Pawlik & Buse, this Volume), self-measurements of various kinds, for example, blood pressure data, and, possibly, ratings of environmental aspects, like ambient noise or temperature. Potential contents of a computer-assisted protocol may further include, for example, individual comments or self-evaluation in connection with events.

The versatility and wide acceptance of computer-assisted data acquisition is evident, although there are limitations and obvious restrictions. All participants of such studies will need sufficient practical training in the basic features of the PC and the program, at least, to avoid malfunctions and missing data. In spite of the obvious increase in computer-literacy within the general population, there are sub-populations which are less familiar with such devices or may experience problems, for example, as in the case of the elderly who were not acquainted with PCs in their job, or in some clinical populations and in patients with sensory or motor disorders. Indeed, the application of questionnaires would likewise prove to be difficult in such samples.

In the past, the issue has been raised whether the use of a hand-held PC will in itself lead to cause a specific method variance. When comparing computer-assisted questioning with paper-and-pencil-type questionnaires, empirical investigations have not confirmed the assumed bias (for example, Finegan & Allen, 1994; Franke, 1998; Hank & Schwenkmezger, 1996). However, the reactivity phenomena may arise in daily life when the participants of such assessments are prompted unexpectedly by a beeper to respond to a number of items; moreover, an enhanced level of self-awareness may be induced by the task of giving self-reports several times during the day.

Outline of MONITOR

Computer-assisted self-reports require a hand-held PC with certain features: a large display, easy handling of basic controls, clock, beeper with volume control, sufficient capacity of storage, low power consumption, and a low weight. For many applications, a comparatively large alphanumeric keyboard (complete QWERTY) is also preferable in order to ease recording and especially, to record verbal responses. The latter may involve, for example, recording reports and comments about specific events, or reporting more precisely the occurrence of physical and psychological symptoms, which in either case hardly fit pre-defined categories. For some applications it may suffice to record only "yes" or "no" responses or numbers (Likert Scale type). In this case, a smaller hand-held PC may be preferable, although small keys may present a problem for some subjects or patients.

The Hand-held (palm-top) computers of the Psion™ Series 3 (Psion PLC, London, England) facilitated the development and application of MONITOR particularly well. The computer, weight 275 g, has sufficient memory capacity (16 bit CPU, RAM 512 K,1 MB ROM, 2 MB RAM, card 1 MB), a clock, a piezoresistive beeper, alphanumeric keyboard, and an operating system that allows flexible programming in OPL. A large LCD (125 x 45 mm, 480 x 160 pixel, that is, 80 symbols x 25 lines) is used to display rating scales, multiple choice items or test items which can be answered by pressing a key or by typing in answers. The Psion™ Revo is a successor of the Series 3 using EPOC Release 5 (36 MHz 32 bit RISC CPU, 8 MB ROM, 8 MB RAM, weight 200 g).

Table 1. MONITOR options for input, control commands, and output

Input	Items, adjective rating scales (various formats), multiple choice items Test responses, performance data Text input Response to specific instructions (tasks) Branching of item sequences, conditional steps (jumps) depending on previously given answers or time (Correction of previous response possible)
Control Commands	Programmed start (fixed schedule, option for individual start time) Various alarm sound (beeper) and timing options Voluntary (Self) start External start (options) Delayed alarm repeat (sleep function) Sleep mode (night) Event/time/contingency sampling
Output	Precise time of alarm, start and duration of input, responses, including test scores, verbal input, etc. ASCII file, ready for transfer to, for example, EXCEL, SPSS, etc.

The MONITOR is a general purpose software which may be used for a variety of applications. In the following, an outline of MONITOR Level 9 is given. MONITOR provides a number of options for input, control commands, and output as depicted in Table 1 (for a detailed description, see the MONITOR Manual, Hüttner, 2001).

MONITOR - an example of its application

A typical assessment may include a setting protocol, a number of self-ratings of subjective state, mental performance tests, and specific questions about aspects of acceptance and reactivity in connection with the prompt-to-respond function of the PC (cf. Fahrenberg, 1996; Heger, 1990; Käppler, 1994). In this example, the setting protocol consists of four questions about location (14 categories), social context (6 categories), posture and motion (4 categories), and present activity (23 categories). The following 14 items relating to subjective state were assessed using seven-point adjective rating scales (from 1 = not at all, to 7 = completely): Is the momentary situation familiar, typical? Is the present situation strenuous, demanding? Is the momentary situation under your control? Do you feel excited, nervous? Is your momentary mood angry, irritated? Is your momentary mood depressed? Do you feel mentally alert? Do you feel weary, exhausted? Do you feel physically well? Did any specific events occur in the preceding interval? (yes – no). Did you experience stress in the preceding interval? When anticipating the outcome of the following tests, how good will your performance be? Having done the tests how good was your actual performance? Was being tested tiresome to you?

Two questions were open, that is, they allowed individual wording of the answer or statement. Following a yes response to whether particular events occurred, the subject was asked to type a short report. When the self-rating indicated that the physical well-being was diminished, that is, a response of 6 or less on the seven-point rating scale, the subject had to specify the complaint or symptom.

Mental performance tests may include tests of attention, for example a Go/No-Go test of reaction time, or a working memory test (adapted by G. Brügner from Zimmermann & Fimm, 1992/93). The Go/No-Go test consists of 60 stimuli. The working memory span test uses 80 stimuli, that is, geometrical symbols: circle, square, diamond, triangle, and cross. The target stimuli was, in each case, the last but one symbol. When a stimulus matched the target stimulus, the subject had to press the key.

MONITOR can be easily adapted to include, for example, retrospective self-ratings for the investigation of recall-error or specific items which relate to the experience of being hindered or distracted by the PC during on-going activities and, as well, of being distracted by external events or persons when responding.

Overview of recent findings

In the following, the findings from a number of recent studies based on MONITOR are reviewed. The hand-held PC is particularly suited to the assessment of diurnal changes in subjective state and performance, for example, in research on aspects of morningness-eveningness. With this methodology an investigation of recall errors with regard to momentary self-ratings and retrospective ratings can be carried out: findings from four studies are available. Repeated ambulatory assessment of behavioral activities and subjective state may contribute to the concurrent validation of psychological tests, for example, measures of personality traits derived from questionnaires.

The MONITOR software was used also in a number of studies reported in this volume (for example, by Käppler & Rieder, by Kubiak & Hermanns, by Schmidt et al.; Stiglmayr et al.).

Mood, attention, and morningness-eveningness

A number of studies have been concerned with the concept of morningness-eveningness. The assumption was that mood, performance, and certain physiological variables like body temperature, skin conductance, and endocrine measures, are dependent on or associated with the individual's basic disposition to exhibit the optimal level of energetic arousal, behavioral activation, and well-being either in the morning or in the evening. A questionnaire to assess this disposition, the Morningness-Eveningness Questionnaire, MEQ, was developed by Horne and Östberg (1976). The empirical findings, however, appear to be rather inconsistent (cf. review by Kerkhof, 1985; Natale & Cigogna, 1996; Tankova, Adan & Buela-Casal, 1994). The circadian regulation of subjective alertness and the individual tendency towards morningness-eveningness may reflect biological rhythms but is also strongly related to socio-cultural factors. Accordingly, sociability and the age-related style of living (life habits) may exert an essential influence on empirical investigations, for example, early and late evening social activities may not only be indicative of eveningness, indeed they may also confound the assessment of mood and performance the next morning.

Nearly all investigations relied on retrospective questionnaires or paper and pencil diaries. Studies that included objective performance tests are an exception. The ambulatory assessment methodology appears to be especially suited to the investigation of the relationships between self-reports on mood, and objective performance tests, morningness-eveningness, and personality dimensions. The present investigation sets its sights on revealing whether morning types and evening types differ in self-reported mood and performance during the course of the day. In particular, it was expected that morning types would exhibit more positive mood and higher performance levels in the morning than evening types (Fahrenberg, Brügner, Foerster & Käppler, 1999).

In this study, 61 university students from various faculties, 24 males and 37 females, participated as paid voluntary subjects. The mean age was 24 years (SD = 3.2, range 20 to 33). In the present study the assessment included: a setting protocol, self-ratings of momentary subjective state, retrospective ratings, and performance in two tests of attention, that is, a Go/No-Go paradigm and a working memory span test (see Section above). The participants received the computer either on Monday or on Wednesday morning at about 9 a.m. and they returned it 48 hours later on Wednesday or Friday morning, respectively. The subjects were trained to operate the PC, paying special attention to the recording of self-ratings according to the different kinds of items and the taking of performance tests. The MONITOR prompted the first and subsequent self-protocols at about 12 a.m., 3 p.m., 6 p.m., and 9 p.m. The data acquisition was automatically resumed at 8 a.m. the following morning.

The participants filled in the adapted German version of the MEQ (Horne & Östberg, 1976). In the present study, two essential items from the MEQ were used instead of the total score of this rather heterogeneous questionnaire. A classification was based on self-ratings of type (Item 17) and statements about "best time of the day" (Item 16): 17 morning types, 24 intermediate types, 20 evening types.

A MANOVA (3 groups, 2 days, 5 protocols) was conducted to test the hypothesis on relationships between morningness-eveningness and the daily course of mood and attention. In this respect, the interaction term (protocols x MEQ) was of special interest. Several significant main effects ($p \leq .01$) were present. *Between days*: 5 items and test scores; *between protocols*: 6 items and 4 test scores. On day 2, participants rated the situation more "familiar", felt less "excited", less "mentally alert", rated their physical well-being and test performance higher, and had better performance scores in both tests of attention. Diurnal changes were evident in items "strenuous, demanding", "angry, irritated", "mentally alert", and "stress", which all showed an inverted U-shape course, and self-rating of test performance, which reflected an increase over protocols. Performance measures like mean reaction time and standard deviations showed a U-shape, that is, decrease and increase during the day. The *interaction terms* morningness-eveningness x protocols were significant for five measures. Significant effects were found for "strenuous, demanding" ($F(8,80) = 2.90$, $p = .007$), "situation under control" ($F(8,80) = 3.32$, $p = .003$), self-rating of performance after testing ($F(8,80) = 2.64$, $p < .05$), irritated by the repeated questioning ($F(8,80) = 3.17$, $p = .004$), and performance index working memory ($F(8,92) = 2.07$, $p < .05$). Morning types and evening types differed as predicted.

Within-subject correlation coefficients, pooled across subjects, were moderate to low, for example between "situation under control", "excited, nervous", "angry, irritated" and "stress since last protocol". With the exception of self-ratings of test performance, not a single relationship ($r > .20$) was found between changes in performance scores and subjective state. This result may be open to question because there were comparatively large intervals, that is, about three hours, between protocols. Furthermore, the statistical distribution of item responses and over-all trends may have affected the results. However, the extension of the assessment over 48 hours and the substantial state variance in most variables appear to support this result.

Discrepancies between subjective state and behavior, although in accordance with many findings in ambulatory assessment research (cf. Fahrenberg & Myrtek, 1996), may not be evident in traditional investigations based on paper-and-pencil questionnaires and retrospective ratings. A direct data acquisition, especially by means of the ecologically more valid ambulatory assessment, is preferable whenever possible.

Negative retrospection effect

The recall-error or retrospection effect has been a methodological issue in several studies. Even though subjects are told to monitor their stress responses, mood and symptoms several times daily, such questionnaire reports are often done from memory. These retrospective ratings are, of course, less accurate. In particular, self-ratings of mood and symptom-reports obtained in the evening may not represent the prevailing state during daytime. A specific retrospection effect may exist when subsequent events and experiences systematically influence and even distort the subjective evaluation and weighting of previous states.

A number of studies have shown discrepancies between actual and retrospective self-ratings. Such discrepancies may be indicative of the subjective evaluation and weighting of previous states, and possibly point to a general response set or bias. (De Beurs, Lange & Van Dyck, 1991; De Longis, Folkman & Lazarus, 1988; De Longis, Hemphill & Lehman, 1992; Hedges, Jandorf & Stone, 1985; Margraf & Jaokobi, 1997; Margraf, Taylor, Ehlers, Roth & Agras, 1987; Shiffman et al., 1997; Smith & Safer, 1993; Stone et al., 1998; Thomas & Diener, 1990).

Käppler, Becker, and Fahrenberg (1993) compared the averages of self-ratings, which were recorded at intervals of about 30 minutes, with the summarizing retrospective ratings, done next morning from memory. The retrospective ratings indicated more negative mood and unease than was to be expected from the actual ratings averaged across the day, that is, a *negative* retrospection bias. The daily course was rated as being more strenuous and the mood more nervous, depressed and weary, , etc., than would have been expected from the averages of repeated self-ratings during the day.

The second study, based on a larger sample of subjects and a 48-hour, allowed for a valid test and generalization of this negative bias in retrospective self-ratings. Sixty-one students participated in this investigation with five self-reports each day for two consecutive days (see morningness-eveningness study). At four particular points of time during the 48 hr monitoring, the subject, after completing the usual protocol, was prompted to provide retrospective ratings about the same set of items, that is, without the performance test, for the whole day. These retrospective summary ratings were obtained in the evening of and in the morning following each of the two days of monitoring.

Once again, a negative bias in self-ratings made in the evening or morning following the day being assessed was evident. The situations were rated as being more strenuous, demanding, less under control, and the mood as being more negative than during the day. These findings substantiated research by De Longis et al. (1988, 1992) and Hedges et al. (1985), and emphasized more clearly the uniformly negative tendency of this retrospection bias. A medium to large effect size was noted here. Hence, the negative retrospection effect, thus, was well replicated. It fits nicely into this construct that a significant correlation between the magnitude of the negative retrospection effect and the personality dimension Emotionality (Neuroticism) was found (Fahrenberg, et al., 1999).

A noteworthy finding was that only one of the ten items, "physical well-being", did not show a significant deviation between daily average and retrospection. It may be speculated that the participants of this study, healthy students, had little variance in their well-being. However, mean and standard deviation were not particularly conspicuous, except for a tendency to exhibit a ceiling effect, indicating well-being (7 = completely). It appeared worthwhile to further investigate the retrospection bias in these positive items. One possible explanation of this effect may concern the distributions and the noticeable tendency to the mean. The retrospective self-ratings were all nearer to the scale midpoint (4) than the means of the momentary ratings. This finding may be interpreted as a regression to the mean because of a less than perfect reliability or as a heuristic used in a decision situation characterized by a context of uncertainty. This radical interpretation does not appear to be compatible with the finding that is also plausible in personality theory, of a correlation between the negative retrospection effect (magnitude of the distortion) and Emotionality. Individuals with a high degree of Emotionality are known to experience depressed mood, many somatic complaints, and a problematic illness behavior as obvious in large scale representative surveys and large-scale investigations (for example, Fahrenberg, Hampel & Selg, 2001; Myrtek, 1998).

A third study was based on a sample of employed persons with a view to testing and generalizing the previous findings. Special care was taken to also include "positive" items, that is, positively worded adjective rating-scales, and to control for the possible inference aspect on the distribution of means and for the tendency towards the mean (Scheibehenne; Saller, Riemann, and Fahrenberg, 2000). A total of 59 participants from different professions (25 m, 34 f), ages from 19 to 58 (M = 34, SD = 10.6) participated in this monitoring study. Most of them worked in an office and had higher education. MONITOR was used to assess (1) setting and activities (4 variables), and (2) the momentary subjective state (14 adjective rating scales) five times during the course of a typical working day.

The findings indicated a highly significant retrospection effect in five of the ten mood items and in four items concerning the situation and distracting influences when responding (Figure 1). In retrospection, the day was valuated more negatively: the situations less familiar, more strenuous, less under control, more distracted; the mood was rated more excited, nervous; angry, irritated; depressed; mentally alert. In eight items, the item means tended toward the scale midpoint ("4"); the only exception was "active, ready to go". The "positive" items, that is, "physical well-being", and the newly included "balanced", "self-confident, self-assured", and "in good mood", showed neither a retrospection effect nor a tendency to the scale midpoint.

The personality trait "Emotionality" (FPI-R, Fahrenberg et al., 2001) was correlated with the magnitude of the retrospection effect in two items: strenuous, demanding $r = .28$ ($p = .03$, $df = 57$) and excited, nervous $r = 0.27$ ($p = .04$). Furthermore, significant correlation coefficients were noted, for example, between questionnaire scales *Physical Complaints* and "mentally alert" 0.35($p = .006$) and "strenuous, demanding" .37 (.004), and FPI-R scale *Strain* and "strenuous, demanding" .44 ($p = .000$) and "excited , nervous" .30 ($p = .023$). Thus, the basic findings of the previous study were replicated. However, the inclusion of more "positive" items was generally not very revealing here. A noteworthy exception was the item "active, ready to go" which exhibited a positive retrospection effect and thereby a large deviation from the scale midpoint. In the retrospective protocol, the participants answered a few questions relating to this task (the distribution of "yes" and "no" are given in parenthesis): Was your retrospective rating guided by your typical answers given during the day ? (46 % yes), by the momentary mood ? (31 % yes), by specific events during the day ? (56 % yes). Are you inclined to evaluate days in retrospection differently ? (39 % yes). The self-rating of being inclined to evaluate days in retrospection differently, concurs with a smaller difference (that is, smaller retrospection effect) in certain items: "excited, nervous", "angry, irritated", "depressed", "tense", and less "balanced" (r significant, $p < .05$). The correlation coefficients indicate that some participants actually were aware of their retrospective interpretation and weighting of daily events.

This series of investigations replicated the previous finding that the recall-error in such self-reports was biased, that is, self-ratings were negatively distorted when summarized in the evening or the following morning. Obviously, neither the average rating nor the retrospective rating can be considered the "true" value since both reflect psychological aspects of state and state change. Nonetheless, the retrospection bias may undermine the validity of self-ratings. A direct data acquisition, espe-

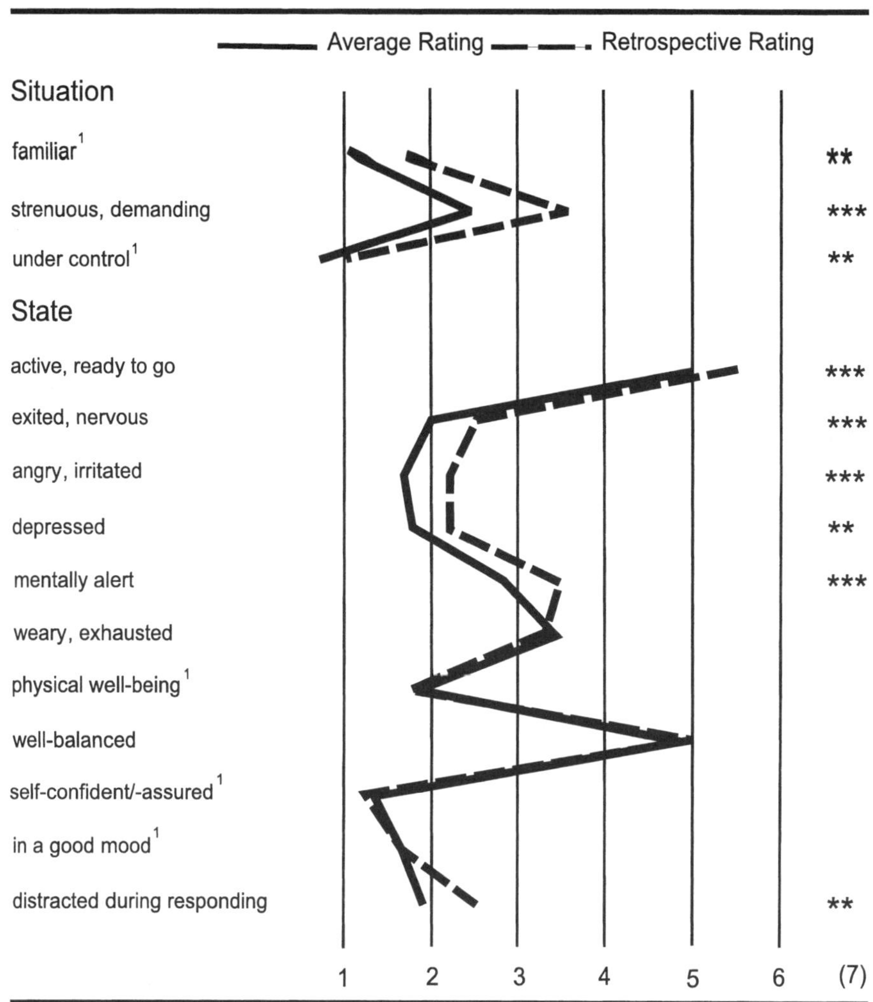

Figure 1. Negative retrospection effect when the retrospective self-rating in the evening is compared to the five momentary ratings averaged across the day.

1) Sign reflected in this Figure. ** $p < .01$; *** $p < .001$, according to t-test and Wilcoxon test, as well.

cially by means of the ecologically more valid ambulatory assessment, is preferable, whenever possible.

Personality questionnaire FPI-R and MONITOR data

Test performance measures and self-ratings of activities and mood, repeatedly assessed by hand-held PC, provide an adequate means of investigating the variability and consistency between and within subjects and between settings. Pawlik and Buse (1982) were the first to utilize the ambulatory assessment methodology in research on the situationism – interactionism – traitism controversy. The previously used data from questionnaires, for example, concerning anxiety responses in various situations (done from memory), may be heavily biased due to recall errors and a general lack of ecological validity.

The feasibility of computer-assisted self-reports on activities and mood in daily life suggests also a new approach in the evaluation of personality tests, especially regarding the concurrent validation of trait scores derived from personality inventories. Preliminary findings on relationships between scores from the *Freiburger Persönlichkeitsinventar* FPI-R and ambulatory monitoring data on subjective state (Fahrenberg et al., 1999; Heger, 1990; Käppler, 1994) led to further investigations. The FPI-R is a German 138-item personality inventory comprising ten personality scales, namely, *Life Satisfaction, Social Orientation, Achievement Orientation, Inhibitedness, Excitability, Aggressiveness, Strain, Somatic Complaints, Health Concern, Frankness, and two further scales, Extraversion* and *Emotionality*, which can be considered to be equivalent to the corresponding scales of the personality questionnaires developed by Eysenck. Normative data are available from a large sample, N = 3740, representative for the German population (Fahrenberg et al., 2001).

An ambulatory monitoring study was designed to investigate the concurrent validity of trait measures and averages of self-ratings level averaged across one day. A total of 59 participants from different professions participated in this monitoring study (sample and general design, see above, study on negative retrospection effect). MONITOR was used to assess: (1) setting and activities (4 variables), and (2) the momentary subjective state (14 adjective rating scales) five times during the course of a typical working day.

The statistical analysis revealed a large proportion of significant ($p < .05$) relationships between personality scores and means of self-ratings: 35 % of a total of 168 coefficients (12 trait scales, 14 state items). Noteworthy was the distribution of these coefficients. Substantial coefficients ($r > .50$) were found, for example, for *Emotionality* and "depressed", *Life Satisfaction* and "well-balanced" and "in a good mood", *Strain* (trait) and experienced "stress" (state), *Health Concern* and "excited, nervous". Most of the significant relationships were with FPI-R Scales *Emotionality, Life Satisfaction, Physical Complaints, Health Concern,* and *Excitability*; only negligible coefficients of correlation were found regarding *Social Orientation, Aggressiveness,* and *Extraversion* (Fahrenberg et al., 2001; Scheibehenne et al., 2000).

Activities and subjective state across the period of one week

A 7-day ambulatory assessment was made to investigate the validity of FPI-R scales to predict the averages and, in particular, the variability of activities and of certain mood items in daily life. An extended monitoring would allow for more data regarding interindividual differences in intraindividual variability. The intention was to replicate the previously observed relationships concerning personality trait scales and item averages and to investigate the predictability of the standard deviation of self-ratings during the week. The hypotheses were, for example, that trait measures of *Emotionality, Strain, Physical Complaints, Health Concern*, would predict the level and, possibly, the variability in the aforementioned items. Furthermore, a 7-day-assessment could be used to test the negative retrospection effect once more, whereby daily and weekly retrospection could be compared.

The participants in this study were 28 first-year students (27 f, 1 m, mean age M = 23.4, SD = 4.6) enrolled in Psychology courses. They received credits for participating in a 7-day monitoring. The data were recorded by MONITOR which was programmed to obtain six records, whereby the first prompt in the morning was timed to occur half an hour after the usual rising time of the subject. MONITOR prompted the subsequent self-protocols at about 11 a.m., 1 p.m., 4 p.m., and 9 p.m. The assessment began at different days of the week in order to balance the assumed weekend effect: 8 subjects began their self-reports on a Monday, 9 subjects on Wednesday, and 11 subjects on Friday. The participants could use the start option, in case they were unable to answer the prompt immediately. Only 3 % of the 28 x 7 x 6 entries were missing. At the beginning, the subjects were given the Freiburger Persönlichkeitsinventar FPI-R (Fahrenberg et al., 2001).

The findings showed relationships between personality measures and weekly averages and variability of several items, for example: *Emotionality* and "excited, nervous" Mean (.52, $p = .004$) and SD (.43, $p = .004$); "depressed" Mean (.47, $p = .01$) and SD (.44, $p= .02$); "weary, exhausted" Mean (.47, $p = .01$); "in a good mood" Mean (-.49, $p = .01$); "physically well" Mean(-.44, $p = .02$). A number of significant relationships were also found between personality trait *Irritability* and items like "angry, irritated", "depressed", and "exhausted"; and for personality traits *Strain*, and *Health Concern*. However, *Extraversion* was only related to the SD of the item "positive changes since previous self-report". It was concluded that the personality test score *Emotionality* predicted the general level and variability of subjective state under naturalistic conditions substantially. The relationship between personality measures and the frequency distributions of certain settings variables, for example, location, social contact, and activities, will be investigated.

As previously noted, a negative retrospection bias was present in 8 of the 10 items used in this study ($p < .01$ in 8 of these items; based on 190, that is 28 x 7, days). The item means changed towards the scale midpoint in 7 items and to the opposite direction in 2 items. The magnitude of this effect was not related to the personality trait *Emotionality* in this study.

Perspectives, developments, and applications

Evaluation and selection of items for diaries

The selection of appropriate items and the psychometric evaluation of the resulting test scales are basic tasks in test construction. This strategy may generally be valid for performance tests used in ambulatory assessment (Buse & Pawlik, 1996; Pawlik & Buse, 1996). However, there are some methodological aspects at issue and, as far as the assessment of subjective state is concerned, there may be essential deviations from the conventional strategies of item analysis and test construction for several reasons: First, an unusually large between- and within-subject variance can be expected for many items assessing state and state change and, therefore, ceiling or floor effects in distributions may often occur; second, the repeated measurement design does not permit the inclusion of more than a minimum of adjective rating scales so that the reliability (consistency), which relates to the concept of parallel measurement and item total correlation coefficients, is hardly practicable; third, since state measures are being sought, retest-reliabilities may be of little value for the evaluation of psychometric properties and the selection of items; fourth, in self-ratings of mood, and especially in performance data, circadian and septemdian (weekly) trends, and moreover, training, satiation and other effects may be obvious; and, fifth, the results of the statistical analyses are subject to controversy, due to such dependencies and the presence of auto-correlation in repeated measurements. Such issues were discussed, for example, by Suen and Ary (1989), Pawlik and Buse (1996), Delespaul (1992), Ott and Scholz (this Volume), Schwartz and Stone (1998), West and Hepworth (1991), and Wilhelm (this Volume).

Even if researchers refrained from performing a statistical test on their hypotheses and were content with descriptive and exploratory analysis, a number of methodological issues nevertheless would persist, especially those dealing with the selection of appropriate items.

Statistical analyses could, however, assist in revealing which items are especially suited to the assessment of *diurnal* changes in subjective state: over-all changes *common to all subjects* and changes *particular to certain subjects*. Other items may be more likely to indicate *habitual* differences in mood. The aforementioned investigation in 61 students may be used as an illustration as to how possible differences in item sensitivity to state changes can be explored.

The 14 items clearly differed in their statistical distributions. Item means ranged between M = 1.85 ("angry, irritated") and M = 5.79 ("situation under control"); SD varied between SD = 1.23 ("depressed") and SD = 1.83 ("testing tiresome"). Accordingly, two items ("situation under control", "physical well-being") showed a ceiling effect and two items ("angry, irritated", "depressed") showed a floor effect. Between days, as revealed by the MANOVA main effect, changes were evident. Participants were more at ease on day 2 and had better performance scores, thus indicating a process of adaptation and training. Significant main effects between protocols indicated that patterns of diurnal changes, common to all subjects, were present (for a further discussion, see Käppler, et al., 2001).

A two-factorial ANOVA (11 protocols x 61 subjects) was used to obtain the relative amount of variance explained by protocols, subjects, and the interaction term protocols x subjects. Between-subject variance was highest, that is, greater than 20 percent, in "situation under control", "angry, irritated", "depressed", "physical well-being", "stress", and "anticipated performance", and was lower, that is, smaller than 10 per cent, in "excited, nervous" and "mentally alert". The between-protocols variance indicating diurnal mood and performance changes common to all subjects was generally low, for example, 3 percent for "strenuous, demanding" and "stress" and even lower for the remaining items.

Substantial interaction variance subjects x protocols was present in most of the items which showed that subjects gave specific self-ratings and performed differently depending on the time of day. The interaction term, which is indicative of diurnal changes specific to individuals, was substantial for "mentally alert" (74 %), "anticipated performance" (75 %), "excited, nervous" (65 %), "testing tiresome" (54 %), and, on the other hand, negligible or low for "under control" (0 %), "depressed" (0 %), and "strenuous, demanding" (12 %). In these items, however, the residual component, which includes higher order interactions that are not separable from error, was substantial.

Coefficients of test-retest reliability (stability) between protocol 1 and protocol 2, of the first day, were between .08 for "strenuous demanding" and .47 for "physical well-being". Such coefficients were of roughly the same range in protocol 1/ protocol 6, that is, the first protocols of each day, and they were slightly higher between protocol 2 and 7, that is, the second protocols of each day. Relationships, of course, were substantially higher when averages, protocol 1 to 5 and protocol 6 to 10, were compared: from .44 "situation under control" to .67 "physical well-being".

Within-subject correlation across protocol averages (pooled for 61 subjects) was obtained to evaluate the covariation of measures. Such coefficients were moderate to low, and there was no indication that certain items from this item pool could be considered redundant, that is, a high ($r^2 > .50$) or very high common variance. None of the items should be eliminated on these grounds.

Based on large-scale assessment studies in students and other populations, Buse and Pawlik (1994; Pawlik and Buse, 1996) developed a battery of performance tests and an item pool suited for ambulatory assessment studies. This may signal the beginnings of the standardization in this domain, possibly based on a core set of normative data. Reference data of this kind could be valuable for many studies. At least, a selection of psychometrically proven items (and item formats) to assess activity level, basic mood dimensions, and workload (job stress) are desirable.

However, the research questions and the applications in many other fields of psychology will require specific assessment strategies in dealing with item contents and sampling (persons, settings, hours, days, etc.) and, therefore, the study protocols, diaries, and symptom reports will remain highly diverse. Thus, the collection of reference data within individual research institutions will be an essential task until cross-institutional standardization is hopefully one day achieved. On the whole, the computer-assisted assessment methodology, appears to be far from standardized, a serious shortcoming compared to conventional psychological testing. The flexibility in programming a PC for recording self-reports, on the other hand, allow for new psychological assessment strategies and other applications of PC technology in daily life.

Compliance and acceptance

Ambulatory assessment by means of hand-held computers is a feasible method. This approach appears to be especially suited to the investigation of diurnal changes and, based on a few items or symptoms only, to long-term assessments extending over many days or weeks.

The assumption, that the general compliance must be perfect because of the computer-assisted method of assessment, may not be true in each participant. The signal can be over-heard, unintentionally or intentionally, so that one or even a number of protocols may be missing. Since the frequency of such missing protocols in a series of studies usually is in the order of a few percent only, a *statistical* analysis exploring such effects and possible relationships with other variables may be pointless. From the protocol provided by means of the hand-held PC, individual differences in the delay in responding (signal compliance) and in duration of input can be noted (or, using MONITOR, also the number of intentional delays when ongoing activities preclude immediate responding).

However, distraction and irritation may be caused by the interruption of the ongoing activity by the beeper signal and the requested responding. This may be disturbing to the participant. Furthermore, an increased state of self-awareness or distinct avoidance behavior, that is, a tendency to evade settings where responding to the items is found to be disturbing for one-self and for others, may occur. The common use of mobile phones will ease much of these reservations. The comments from participants of such monitoring studies indicate that the primary complaint was the frequency of protocols requested by this methodology. The acceptance and compliance will depend also on the number of items, protocols, and the length of study (days). From a series of such studies it may be concluded that the motivation may differ between student subjects (with and without credit points or financial rewards) and patients. Patients can be highly motivated, when there is an evident relationship between the assessment and clinical diagnosis or treatment evaluation.

There are two practical approaches to obtaining evaluating comments from participants: A post-monitoring interview or questionnaire and the use of specific questions to be included in the item pool for concurrent responses during the ongoing monitoring protocol.

A written post-monitoring interview was regularly used in our monitoring studies. For example, in one study, 61 students were given a 17-item questionnaire after returning on the third day asking them about compliance, acceptance, possible reactivity induced by such monitoring, and general criticism about this investigation, and a self-evaluation concerning both the role of distracting events during responding and enhanced states of self-awareness. The participants gave their evaluation of the investigation on seven point rating scales (1 = not at all, 7 = completely). Interest in the present study, for example, was rated at 4.9 on average, typicality of the two days compared to one's usual life at 4.8, interference of repeated self-ratings with daily routine at 3.2, enhanced self-awareness at 3.6, and method-dependent (reactive) changes in behavior at 2.3. Nearly all of the subjects were willing to participate in subsequent studies. Corresponding ratings obtained from the study of 59 employed persons showed very similar results. These subjects were asked whether they noticed a heightened awareness of their behavior on that same day (17 % yes) and whether they had modified their daily routine to adapt to and cope with the monitoring (3 % yes). In general, all of the participants volunteered for another ambulatory monitoring.

In two recent studies, specific items were included in MONITOR concerning the role of distracting events during responding. Commencing the list of items, the participant was asked whether distracting or irritating influences were present during answering. The responses indicated some effects (M = 1.98, SD = 1.46), the mode = 1 showed, however, that in most instances there was no distraction present. For this item, there were no relationships found with the personality measures (FPI-R), however, small coefficients of correlation with concurrent self-ratings "active, ready to go" (r = .27, pooled across subjects, df = 57), "mentally alert" (.23), "excited, nervous" (.22), and "stress" during past period (.21). In the 7-days monitoring study with 28 participants, correlation coefficients between the 42 momentary ratings (M and SD) of being disturbed by the beeper and personality measures from the FPI-R were insignificant.

The compliance and the generally positive attitude seen in participants were noteworthy, but it should be taken into account that in many investigations they were paid volunteers. However, an outstanding degree of compliance in such ambulatory assessment has also been reported in patient groups and other populations (cf. Fahrenberg & Myrtek, 1996).

Conclusions

Ambulatory assessment of subjective state, symptom reports, or job stress by hand-held PCs (PDAs, "electronic diaries") appears to have many advantages compared to the Experience Sampling Method ESM (de Vries, 1992), which used a beeper and a booklet, that is, paper-and-pencil method. Reviews on self-report and self-monitoring methodologies indicate that questionnaires and diary forms seem to be still the standard methodology to assess self-reports. However, the shortcomings of these methods are also acknowledged (Pawlik & Buse, 1996; Perrez, 1994; Stone et al., 2000; Suls & Martin, 1993; Wheeler & Reis, 1991; Wilz & Brähler, 1997; Hank, Schwenkmezger & Schumann, this Volume).

The present volume contains a number of investigations which likewise used a computer-assisted methodology to assess psychological data, that is subjective state or behavioral reports, in daily life. Noteworthy applications have been reported in clinical psychology and at the workplace. Data acquisition software like MONITOR will be of practical use. It became evident that computer-assisted methodologies enable innovative strategies in self-monitoring of job stress and of symptoms. Further developments may include new strategies in health care and self-management, for example, of conditions of chronic illness.

Acknowledgements

This research was supported by the Deutsche Forschungsgemeinschaft. We thank Marcus Cheetham for improving the English version of this Chapter. We acknowledge Miriam Jakob, Benjamin Scheibehenne, Thomas Saller, and Andreas Sieburg, psychology students, for their assistance, especially in the acquisition of data.

References

Brügner, G. (1998). MONITOR: Ein flexibles Programm zur Datenerhebung mittels Pocket-PC. *Zeitschrift für Differentielle und Diagnostische Psychologie, 19,* 145–147.

Buse, L. & Pawlik, K. (1994). Differenzierung zwischen Tages-, Setting- und Situationskonsistenz ausgewählter Verhaltensmerkmale, Maßen der Aktivierung, des Befindens und der Stimmung in Alltagssituationen. *Diagnostica, 40,* 2–26.

Buse, L. & Pawlik, K. (1996). Ambulatory behavioral assessment and in-field performance testing. In J. Fahrenberg & M. Myrtek (Eds.). *Ambulatory Assessment: computer-assisted psychological and psychophysiological methods in monitoring and field studies* (pp. 29–50). Seattle, WA: Hogrefe & Huber.

De Beurs, E., Lange, A. & Van Dyck, R. (1991). Self-monitoring of panic attacks and retrospective estimates of panic: Discordant findings. *Behaviour Research and Therapy, 30,* 411–413.

Delespaul, P.A.E.G. (1992). Technical note: devices and time-sampling procedures. In M. de Vries (Ed.), *The experience of psychopathology. Investigating mental disorders in their natural settings* (pp. 363–373). Cambridge: Cambridge University Press.

de Vries, M.W. (Ed.). (1992). *The Experience of Psychopathology. Investigating Mental Disorders in their Natural Settings.* Cambridge: Cambridge University Press.

DeLongis, A., Folkman, S. & Lazarus, R.S. (1988). The impact of daily stress on health and mood: Psychological and social resources as mediators. *Journal of Personality and Social Psychology, 54*, 486–495.

DeLongis, A., Hemphill, K.J. & Lehman, D.R. (1992). A structured diary methodology for the study of daily events. In F.B. Bryant, J. Edwards, R.S. Tindale, E.J. Posavac, L. Heath, E. Henderson, & Y. Suarez-Balcazar (Eds.), *Methodological Issues in Applied Social Psychology. Social Psychological Applications to Social Issues.* (Vol. 2, pp. 83–109). New York: Plenum.

Fahrenberg, J. (1996). Ambulatory Assessment: Issues and perspectives. In J. Fahrenberg & M. Myrtek (Eds.). *Ambulatory Assessment: computer-assisted psychological and psychophysiological methods in monitoring and field studies* (pp. 3–20). Seattle, WA: Hogrefe & Huber.

Fahrenberg, J., Brügner, G., Foerster, F. & Käppler, C. (1999). Ambulatory assessment of diurnal changes with a hand-held computer: Mood, attention, and morningness – eveningness. *Personality and Individual Differences, 26*, 641–656.

Fahrenberg, J., Hampel, R. & Selg, H. (2001). *Freiburger Persönlichkeitsinventar FPI-R* (7th ed.). Göttingen: Hogrefe.

Fahrenberg, J., Foerster, F., Schneider, H.J., Müller, W. & Myrtek, M. (1984). *Aktivierungsforschung im Labor-Feld-Vergleich.* München: Minerva.

Fahrenberg, J. & Myrtek, M. (Eds.) (1996). *Ambulatory Assessment: computer-assisted psychological and psychophysiological methods in monitoring and field studies.* Seattle, WA: Hogrefe & Huber.

Fahrenberg, J. & Myrtek, M. (2001). Ambulantes Monitoring und Assessment. In F. Rösler (Ed.), *Enzyklopädie der Psychologie: Themenbereich C Theorie und Forschung, Serie 1 Biologische Psychologie, Band 4 Grundlagen und Methoden der Psychophysiologie (pp. 657–798).* Göttingen: Hogrefe.

Finegan, J.E. & Allen, N.J. (1994). Computerized and written questionnaires: Are they equivalent? *Computers in Human Behavior, 10*, 483–496.

Franke, G.H. (1998). *Computerunterstützte klinisch-diagnostische Selbstbeurteilungsverfahren im Äquivalenztest. Experimentelle Studien.* Lengerich: Pabst Science Publishers.

Hank, P. & Schwenkmezger, P. (1996). Computer-assisted versus paper-and-pencil based self-monitoring: An analysis of experimental and psychometric equivalence. In J. Fahrenberg & M. Myrtek (Eds.), *Ambulatory Assessment. Computer-assisted psychological and psychophysiological methods in monitoring and field studies* (pp. 85–99). Seattle, WA: Hogrefe & Huber Publishers.

Hedges, S.M., Jandorf, L. & Stone, A.A. (1985). Meaning of daily mood assessments. *Journal of Personality and Social Psychology, 48,* 428–434.

Heger, R. (1990). *Psychophysiologisches 24-Stund en-Monitoring. Methodenentwicklung und erste Ergebnisse eines multimodalen Untersuchungsansatzes bei 62 normotonen und blutdrucklabilen Studenten.* Frankfurt. a. M.: Lang.

Horne, J.A. & Östberg, O. (1976). Individual differences in human circadian rhythms. *Biological Psychology, 5,* 179–190.

Hüttner, P. (2001). *MONITOR Manual.* Forschungsgruppe Psychophysiologie. Department of Psychology. University of Freiburg, Germany.

Käppler, C. (1994). *Psychophysiologische Bedingungsanalyse von Blutdruckveränderungen im alltäglichen Lebenskontext.* Frankfurt a. M.: Lang.

Käppler, C., Becker, H.-U. & Fahrenberg, J. (1993). Ambulantes 24-Stunden-Monitoring als psychophysiologische Assessmentstrategie: Reproduzierbarkeit, Reaktivität, Retrospektions-effekt und Bewegungskonfundierung. *Zeitschrift für Differentielle und Diagnostische Psychologie, 14,* 235–251.

Käppler, C., Brügner, G. & Fahrenberg, J. (in press, 2001). Computer-unterstütztes Assessment mit MONITOR: Befindlichkeit und Aufmerksamkeit im Alltag. *Zeitschrift für Differentielle und Diagnostische Psychologie.*

Kerkhof, G.A. (1985). Inter-individual differences in the human circadian system: A review. *Biological Psychology, 20*, 83–112.

Margraf, J. & Jacobi, F. (1997). Marburger Angst- und Aktivitätstagebuch. In G. Wilz & E. Brähler (Eds.), *Tagebücher in Therapie und Forschung. Ein anwendungsorientierter Leitfaden* (pp. 139–153). Göttingen: Hogrefe.

Margraf, J., Taylor, C.B., Ehlers, A., Roth, W.T. & Agras, W.S. (1987). Panic attacks in the natural environment. *Journal of Nervous and Mental Disease, 175*, 558–565.

Myrtek, M. (1998). *Gesunde Kranke – kranke Gesunde.* Bern: Huber.

Myrtek, M., Brügner, G., Fichtler, A., König, K., Müller, W., Foerster, F. & Höppner, V. (1988). Detection of emotionally induced ECG changes and their behavioral correlates: A new method for ambulatory monitoring. *European Heart Journal, 9* (Supplement N), 55–60.

Myrtek, M., Brügner, G. & Müller, W. (1996). Interactive monitoring and contingency analysis of emotionally induced ECG changes: Methodology and applications. In J. Fahrenberg & M. Myrtek (Eds.). *Ambulatory Assessment: computer-assisted psychological and psychophysiological methods in monitoring and field studies* (pp. 115–127). Seattle, WA: Hogrefe & Huber.

Natale, V. & Cigogna, P. (1996). Circadian regulation of subjective alertness in morning and evening "types". *Personality and Individual Differences, 20*, 491–497.

Pawlik, K. (1995). Persönlichkeit und Verhalten: Zur Standortbestimmung von differentieller Psychologie. In K. Pawlik (Ed.), *Bericht über den 39. Kongreß der Deutschen Gesellschaft für Psychologie in Hamburg 1994* (pp. 31–49). Göttingen: Hogrefe.

Pawlik, K. & Buse, L. (1982). Rechnergestütze Verhaltensregistrierung im Feld: Beschreibung und erste psychometrische Überprüfung einer neuen Erhebungsmethode. *Zeitschrift für Differentielle und Diagnostische Psychologie, 3,* 101–118.

Pawlik, K. & Buse, L. (1996). Verhaltensbeobachtung in Labor und Feld. In K. Pawlik (Ed.), *Enzyklopädie der Psychologie. Differentielle Psychologie und Persönlichkeitsforschung. Band 1. Grundlagen und Methoden der Differentiellen Psychologie* (pp. 359–394). Göttingen: Hogrefe.

Perrez, M. (1994) Felddiagnostik mit besonderer Berücksichtigung der computerunterstützten Diagnostik. In R.-D. Stieglitz & U. Baumann (Eds.), *Psychodiagnostik Psychischer Störungen* (pp. 149–161). Stuttgart: Enke.

Scheibehenne, B. Saller, T., Riemann, D. & Fahrenberg, J. (2000). Befinden im Tageslauf. Zwei Untersuchungen mit MONITOR. Research Reports. Institute of Psychology, University of Freiburg, Germany.

Schwartz, J.E. & Stone, A.A. (1998). Strategies for analyzing ecological momentary assessment data. *Health Psychology, 17,* 6–16.

Shiffman, S., Hufford, M. Hickcox, M., Paty, J.A., Gnys, M. & Kassel, J.D. (1997). Remember that? A comparison of real-time versus retrospective recall of smoking lapses. *Journal of Consulting and Clinical Psychology, 65,* 292–300.

Smith, W.B. & Safer, M.A. (1993). Effects of present pain level on recall of chronic pain and medication use. *Pain, 55,* 355–361.

Stone, A.A. & Shiffman, S. (1994). Ecological momentary assessment (EMA) in behavioral medicine. *Annals of Behavioral Medicine, 16,* 199–202.

Stone, A.A., Schwartz, J.E., Neale, J.M., Shiffman, S., Marco, C.A., Hickcox, M. & Paty, J. (1998). A comparison of coping assessed by ecological momentary assessment and retrospective recall. *Journal of Personality and Social Psychology, 74,* 1670–1680.

Stone, A.A., Turkhan, J.S., Bachrach, C.A., Jobe, J.B., Kurtzman, H.S. & Cain, V.S. (2000). The science of self-report. Implications for research and practice. Mahwah, N.J.: Lawrence Erlbaum.

Suen, H.K. & Ary, D. (1989). *Analyzing quantitative behavioral observational data.* Hillsdale, N.J.: Lawrence Erlbaum.

Suls, J. & Martin, R.E. (1993). Daily recording and ambulatory monitoring methodologies in behavioral medicine. *Annals of Behavioral Medicine, 15,* 3–7.

Tankova, I., Adan, A. & Buela-Casal, G. (1994). Circadian typology and individual differences: A review. *Personality and Individual Differences, 16,* 671–684.

Thomas, D.L. & Diener, E. (1990). Memory accuracy in the recall of emotions. *Journal of Personality and Social Psychology, 59,* 291–297.

West, S.G. & Hepworth, J.T. (1991). Statistical issues in the study of temporal data: Daily experiences. *Journal of Personality, 59,* 609–662.

Wheeler, L. & Reis, H.T. (1991). Self-recording of everyday life events: Origins, types, and uses. *Journal of Personality, 59*, 339–354.

Wilz, G. & Brähler, E. (Eds.) (1997). *Tagebücher in Therapie und Forschung. Ein anwendungsorientierter Leitfaden.* Göttingen: Hogrefe.

Zimmermann, P. & Fimm, B. (1992/93). *Testbatterie zur Aufmerksamkeitsprüfung TAP. Department of Psychology. University of Freiburg*: Psytest.

Chapter 6

Does the Retrospection Effect Hold as a Stable Phenomenon? – First Results from a Trans-Cultural Self-Monitoring Study of Mood and Cognitive States in Brazil and Germany

Christoph Käppler and Stephan Rieder
Department of Psychology, University of Freiburg, Germany, and Universidade Federal de Minas Gerais, Belo Horizonte, Brazil

Introduction

The assessment of subjective states, cognitive functions and clinical symptoms is one of the main objectives in psychology and medicine. In evaluating psychological condition, the application of hand-held computers can be considered to be a new and important supplement to the traditional forms of paper-and-pencil procedures such as questionnaires, diaries, and interviews that normally yield summarized information. However, these retrospective ratings cannot illustrate the dynamics of psychological changes in daily life. Furthermore, it is unknown exactly how subjects aggregate and weight their experiences. Even if they are asked to monitor their mood and symptoms several times a day, the reports are often done from memory, which can not be ascertained without the time-control functions of a pocket-computer.

Several empirical studies have already reported the (non-)reliability of retrospectively answered questionnaires and diary entries (Biemer, Groves, Lyberg, Mathiowetz & Sudmann, 1992; Kahneman & Tversky, 1982; Schwarz, 1990; Wheeler & Reis, 1991). A systematic shift in retrospectively rated moods was already described by Hedges, Jandorf and Stone (1985). In our first study (Käppler, Becker & Fahrenberg, 1993; Käppler, 1994), we used pocket-computers to compare actual and retrospective self-ratings systematically. We found a negative bias in retrospective self-ratings at the end of a 24-hour monitoring period. In a second study (Fahrenberg, Brügner, Foerster & Käppler, 1999; Käppler, Brügner & Fahrenberg, in press), we used PSION hand-held computers and the MONITOR software

(Brügner, 1998) to investigate the variability of mood and cognitive performance in daily life during two consecutive days. The negative bias in retrospective self-ratings was proven and replicated several times; the retrospection effect was evident in the evening and next morning of each day. In the third project, we have now had the opportunity to replicate the former study in a different cultural context in Brazil. The study was based on three main objectives:

- To examine whether ambulatory assessment with pocket-computers is an applicable research strategy in (culturally) different populations;
- To compare the variability of mood and attention in daily life for both a Brazilian and German samples; and,
- To discover whether the negative retrospection effect holds in different cultural contexts or is unique to some populations (that is, German).

The present paper reports – in the style of a research note – the first results of this trans-cultural comparison.

Methods

Pocket-computer and Software

A suitable pocket-computer was selected according to the criteria size, weight, running time, memory capacity, and resolution characteristics of the screen. We used PSION hand-held computers (PSION Series 3a, PLC, London, England) and the MONITOR software (Brügner, 1998). MONITOR is a flexible program with an extensive repertoire of features: functions to control program course (for example, prompting by beeper or self-activation of the computer, etc.) and presentation of items in different input formats (for example, rating scales, multiple choice, free text, etc.). Adaptations are easily achieved by researchers according to their interests.

The participants received the computer either on Monday or on Wednesday morning at about 9 a.m. and they returned it 48 hours later on Wednesday or Friday morning, respectively. According to an acoustic signal, participants had to run the program five times a day (8:00, 12:00, 15:00, 18:00, 21:00h). The items were presented in sequence on the LCD-screen and could be answered by typing in a response (in most cases numbers). Each time, subjects were prompted to rate current setting features, such as, location and social context, and momentary subjective state. Furthermore they completed two psychometric tests of attention – a Go/NoGo-paradigm and a working memory test, derived from the TAP (Testbattery for Attentional Performance, Zimmermann & Fimm, 1992/93) – in order to analyse the daily course of these cognitive functions. The translation and adaptation of the self-report items and the test instructions was done by an expert group of five professionals (including a linguist). Each of them speaks both German and Portuguese languages and is native speaker in one of them.

At four particular points of time during the 48-hr monitoring period, the subjects, after completing the regular protocol, were prompted to provide retrospective ratings using the same item set for the entire day. These retrospective summary ratings were obtained in the evening and again in the morning, following each day of monitoring. After returning on the third day, a 17-item questionnaire was given to the participants asking them about their compliance, acceptance, possible reactivity phenomena induced by the monitoring procedure, and some general suggestions and critics.

Samples

The Brazilian sample consisted of 40 voluntary university students, 19 males and 21 females, from different faculties of the Federal University in Belo Horizonte. They were motivated by the offer of lottery tickets for their participation. Their mean of age was 24 years (SD = 4.8, ranging from 18 to 38 years).

In the German sample, 61 students of the University of Freiburg, 24 males and 37 females, also from various faculties, participated as paid voluntary subjects. Their mean age of 24 years was equivalent to their Brazilian counterparts (SD = 3.2, range 20 to 33 years). The whole sample of 101 participants was informed that the computer-assisted ambulatory assessment referred to differences in diurnal changes of mood and test performance. Written consent was obtained.

Results

Compliance and acceptance

Referring to the compliance of the participants, the German sample appeared to be more accurate. The number of subjects with incomplete data sets – lack of entire protocols or retrospective ratings or lack of response within an interval of one hour around the protocol times – was much higher for the Brazilian group. For this reason the number of subjects in the two samples is not equal, as was intended.

The evaluation of the monitoring study according to the questionnaire was generally positive in both samples. For the Brazilians it was even better in some respects (Table 1).

In comparison to the German group, the Brazilian students showed a higher interest in the study, rated the two monitoring days as more "typical" (representative) and the self-report items as more appropriate to express their feelings. They also reported an increased self-observation of their psychological state during the study, but felt less tired by the self-ratings. The interference of their daily routines by repeated self-ratings was lower than that assessed by the German students. In general, the acceptance of the "electronic diary" used in this study was, without doubt, satisfying for the entire sample.

Table 1. Method acceptance, reactivity and load evaluated by participants

Item		German sample (N = 61)	Brazilian Sample (N = 40)	t	p
Representativeness	M	4.82	5.51	-2.24	.027
of the 2 days assessed	SD	1.60	1.35		
Suitable items of locations and activities	M	5.43	5.31	0.41	.683
for assessment of daily life situations	SD	1.16	1.67		
Possibility to express the authentic	M	3.79	5.13	-4.32	.000
feelings using the given self-ratings	SD	1.47	1.58		
Interest in the study	M	4.90	6.18	-4.92	.000
	SD	1.40	1.02		
Increased self-observation of	M	2.67	4.21	-3.96	.000
psychological state during the study	SD	1.78	2.05		
Temporary changes of behavior induced	M	2.34	2.13	0.63	.519
by the study methodology	SD	1.64	1.61		
Disturbance by completing the protocols	M	3.18	2.54	2.36	.020
	SD	1.25	1.45		
Number of protocols too much	MW	2.43	2.64	-0.55	.564
	SD	1.73	1.77		
Tiresomeness of self-ratings	M	2.38	1.77	2.28	.025
	SD	1.32	1.27		
Tiresomeness of attention test	M	2.08	2.03	0.21	.836
	SD	1.41	1.27		
Tiresomeness of working memory test	M	3.48	2.82	1.85	.067
	SD	1.72	1.73		

Note: The items were seven-point rating scales (from 1 = not at all to 7 = completely).

Variability of mood and attention

In the entire sample, the ratings representing momentary state and the various scores derived from the performance tests clearly differed in their statistical distribution. Item means ranged from M = 1.65 ("angry, irritated") to M = 6.01 ("situation under control"). The standard deviations varied between SD = .70 ("depressed") and SD = 1.64 ("situation typical"). The item "situation under control" showed a ceiling effect, the number of false responses in the Go/NoGo-test presented a floor effect.

In the Brazilian sample (the results referring to the German sample are described in detail in Fahrenberg et al., 1999), diurnal changes in mood were observed in the items "mentally tense" and "situation strenuous, demanding" according to a MANOVA (2 days, 5 protocols). The profiles could be described by an inverted U-shape. In contrast, the item "situation under control" showed the course of a U. The main effects of protocol times were also evident in the items "angry, irritated", "weary, exhausted" and "stress", as well as in performance scores of both attention tests, which could all be classified as increasing tendency. The main effects between days revealed that on the second day the Brazilian students felt less excited, less mentally tense, rated their physical well-being as higher, and had better performance scores in the tests, especially in the working memory test.

Some trans-cultural differences concerning mood and attention could be found using a MANOVA (2 groups, 2 days, 5 protocols) and subsequent t-tests (for single protocols). To give an example (Figure 1) the group x protocols interaction term was significant in the item "weary, exhausted" (F = 7.24, p = .000).

Whereas the curve of the German sample does not show a special shape over protocols and days, a daily course can be seen in the Brazilian students. They felt less "weary, exhausted" in the morning (8:00 a.m.) – compared to the Germans sig-

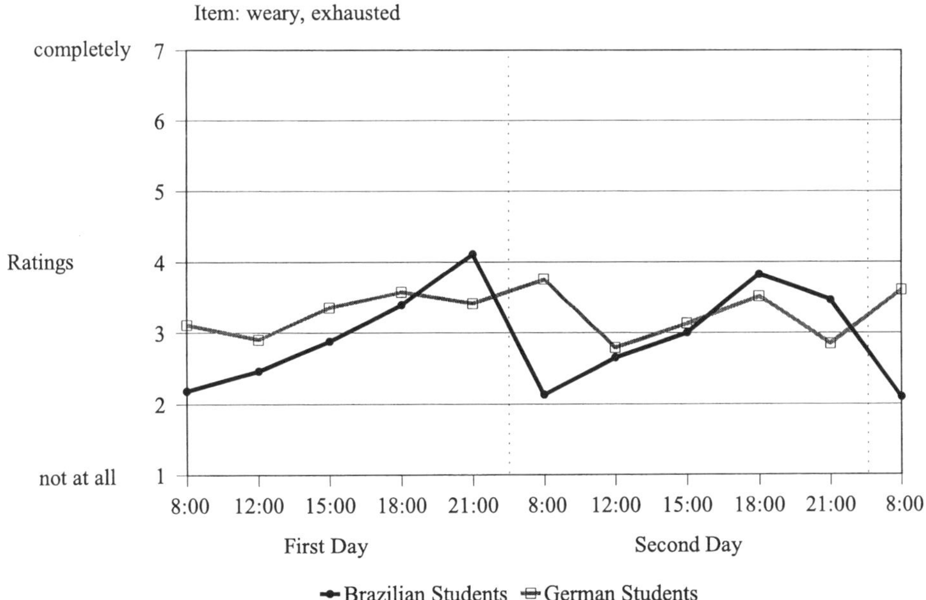

Figure 1. Diurnal changes in average responses of Brazilian and German students to the item "weary, exhausted" across 11 protocols.

nificant in both days (t-tests, $p \leq .001$) – with an increasing tendency over the day.

The second example refers to the averaged reaction times of correct responses in the Go/NoGo-test (Figure 2), in which the interaction term between protocols and group also was significant ($F = 4.08$, $p = .003$).

This time the Brazilian group does not show a special profile, so the performance seems to be stable. However the reaction time of correct responses in the Go/NoGo-test in the German sample increased over time and was significantly higher in the evening of day 1 (t-test, $p \leq .05$). The results shown of these preliminary analyses tend to illustrate that the methodology is appropriate for the evaluation of diurnal variability in mood and attention and can reveal interesting (even trans-cultural) effects.

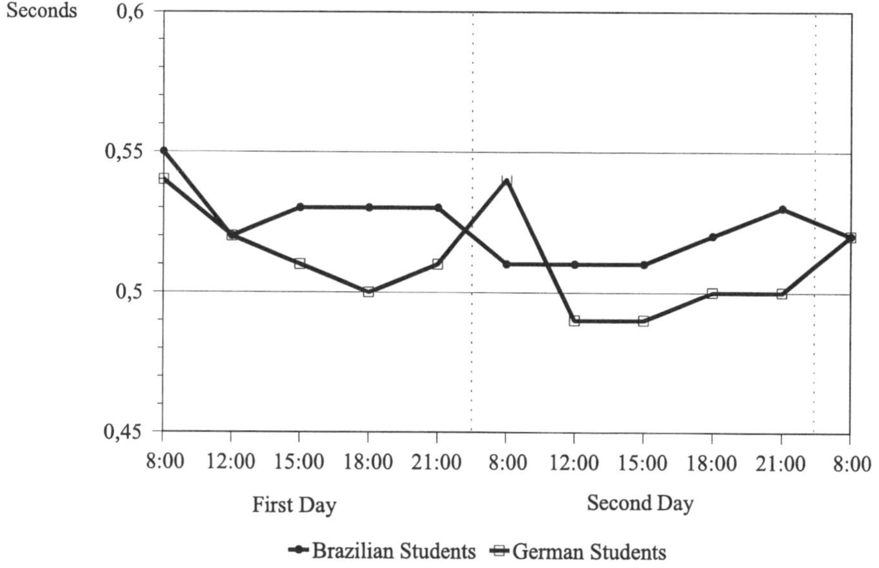

Figure 2. Diurnal changes in average reaction times of correct responses of Brazilian and German students in the concentration test (go/no go) across 11 protocols.

Retrospection effect

The negative bias in retrospectively reported mood was a main finding in the first study with a German sample. In the replication study in Germany, this retrospection effect – comparing the averages of momentary and retrospective ratings – was significant in nine of the ten items (without the item "physical well-being", see Figure 3), whereby parametric and non-parametric tests yielded convergent findings.

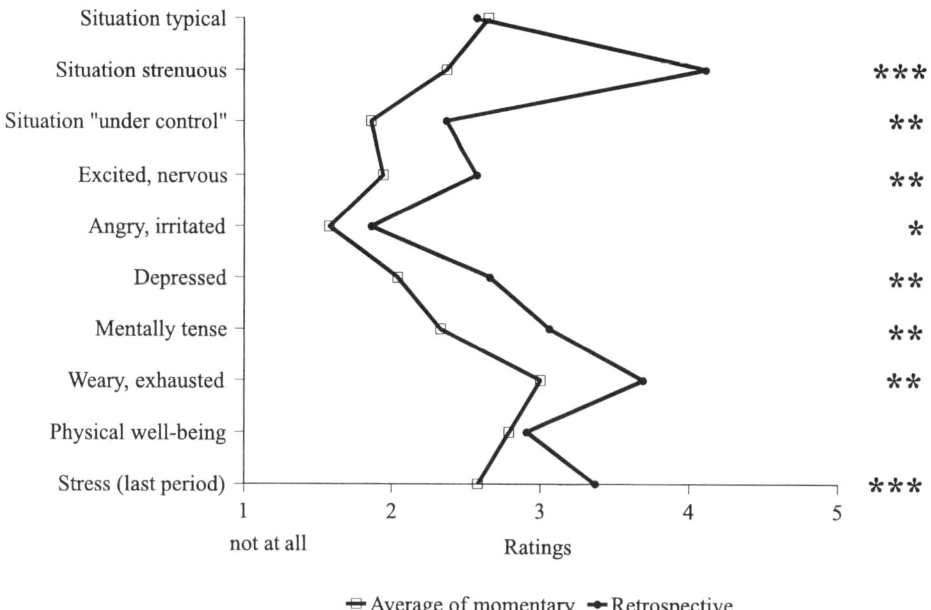

Figure 3. Retrospection effect in self-ratings of German students. The profiles represent averages of five protocols (first day) and the retrospective summary ratings obtained in the evening, compared by t-tests for dependent samples (* $p \leq .05$, ** $p \leq .01$, *** $p \leq .001$). The items were based on seven-point rating scales.

The retrospection effect showed again a negative tendency in each case (when the polarity was taken into account for the positive items, that is, "situation under control"; for the same reason these items were inverted in sign for the graphical presentations).

In this study, we could now replicate the effect in a culturally different sample. As the main result, an almost identical pattern occurred in retrospective reported mood with the Brazilian sample (Figure 4).

The Brazilian students rated the situations as more "strenuous, demanding", less "under control", described themselves retrospectively as more "excited, nervous", "angry, irritated", "depressed", "mentally tense", "weary, exhausted" and "stressed" than could be expected from the averages of repeated self-ratings during the day. Again, no difference was evident in the item "physical well-being". Additionally, the item "situation typical" did not show a significant deviation between daily average and retrospection. Again, comparing all four retrospective protocols (in the evening and next morning for both days), the pattern of a negative bias appeared in most items as a stable retrospection effect. The effect size was not different between the German and Brazilian sample.

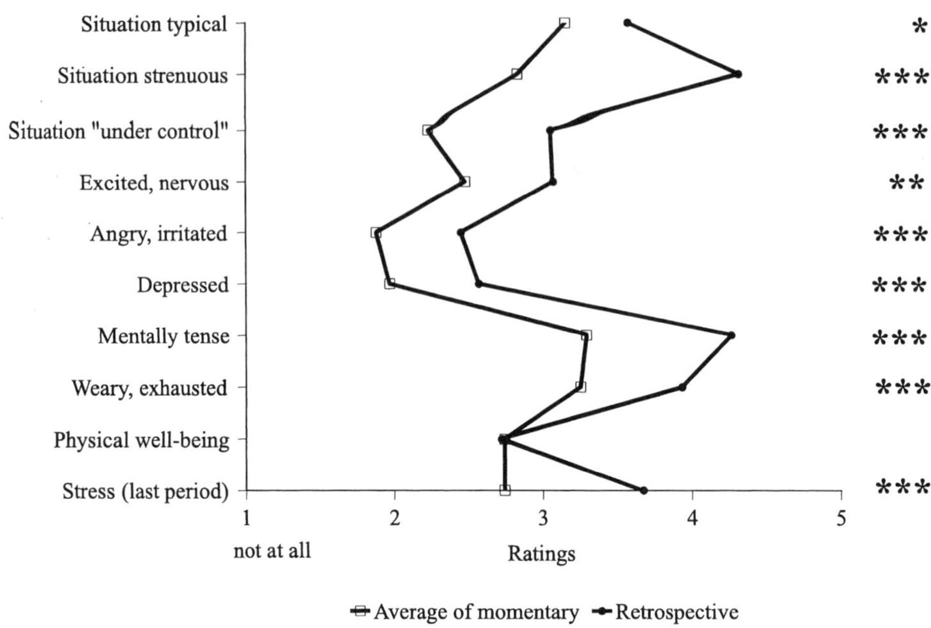

Figure 4. Retrospection effect in self-ratings of Brazilian students. The profiles represent averages of five protocols (first day) and the retrospective summary ratings obtained in the evening, compared by t-tests for dependent samples (* $p \leq .05$, ** $p \leq .01$, *** $p \leq .001$). The items were based on seven-point rating scales.

Discussion

Ambulatory assessment by means of hand-held computers appears to be specially suited to the investigation of psychologically relevant diurnal changes of subjective and objective states, and the evaluation of retrospective self-ratings, that is, research on recall-errors and biases in psychological data. In combination of the PSION pocket-computer and the MONITOR software, the methodology of ambulatory assessment – already used in various studies in Germany – was adapted and applied successfully in the different cultural context of Brazil.

The evaluation of the compliance in the Brazilian study has to consider various aspects: On the one hand, more than 50 percent of the participants did not answer at least ten protocols within a period of one hour before or after the given time points. This could be due to a different attitude towards commitments in general, but also to factors such as a higher level of ambient noise in Brazil, which makes it easier to miss the acoustic signal of the PSION, as reported by some subjects. On the other hand, the answers in the questionnaire given after the 48-hour monitoring period show an even better acceptance by the Brazilians, in comparison to the

German sample. However, a response set with a general tendency to more positive ratings was not found in the Brazilian sample.

Diurnal changes in mood and attention of Brazilian and German students were evident in a number of items as well as in the performance scores. In the case of test results, better scores of both samples on the second day could be explained by training effects. Preliminary trans-cultural comparisons concerning mood and attentional performance yielded some differences in diurnal changes. Our data do not offer an extensive basis for hypotheses about influencing factors, that is, socially anchored rules of mood expression, attribution stiles etc. However, mood and attention are central concepts in psychology, and, therefore, observable differences between populations should be considered in future research.

The main question of the present study refers to the negative bias in retrospective self-ratings found in previous research. The results show an almost identical pattern in the German and Brazilian samples. Thus, the retrospection effect could be replicated not only in different study samples but also in different cultural contexts. It seems to be a stable psychological bias in self-reporting of mood states. A wider discussion of possible hypotheses that could explain this phenomenon – ranging from a "psychometric" explanation such as a tendency toward the mean, over co-variations found with personality traits (emotional lability/stability) to corresponding clinical experience with depressive or panic patients – cannot be presented here (see Fahrenberg et al., 1999; Käppler et al., in press). In any case, it seems to be clear, that the negative retrospection effect is a common phenomenon, and has an important impact on the assessment and interpretation of psychological data in research and applied areas.

References

Biemer, P.P., Groves, R.M., Lyberg, L.E., Mathiowetz, N.A. & Sudman, S. (Eds.) (1992). *Measurement errors in surveys.* New York: John Wiley & Sons.

Brügner, G. (1998). MONITOR: Ein flexibles Programm zur Datenerhebung mittels Pocket-PC. *Zeitschrift für Differentielle und Diagnostische Psychologie, 19*, 145–147.

Fahrenberg, J., Brügner, G., Foerster, F. & Käppler, C. (1999). Ambulatory assessment of diurnal changes with a hand-held computer: Mood, attention, and morningness – eveningness. *Personality and Individual Differences, 26*, 641–656.

Hedges, S.M., Jandorf, L. & Stone, A.A. (1985). Meaning of daily mood assessments. *Journal of Personality and Social Psychology, 48*, 428–434.

Kahneman, D. & Tversky, A. (Eds.) (1982). *Judgment under uncertainty: heuristics and biases.* New York: Cambridge University Press.

Käppler, C. (1994). *Psychophysiologische Bedingungsanalyse von Blutdruckveränderungen im alltäglichen Lebenskontext.* Phil. Diss. Universität Freiburg i. Br.. Frankfurt a.M.: P. Lang.

Käppler, C., Becker, H.-U. & Fahrenberg, J. (1993). Ambulantes 24-Stunden-Monitoring als psychophysiologische Assessmentstrategie: Reproduzierbarkeit, Reaktivität, Retrospek-tionseffekt und Bewegungskonfundierung. *Zeitschrift für Differentielle und Diagnostische Psychologie*, *14*, 235–251.

Käppler, C., Brügner, G. & Fahrenberg, J. (in press). Pocketcomputer-unterstütztes Assessment mit MONITOR: Befindlichkeit und Aufmerksamkeitsverlauf im Alltag und die Replikation des negativen Retrospektionseffektes. *Zeitschrift für Differentielle und Diagnostische Psychologie.*

Schwarz, N. (1990). Assessing frequency reports of mundane behaviors: Contributions of cognitive psychology to questionnaire construction. In C. Hendrick & M.S. Clark (Eds.), *Research methods in personality and social psychology*, (pp. 98–119). Newbury Park, CA: Sage.

Wheeler, L. & Reis, H.T. (1991). Self-recording of everyday life events: Origins, types, and uses. *Journal of Personality*, *59*, 339–354.

Zimmermann, P. & Fimm, B. (1992/93). *Testbatterie zur Aufmerksamkeitsprüfung TAP*. Psychologisches Institut der Universität. Freiburg: Psytest.

Chapter 7
Ambulatory Monitoring of Diurnal Changes in Pain in Chronic Pain Disorder, Migraine and Rheumatoid Arthritis

Guido L.R. Godaert[1], Marjolijn J. Sorbi[2], Madelon Peters[2],
Caroline Dekkers[1], and Rinnie Geenen[1]
[1]*Department of Health Psychology, Faculty of Social Sciences, Utrecht University, Nl.*
[2]*Department of Medical, Clinical and Experimental Psychology, Maastricht University, Nl.*

Introduction

Pain has been shown to be affected by a wide range of physiological, affective and cognitive behavioral apects (Loeser & Melzack, 1999). The severity and quality of pain may be expected to differ as a function of several variables among which the persistence of the pain and the underlying pathophysiology. For instance, physical deconditioning and accompanying neuroendocrine changes may increase with longer persistence of pain, and affect pain.

This study explores fluctuations of pain across the day in three groups: patients with chronic pain disorder (CPD), migraine (specifically migraine without aura), and rheumatoid arthritis (RA). It is likely that distinct mechanisms determine and modulate pain in these different groups. In CPD no clear pathophysiology or nociception has been proven. It has been suggested that the intensity of pain report could be related to hypervigilance or increased sensitivity to sensory cues (Chapman, 1979; McCracken, 1997). Migraine is a complex neurovascular response to sudden in- or external changes. The pain is attributed to extra- but also intracranial vasodilatation, neurogenic inflammation, central pain sensitization, and a cascade of biochemical changes (Lance & Goadsby, 1999; Olesen & Edvinsson, 1997). In RA, among several factors that are shared with other pain syndromes, inflammation and tissue destruction cause pain (Rice & Pisetsky, 1999).

The course of pain accross the day may depend on these disturbed underlying processes as well as on a wide range of other factors that may differ for these syndromes such as sleep and mood disturbances, circadian physiological variations, and fatigue during the day. If this assumption holds, patient groups differing in pain mechanisms will show a different course of pain during the day. The first aim of our study was to visualize and compare the course of pain of three patient groups.

Additionally, we explored whether the diurnal course within two of these groups might be related to other important characteristics of that specific group. In CPD it was investigated whether patients differing in pain persistence show different profiles during the day, for example, a "flattening"of the curve in patients with a longer pain history. In RA, the pain curve is compared to simultaneously obtained salivary cortisol. Cortisol has been shown to vary as a function of inflammation (Dekkers, Geenen, Godaert, Van Doornen & Bijlsma, 2000a) and could thus be related to the pain. Considering the exploratory nature of this investigation, and because somewhat different procedures were used in the primary three studies, we will suffice with graphical presentation of the results.

Methods

Data from three different but related studies were included. *CPD*: Eighty patients (age 18–60) reporting pain without an established cause for at least 6 weeks were included in the CPD group. Data were collected for 4 weeks with a palmtop computer, which randomly prompted the patients to record pain intensity within 4 predetermined time frames between 08:00 am and 9.30 pm. Z score transformations of the pain intensity scores correspond to hourly averages. Three matched patient groups suffering from CPD for, respectively, 3–6 months (N=15), 6–12 months (N=25) and >12 months (N=40) were compared (Peters, Sorbi, Kruise, Kerssens, Verhaak & Bensing, 2000). *Migraine.* This study was conducted in 56 female patients (age 18–65) selected strictly following the International Headache Committee classification criteria for migraine without aura. Data on pain and accompanying symptoms were collected for 10 weeks with the same electronic diary as was employed in the CPD study but within 6 predetermined time-frames between 08:30 am and 11:00 pm. Fifty-four attacks that had started in the early morning between waking-up and the first beep diary were selected. Z-score transformations of the pain intensity scores correspond to the *actual* time of recording (Honkoop, Sorbi, Godaert & Spierings, 1999). *RA*: Twenty-five patients recently diagnosed as having RA (age 30–78) and 28 healthy controls (age 26–76) completed two consecutive days of pain reporting, using a paper and pencil booklet, being prompted 4 times in the first hour after awakening and 5 times between 10.00 am and 7.30 pm by a wrist watch controlled beep. Pain was rated on a Likert scale labeled 1 (not at all) to 5 (extremely) (Dekkers, Geenen, Godaert, Van Doornen & Bijlsma, 2000b).

Results

The three groups showed a different diurnal course of self reported pain over the day. (Figure 1). CPD subjects reported steadily increasing pain; in migraine the pain fluctuated heavily but clearly decreased during the day; in RA we saw a rather flat diurnal curve, interrupted by a small increase in the late afternoon.

Exploring the effects of important within group characteristics, we observed no

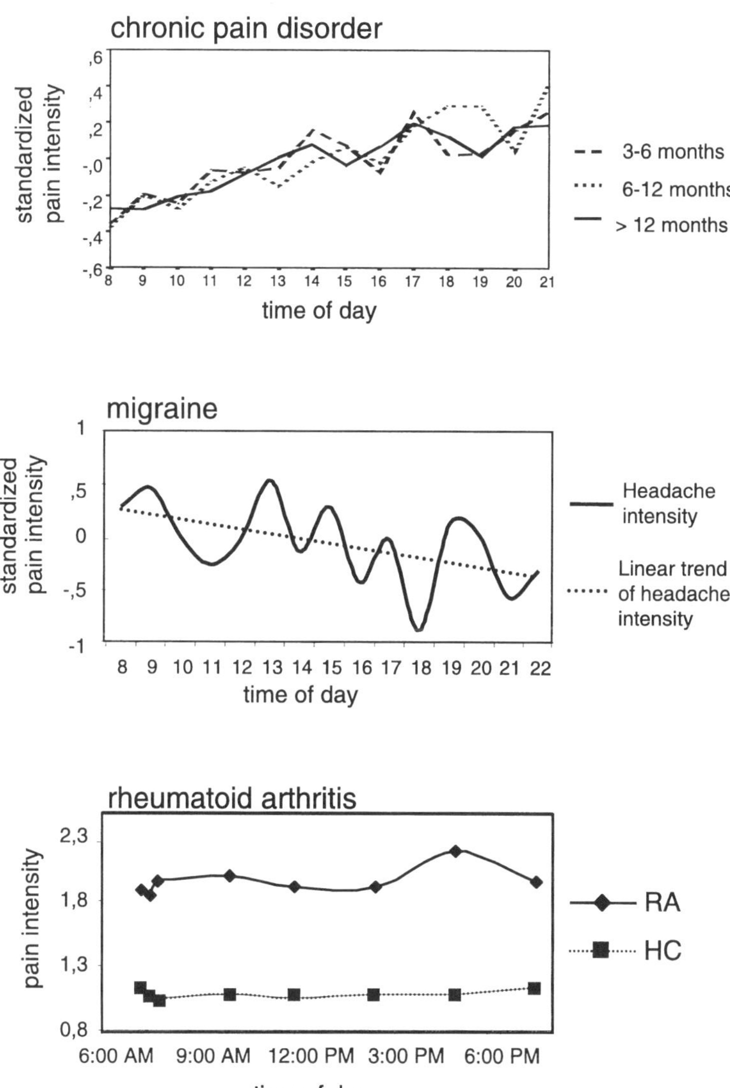

Figure 1. Diurnal changes in pain in patients with chronic pain disorder, migraine, and rheumatoid arthritis.

noticable effect of persistence of the CPD on the slope of the diurnal curve. Figure 2 reveals a different course of cortisol for patients reporting pain and patients not actually having pain. Cortisol was clearly elevated in the afternoon for the pain patients. The cortisol curve of patients without pain was identical to that of healthy controls.

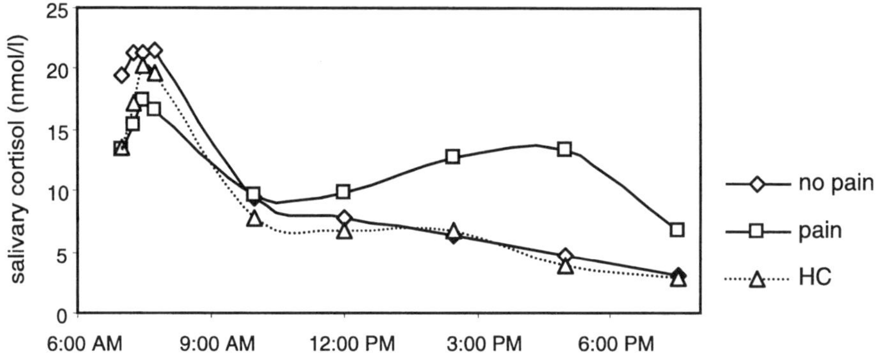

Figure 2. Diurnal course of salivary cortisol of patients with rheumatoid arthritis actually reporting pain or no pain, and healthy controls.

Discussion

Visual inspection of data from three distinct studies suggests that the daily course of pain differed between patient groups. Differences in study design did not allow a statistical comparison of data, but our results are provocative in that they show the importance of comparing momentary pain across the day between patient groups. This holds promise to yield new information regarding the differential determinants or concommitants of experienced pain.

The different profiles challenge to propose possible mechanisms involved. In CPD, due to hypervigilance and increased sensitivity, normal sensory, for example, proprioceptive sensations associated with increasing muscular fatigue during the day may be amplified and perceived as increasing pain. Physical deconditioning may emphasise this process. Interestingly, patients differing in pain persistence had the same, increasing pain profile. If the proposed explanation holds, this would imply that these mechanisms are already present in an early stage of CPD and still keep their grip on pain perception months or years after diagnosis.

In contrast, migraine is typically characterized by intermittent pain episodes of 4 to 72 hours taking turns with clear pain-free episodes. The study depicted the first and most erratic part of this process. The neurovascular reaction is in part self-regulatory, contributing to pain oscillation. It depends also on external aggravating factors and patient behavior. This latter includes the use of potent vasoconstrictive medication, which may temporarily but effectively suppress the pain or cut down the attack alltogether.

In patients with rheumatoid arthritis experiencing a pain episode at the time of the ambulatory assessment, the level of cortisol in the afternoon is clearly higher than in their fellow patients not actually reporting pain, the peak of cortisol roughly corresponding to the pain peak. This might give us a clue as to what happened. The level of cortisol in the afternoon has been shown to be associated with ongoing inflammation, that is, the organism reacts to inflammation with an increase in cortisol (Dekkers et al., 2000a). Since pain occurs also as a consequence of inflammation, the scenario we propose is that in patients with a flare up of inflammation, both the pain sensation and the cortisol production increase.

This study was exploratory. Patient groups were not matched for age and procedures differed regarding the duration of the recording and the specific instrument to assess the amount of pain. These differences prohibit a straightforward quantitative analysis. However, our results instigate to design a study that directly compares the diurnal variations in pain in the three different groups. Studies specifically elucidating the suggested processes affecting the daily course of pain within the different groups should also be welcomed. Fear of pain, hypervigilance, and the contribution of simultaneous pain inhibitory and excitatory physiological processes may be considered as candidates.

In conclusion, this study suggests that patients with distinct chronic pain disorders experience a different course of pain across the day and that within group characteristics may affect this pain profile as well. This implies that extracting information from the dynamics of ambulatory measurement has potential value for improved understanding of the physiological and experiential mechanisms that modulate temporal changes in pain severity.

References

Chapman, R. (1979). Pain, Perception and Illness. In R.A. Sternbach (Ed.), *The Psychology of Pain.* New York: Raven Press.

Dekkers, J.C., Geenen, R., Godaert, G.L.R., Van Doornen, L.J.P. & Bijlsma, J.W. J. (2000a). Diurnal rhythm of salivary cortisol in patients with recent-onset rheumatoid arthritis. *Arthritis & Rheumatism, 43*, 465–467.

Dekkers, J.C., Geenen, R., Godaert, G.L.R., Van Doornen, L.J.P. & Bijlsma, J.W.J. (2000b). Diurnal courses of cortisol, pain, fatigue, negative mood, and stiffness in patients with recently diagnosed rheumatoid arthritis. *International Journal of Behavioral Medicine, 7*, 353–371.

Honkoop, P.C., Sorbi, M.J., Godaert, G.L.R. & Spierings, E.H.L. (1999). High-density assessment of the IHS classification criteria for migraine without aura: a prospective study. *Cephalalgia, 19,* 201–206.

Lance, J.W. & Goadsby, P.J. (1999). *Mechanisms and Management of Headache.* (6th ed.). Oxford: Butterworth-Heinemann.

Loeser, J.D. & Melzack, R. (1999). Pain: an overview. *Lancet, 353*, 1607–1609.

McCracken, L.M. (1997). "Attention" to pain in persons with chronic pain: A behavioral approach. *Behavior Therapy, 28*(2), 271–284.

Olesen, J. & Edvinsson, L. (1997). *Headache pathogenenesis. Monoamines, Neuropeptides, Purines, and Nitric Oxide.* New York: Lippincot-Raven.

Peters, M.L., Sorbi, M.J., Kruise, D.A., Kerssens, J. J., Verhaak, P.F.M. & Bensing, J.M. (2000). Electronic diary assessment of pain, disability and psychological adaptation in patients differing in duration of pain. *Pain, 84*, 181–192.

Rice, J.R. & Pisetsky, D.S. (1999). Pain in the rheumatic diseases. Practical aspects of diagnosis and treatment. *Rheumatic Disease Clinics of North America, 25*(1), 15–30.

Chapter 8
Development and User's Acceptance of the General Electronic Psychotherapy Diary

Michael Hinkel and O. Berndt Scholz
Department of Psychology, University of Bonn, Germany

Introduction

Current diary research in psychology is mostly concerned with paper-pencil diaries (PP; Schandry & Leopold, 1996; Taylor, Fried & Kenardy, 1990). PP have several limitations which can be eliminated by the use of computerized diaries (different kind of usages are presented by Fahrenberg & Myrtek, 1996). Nowadays one of the main reasons for the seldom use of electronic diaries is the expense of purchasing mobile computer devices (MCD) and developing a customized diary software (Buse & Pawlik, 1996). So far various research teams used a combination of soft- and hardware, which was on the one hand adapted to their needs but on the other hand not very flexible (Fahrenberg & Myrtek, 1996). Additionally, the utilized MCDs had either a good performance, sufficient memory, but were of large size and heavy weight (for example, Baumann, Thiele, Laireiter & Krebs, 1996; Bolten, Emmerich, Weber & Faßmeyer, 1991; Finkelstein, Hripcsak & Cabrera, 1998) or they were technically restricted, but in return of a small size and light weight (for example, Perrez & Reicherts, 1996; Lewis, Lewis & Cumming, 1995).

In this paper the generalized electronic psychotherapy diary (GEPD) will be introduced. It gives the interested scientist the opportunity to generate a wide range of different electronic diaries simply by entering the diary-questionnaire and selecting the appropriate answer types. The evaluation of the obtained data is automated in combination with an ordinary personal computer (PC).

Characteristics of the GEPD

The GEPD was implemented on a "palm computing device" (OS version 3.x). This MCD is pocket-sized (7.7 x 12.2 x 1.7 cm^3), light (155 g), with a battery life of about 10 h, and a minimal random access memory (RAM) of 2 MB (models with up to 8 MB RAM are available). The device is usually operated by tapping its touchscreen with a special pen.

The diary software was developed using an adapted version of the GNU C++-Compiler (PRC-tools 0.5.0; http://www.palm.com) and IBM's 'DB2everywhere'

SQL database engine (version 1.2) for the palm computing device (http://www.ibm.com). Data transfer to the PC is done by using a docking station (called cradle) and the data ara evaluated with a combination of Microsoft's Access and Excel (both of version 2000).

The GEPD was developed to provide a maximum of flexibility to the user. It has a built-in database of patients and can hold a large number of different diary questionnaires as well as diary entries (limited only by the device's RAM). Each diary consists of one or more categories, which contain the diary items. The categories can be linked to each other (that is, if the category "noon" is linked to "morning" then "noon" is only available after all questions of "morning" were completely processed) and/or activated by a timer (at one or more fixed or random times). Timer activated categories are announced by a signal sound that is repeated several times if no action is taken. Each diary item contains a question text (max. 200 characters) and an answer type, which can be one of the following: rating scale, bipolar rating scale (both are free configurable concerning the scale description, rating range, step width, display of units and scale division), yes/no-answer, frequency, and text. Skipping of unanswered questions and recalling of previous ones can be disabled.

After setting up the GEPD (that is, entering the patients data and the desired diary questionnaire), the data collection mode (DCM) is activated by selecting the patient and a diary. In order to perform a diary entry, the patient has to turn on the device and select the appropriate category. He has no chance to manipulate the DCM as this mode is protected by a password. The questions are answered by tapping the corresponding areas of the touchscreen. After all queued questions had been answered, the patient simply turns off the device.

Investigating the usability and acceptance of the GEPD

Subjects

A total of 40 adult subjects (31 females and 9 males) with an average age of $M = 24.2$ years ($SD = 6.2$ years) attended this study. These subjects were recruited by an announcement at the university and received a participation certification.

Procedure and Design

The entire course of the investigation consisted of a training trial, PP and GEPD entries, and a final evaluation of the GEPD. The sequence of PP and GEPD entries was counterbalanced and the subjects were randomly assigned to the testing order (PP first vs. GEPD first). To cover a wide variety of possible diary questions, each diary entry trial (PP and GEPD) consisted of five sleeping disorder and five panic disorder entries. Since this was a laboratory study, imaginary situations were presented and had to be read once before each entry. As diary inventory a slightly modified version of the Marburger Angsttagebuch by Margraf and Schneider (1990) and a sleeping-disorder diary by Scholz (1983) were used.

Before starting the data acquisition with the GEPD, the subjects had to read a short user's manual and take a training trial, which consisted of ten everyday-life questions where each answer type was used twice altogether.

Variables

A questionnaire was developed to evaluate the usability and acceptance of the GEPD. To judge the readability, general usability and the different answer types as well as to state a preference of either the PP or the GEPD, a 3-point rating scale was used ("good" – "acceptable" – "bad" or "GEPD" – "indifferent" – "PP", respectively).

Results

Main results: The main results are presented in Figure 1. Readability and general usability were well accepted. Between 75 % and 95 % of the subjects judged the GEPD's rating scale, frequency- and yes/no-answers as good. Text- and time-answers were not entirely considered good, but only 10 % (time) or 22.5 % (text) gave a negative rating, respectively. If no text-answers were asked for 72.5 % preferred the GEPD (PP: 10 %). If a diary contains a lot of text-answers the distribution of the ratings is nearly even to both sides (GEPD: 47.5 %, PP: 42.5 %).

Additional results: On the GEPD each subject answered a total of 75 questions. As in this study only one MCD was used, a total of 3,000 answers were stored on a single device and occupied 109 KB of RAM. The batteries needed to be changed after 10.5 h of operation. At this time more than 2,000 diary questions had been answered with one set of batteries.

Summary

The GEPD was developed to provide the psychotherapist with a multifunctional electronic diary. The device is pocked-sized, light, and can be regarded as cheap as compared to other MCDs. The diary-software offers a great extend of flexibility, has a low memory usage, is reliable, and performs no malfunction. Subjects emphasized the usability of the well-designed user-interface – particularly of rating-, frequency-, and yes/no-answers – and stated a clear preference towards the GEPD as opposed to the PP, if no text-answers were asked for. Otherwise the subject's preference was well-balanced.

In future investigations the GEPD should be given to patients who keep the diary for at least two or three weeks. In these studies the GEPD should be compared with

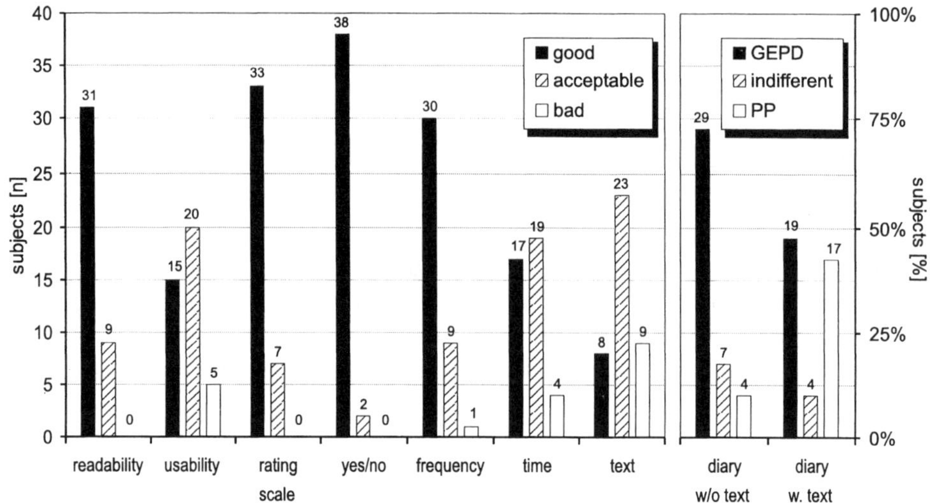

Figure 1. Subjects differentiated evaluation of the GEPD (left) and preference of a diary method, depending on the kind of the diary (right).

PP concerning its psychometric quality as well as the patient's acceptance in everyday life. Furthermore, efforts should be taken to generalize the psychometric quality for each answer-type in order to get provisional estimates of future diaries.

References

Baumann, U., Thiele, C., Laireiter, A.-R. & Krebs, A. (1996). Computer-assisted interaction diary on social networks, social support, and interpersonal strain. In J. Fahrenberg & M. Myrtek (Eds.), *Ambulatory assessment: computer-assisted psychological and psychophysiological methods in monitoring and fields studies* (pp. 69–83). Seattle, WA: Hogrefe & Huber Publishers.

Bolten, W., Emmerich, M., Weber, E. & Faßmeyer, N. (1991). Validierung elektronischer Tagebücher an konventionellen Schmerztagebüchern. *Zeitschrift für Rheumatologie*, *50*, 55–64.

Buse, L. & Pawlik, K. (1996). Ambulatory behavioral assessment and in-field performance testing. In J. Fahrenberg & M. Myrtek (Eds.), *Ambulatory assessment: computer-assisted psychological and psychophysiological methods in monitoring and fields studies* (pp. 29–50). Seattle, WA: Hogrefe & Huber Publishers.

Fahrenberg, J. & Myrtek, M. (Eds.). (1996). *Ambulatory assessment: computer-assisted psychological and psychophysiological methods in monitoring and fields studies*. Seattle, WA: Hogrefe & Huber Publishers.

Finkelstein, J., Hripcsak, G. & Cabrera, M. (1998). Telematic system for monitoring of asthma severity in patients' homes. *Medinfo*, *9*, 272–276.

Lewis, B., Lewis, D. & Cumming, G. (1995). Frequent measurement of chronic pain: an electronic diary and empirical findings. *Pain*, *60*, 341–347.

Margraf, J. & Schneider, S. (1990). *Panik: Angstanfälle und ihre Behandlung* (2. Aufl.). Berlin: Springer.

Perrez, M. & Reicherts, M. (1996). A computer-assisted self-monitoring procedure for assessing stress-related behavior under real life conditions. In J. Fahrenberg & M. Myrtek (Eds.), *Ambulatory assessment: computer-assisted psychological and psychophysiological methods in monitoring and fields studies* (pp. 51–67). Seattle, WA: Hogrefe & Huber Publishers.

Schandry, R. & Leopold, C. (1996). Ambulatory assessment of self-monitored subjective and objective symptoms of diabetic patients. In J. Fahrenberg & M. Myrtek (Eds.), *Ambulatory assess-*

ment: computer-assisted psychological and psychophysiological methods in monitoring and fields studies (pp. 393–402). Seattle, WA: Hogrefe & Huber Publishers.

Scholz, O.B. (1983). Schlafstörungen im Alter und deren Behandlung. In J. C. Brengelmann & G. Bühringer (Eds.), *Therapieforschung für die Praxis* (pp. 167–182). München: Röttger.

Taylor, C. B., Fried, L. & Kenardy, J. (1990). The use of a real-time computer diary for data acquisition and processing. *Behavior Research and Therapy*, *28*, 93–97.

Chapter 9
States of Aversive Tension in Patients with Borderline Personality Disorder: A Controlled Field Study

Christian Stiglmayr[1], Tanja Grathwol[2], and Martin Bohus[3]
[1]Department of Psychology, Free University Berlin, [2]Michael-Balint-Klinik, Königsfeld and [3]Department of Psychiatry and Psychotherapy, University of Freiburg, Germany

Introduction

Clinical observations indicate that patients with borderline personality disorder (BPD) suffer from sudden attacks of intense states of tension, which they subjectively describe as extremely unpleasant and which often cannot be otherwise terminated than to employ some means of dysfunctional behavior such as injuring oneself. The current study uses hand-held PCs to examine the course of states of aversive tension in female patients with BPD as compared to healthy female controls over a 48-hour period. In accordance with assumptions on the course of emotional arousal in patients with BPD (Linehan, 1993/1996), the study tested the following hypotheses: patients with BPD reported a generally greater level of experienced aversive tension than did healthy controls (Hypothesis 1), which was triggered more frequently (Hypothesis 2), rose more rapidly (Hypothesis 3) and persisted for a longer period of time (Hypothesis 4).

Method

Subjects

A hand-held PC (PSION 3a) was distributed for a 48-hour period to 63 female borderline patients and 40 age-matched controls, who entered self-ratings of tension in response to an hourly beeper signal.

Between December 1997 and August 1999, patients were recruited within the framework of a large-scale psychotherapy study funded by the Deutsche Forschungsgemeinschaft (DFG) and carried out by the Department of Psychiatry and Psychotherapy at the University Hospital Freiburg, Germany. All patients - 32 outpatients (50.79%) and 31 inpatients (49.21%) - fulfilled the DSM-IV criteria (American Psychiatric Association, 1994) for a borderline personality disorder

(Structured Clinical Interview for DSM-IV for Axis II: Personality Disorders. SCID-II; First, Gibbon, Spitzer, Williams & Benjamin, 1997a) and achieved a minimum score of 8 points on the DIB-R (Diagnostic Interview for Borderlines. Revised version: Gunderson & Zanarini, 1983/1990). The lifetime exclusion criteria - schizophrenia, Bipolar I and alcohol, respectively drug dependence - were controlled for by means of the SCID-I (Structured Clinical Interview for DSM-IV Axis I; First, Spitzer, Gibbon & Williams, 1997b). There were no restrictions with regard to the intake of psychotropic drugs; however, such use was recorded in the protocols.

Controls were recruited from the resident register of the City of Freiburg. Exclusion criteria constituted the diagnosis of a borderline personality disorder (DSM-IV criteria, DIB-R), an axis-I disorder (SCID-I), one or more first-degree relatives with a mental disorder, or current psychotherapeutic treatment for the potential control. Of the 67 individuals who responded by telephone to the original written contact, 40 mentally healthy controls participated.

The average age of the patients was 27.44 years (SD = 6.63; Minimum = 17 years; Maximum = 46 years), that of the controls 27.75 years (SD = 7.40; Minimum = 19 years; Maximum = 43 years). The statistical test yielded no significant difference with regard to age ($t = -.22$; $df = 101$; $p = .828$). But the controls were significantly better educated than the patients ($\chi^2 = 9.96$; $df = 1$; $p < .01$).

The MONITOR Program

With the aid of a hand-held PC PSION 3a equipped with the MONITOR program (Brügner, 1998), the subjective state of aversive tension was monitored hourly. Patients could enter their responses according to a 9-step scale ranging from "0"/"not observed" to "9"/"very severe". By means of an acoustic signal, the PC reminded its carrier to enter data, where the "tension question" in all cases referred to the time period immediately preceding the acoustic signal. No monitoring was carried out during the individually set night rest. In the morning the PC signaled the participants at the agreed-upon time. Participants operated the PC by means of the numeric and enter keys exclusively.

In addition to the data entered by the study participants, the PC automatically recorded the date, time of the initial reminder to enter data, the time span that elapsed between the initial reminder and begin of actual data entry, as well as the length of time needed to respond to the questions. If, in comparison to the previous data entry period, tension had risen by three or more points (definition of a tension increase), the PC requested the participant to enter how quickly tension had increased by means of a second 9-step scale ("0"/"not present" – "9"/"sudden increase"). This did not apply if such an increase in tension had occurred during the night or in the case of one or more "missing" periods where data failed to be entered (see Figure 1).

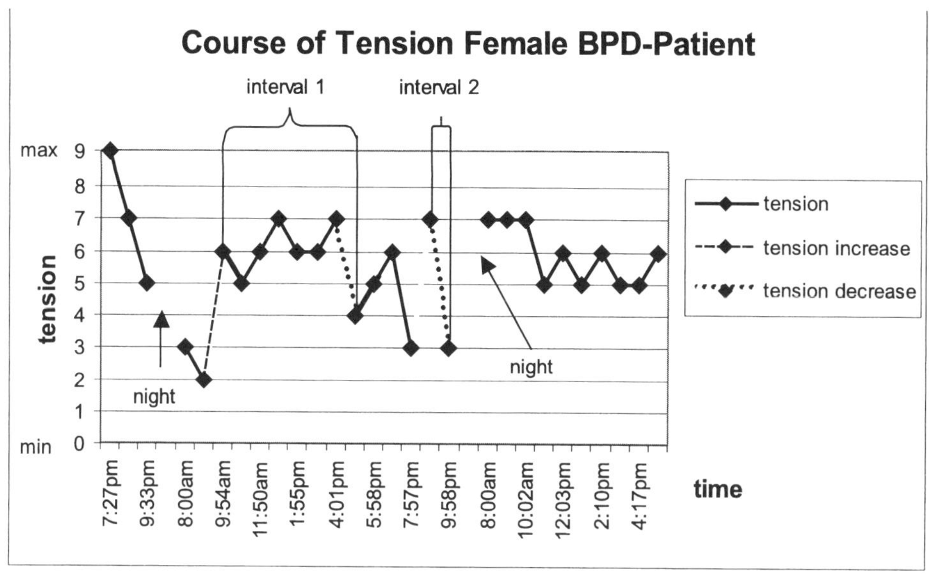

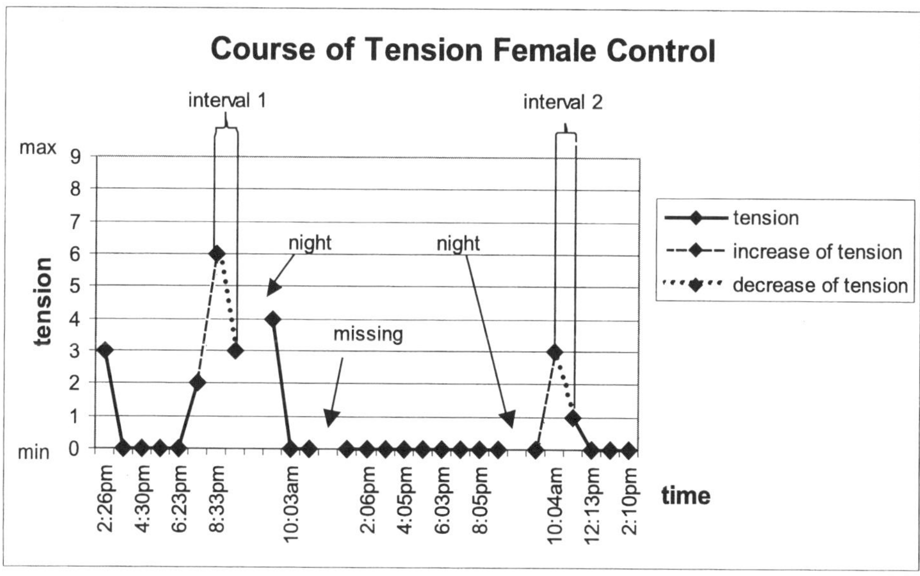

Figure 1. Course of tension of a female BPD-patient and a female control

Procedure

The hand-held PC was distributed on different days of the week. For training purposes a test run using the PSION 3a was carried out with each participant. Upon completion, each participant answered a questionnaire to control for possible effects of study conditions on the subjective tension scores, responding to the following questions:

"How bothersome was the self-evaluation by means of the hand-held PC? "
"Were there too many response time points? "
"Were the reactions to the study in your environment unpleasant? "

Participants entered their responses according to a 9-step scale analogous to those used to assess the severity of the aversive tension.

Inference statistical tests were carried out at the parametric level. Confounding variables were tested for using a two-tailed test, the hypotheses were tested using a one-tailed test. The level of significance for all statistical tests was $\alpha = .05$.

Results

The average number of responses entered by patients amounted to 25.90 (SD = 3.96) and by controls to 25.88 (SD = 3.28). Patients required an average of 2:53 minutes (SD = 0:49 minutes) to enter their scores, while controls required 2:18 minutes (SD = 0:42 minutes). Patients began entering data on the average at 8.15 h (SD = 1:06 hours), the controls at 8.41 h (SD = 0:54 hours). Patients stopped entering data evenings at an average of 22.20 h (SD = 0:56 hours), controls at 21.55 h (SD = 1:14 hours). The percentage of missing data periods in relation to the respective number of entries amounts to an average of 11.34% (SD = 11.64%) among patients, and to 6.14% (SD = 6.08%) among controls.

Controlling for confounding variables

The patients experienced the self-evaluation by means of the PC as more bothersome ($t = 5.84$; $df = 100$; $p < .001$; $n_{Pat} = 62$, $n_{con} = 40$), thought there were too many monitoring time points ($t = 5.90$; $df = 100$; $p < .001$; $n_{Pat} = 62$, $n_{con} = 40$) and the reactions by those in their environment more unpleasant ($t = 4.33$; $df = 99$; $p < .001$; $n_{Pat} = 61$, $n_{con} = 40$). None of these variables had to be controlled for when testing the hypotheses, since they failed to correlate with the experienced aversive tension in either the patient or the control group. The same applies to the variable level of education and within the patient group, to the variable intake of medication as well (0, 1 or 2 medications). Finally there were no significant differences between outpatients and inpatients with regard to the tension recorded.

Hypothesis I

The results point in the expected direction: patients experience an average level of tension clearly higher than that experienced by healthy controls ($t = 13.97$; $df = 101$; $p < .001$). The average tension level among patients is 4.45 (SD = 2.15), among controls 0.55 (SD = 0.54).

Hypothesis II

Three patients who exhibited tension scores > 7 were excluded from the inference statistical test of this hypothesis. Given the gradients on the tension scale of 0 to 9, tension among these patients could go no higher (ceiling effect). In 9.57% of the entries patients recorded a rise in tension (SD = 7.80%), while controls recorded only 3.59% (SD = 4.75%). This difference is statistically significant ($t = 4.76$; $df = 98$; $p < .001$).

Hypothesis III

Patients experience increases in tension as being clearly more rapid, respectively more sudden than do controls ($t = 3.94$; $df = 64$; $p < .001$). The mean for patients is 6.81 (SD = 1.66; $n_{Pat} = 48$), for controls 4.40 (SD = 2.39; $n_{Kon} = 18$).

Hypothesis IV

The length of a tension interval refers to the time span between the point of tension increase and the subsequent drop in tension by two or more points (definition of a tension decrease). The tension interval can also be terminated by a missing data entry, the onset of night rest, or the end of data entry. In addition, a decrease in tension exists if there is a slow decline over several monitoring time points; the tension interval is regarded as being over once the baseline value is fallen short of by two points (see Figure 1). The average tension interval among patients amounts to 1.98 monitoring time points (SD = 1.06; $n_{Pat} = 48$), among controls to 1.10 (SD = 0.26; $n_{Kon} = 18$). This difference is statistically significant ($t = 5.30$; $df = 64$; $p < .001$).

Discussion

According to the results of this study, patients with a borderline personality disorder experience the extent of their level of aversive tension as being much higher than that of mentally healthy controls. Over a two-day period patients experience almost three times more states of aversive tension, lasting an average of 2 hours - almost twice as long as the states reported by controls. At the same time the patients experience the rise in tension as having appeared far more suddenly, which severely limits their subjective feeling of being able to control the occurrence of such states. Against this background, the severity of the impairment experienced by patients with BPD as opposed to mentally healthy controls is considerable, which is in agreement with clinical findings.

The current study introduces a relatively recent method - ambulatory monitoring by means of a hand-held PC. Particularly in the field of psychiatric research, ambulatory monitoring still represents a relatively little-used method. Many of the data collected in this study could only be collected by means of a computer, for example, responses to the conditional question regarding the rapidity of the tension increase. The detailed record also allows data to be analyzed and used with much greater efficiency, for example, in planning therapy. A knowledge of the average length of such states of tension can be used to counteract the catastrophic trends that frequently occur in conjunction with states of highly severe aversive tension. The flexible programming makes far more complex monitoring scenarios conceivable (for example, monitoring with regard to events preceding an increase or decrease in tension). The possibility of interactive application in a therapy setting opens a whole new horizon of potential applications. Promising among them would be the display of tension reduction techniques once a particular level of tension has been reached.

Worthy of mention is the good compliance on the part of the participants both with regard to their willingness to participate - only two patients declined to do so - as well as with regard to the study proper. This agrees with the findings of other studies that employed ambulatory monitoring (Fahrenberg & Myrtek, 1996). Critical is the retrospective collection of variables to control for possible confounding variables; actual effects can thus be reported only with reservations. Another critical issue is the fact that frequent monitoring can increase the awareness of a phenomenon, which could result in biased results (for example, suitable tension reduction techniques might be employed earlier than otherwise, or tension might increase as a result of the focussing).

Nonetheless the advantages of data collection over a longer period of time, the "naturalistic" approach, and the expected greater external validity have already been emphasized in a number of studies (survey: Suls & Martin, 1993). As these studies have demonstrated, there are indeed practice-relevant research issues that would lend themselves to data collection in an every-day situation. Given the active participation by patients, essential and novel insights into self-monitoring and perhaps even into the self-management of specific symptoms could be found.

References

American Psychiatric Association. (1994). *Diagnostic and statistical manual of mental disorders* (4th ed.). Washington, DC: American Psychiatric Association.

Brügner, G. (1998). MONITOR: Ein flexibles Programm zur Datenerhebung mittels Pocket-PC. *Zeitschrift für Differentielle und Diagnostische Psychologie, 19*, 145-147.

Fahrenberg, J. & Myrtek, M. (Eds.) (1996). *Ambulatory assessment: computer-assisted psychological and psychophysiological methods in monitoring and field studies.* Göttingen/Seattle: Hogrefe & Huber Publishers.

First, M.B., Gibbon, M., Spitzer, R.L., Williams, J.B.W., Benjamin L. *User's Guide for the Structured Clinical Interview for DSM-IV Axis II Personality Disorders (SCID-II).* Washington, DC: American Psychiatric Press, 1997a. [Translated into German as SKID. Strukturiertes Klinisches Interview für DSM-IV. Achse II. (1997a). (H.-U. Wittchen, M. Zaudig & T. Fydrich). Göttingen: Hogrefe.]

First, M.B, Spitzer, R.L, Gibbon, M., Williams, J.B.W. *User's Guide for the Structured Clinical Interview for DSM-IV Axis I Disorders (SCID-I) – Clinician Version.* Washington, DC: American Psychiatric Press, 1997b. [Translated into German as SKID. Strukturiertes Klinisches Interview für DSM-IV. Achse I. (1997b). (H.-U. Wittchen, U. Wunderlich, S. Gruschwitz & M. Zaudig). Göttingen: Hogrefe.]

Gunderson, J.G., Zanarini, M.C. *Revised Diagnostic Interview for Borderlines (DIB-R).* Modified: February, 1992. McLean Hospital, Harvard Medical School, Belmont/Massachusetts, 1983. [Translated into German as Diagnostisches Interview für Borderline-Patienten - revidierte Fassung (DIB-R). In: C. Rohde-Dachser (Ed.). Das Borderline-Syndrom. Göttingen: Huber, 1990, modified 1995. pp. 224-238.]

Linehan, M. (1993). *Cognitive-Behavioral Treatment of Borderline Personality Disorder.* New York: Guilford. [Translated into German as Dialektisch-Behaviorale Therapie der Borderline-Persönlichkeitsstörung (1996). (M. Linehan.) München: CIP-Medien.]

Suls, J. & Martin, R. E. (1993). Daily recording and ambulatory monitoring methodologies in behavioral medicine. *Annals of Behavioral Medicine, 15*, 3-7.

Chapter 10
Daily Mood Reports in Hindsight: Results of a Computer-Assisted Time Sampling Study

Petra Hank, Peter Schwenkmezger, and Jens Schumann
Department of Psychology, University of Trier, Germany

Introduction

Statements about a person's own mood are typically made on the basis of a retrospective self-judgment made over a more or less precisely defined period of time. Self-judgments of mood are frequently collected using (partially) standardized observation inventories or questionnaires, either in a conventional paper and pencil or computer format. But how does this reflection on one's own mood come about? How are the different mood states which arise during any given time period recollected and evaluated? Or put in another way: how reliable are these data, and do they really allow valid conclusions to be drawn about how people feel from day to day?

Numerous research findings urge caution here, and demonstrate impressively that retrospective overall judgments are tainted with cognitive errors (Clark & Teasdale, 1982; Käppler, Becker & Fahrenberg, 1993; Kahneman & Tversky, 1982), and only shorter review times, if any, can be justified (Parkinson, Briner, Reynoldts & Totterdell, 1995). This has been shown when a comparison is made between the mood reported at different points during the period of time being measured and the overall judgment made in hindsight: Whereas some momentary moods are no longer remembered, for example, because the memory trace has been destroyed by subsequent information, other *salient moments of experience* are much more strongly integrated into the overall judgment. Hedges, Jandorf, and Stone (1985) report such peak effects. They telephoned people four times a day on 14 successive days to ask how they were feeling at that moment. In addition, the subjects submitted an evaluatory summary of each day. They found that the best predictor of the retrospective daily summary proved to be the peak momentary mood. Similar findings have been reported by Kahneman's group (Fredrickson & Kahneman, 1993; Varey & Kahneman, 1992). Moreover, these results prove that the ability to remember something is dependent on the *time positioning* of the mood which is to be remembered. More recent moods tend to be taken into consideration more when a retrospective general evaluation is made, a phenonemon which can be seen as a primary-recency effect (Fredrickson & Kahneman, 1993; Hank, 1994; Hedges, Jandorf & Stone, 1985; Varey & Kahneman, 1992).

If the retrieval does not succeed because the corresponding episodic memory is missing, the subject will try to actively reconstruct their mood. In the process, they resort to idiosyncratic inference strategies (cf. Stahlberg & Maass, 1997; Strack & Förster, 1998). One strategy may consist of recapitulating the course of one's mood over a period of time, using the mood which is closest in time to the summary report as an anchor for a judgment of one's subsequent mood. This strategy is seen in the so-called recency effect or end effect, which has been described, among others, by Fredrickson and Kahneman (1993) in the case of healthy subjects and Redelmeier and Kahneman (1996) in a medical context. Patients undergoing colonoscopy and lithotripsy recorded in real-time every sixty seconds the intensity of pain they were feeling. In addition, they evaluated retrospectively the pain they had experienced immediately after the examination was completed. Apart from the greatest intensity of pain, the level of pain at the end of the examination correlated most strongly with the overall retrospective judgment. The absolute length of the examination, which varied from 4 minutes to 69 minutes, had, on the other hand, no effect on the retrospective evaluation. Ruoss (1997) reported similar results. Fredrickson and Kahneman (1993) evaluate this as proof that emotional experiences are remembered as snap shots, neglecting duration of moods, rather than chronologically over time.

Support for this kind of retrospective extrapolation is provided by the results of our own computer supported laboratory and field experiment, with 40 participants (Post, 1999; Schönfeld, 1999). In the laboratory part, positive or negative moods were inducted by the presentation of a balanced sequence of positive or negative pictures, which could be viewed for either a short or a long period of time. The subjects assessed their mood immediately after viewing each of the pictures, as well as retrospectively at the end of a sequence of pictures. In the subsequent field experiment, the subjects recorded their current mood states on a palmtop computer at 10 randomly selected points in time on each of two successive days. Subsequent to the last measurement on the first and second days, they retrospectively evaluated their mood during the day that had just ended. The results of this experiment can be summed up as follows: Both the extreme manipulation of mood and the absolute length of the experienced mood were relatively poor predictors of the retrospective judgment, at least for this sample. Retrospective judgments of one's mood are, to a high degree, determined by average momentary moods, and, beyond this, they are modulated by the mood predominating at the time of the review. Significant mean differences between the momentary mood reports and the mood review combined with the positive correlation between both variables point to a linear relationship. This shows that people remember the moods they have experienced on the basis of a "relative precision" (Thomas & Diener, 1990). Taken together these results provide a hint for memory distortion during the encoding process.

A further source of information for a retrospective judgment of one's mood can be contextual information. In an attempt to come up with an overall judgment, the person tries to remember the contexts surrounding the mood they are looking for. In this process, the predominant mood at the time of a summary mood judgment in retrospect makes a momentary mood or context information with a congruent mood easier to remember; and so, as Nasby and Yando (1982) have shown, they contribute excessively to an overall judgment, whereas other – mood incongruent - information is left behind. Furthermore, a retrospective look back can also be skewed even when the necessary context information is more or less available but has been evaluated in a different way regarding its significance for the mood experience. In other words, it may carry a different weight for the retrospective review than it did for the original emotional experience.

Apart from these strategic inference processes, Werth (1998) points out the importance of socially conveyed knowledge in forming a judgment. According to this theory, a retrospective judgment (about one's mood) is the result of a socially influenced process, when the low confidence and skills of the interviewee are combined with the assessment of a very confident and knowledgeable interviewer.

So much for the possible cognitive and social factors influencing retrospective judgments of one's mood. Further, since such a review cannot be carried out detached from a person's habitual personal characteristics, numerous research findings allow one to presume a connection between different personality characteristics and average mood levels. For example, there are substantial positive correlations between extraversion and other related constructs, such as sociability and positive states of feeling. In contrast, neuroticism and similar constructs (such as, for example, trait anger) only correlate positively with negative states of feeling (cf. Post, 1999). Furthermore, these characteristics have been connected with a tendency toward mood swings. Hepburn and Eysenck (1989) have been able to show that extraversion correlates positively with swings toward both positive and negative states of feeling and with average variability, whereas for neuroticism, positive correlations with swings only toward negative feeling states have been reported.

Along with such habitual personal characteristics, there are also self-presentation strategies to consider. A series of research findings points to the fact that judgments of one's mood are modulated by presentation strategies which serve one's own self-worth (Fredrickson & Kahneman, 1993; Nasby & Yando, 1982; Taylor & Brown, 1988). In an effort to present oneself in a good light, a retrospective overall judgment is corrected in a positive way. But the opposite direction, namely the evaluation of one's mood more negatively with hindsight than was actually experienced, has also been repeatedly observed by Käppler, Brügner, and Fahrenberg (1998). Under everyday conditions, they asked 61 students for a self-judgment of their mood on two days for five time samples. Additionally, an evening and morning review, that is, an overall judgment of the days in question was recorded. In retrospect, the subjects judged their mood more negatively than was to be expected from the average values of the individual records. Interindividual differences in the ability to control the expression of one's emotions or in self-monitoring following Snyder (1987) underlie this selective management strategy. Closely connected to this is the self-consciousness construct in the sense of an increased consciousness of one's own person (private self-consciousness; Buss, 1980). According to various research findings, this condition of being privately self-conscious leads to an intensification of both positive and negative states of feeling and sensitizes physiological reactions. As a result, people with a higher self-consciousness differently perceive moods which are provoked and tend to less false attribution than people with a lower self-consciousness. Might this have, as a consequence, that private self-consciousness prevents one from errors in review?

What must be stressed here, is that retrospective judgments of one's mood seem to have more to do with memory and reconstruction errors than with a complete, reliable, and undistorted review, which is not surprising, since these memory achievements do not just passively filter into the consciousness but are rather constructed ad hoc. What aspects of memory and reconstruction or motivational processes underlie errors made when reviewing the past, and do they apply to everyone in the same way or can interindividual differences be assumed? To proceed, questions about the type and content of the cognitive and motivational processes involved must be posed.

Attempts at explanation which have been made from the area of emotional psychology are unsatisfactory because they merely establish the retrospective errors in a descriptive way. More useful are rather the approaches from cognitive psychology, that are used in the following research: the effect of retrospection is understood as an expression of the so-called knew-it-all-along-effect (Fischhoff, 1975; Wood, 1978) or hindsight bias (Dehn & Erdfelder, 1998; Hell, 1993; Pohl, 1996). This phenomenon, which has been shown to be relatively robust, states that an earlier opinion or prediction aligns itself with results which subsequently become known. Applied to the present context, it means that each information about one's emotional state available at one particular time changes one's memory of earlier moods in the past. As a consequence, judgments of one's mood adjust themselves to one's present mood. From this point of view, present mood serves as a source of feedback the subjects rely on, when they try to rate their mood in retrospect.

To explain this mistaken view of the past, recollection and reconstruction processes are postulated (Hawkins & Hastie, 1990). Concerning recollection processes, Hell, Gigerenzer, Gauggel, Mall, and Müller (1988, p. 536–537) postulated the so-called memory-trace strength hypothesis. According to this hypothesis a weaker or less elaborate memory trace for the original momentary mood rating, given a fixed trace strength for feedback information about mood, should enhance the probability of distorted retrospective mood ratings. Hence, an important variable in this process is encoding depth. Dehn and Erdfelder (1998) focus to another crucial variable in this process: the similarity between the original (past) mood and that of present mood. It has been hypothesized that the less distinct two memory traces representing original and feedback answer are, the higher is the probability that (1) thc two traces merge (c.f. Fischhoff, 1975; Pohl & Gawlik, 1995), (2) one superimposes the other (c.f. Hasher, Attig & Alba, 1981; Schkade & Kilbourne, 1991) or (3) that both become indistinguishable during recall (Kohnert, 1996). So, memory trace may either be completely distorted by feedback information or may be reduced in its accessibility.

Goals of the present research

The aim of the present field study is to identify the cognitive processes involved in retrospective mood reports, and to separate recollection and reconstruction biases. In order to do so, the study is restricted to memory design. Two variables which have been proved, among others, to be important in the discrimination between actual mood reports and retrospective mood reports, depth of processing during encoding and the similarity of the original answer and the feedback answer are experimentally manipulated. According to the theoretical considerations outlined above, we assume that mood report in hindsight will be stronger biased when

- encoding depth for momentary mood reports is reduced and
- the subjects are provided with feedback about their average mood for the entire day.

Beyond this, the effect of private self consciousness on retrospective mood judgments is analysed.

Method

Subjects

A total of 44 subjects (22 male, 22 female) aged between 18 and 62 years (M = 33.5, SD = 10.3 years) took part in the experiment. They were recruited through personal contact and received 100 DM for their participation.

Materials

Variables at state level. The current mood state was ascertained using the multidimensional mood questionnaire (MDBF; Steyer, Schwenkmezger, Notz & Eid, 1997) with the dimensions: good-bad mood (GB), alertness-tiredness (AT), and calmness-agitation (CA). The procedure is in two parallel forms with 12 adjectives (in each case four per mood dimension) to be answered on a five-point rating, ranging from not at all (1) to very (5), corresponding to the intensity experienced. The estimated consistency of the scales range from .73 to .88, and the stability coefficients are small, as is expected. This questionnaire was put on the palmtop computer HPLX 200.

Variables at trait level. Private self-consciousness was measured using the scale for measuring dispositional self-consciousness developed by Filipp and Freudenberg (1989). The 13 items on this scale, with a test bisection reliability of r =.77, relate both to public behavioral patterns and self-reflective thoughts or hidden behavioral patterns and are assessed by the subject according to how often they appear on a five-point scale.

Procedure

The study consisted of three phases. In the first phase, the subjects were told about the aim of the study, and they were explicitly informed about the amount of time to be taken for data collection in the second phase. Additionally, the subjects were provided with the scale of private self-consciousness and trained in the use of the handheld computer.

In the computer-assisted field study (second phase of the study) which began the next day, the subjects self-recorded their mood states using the handheld computer HP LX 200. Two types of mood reports were made, momentary and daily, according to the following time schedule: On three successive days, the subjects had to self-report their momentary mood eight times a day with four observation times in the morning between 9.00 a.m. and 12.00 a.m. and another four observation times in the afternoon between 2.00 p.m. and 5.00 p.m. The observation times in the morning and afternoon sequences followed each other randomly with a minimum time interval of 45 minutes between occasions. After the eight momentary ratings, the subjects were provided with feedback information allegedly "original" momentary mood ratings on average. At least one hour later, the subjects were requested to give a retrospective mood report for the entire day (daily report). When the subjects provided a momentary report, their instructions were to describe their mood at the moment they were being asked. Daily mood reports were taken by asking subjects to rate their mood for the entire day.

In the third phase of the study, the computers were collected from the subjects, they reported on their experiences in a written form and were finally paid for their cooperation.

Design

The experiment is designed with two independent variables: depth of encoding and type of feedback. Each variable has three levels, the second being repeatedly measured.

Encoding depth. Encoding depth was varied on three levels: deep encoding, shallow encoding, and natural encoding. Deep encoding was implemented by instructing the subjects to focus attention on themselves. For shallow encoding, the subjects were provided with news which should be evaluated. In addition to these experimental conditions, there was a control condition without any manipulation of encoding. The subjects were randomly assigned to one of these conditions. Encoding depth was manipulated each time before a momentary rating was collected.

Type of feedback. The difference between the original momentary mood rating (OMR) and the feedback mood rating (FMR) was varied on three levels differing in the absolute value and direction of deviation. The subjects were either provided with feedback information one standard deviation above the averaged momentary ratings (positive feedback) or below the averaged momentary ratings (negative feedback). In the control condition subjects were provided with feedback equal to the average of momentary mood ratings.

Dependent variables. The deviation between the daily mood reports (DMR), in terms of averaged original mood rating subtracted from retrospective mood rating (RMR – OMR) was chosen as an indicator of the size of hindsight bias. This difference variable was computed for each of the collected mood dimensions (good mood – bad mood, alertness – tiredness, and calmness – agitation).

Results

Data analysis is based on the time samples of 44 subjects with 16 subjects in each treatment group (shallow vs. deep encoding) and 12 subjects in the control group.

The subjects responded on average to 93.8 percent of the 27 sampling points. In detail, 22.6 daily time samples were gathered by each subject and 2.7 ratings covering the whole day in retrospect. This corresponds to response rates of 94.3 percent and 90.0 percent, respectively. In general, it took subjects about 2 minutes to complete one mood rating.

How do subjects arrive at an average daily mood rating? In order to answer this question, each subjects' original mood ratings were averaged across the eight times of momentary self-recording, yielding three means for the dimensions good mood – bad mood (OMR_{GB}), alertness – tiredness (OMR_{AT}), and calmness – agitation (OMR_{CA}), respectively. As an indicator of hindsight bias each of these means was subtracted from its corresponding retrospective mood rating for the entire day (RMR_{GB}, RMR_{AT}, RMR_{CA}). Hence, mean RMR – OMR deviations (deviated mood rating) equal to zero mean that daily mood reports reflect mood throughout the day with accuracy. A positive difference indicates that looking back at the mood of an entire day, the day appeared to be more positive than it actually had been experienced, whereas a negative difference indicates that the day in retrospect is evaluated worse than it was.

These RMR – OMR deviations were statistically analyzed using the MANOVA approach to repeated measures designs (O'Brien & Kaiser, 1985).

Concerning *good mood – bad mood*, a 3 (encoding depth) by 3 (feedback sequence) by 3 (feedback type) repeated measures MANOVA of the RMR – OMR deviations revealed a significant main effect of the feedback type (Pillai's V = 0.42, F (2,19) = 7.00, $p \leq .01$). There was neither a main effect of the encoding depth nor of the feedback sequence. Additionally, all interactions proved to be statistically insignificant.

As can be seen from Figure 1, there is a negative deviation in the case of correct feedback (M = -.19, SD = .49), indicating that the subjects feel worse than they actually felt throughout the day when they rate their mood in retrospect. Providing the subjects with either positive or negative feedback yields almost accurate mood reviews. The corresponding means are 0.07 (SD = .32) for positive feedback and 0.03 (SD = .50) for negative feedback.

With regard to the dimension *alertness – tiredness*, the MANOVA shows a significant effect of feedback sequence (Pillai's V =0.50 , F (5,19) = 3.80, $p < .02$). Post hoc comparisons according to the modified least significant difference approach reveal that this effect is attributable to significant group differences when subjects are either provided with positive or negative feedback. No differences between the groups

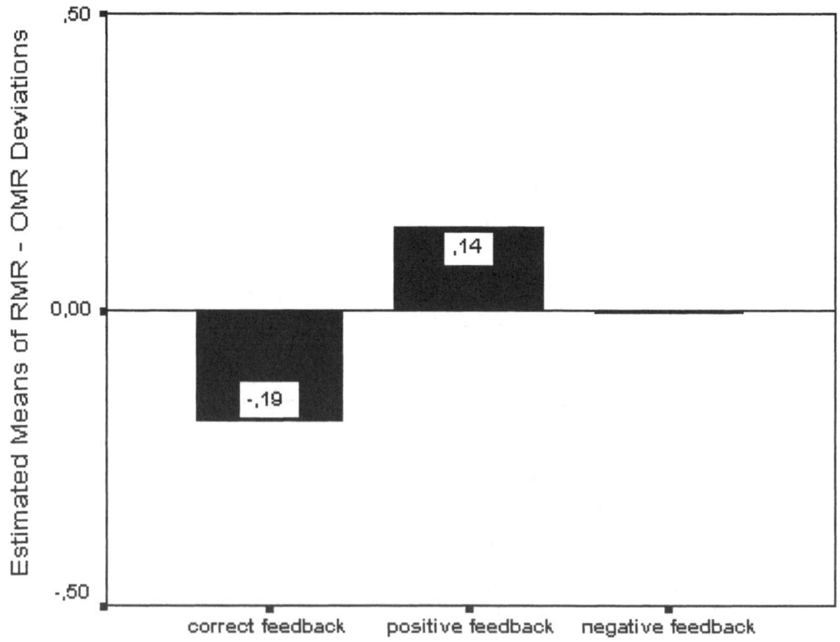

Figure 1. Estimated means of deviations between retrospective and momentary mood ratings for the dimension good mood - bad mood as an effect of feedback type.

are seen when correct feedback is given. Because this effect is of no theoretical interest per se, it is not examined in further analyses.

Concerning the dimension *calmness – agitation*, the interaction feedback type x feedback sequence reaches significance (Pillai's V = .93, F (10,40) = 3.50, $p \leq 0.01$; see Figure 2). In order to get some detailed information about this effect a multivariate ANOVA was computed with the between-subject factor feedback sequence and the dependent variables RMR – OMR deviation for correct, positive, and negative feedback, respectively. It revealed a significant main effect of feedback sequence (Pillai's V = .80, F (19, 90) = 2.16, p = .01) combined with a significant interaction of feedback sequence x positive feedback (F (5,36) = 7.10, $p \leq .00$; see Figure 3).

With regard to either correct feedback or negative feedback, feedback sequence seems to be of no importance.

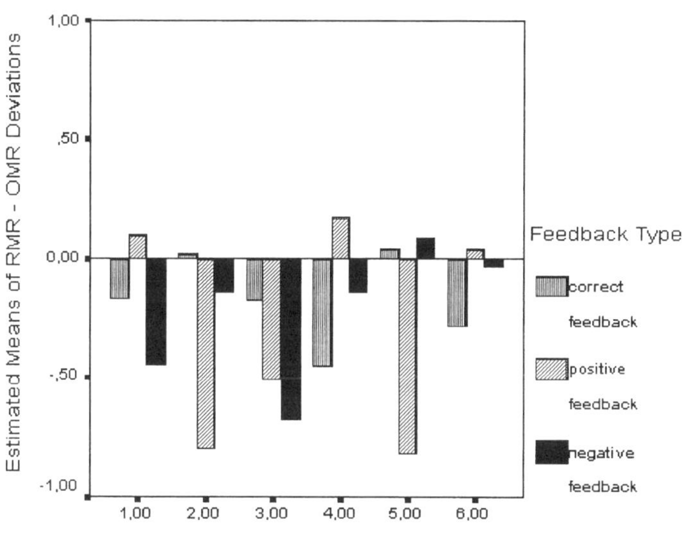

Feedback sequence	Recording day 1	Recording day 2	Recording day 3
1	Correct feedback	Positive feedback	Negative feedback
2	Correct feedback	Negative feedback	Positive feedback
3	Positive feedback	Correct feedback	Negative feedback
4	Positive feedback	Negative feedback	Correct feedback
5	Negative feedback	Correct feedback	Positive feedback
6	Negative feedback	Positive feedback	Correct feedback

Figure 2. Estimated means of deviations between retrospective and momentary mood for the dimension calmness - agitation as an interaction effect of feedback type by feedback sequence.

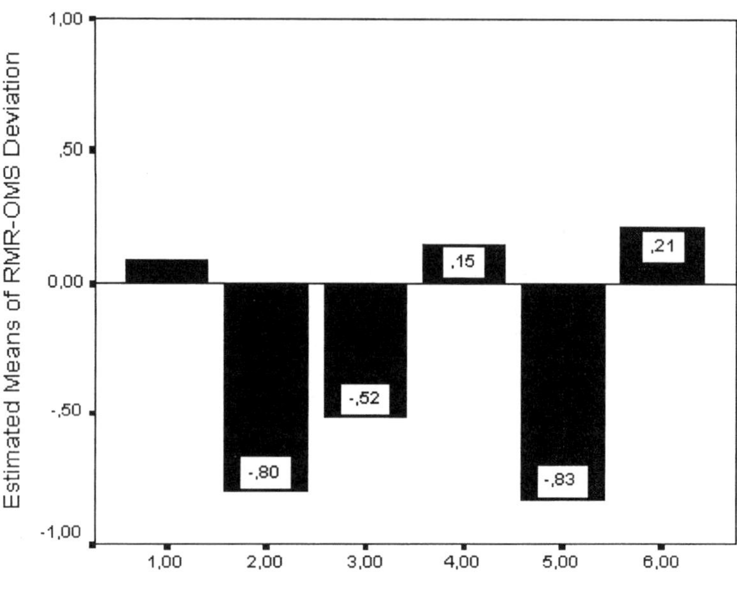

Feedback sequence	Recording day 1	Recording day 2	Recording day 3
1	Correct feedback	Positive feedback	Negative feedback
2	Correct feedback	Negative feedback	Positive feedback
3	Positive feedback	Correct feedback	Negative feedback
4	Positive feedback	Negative feedback	Correct feedback
5	Negative feedback	Correct feedback	Positive feedback
6	Negative feedback	Positive feedback	Correct feedback

Figure 3. Estimated means of deviations between retrospective and momentary mood for the dimension calmness - agitation as an interaction effect of feedback type by feedback sequence in case of positive feedback

There was no effect of private self-consciousness for any of the dependent variables.

Discussion

The present research aimed at exploring the nature of retrospective mood judgments within the context of theories to the phenomenon of hindsight bias, stressing the aspect of recollection in this process. According to the memory trace strength hypothesis, it was hypothesized that manipulation of the encoding depth and the similarity between the memory trace of past or original mood and that of (present) mood at the time of recall should enhance mood recollection biases.

In particular, a linear relationship between encoding depth and accuracy of mood recall was postulated. This hypothesis did not withstand empirical results. There was no significant effect of encoding depth for any of the mood dimensions analyzed. So it appears that encoding depth can be discounted as influential factor on daily mood records.

With regard to the second variable, it was assumed that the degree of similarity between memory trace for original mood and that for present mood should influence the degree of distorted mood ratings in hindsight. This effect was only found for the dimension good mood – bad mood – but the expected mean shift toward feedback value, commonly known as „hindsight bias" was only found when the subjects were provided with positive feedback. Just in contrast to our expectation, daily mood reports reflect mood throughout the day with reasonable accuracy, when negative feedback is given. In the case of correct feedback the subjects shift in a negative direction when looking back at the mood of an entire day. This result is in line with those reported by Fahrenberg's group, referred to above.

Furthermore, the significant interaction between feedback sequence and feedback type concerning the mood dimension calmness – agitation needs mentioning. With regard to positive feedback, it seems to be important in which sequence feedback is provided. But again, daily mood reports do not deviate in a consistent direction. Only half of them show a mean shift towards the feedback value as expected.

No effect was found for the influence of private self-consciousness on daily mood report.

Taken together, what tell us these results concerning the processes involved in reporting on mood in hindsight? Giving a satisfactory answer to this question is somewhat difficult, as there is no consistent result pattern across the analysed mood dimensions. A possible post hoc explanation may be to assume some evaluative stage in the process of retrospective mood report. According to Pohl and Eisenhauer (1997; see also Strack & Mussweiler, 1997) the feedback value is compared against a mood-specific knowledge base. In this stage of the process, the plausibility of the feedback value is checked. As in the present research, the feedback value was about one standard deviation above or below the averaged momentary mood ratings, it seems plausible to assume that the subjects doubted its credibility. As a consequence, feedback might have been rejected as useful information for a retrospective mood report. Instead, the subjects seem to have consciuosly tried to recollect mood throughout the day, resulting in a precise daily report. Other subjects might have been surprised by the feedback and reacted with counterfactual reasoning, so that hindsight bias was reduced, eliminated, or even reversed. On the other hand, if feedback value falls within a plausible range as in the case of correct feedback, the automatic recollection processes should not be disrupted, resulting in daily mood reports which are negatively biased.

As the present research was intended to experimentally enhance the probability of recollection biases, the results tell us little about the causes of any "natural" hindsight bias in retrospective mood reports with less extreme conditions. But nevertheless, these results pose a problem for theories that assume purely automatic processes like immediate assimilation (Fischhoff, 1975) or anchoring and adjustment (Tversky & Kahneman, 1974). In line with Hawkins and Hastie (1990) it is to be stated that "composite, multifactor explanations will be required to provide complete accounts for any of the behavioral phenomena" (Hawkins & Hastie, 1990, p. 324). In order to identify and deconstruct these processes future research should be directed to the multinomial model suggested by Erdfelder & Buchner (1998). It allows assumptions about the processes underlying hindsight bias to be formulated and empirically analyzed so that the stochastic connections between manifest retrospective judgments of one's mood and their latent cognitive processes may be revealed.

References

Buss, A.H. (1980). *Self-consciousness and social anxiety*. San Francisco: Freeman.

Clark, D.M. & Teasdale, J.D. (1982). Diurnal variation in clinical depression and accessibility of memories of positive and negative experiences. *Journal of Abnormal Psychology, 91*, 87–95.

Dehn, D.M. & Erdfelder, E. (1998). What kind of bias is hindsight bias? *Psychological Research, 61*, 135–146.

Erdfelder, E. & Buchner, A. (1998). Decomposing the hindsight bias: An integrative multinomial processing tree model. *Journal of Experimental Psychology: Learning, Memory, and Cognition, 24*, 387–414.

Filipp, S.-H. & Freudenberg, E. (1989). SAM: *Fragebogen zur Erfassung dispositionaler Aufmerksamkeit* [SAM: Questionnaire to assess dispositional self-consciousness]. Göttingen: Hogrefe.

Fischhoff, B. (1975). Hindsight ? foresight: The effect of outcome knowledge on judgment under uncertainty. *Journal of Experimental Psychology: Human Perception and Performance, 1*, 288–299.

Fredrickson, B.L. & Kahneman, D. (1993). Duration neglect in retrospective evaluation of affective episodes. *Journal of Personality and Social Psychology, 65*, 45–55.

Hank, P. (1995). *Ärgererleben und Ärgerverarbeitung im Alltag: Ergebnisse zweier Felduntersuchungen mittels Zeit- und Ereignisstichprobentechnik* [Experience and expression of anger during daily life: Results of two fieldstudies by means of time- and experience sampling method]. Hamburg: Dr. Kovac.

Hasher, L., Attig, M.S. & Alba, J.W. (1981). I knew it all along: Or, did I? *Journal of Verbal Learning and Verbal Behavior, 20*, 86–96.

Hawkins, S.A. & Hastie, R. (1990). Hindsight: Biased judgments of past events after the outcomes are known. *Psychological Bulletin, 107*, 311–327.

Hedges, S.M., Jandorf, L. & Stone, A.A. (1985). Meaning of daily mood assessments. *Journal of Personality and Social Psychology, 48*, 428–434.

Hell, W. (1993). Gedächtnistäuschungen [memory distortions]. In W. Hell, K. Fiedler & G. Gigerenzer (Eds.). *Kognitive Täuschungen*, (pp. 13–38) [Cognitive distortions]. Heidelberg: Spektrum.

Hell, W., Gigerenzer, G., Gauggel, S., Mall, M. & Müller, M. (1988). Hindsight bias: An interaction of automatic and motivational factors? *Memory and Cognition, 16*, 533–538.

Hepburn, L. & Eysenck, M.W. (1989). Personality, average mood, and mood variability. *Personality and Individual Differences, 10*, 975–983.

Kahneman, D. & Tversky, A. (Ed.) (1982). *Judgment under uncertainty: Heuristics and biases.* New York: Cambridge University Press.

Käppler, C., Becker, H.-U. & Fahrenberg, J. (1993). Ambulantes 24-Stunden-Monitoring als psychophysiologische Assessmentstrategie: Reproduzierbarkeit, Reaktivität, Retrospektionseffekt und Bewegungskonfundierung [Ambulatory 24-hour monitoring as psychophysiological assessment strategy: replicability, reactivity, retrospection effect, and movement confoundation]. *Zeitschrift für Differentielle und Diagnostische Psychologie, 14*, 235–251.

Käppler, C., Brügner, B. & Fahrenberg, J. (1998). Pocketcomputer-unterstütztes Assessment mit MONITOR: Befindlichkeit und Aufmerksamkeitsverlauf im Alltag, Methodenakzeptanz und die Replikation des Retrospektionseffektes [Pocketcomputer-based assessment using MONITOR: Changes of mood and attention in daily life, compliance, and replication of the retrospection bias]. *Diagnostica, 22*

Kohnert, A. (1996). *Grenzen des Rückschaufehlers: Die Verzerrung von Erinnerungen an früheres Wissen durch neue Informationen [Limitations of hindsight bias: The distortions of recollections of earlier knowledge through new information]*.. Bonn: Holos.

Nasby, W. & Yando, R. (1982). Selective encoding and retrieval of affectively valent information: Two cognitive consequences of children's mood states. *Journal of Personality and Social Psychology, 43*, 1244–1253.

O'Brien, R.G. & Kaiser, M.K. (1985). MANOVA method for analyzing repeated measures designs: An extensive primer. *Psychological Bulletin, 97*, 316–333.

Parkinson, B., Briner, R.B., Reynolds, S. & Totterdell, P. (1995). Time frames for mood: Relations between momentary and generalized ratings of affect. *Personality and Social Psychological Bulletin, 21*, 331–339.

Pohl, R.F. (1996). Der Rückschaufehler – eine systematische Verfälschung der Erinnerung [Hindsight bias – a systematic distortion of recollection]. *Report Psychologie, 21*, 596–609.

Pohl, R.F. (1998). The effects of feedback source and plausibility of hindsight bias. *European Journal of Cognitive Psychology, 10*, 191–212.

Pohl, R.F. & Eisenhauer, M. (1997). Ein kognitives Prozeßmodell zur Erklärung systematisch verzerrter Urteile und Erinnerungen [A cognitive process model to explain systematically distorted judgment and recall]. In H. Mandl (Ed.), *Bericht über den 40. Kongreß der Deutschen Gesellschaft für Psychologie in München 1996* (pp. 805–812) [Proceedings of the 40th Congress of the German Society of Psychology, Munich 1996]. Göttingen: Hogrefe.

Pohl, R.F. & Gawlik, W. (1996). No reduction of hindsight bias with complete information and repeated testing. *Organizational Behavior and Human Decision Processes, 67*, 49–58.

Post, Y. (1999). *Wie wird Befindlichkeit erinnert? Eine Untersuchung der bei Retrospektionen auftretenden Effekte anhand einer experimentellen Induktion von Befindlichkeit* [How is mood recalled? An analysis of the retrospection effect by experimentally inducing mood]. Unveröffentlichte Diplomarbeit [Unpublished master's thesis]. University of Trier, Trier.

Redelmeier, D.A. & Kahneman, D. (1996). Patients' memories of painful medical treatments: real-time and retrospective evaluations of two minimally invasive procedures. *Pain, 66*, 3–8.

Ruoss, M. (1997). Schmerzpatienten zeigen einen höheren Hindsight Bias [Patients with chronical pain display a greater hindsight bias]. *Zeitschrift für Experimentelle Psychologie, 19*, 561–588.

Schkade, D.A. & Kilbourne, L.M. (1991). Expectation-outcome consistency and hindsight bias. *Organizational Behavior and Human Decision Processes, 49*, 105–123.

Schönfeld, A. (1999). *Ist Stimmung Bestimmung? Alltagsbefindlichkeit in Situation und Erinnerung und ihr Zusammenhang mit Persönlichkeitsmerkmalen* [Is mood ? daily mood at present and in hindsight and the relationship of daily mood to personal dispositions]. Unveröffentlichte Diplomarbeit [Unpublished master's thesis]. University of Trier, Trier.

Snyder, M. (1987). *Public appearances, private realities: The psychology of self-monitoring.* New York: Freeman & Co.

Stahlberg, D. & Maass, A. (1997). Hindsight bias: Impaired memory or biased reconstruction? In W. Stroebe & M. Hewstone (Eds.). *European Review of Social Psychology, 8,* 105–132. New York: Wiley & Sons

Steyer, R., Schwenkmezger, P, Notz, P. & Eid, M. (1997). *Handanweisung zum Mehrdimensionalen Befindlichkeitsfragebogen (MDBF)* [Manual of the multidimensional mood questionnaire (MDBF)]. Huber: Bern.

Strack, F. & Förster, J. (1998). Self-reflection and recognition: The role of meta-cognitive knowledge in the attribution of recollective experience. *Personality and Social Psychology, 2*, 111–123.

Strack, F. & Mussweiler, T. (1997). Explaining the enigmatic anchoring effect: Mechanisms of selective accessibility. *Journal of Personality and Social Psychology, 73*, 437–446.

Thaylor, S.E. & Brown, J.D. (1988). Illusion and well-being: A social psychological perspective on mental health. *Psychological Bulletin, 103*, 193–210.

Thomas, D. & Diener, E. (1990). Memory accuracy in the recall of emotions. *Journal of Personality and Social Psychology, 59*, 291–297.

Tversky, A. & Kahneman, D. (1974). Judgment under uncertainty: Heuristics and biases. *Science, 185*, 1124–1131.

Varey, C. & Kahneman, D. (1992). Experiences extended across time: Evaluation of moments and episodes. *Journal of Behavioral Decision Making, 5*, 169–186.

Werth, L. (1998). *Ein inferentieller Erklärungsansatz des Rückschaufehlers* [An inferential explanation of hindsight bias]. Hamburg: Dr. Kovac.

Wood, G. (1978). The "knew-it-all-along" effect. *Journal of Experimental Psychology: Human Perception and Performance, 4*, 345–353.

Chapter 11
Time-Series Analysis of Diary Data

Ralf Ott and O. Berndt Scholz
Department of Psychology, University of Bonn, Germany

Time series analysis of diary data

Virtually all scientists and especially behavioral scientists have attended at least one course in research methods, in which they learned a little about experimental design. The overwhelming majority of time spent on design probably involved discussion of "group design" in which researchers group *n* subjects within *k* different conditions or "treatments". Only a few scientists and clinicians were exposed to an alternative paradigm of experimental design – single-case research. The use of such designs has a long history (see, Ittenbach & Lawhead, 1996), nevertheless, today such designs are still widely not acknowledged in behavioral sciences.

Behavioral researchers have long relied on the use of self-report diaries for collection of information on many subjective and behavioral variables relevant for clinical and research practice. A variety of diaries for measuring such variables on a self-report basis are currently at hand, an overview is provided by Seemann (1997), see also the chapters by Baumann et al., Perrez at al., and Godaert et al. in this Volume. Recent developments focus on electronic applications, however, some methodological problems such as the comparability of electronic and paper-pencil diaries are not yet solved (Hank & Schwenkmezger, 1996). These diaries all share one common characteristic, they all provide short time-series data mostly under $t = 100$ with single or multiple baselines to which standard statistical time-series analysis such as ARIMA models can not be applied.

The aim of this paper is to provide an overview of statistical procedures for typical diary data from short time-series designs. After presenting a framework with different statistical strategies, the second part gives two brief examples, one using an interrupted time-series analysis to test treatment effects, the other using lag sequential analysis to determine covariations and serial dependencies between different variables over time. Note, because of space limitations most statistical ideas are only covered briefly and corresponding authors are referenced for more detail.

Potential strategies for the analysis of diary data

Analyzing diary data: A framework

Essentially, the question here is what to do with the raw data once they have been collected. A general framework is provided by Scholz (1995), who distinguished between primary data, which may be analyzed by visual inspection and secondary data, such as agglomeration data, variability and covariation measures (see Figure 1).

The first evaluation step includes the visual analysis of the primary data. This provides an overview of the process of the diary variables. The secondary data can be subdivided into agglomeration, variability, and covariation data. Agglomeration data such as *range* or *mean* of the time-series are first quantitative benchmarks of the underlying process. Additionally, these data should be completed by variation measures to characterize the data with regard to their variability. A common statistic within this step is the mean square successive difference (MSSD, Neumann, Kent & Bellison, 1941). A small MSSD indicates a relative constant course of the diary variable, whereas a large MSSD indicates an instable course. Terms and examples may be found in Scholz (1995). Moreover, the variability of the data can be analyzed by *trend coefficient* and *time-series analysis*. Finally, the use of correlation statistics is useful to reveal important relationships between different diary variables. In this chapter we will describe a modified version of the *lag sequential analysis* by Faraone and Dorfman (1987), which allows to determine cross-dependencies over time between diary variables.

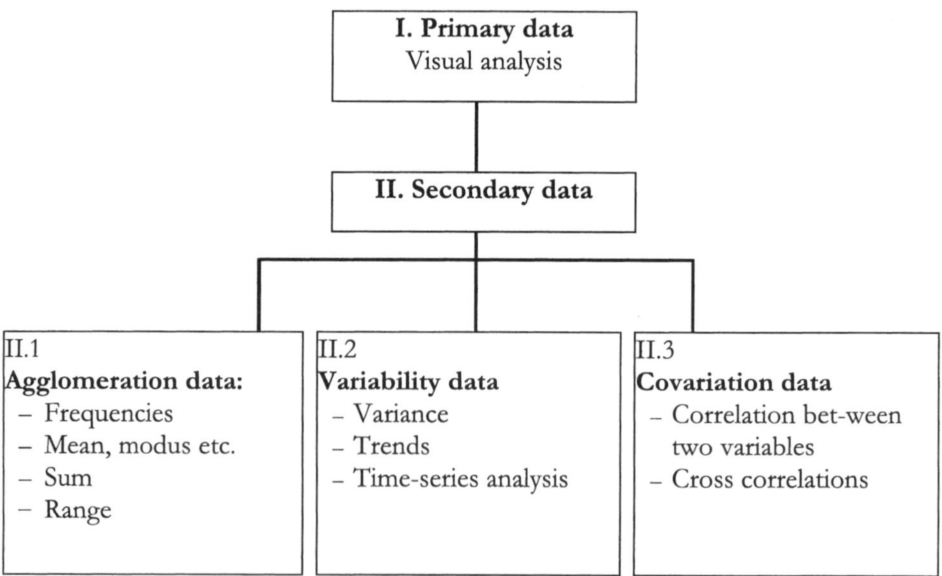

Figure 1. A general framework for the analysis of diary data (Scholz, 1995)

Serial dependence and short time-series

The presence of serial dependence in single-case data has implications for both visual and statistical analyses of such data. Matyas and Greenwood (1990) reviewed on visual analysis of original data and demonstrated that they were affected by serial dependence. Statistical analysis is also influenced by the presence of serial dependence. Use of the *t* and *F* distributions has been widely criticized (for example, Kazdin, 1982) because the presence of serial dependence, if ignored, can lead to considerable misestimations of the Type I error rate. To overcome the problem of serial dependence, some parametric and nonparametric approaches have been recommended. Table 1 gives an overview of the prominent class of parametric approaches. More detailed discussion may be found in the comprehensive reader by Franklin, Allison, and Gorman (1996), focusing on all aspects of design and analysis of single-case research – including also the issues of meta-analysis, cyclicity and statistical software.

Parametric approaches all start with an evaluation of autocorrelation in the data. They then proceed to an identification of appropriate stochastic models that might be used to transform the data such as to remove serial dependence. Finally, to test the success of the model, they then need to test for the presence of autocorrelation in the residual time-series. *Moving-average models* (ARIMA), following Box and Jenkins (1970), are mathematically sophisticated but they require intensive labour and many observations. However, most applied studies like diary examinations have very few baseline measures and very few post-intervention measures. Matyas and Greenwood (1991) found that overfitting inflated the values of *t*-test and *F*-ratios in ARIMA models with short time-series ($t < 20$).

Table 1. Possible parametric time-series techniques in single-case research

Method	General idea	Reference
Least-squares regression discontinuity models	Comparison of pre- and posttest regression models. Given an effect the series might change in trend, periodicity, and / or level	Campbell (1963)
Generalized least-squares models	Same general idea as above, incorporating autocorrelation effects	Ostrom (1978)
Box-Jenkins ARIMA models	Incorporating autoregressive and moving average, trend effects	Box & Jenkins (1976)
Interrupted time series analysis (ITSA)	Unlike ARIMA uses least-squares methods, like ARIMA uses autocorrelation and trend information	Glas, Wilson and Gottman (1975)
ITSACORR	ITSA model with modified lag-1 autocorrelation estimations	Crosbie (1993)

Fortunately, there are some least-squares methods that combine the best of the ARIMA and regression approaches. Glas, Wilson and Gottman (1975) proposed the *interrupted time-series* analysis (ITSA) using autoregressive, integrated, moving-average models to analyze the time-series, which show less vulnerability in short series.

A variety of nonparametric approaches, loosely called *randomization test*, can also often work effectively with time-series designs. These tests also dispense with some restrictive assumptions of ordinary *t*-test and ANOVA analyses, particularly those of normality of distributions. With this relative freedom from restrictions of distributional forms and random selection, one might at first glance suspect, that these nonparametric test might also be free from assumptions about autocorrelated processes. Nevertheless, simulation studies (Allison, Faith & Gorman, 1995) strongly suggested that, as in their parametric counterparts, true significance probability values are underestimated for positive autocorrelated residuals. The opposite effect occurs in the presence of negatively autocorrelated residuals, in which the obtained significance values are overestimates of the true values. Overviews are provided by Bortz, Lienert and Boehnke (2000) and Edgington (1987).

Meta-analysis of single-case results

Single-case research has traditionally been neglected in meta-analytic reviews. Nevertheless, meta-analyzing single-case research seems essential for two reasons: First, many treatments, particularly behavioral treatments, have been tested primarily in single-case designs. Therefore, evaluation of these treatments necessitates meta-analysis of single-case literature. Second, single-case research frequently leaves readers wondering whether observed treatment effects would generalize to individuals other than the one being studied. By meta-analyzing data from many individuals, one obtains a better picture of the expected average effect than by computing arithmetic means and other group average parameters. Meta-analysis techniques allow the combination of group and single-case studies, one can conduct parallel analyses within each type of study and compare the results. In case of diary data, meta-analysis offers a stringent solution to finally pool variability data and thus make conclusions about the *average variability*.

Some issues, like regression-based effect sizes or weighting effect sizes, have still to be solved. A more detailed introduction may be found in Faith, Allison and Gorman (1996).

Study 1: Variability data "Effectiveness of tape-based hypnotherapy in insomnia"

This study (Scholz & Ott, 2000) examines the efficacy of hypnotherapeutic audio tapes with consecutive 21 patients suffering from chronic insomnia. The sample was enrolled in a prospective two-period treatment protocol. Following a 7-day conventional baseline phase, a supplemental tape-based hypnotherapeutic treatment was administered for the following three weeks. Patients kept a sleep diary that recorded several sleeping parameters for the whole period of 28 days.

The main aim of this study was not only to determine the effectiveness of tape based hypnotherapy, but to demonstrate the effectiveness of different types of hypnotherapeutic metaphors. Construction of the metaphors and discussion of the methodological reservations concerning the validity of sleep diary items may be found in the original paper by Scholz and Ott (2000).

Method

Procedure: The patients were recruited consecutively from two medical doctors in general practice. In addition to the initial interview, patients underwent several psychometric measurements and interviews (see Scholz & Ott, 2000) to determine their clinical status and complaints accompanying their sleep disorders. They were then instructed how to fill in the sleep diary. The patients received the first cassette after they had kept their diary for one week. The patients were not given any additional medical or psychotherapeutic treatment during the course of this study.

Subjects: Twenty-one patients, 13 men and 8 women, took part in the study (age: M = 47.38, SD = 13.18 years). Their sleep disorders had already lasted an average of 3.90 (SD 4.86) years, with a minimum length of 6 months and a maximum length of 20 years.

Sleep diary: Each patient kept a sleep diary for 28 days. Five variables were extracted 1. latency of sleep (in min), 2. number of awakenings, 3. time spent lying awake (in min), 4. feeling of recovery, and 5. sleep duration (in h). The diary was administered as paper pencil version, however, it should be noted that an electronic version is at hand (see the Hinkel and Scholz chapter within this volume).

Data Analysis

Time-series analysis of the five diary variables were calculated for each individual patient. An AB design was used. The diary entries for the first seven days served as baseline measurements, while days 8 to 28 served as the treatment phase. Because of the short time period with $t = 28$, an *interrupted time-series analysis* (ITSACORR, Crosbie, 1993) was calculated. ITSACORR tests for variability between baseline and treatment phase by comparing intercept and slope, both corrected for lag-1 autocorrelation between the two phases. In order to be able to make a comparison with the group analysis, we also performed *meta-analysis* (Stouffer method, see Rosenthal, 1984) to agglutinate the data of the single cases. The *p*-values resulting from time-series analysis were agglomerated for all five sleep diary variables. The calculations were made with the help of the Meta-Analysis program (Schwarzer, 1989).

The *slope* is represented by a positive or a negative number. It describes an increase or decrease in the respective parameter in the specific phase. Furthermore, it indicates the velocity of the change. Improvement is shown if the slope changes from a negative number in the baseline to a positive number in the treatment phase or if it increases from a small positive number in baseline to a larger positive number in the treatment phase. The *intercept* describes the level of a series over a given length of time. Improvement is shown if there is a change in intercept from baseline to treatment phase.

Table 2. Single-case comparison baseline versus treatment for the 5 sleep diary variables from Interrupted Time-series Analysis (ITSACORR)

Ss		Sleep duration			Sleep recovery			Time lying awake			Number of awakenings			Latency of sleep		
		Base line	Treat ment	p	Base line	Treat ment	p	Base line	Treat ment	p	Base line	Treat ment	p	Base line	Treat ment	p
01	I	7.9	5.9	.16	2.2	4.3	.07	0.91	0.99	.94	0.33	0.58	.75	- 0.92	0.00	.95
	S	- 0.71	.03	.03	.4	- .06	.11	.01	.01	.96	.14	.02	.48	.85	.03	.05
02	I	6.0	6.6	.41	5.2	5.1	.86	0.70	1.29	.38	1.03	0.90	.87	0.15	0.34	.79
	S	.18	.01	.38	.16	- .06	.39	.01	- .07	.58	.31	- .03	.34	.15	- .01	.14
03	I	7.3	7.4	.90	3.5	4.0	.37	1.27	0.23	.18	1.43	2.66	.20	0.22	0.09	.61
	S	- .31	- .01	.17	.25	- .06	.03	- .01	.00	.56	- .08	- .07	.01	.01	- .01	.84
04	I	6.6	6.6	.89	3.4	2.9	.60	1.59	0.87	.15	2.07	1.01	.29	- 0.07	0.86	.55
	S	- .24	.01	.46	.09	.00	.64	- .03	- .03	.92	- .14	- .04	.66	.06	- .05	.65
05	I	4.7	5.0	.77	2.4	3.6	.54	0.60	- 0.05	.15	2.40	1.09	.15	0.89	0.62	.10
	S	- .16	.04	.38	.35	- .06	.17	.02	.03	.93	- .11	- .03	.66	- .05	- .02	.44
06	I	6.2	4.4	.21	5.0	3.9	.04	0.03	0.17	.45	0.23	0.17	.79	0.56	0.83	.42
	S	- .26	.06	.32	- .10	- .10	.95	- .02	.01	.54	- .02	- .01	.87	- .05	.04	.26
07	I	7.9	7.9	.95	2.0	3.2	.47	0.26	0.56	.49	0.05	0.83	.20	0.45	1.18	.37
	S	- .05	- .03	.92	.54	.05	.14	.07	- .02	.39	.18	- .03	.14	.17	.01	.39
08	I	3.9	4.1	.93	4.5	4.3	.66	3.65	3.09	.73	1.13	1.37	.69	0.81	0.87	.91
	S	.54	.12	.39	.00	- .07	.49	- .55	- .14	.18	- .08	- .02	.65	- .04	- .04	1.00
09	I	8.6	8.8	.72	5.4	4.7	.06	0.00	0.01	.77	0.00	0.06	.77	4.65	0.20	.00
	S	- .16	- .01	.35	- .30	- .01	.03	.00	.00	.98	.00	- .01	.98	- .96	.00	.00
10	I	7.0	7.1	.90	2.8	3.1	.92	2.26	0.73	.00	2.36	1.20	.12	0.95	0.52	.40
	S	- .26	- .06	.18	.07	- .08	.61	- .32	- .04	.00	- .09	- .07	.87	.04	- .02	.54
11	I	2.8	5.7	.01	5.1	3.3	.17	3.56	2.69	.56	3.36	1.99	.37	0.46	0.98	.32
	S	.87	.00	.00	- .26	.02	.33	- .33	- .04	.41	- .25	- .03	.54	- .04	- .05	.97
12	I	9.6	7.7	.23	2.4	2.0	.24	0.86	0.90	.99	1.64	1.94	.75	- 0.03	1.31	.17
	S	- .65	- .05	.16	- .08	.01	.27	.15	- .05	.36	.03	- .04	.74	.22	- .03	.23

Ss		Sleep duration			Sleep recovery			Time lying awake			Number of awakenings			Latency of sleep		
		Base line	Treat ment	p	Base line	Treat ment	p	Base line	Treat ment	p	Base line	Treat ment	p	Base line	Treat ment	p
13	I	6.4	7.2	.50	4.2	2.0	.25	0.87	0.54	.68	2.72	2.00	.23	1.78	0.73	.00
	S	.00	- .01	.97	- .20	.04	.52	- .07	- .01	.69	- .06	.01	.62	- .16	- .01	.06
14	I	6.6	6.8	.85	6.0	4.3	.04	1.71	0.05	.05	4.47	0.09	.04	0.48	0.36	.51
	S	- .14	- .01	.77	- .34	.01	.05	- .32	.04	.04	- .81	.07	.06	- .04	.00	.28
15	I	8.3	7.7	.36	4.6	3.6	.29	– a			2.86	1.40	.01	0.20	0.13	.11
	S	- .09	.00	.57	.13	.05	.71				- .34	- .01	.01	- .01	.00	.25
16	I	5.6	7.3	.41	1.9	3.0	.02	0.67	0.47	.79	1.63	2.08	.23	0.06	0.39	.05
	S	.54	.00	.19	.36	- .01	.05	.00	- .01	.93	.03	- .06	.36	.01	- .01	.76
17	I	5.6	7.2	.10	2.6	3.3	.11	2.69	0.77	.03	0.41	0.22	.06	0.61	0.30	.40
	S	.44	.08	.12	- .08	.02	.36	- .45	- .04	.04	- .11	.02	.35	- .01	- .01	.99
18	I	9.0	7.8	.01	3.3	4.6	.44	- 0.75	0.08	.47	- 0.82	0.36	.58	0.10	0.35	.48
	S	- .19	.05	.04	.00	.01	.99	.18	.02	.39	.25	.05	.54	.08	.00	.33
19	I	3.6	2.7	.43	3.3	4.6	.43	0.36	1.24	.39	0.77	0.98	.82	3.59	1.74	.21
	S	.25	.03	.49	.00	.01	.99	.18	.01	.49	.00	.03	.90	- .29	.01	.33
20	I	5.9	6.6	.67	3.6	3.4	.68	1.21	0.24	.10	2.63	0.32	.00	1.31	0.78	.20
	S	- .02	.05	.82	.10	- .04	.45	- .12	- .01	.19	- .25	- .01	.13	- .15	- .02	.16
21	I	4.7	5.6	.65	5.5	3.6	.36	1.26	1.00	.19	2.79	2.23	.36	0.37	0.12	.45
	S	.35	.09	.55	-.50	- .06	.27	- .04	- .04	.86	-.22	- .05	.24	- .07	.00	.29

Notes: I = steady state intercept of time-series, intercepts characterize the average level within the baseline and the treatment phase; S = steady state slope of time-series, slopes characterize the velocity of the hypnotherapeutic process portrayed by the diary, [a] = time-series could not be computed because of autocorrelation = 1

Results

Effects in interrupted time-series

ITSACORR was applied to the diary data of all five dependent variables with a $p <$ .10. ITSACORR uses autocorrelation information to obtain least-squares estimations of phase 1 and 2 intercept and slope. Univariate variabilities in intercept/slope are then compared by *t*-test. Table 2 provides an overview of all interrupted time-series results for the intercept comparisons. The complete results are described in Scholz and Ott (2000).

Only 2 patients showed a significant improvement in the intercepts (1 patient in a variability of slope) for "sleep duration", expected improvement in "sleep recovery" could be found in only 4 patients (3 for slopes), "time lying awake" was significantly decreased in only 4 patients (3 for slopes), "number of awakenings" was reduced in 4 patients (3 in slopes) and "latency of sleep" decreased significantly in 5 patients (3 in slopes).

Meta-Analysis of time-series results

To account for the overall significance of these results, all of the *p*-values for each of the comparisons of the intercepts were then agglomerated using meta-analysis (Stouffer method). Those *p*-values which had significant results in a direction contrary to that which was expected (for example, a decrease in sleep duration) were marked with a minus sign. The results are summarized in Table 3.

Table 3. Meta-Analysis of time-series results for the diary variables

	Weighted Z	p	Effect Size r	Homogeneity
Latency of sleep	1.95	.03	.08	χ^2 (20) = 37.6, s.
Time lying awake	2.27	.01	.10	χ^2 (20) = 28.6, ns.
Number of awakenings	2.40	.01	.10	χ^2 (20) = 29.0, ns.
Sleep recovery	0.45	.32	.02	χ^2 (20) = 22.2, ns.
Sleep duration	- 2.49	.01	-.10	χ^2 (20) = 20.7, ns.

Notes: p-values were combined using the Stouffer method. Weighted solutions, more rigid statistical tests, were preferred because of results in unexpected directions. Significant χ^2-tests indicate that the underlying data set is not sufficiently homogeneous

Three out of the five diary variables – latency of sleep, number of awakenings and time spent lying awake – showed significant overall improvement between baseline and treatment phases as a result of hypnotherapy. Striking results were found for the variable "sleep duration". Although a hypnotherapeutic treatment effect is evident and data are homogeneous, the negative *Z* value indicates a finding contrary to expectations – sleep duration actually decreases from baseline to treatment.

Impact of cyclic processes in group analysis

It is noteworthy that not reported group analysis revealed more convincing evidence. MANOVA showed a significant overall effect. Furthermore, all five sleep variables showed significant improvement in the corresponding univariate analyses. However, group analysis does not account for periodic or cyclical changes in the data, which are not attributable to the treatment itself. This fact is well demonstrated in a simple visual and statistical analysis of two time-series examples. Figure 2 shows the time-series for the diary variable "sleep duration" in patients 16 and 17.

Given the nearly congruent intercepts of patient 16 (baseline: 5.6, treatment: 7.3) and patient 17 (baseline: 5.6, treatment: 7.2, see Table 3), the visual information provided by the graph does not permit us to make an decision which patient benefited more from hypnotherapy. One might easily conclude that both time-series exhibit a significant improvement from baseline to treatment phase. In repeated measurement group designs, these two time-series will both contribute to significant change over time.

ITSACORR was then performed on both of these time-series data with a $p < .10$

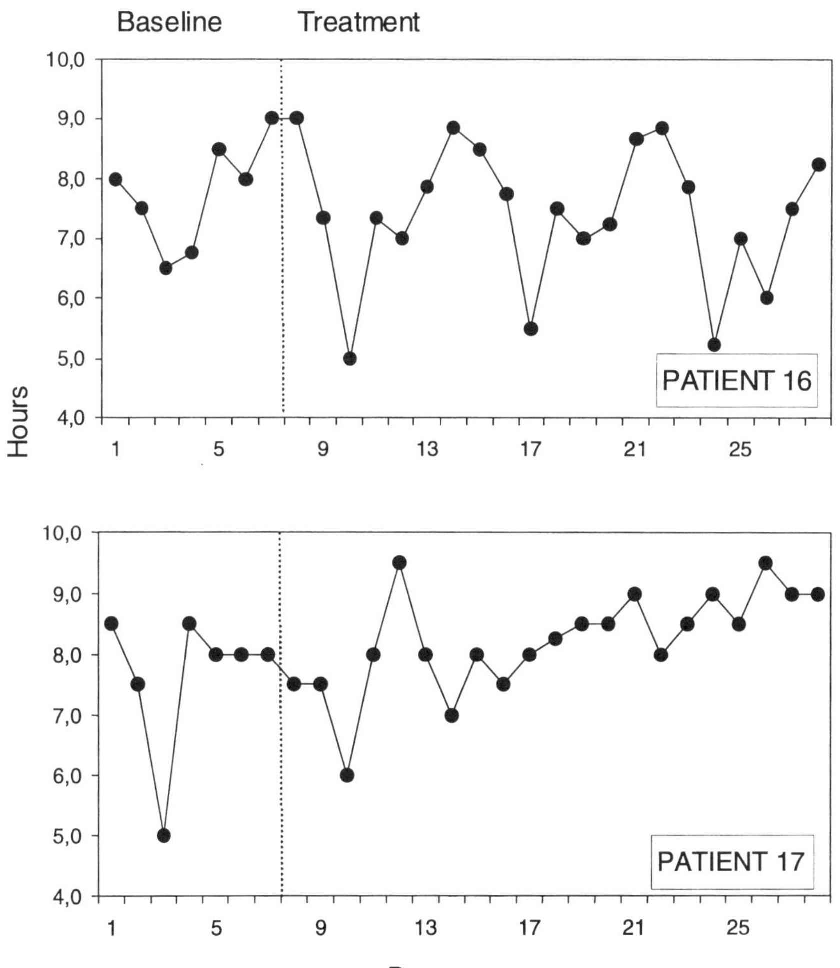

Figure 2. Single time-series of "sleep duration" for patients 16 and 17 over baseline (day 1 to 7) and treatment phase (days 8 to 28).

significance level. There was no increase in intercept for patient 16 [t (23) = 0.85, p = .41]. For Patient 17, there was significant increase in intercept [t (23) = 1.72, p = .10]. Patient 16 provides a good example of the problems which arise when a group analysis of these data is performed. Even though the time-series seems to be increasing, this trend is *not* attributable to the change of phases, that is, Patient 16 shows a cycle in sleep duration, which is continued over phases and does not change because of the treatment.

Especially in cases of insomnia one should not neglect the cyclic nature of the disease. Insomnia patients typically report periods of both improvement and gradual decline in sleep within the normal course of their sleep disorder.

Study 2: Covariaton Data
"Potential lags in pain diary variables"

The aim of this study was to examine the sequential dependencies between intensity of pain and sleep duration in a consecutive sample of 13 patients with pain disorders. Patients filled in the Electronic Bonn Pain Diary (Ott, Hinkel & Scholz, 2000; Ott & Scholz, 1999) during the initial phase of a ambulant behavioral therapy. Lag sequential analysis, an approach introduced by Sackett (1979), was used to determine sequential covariations between the variables.

Method

Subjects: Thirteen patients, 8 women and 5 men, took part in the study (age: M = 44.11, SD = 11.76 years). Nine patients fulfilled the diagnostic criteria for persistent somatoform pain disorders (ICD-10: F45.4), the other patients with migraine headache fulfilled the diagnostic criteria for psychological and behavioral factors associated with disorders or diseases classified elsewhere (ICD-10: F54, G43). During a standardized instruction session, patients were introduced how to keep the Pain Diary. None of the patients received psychotherapeutic treatment during the initial phase of the behavioral therapy.

Electronic Bonn Pain Diary: Each patient kept a diary for 14 days. From the data only two variables were selected, firstly the amount of sleep (in hrs) and secondly the rated pain intensity. A complete description of all items and variables may be found in Ott and Scholz (1999).

Data Analysis

Data analysis in time-series experiments requires several steps. First, both variables were dichotomized based on the intercepts of the individual times-series. Second, *modified lag sequential analysis* (LSA, Faraone & Dorfman, 1984) was used in order to detect serial dependence within the data-points of the individual time series. LSA tests for auto- and cross-correlations over different time periods were applied to specified time lags. In this study we chose lag -1, lag 0, lag 1. In order to finally make inferences, what lag is most influential in the data, three *meta-analyses* (Stouffer method, see Rosenthal, 1984) were performed. The *p*-values resulting from the cross-correlations were agglomerated for the three lags. The calculations were made with the help of the Meta-Analysis program (Schwarzer, 1989).

Results

Table 4 presents the cross-correlations between pain intensity and sleep duration and their corresponding *z*- and *p*-values for each patient on the same day (lag 0) as well as on the preceding day (lag -1) and on the following day (lag 1), based on the individual time-series over 14 days.

Inspecting the results of a single-case LSA, one might easily conclude which patient shows what kind of serial dependencies. For example, patient A's current pain intensity was influenced by the sleep duration he had the day before (cross-correlation .59, lag -1). Patient D showed a different pattern. Here, the cross-correlation for lag 1 turned out to be the biggest of all three cross-correlations, which means, that his sleep duration is influenced by the pain intensity he experienced the day before.

To account for an overall comparison of the serial dependence between sleep duration and pain intensity, all of the *p*-values from the single-cases were then pooled using meta-analysis (see Table 4). Meta-analysis over the lag 0 results turned out to show the highest *Z*. Furthermore, pooled lag -1 data reached statistical significance, pooled lag 1 analysis did not. Thus, with regard to the whole sample, the analysis revealed a serial dependence – sleep duration did influence pain intensity of the following day. Vice versa serial dependence, that is, pain intensity influences the sleep duration of the following night, could not be found. A discussion of the clinical and practical impact of these results lies beyond the scope of this chapter.

Discussion

In this chapter we have focused on application-oriented robust methods for the analysis of short time-series like they typically result from diary studies. Following a framework introduced by Scholz (1995), a distinction between research questions about change within a single baseline design and covariation in a multiple baseline design is made. Data analysis for both cases was then illustrated in two examples. The use of time series methodology ensures that revealed effects could not be due to random variation, seasonal cycles, or long-term trends.

Both single-case and group-based designs have their advantages and disadvantages, with neither being universally better than the other. Rather, strategy of data analysis must be assessed by an investigator according to the parameters of a par-

Table 4. Results from modified lag-sequential analysis by Faraone and Dorfman (1987) for the diary variables pain intensity and sleep duration and succeeding meta-analysis

Patient	Crosscorrelations pain intensity today and sleep duration			z-values (and p-values) for the crosscorrelations pain intensity today and sleep duration		
	yesterday (lag -1)	today (lag 0)	tomorrow (lag 1)	yesterday (lag -1)	today (lag 0)	tomorrow (lag 1)
A	.59	.50	-.22	2.53 (.01)	2.13 (.02)	- 0.96 (.83)
B	-.30	.12	-.07	-1.33 (.90)	0.55 (.29)	- 0.31 (.62)
C	.04	-.12	.13	0.17 (.43)	-.55 (.70)	0.60 (.28)
D	.09	.29	.38	0.39 (.35)	1.21 (.11)	1.56 (.06)
E	.09	.40	.25	0.38 (.35)	1.69 (.05)	1.04 (.15)
F	.47	.54	.30	1.61 (.05)	1.84 (.03)	1.02 (.15)
G	.30	.49	.44	1.24 (.11)	1.99 (.02)	1.79 (.03)
H	.30	.47	.11	1.03 (.15)	1.64 (.05)	.38 (.35)
I	-.07	-.31	-.22	-.29 (.61)	-1.34 (.91)	-.98 (.84)
K	.09	-.34	-.49	.39 (.35)	-1.41 (.92)	-2.05 (.98)
L	.13	.28	.14	.58 (.28)	1.23 (.11)	.60 (.27)
M	.10	.33	-.11	.46 (.32)	1.57 (.06)	-.54 (.70)
N	.32	.00	-.25	1.33 (.09)	.02 (.50)	-1.01 (.85)
Meta-analysis			Z =	2.47	2.87	-0.04
			p =	.01	.00	.52

Notes: p-values were combined using the Stouffer method. Weighted solutions, more rigid statistical tests, were preferred because of results in unexpected directions.

ticular study. However, techniques for single-case analysis are far less well developed and promoted, and researchers tend to fall back on aggregating their data in a way enabling them to perform conventional group analysis, or to present arbitrarily chosen individual cases. In other words, we tend to choose between either losing all the detail we have, or seeing just the individual trees but no wood if we are only focusing on quantitative single-case data analyses.

Single-case designs may be preferable and generally present advantages in three occasions. First, research funds sometimes turn out to be scarce, especially for people working in private practice. Nevertheless, many clinicians pursue a scientist-practitioner model, or at least would like to pursue. Second, single-case designs are helpful when one whishes to intensively study the *process* of change. By taking many measurements over time, the single-case researcher can observe dynamic aspects of change over time. Third, in much clinical work the crucial question is "Does the treatment work for *this patient*," – but not – "Does the treatment work for the *average* patient". Group designs, well suited to answering the latter question, ignore the former. Only single-case designs allow rigorous objective experimental assessment of the efficacy of treatment for the individual.

There are many statistical alternatives available to single-case researchers and practitioners. Some of them have been described or illustrated within this chapter. A detailed description and evaluation of these and other statistical models is done by Franklin et al. (1996). However, even if we could not focus on the basic statistics behind these models, it should be stressed, that each technique has its inherent assumptions and limitations. For example, there is still an ongoing discussion about how to create test-statistics for testing cross-dependence and especially how to estimate confidence intervals in lag sequential analysis. The approach by Faraone and Dorfman (1987) used in study 2 has become very prominent in psychology research, although it has of course not been undefeated and replaced by other approaches in special data situations (for example, Bakeman & Quer, 1995). Preparing single-case research, therefore, also needs inspection of recent state-of-the-art in time-series analysis.

Although some analysis methods favor small-sample properties more than others, all techniques are severely limited by small sample-sizes. As Allison, Silverstein, and Gorman (1996) concluded by discussing power analysis in time-series models, all statistical techniques, whether parametric or nonparametric, will produce more precise estimates when sample size increases. However, most single-case studies lack the number of observations needed to achieve a robust power. Therefore, single-case studies are often restricted to test research hypotheses or establish the boundaries of parameter estimates more precisely. But single-case studies can ask in detail about the validity of established hypotheses. Perhaps the strongest suggestion to be made is that researchers should collect a greater number of observations, that is, focus on statistical power *before* designing diary studies.

When we started to work with time-series analysis of diary data several years ago, we were far more optimistic about the ease with which we could draw valid conclusions. We thought that if we had state-of-the-art statistical techniques single-case analysis should present no more, and possibly even fewer problems than should multi-subject designs. Somewhat foolishly we rushed to accumulate time-series results with a bunch of statistical procedures without any limitations. We are more cautious now but we are not pessimistic. Rather we believe that with better research designs and with the discovery of new statistical techniques, we can profit from the rich source provided by diary data.

References

Allison, D.B., Faith, M.S. & Gorman, B.S. (1995, August). *Type-I error in autocorrelated time series analyzed by randomization tests.* Paper presented at the American Psychological Convention, New York.

Allison, D.B., Silverstein, J.M. & Gorman, B.S. (1996). Power, sample size estimation, and early stopping rules. In R.D. Franklin, D.B. Allison & B.S. Gorman (Eds.), *Designs and analysis of single-case research* (pp. 335–372). Mahwah, New Jersey: Lawrence Erlbaum Associates.

Bakeman, R. & Quera, V. (1995). Log-linear approaches to lag-sequential analysis when consecutive codes may and cannot repeat. *Psychological Bulletin, 118*, 272–284.

Bortz, J., Lienert, G.A. & Boehnk, K. (2000). Verteilungsfreie Methoden in der Biostatistik (2. erw. Ausgabe). Berlin: Springer.

Box, G.E.P. & Jenkins, G.M. (1970). *Time series analysis: Forecasting and control.* San Francisco: Holden-Day.

Campbell, D.T. (1963). From description to experimentation: Interpreting trends as quasi-experiments. In C.W. Harris (Ed.), *Problems of measuring change* (pp. 163–198). Madison: University of Wisconsin Press.

Crosbie, J. (1993). Interrupted time-series analysis with brief single-subject data. *Journal of Consulting and Clinical Psychology, 61*, 966–974.

Edgington, E.S. (1987). *Randomization tests* (2nd ed.). New York: Marcel Dekker.

Faith, M.S., Allison, D.B. & Gorman, B.S. (1996). Meta-analysis of single-case research. In R.D. Franklin, D.B. Allison & B. S. Gorman (Eds.), *Designs and analysis of single-case research* (pp. 245–278). Mahwah, New Jersey: Lawrence Erlbaum Associates.

Faraone, S.V. & Dorfman, D.D. (1987). Lag sequential analysis: Robust statistical methods. *Psychological Bulletin, 101*, 312–323.

Franklin, R.D., Allison, D.B. & Gorman, B.S. (Eds.) (1996). *Designs and analysis of single-case research.* Mahwah, New Jersey: Lawrence Erlbaum Associates.

Hank, P. & Schwenkmezger, P. (1996). Computer-assisted versus paper-and-pencil based self monitoring: An analysis of experimental and psychometric equivalence. In J. Fahrenberg & M. Myrtek (Eds.), *Ambulatory assessment: computer-assisted psychological and psychophysiological methods in monitoring and field studies* (pp. 85–99). Toronto: Hogrefe & Huber.

Faraone, S.V. & Dorfman, D.D. (1987). Laq sequential analysis: Robust statistical methods. *Psychological Bulletin, 101*, 312–323.

Glass, G.V., Willson, V.L. & Gottman, J.M.. (1978). *Design and analysis of time-series experiments.* Boulder: Colorado Associated University Press.

Ittenbach, R.F. & Lawhead, W.F. (1996). Historical and philosophical foundations of single-case research. In R.D. Franklin, D.B. Allison & B.S. Gorman (Eds.), *Designs and analysis of single-case research* (pp. 159–214). Mahwah, New Jersey: Lawrence Erlbaum Associates.

Kazdin, A.E. (1982). *Single-case research designs: Methods for clinical and applied settings.* New York: Oxford University Press.

Neumann, J. von (1941). Distribution of ratio of the mean square successive difference to the variance. *Annals of Mathematical Statistics, 12*, 367–379.

Matyas, T.A. & Greenwood, K.M. (1990). The effect of serial dependence on visual judgment of single-case charts: An addendum. *Occupational Therapy Journal of Research, 10,* 208–220.

Matyas, T.A. & Greenwood, K.M. (1991). Problems in the estimation of autocorrelations in brief time series: some implications for empirical data. *Behavioral Assessment, 13,* 137–157.

Ostrom, C.W. (1978). *Time series analysis: regression techniques.* Beverly Hills: Sage.

Ott, R., Hinkel, M. & Scholz, O.B. (2000). Das Elektronische Bonner Schmerztagebuch (EBST): Vorstellung einer PC Desktop Version für den stationären Bereich [The Electronic Bonn Pain Diary: A desktop version for the inpatient setting]. *Verhaltenstherapie, 10*, 160–165.

Ott, R. & Scholz, O.B. (1999). Das Elektronische Bonner Schmerztagebuch (EBST): Vorstellung eines computergestützten Verfahrens zur Schmerzdiagnostik [The Electronic Bonn Pain Diary: Proposal for a computer-aided method of pain diagnosis]. *Zeitschrift für Klinische Psychologie, Psychiatrie und Psychotherapie, 47,* 191–206.

Rosenthal, R. (1984). *Meta-analytic procedures for social research.* Beverly Hills, C.A: Sage.

Sackett, G.P. (1979). The lag sequential analysis of contingency and cyclicity in behavioral interaction research. In J.D. Osofsky (Ed.), *Handbook of infant development* (pp. 623–649). New York: Wiley.

Scholz, O.B. (1995). Was leisten Schmerztagebücher? Vorzüge und Grenzen ihrer Anwendung unter besonderer Berücksichtigung einzelfallbezogener Auswertung [What can pain diaries achieve? Advantages and limitations of their use with reference to single case evaluation]. *Der Schmerz, 9,* 107–116.

Scholz, O.B. & Ott, R. (2000). Tape based hypnotherapeutic treatment in sleep disorders: time series data from sleep diaries. *Australian Journal of Clinical Hypnotherapy and Hypnosis, 21,* 96–114.

Seemann, H. (1997). Tagebuchverfahren – Eine Einführung. In G. Wilz & E. Brähler (Eds.), *Tagebücher in Therapie und Forschung* [Diaries in research and practice] (pp. 13–33). Göttingen: Hogrefe.

Schwarzer, R. (1989). *Meta-Analysis* (Version 5.3) [Computer Software]. Freie Universität Berlin, Germany: Department of Psychology.

Chapter 12
A Multilevel Approach to Analyze Ambulatory Assessment Data: An Examination of Family Members' Emotional States in Daily Life

Peter Wilhelm
Psychology Department, University of Fribourg, Switzerland

Introduction

Ambulatory assessment research leads to data sets that usually have two main sources of variation: *Variation between persons*, due to stable individual characteristics (traits) and *variation within persons* due to states or circumstances that change within the timeframe of the observation period, the latter being nested within the former. This specific structure of the data allows researchers to answer interesting questions about the influence of a) traits, b) states (or situations) and c) the interaction between traits and states (or situations), but it also complicates the statistical analysis (see Larson & Delespaul, 1992; Schwartz & Stone, 1998). One major problem for data analysis is, that the particular observations within a person are interrelated and often show patterns over time. Common approaches to control dependence within the framework of conventional statistical methods often eliminate undesired variation.

Thus, researchers interested in situation or state effects, have eliminated the entire between subject variation by introducing a set of N-1 "person" dummy variables as covariates into a regression analysis or using other techniques. This approach ignores individual differences and has several other disadvantages (see Larson & Delespaul, 1992; Schwartz & Stone, 1998).

Other investigators prefer to keep the between person variation and eliminate undesired within person variation by aggregation. Computing for each person the average over different types of situations allows the comparison of these situations as well as the analysis of trait effects and the trait by situation interaction with repeated measurement ANOVA. This data analytic strategy is rather easy to apply and to communicate, but it has also several disadvantages such as reduction of power, varying reliability of the aggregated measures due to a different amount of observations per person, loss of a whole case when a particular situation type is missing and limited possibilities to control other effects.

Others have applied two stage procedures, some of them using time-series approaches to investigate individual processes in a first step and then taking the results of the separate individual analysis in a second step to further analyze them in a meta-analytic fashion (for example, Pawlik & Buse, 1994; Pihet, 2000; Reicherts & Pihet, in press). However, this approach also has to deal with problems (for example, sufficient number of observations, unequal spacing between observations, missing observations, necessity to check for trends, cyclical components, and serial dependencies, difficulty of comparing single case parameters if they rely on different combinations of control variables; Suen & Ary, 1989; West & Hepworth, 1991).

Troubles become worse if one has to treat self-monitoring data gathered from family-members (or individuals belonging to the same group, such as work teams, etc.). In this situation a further level of dependence occurs, because family-members are in many aspects more similar than randomly sampled individuals. Ignoring existing similarity and just analyzing the data on the individual level may invalidate significance testing, because the true alpha error is usually inflated (Kenny, Kashy & Bolger, 1998). Different conceptual and statistical models to disentangle the structure of within and between group variation were proposed (for example, Gonzales & Griffin, 1999; Kenny, 1996; Kenny et al., 1998), but they are not conceptualized to deal with complex within subject variation.

A solution for the data analytic problems discussed here is available in the framework of the multilevel approach. The purpose of this contribution is to show the usefulness of multilevel modeling for the analysis of data, as they are gathered when one uses ambulatory assessment methods. After a short introduction into basic concepts of multilevel analysis, an example of its application to family-self-observation data is given.

The multilevel approach

Multilevel models have been developed in the context of educational research in the 80ies (Goldstein, 1995), and have been spread out into many research areas of medical and social sciences in recent years (for example, Hedeker & Gibbons, 1996; Jones, 1993; Kenny et al., 1998; Langford, Bentham & McDonald, 1998; Raudenbush, Brennan & Barnett, 1995; Schwartz, Warren & Pickering, 1994; Snijders & Kenny, 1999). Because different authors work in the field, different terms exist, to name essentially the same type of statistical models: for example, *mixed-effects regression models, random-effects models, hierarchical linear models, empirical Bayes models* (see Hedeker & Gibbons, 1996). The multilevel approach is an extension of the multiple regression/correlation analysis (Cohen & Cohen, 1983) that allows to treat data, that are nested within a hierarchical structure (such as repeated observations, that are nested within individuals, that are nested within families or groups).

Multilevel analyses provide intercept and slope parameters that are similar to the unstandardized coefficients in an ordinary multiple regression analysis. These parameters are called *fixed parameters*. All of them or only a selection can vary at the different levels of the hierarchy. For each fixed parameter that is allowed to vary a variance component is computed, that is regarded as an estimation of the variance in the underlying population. If more than one parameter is allowed to vary the covariances are estimated as well. The variance and covariance estimates are called *random parameters*. Modeling at least the variation of the intercept at each level of the hierarchy is the way to adjust the parameter estimates and their standard errors for the amount of dependency that is due to the hierarchical structure of the data. Thus, there is no need for aggregation. Data can be analyzed at the level of the single observations, keeping all the original information, providing high power for the significance testing and allowing the control of many other variables simultaneously. Furthermore, multilevel models do not need balanced data sets. Every person (case) that provides at least one valid observation is going to be analyzed.

There are various software packages available (see Snijders & Bosker, 1999). We use *MLwiN*, which was developed by the Multilevel Models Project at the University of London (Rasbash, Browne, Goldstein, Yang, Plewis, et al., 2000; actual information can be obtained from the web side: *http://www.ioe.ac.uk/MLwiN/*). *MLwiN* uses an iterative generalized least square (IGLS) algorithm to get estimates of the parameters. At convergence these estimates are maximum likelihood (for computational details, see Goldstein, 1995). The procedure computes a measure that is called deviance, which indicates how well the specified model fits the data. If two models are nested, the difference of their deviances has a χ^2 distribution with degrees of freedom that are equal to the difference in the number of parameters estimated in the two models. This statistic can be used to test if a new model has a significant better data fit.

The multilevel framework is a large and quite complex family of statistical tools that can be fitted to a broad range of applications. For further conceptual as well as mathematical details, the reader is referred to the literature (for example, Goldstein, 1995; Snijders & Bosker, 1999; a short and comprehensible introduction is given by Jones, 1993).

A multilevel analysis of the emotional state in families daily life

In this chapter a multilevel analysis is applied to investigate the influence of basic situational factors, like time of the observation, local setting, social contact, and current activity on the emotional state of family members. The data were gathered in the Fribourg Family Project. 314 mothers, fathers, and their adolescent children from 96 families reported their emotional state and additional information six times a day over the course of a week, using a computerized self observational system (FASEM-C; see Perrez, Wilhelm, Schoebi & Horner, in this book). Therefore the data matrix should contain 314 * 6 * 7 = 13188 single observations. A part of the observations was missing (about 7 percent), therefore the number of single observations that could be analyzed was 12278. The emotional state was measured as the average score over eight bipolar items that have been found to create a common factor and have a high situation specific reliability (Cronbach's alpha = .95; see Perrez, Schoebi & Wilhelm, 2000). To make small effects better interpretable, the original six point scale was transformed to a scale that ranges from 0 (very bad) to 100 (very good).

Decomposition of the total variance

First we set up different models without any explanatory variables (intercept-only-models) to decompose the total variance. This gives us information about how much variance exists at each level and how many levels we should use to model the hierarchical structure of our data. The different variance estimates can also be used to calculate intra-class-correlation-coefficients (ICC), which are measures for the amount of similarity in terms of shared variance between the single units belonging to a certain level (see Snijders & Bosker, 1999, for computational details). The initial steps showed that the data structure was best represented by a four level model (*model-1)*, where the single observations (level 1) were nested within days (level 2), that were nested within individuals (level 3), who were nested within families (level 4).

The decomposition of the total variance of 293.9, showed that 16.2 percent of the total variation is accounted for by family membership (level 4), 28.6 percent is due to differences between individuals within families (level 3), 12.7 percent is variation between days within family-members (level 2) and 42.5 percent is variation of the single observation within days within family-members (level 1). Thus, 55.2 percent of the total variability is variation within individuals and 44.8 percent between them. The average amount of similarity between two emotional state ratings within an individual is given by the corresponding ICC = (44.8 / (44.8 + 55.2)) = .448. The ICC for general mood in family-members is (16.2/(16.2 + 28.6)) = .362, indicating that about 36 percent of the inter-individual variation in mood is due to family membership. This shows that the emotional climate in the family has quite a substantial impact on how people feel.

Time related effects

The aim of the next steps was, to model the time dependent structure of the data. We began with a composition of the fixed part: Mean differences in the *emotional* *state between days of the week* were estimated for Friday, Saturday and Sunday (dummy coded, with Monday to Thursday as the reference category). To model changes in the *emotional state within days* from morning to evening, the linear, quadratic and cubic trend was estimated (coded as orthogonal polynomials). These trends were supposed to be different on Friday, Saturday, and Sunday (3 * 3 interaction effects between the days mentioned and the trend components). In the random part the intercept was allowed to vary at each of the four levels. This *model-2* had a much better data fit than model-1 (reduction in deviance: $\chi^2_{(15)} = 217.8$; $p < .000001$). Removing six of the nine interaction effects that were far from being significant (alpha = .05 two tailed, according to the Wald-test, which is a t-ratio, that can be obtained by dividing the parameter estimate through it's associated standard error) simplified the new *model-3* without loosing much information ($\chi^2_{(6)} = 8.2$; $p > .20$). Previous analysis had shown that people generally tend to report better emotional states in the last days of the self observation than in the first days (Perrez et al., 2000). To take this *reactivity* effect into account a linear and quadratic trend for the rank-order of the observation days (coded as orthogonal polynomials) was added, resulting in a significantly better fitting new *model-4* ($\chi^2_{(2)} = 18.8$; $p < .0001$). Because some families had an *official holiday* during their observation week, a dummy variable was further introduced to control for that influence (*model-5*). This last step did not result in a significant improvement of the model fit ($\chi^2_{(1)} = 1.6$; $p > .20$). The fixed parameter estimates of model 5 are shown in Table 1 and it's random parameter estimates in Table 2.

Elaboration of the random part of the model

In the models estimated so far, only the intercept was allowed to vary at each level. Especially for the within subject part, these models are probably too restrictive. They assume implicitly that the variance for every observation and the covariance between each pair of observations within a day is equal and that the same is true for the variance and covariance of the days of the week. Usually repeated measurement data have a more complex covariance structure. They often show patterns of serial autocorrelation. Also the variances might be different for different points in time. Taking such patterns into account for the within subject error part is necessary, because an inadequate specification of the error part, can lead to unreliable standard errors for the fixed effect estimates.

One way to reduce the amount of autocorrelation in the within subject error part, is to allow not only the intercepts but also the slopes of the time related effects to vary. This has the consequence, that these effects can be better adapted to existing differences between persons. If the estimated effects are closer to the individual data, the absolute amount of error at the lower level as well as the autocorrelation at this level will be reduced (see Snijders & Bosker, 1999).

Therefore the random part of model-5 was elaborated further. We allowed the three within day trend components to vary over days (level 2) as well as over individuals (level 3). Individual differences were further modeled for the linear and quadratic component of the reactivity effect and for differences between weekend and weekdays (dummy coded). The deviance of this *model-6* was reduced to a large extend ($\chi^2_{(36)} = 730.4; p < .000001$). In order to keep the random part as simple as possible, non-significant variance or covariance estimates were constrained to be zero in the next analysis. The resulting *model-7* fit's the data not significantly worse than model-6 ($\chi^2_{(20)} = 12.6; p > .20$), but is much simpler.

Interpretation of the time related fixed effects

The *intercept* of model-7 (Table 1) represents the emotional state, for a normal day of the week between Monday and Thursday, of an average person, in an average family, when reactivity effects are controlled. The value of 76.4 indicates that people in general feel quite well. There are significant *weekend effects* and also during *holidays* the emotional state is above the mean of the weekdays, but it fails to become significant, because of its low frequency. Only the linear *reactivity*-trend is significant, indicating a linear increase of the emotional state of about 2.59 units (7 * 0.37) between the first and the last observation day.

Within a day the emotional state increases usually from morning to evening, with two turning points (significant linear and cubic trend) (see Figure 1, where the observed and estimated emotional state over the course of the week is shown). On Friday, the increase from morning to evening is twice that of the other days. For

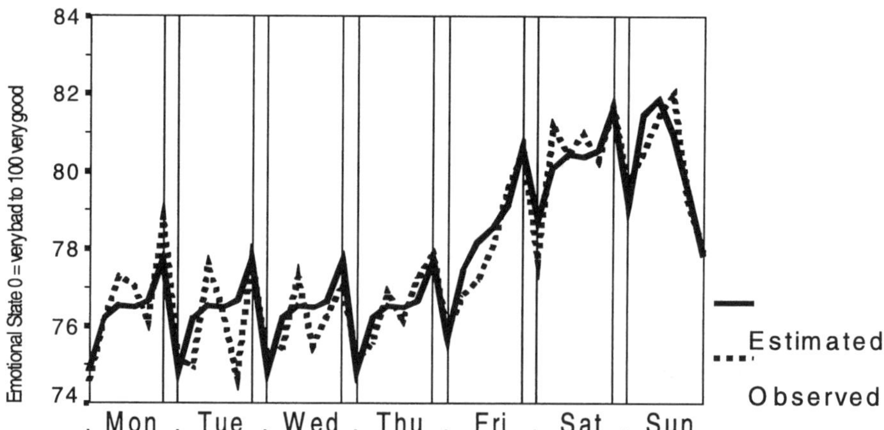

Figure 1: Estimated and observed emotional state over the course of the week.
Notes: The estimated emotional state is based on the parameters of model-7. The observed emotional state represents the mean of each single observation computed overall the persons. The double lines between two days indicate the night period without observations.

Table 1. Fixed parameter estimates of the different models

	model-5		model-7		model-11		model-14		model-17	
	param.	SE	param.	SE	param.	SE	param.	SE	param.	SE
Intercept	76.42	(0.90)f	76.40	(0.89)f	75.16	(1.19)f	76.00	(1.22)f	75.60	(1.10)f
Adolescent (=1, par.= 0)					1.85	(1.55)	1.42	(1.55)	2.27	(1.42)
Female (=1, masc.= 0)					1.35	(1.35)	1.13	(1.34)	0.56	(1.23)
Female * Adolescent					-0.64	(2.34)	-0.49	(2.34)	-0.67	(2.14)
Weekdays (0=Mon-Thu)										
Friday	1.77	(0.48)c	1.88	(0.42)e	1.84	(0.41)e	1.70	(0.41)d	1.47	(0.38)d
Saturday	4.07	(0.48)f	3.91	(0.49)f	3.82	(0.49)f	3.40	(0.49)f	2.77	(0.45)f
Sunday	3.60	(0.48)f	3.71	(0.49)f	3.87	(0.49)f	3.47	(0.49)f	3.07	(0.45)f
Holiday (=1, other=0)	2.47	(1.95)	2.32	(1.84)	1.90	(1.79)	1.29	(1.79)	1.29	(1.65)
Reactivity										
Linear trend	0.31	(0.08)c	0.37	(0.11)c	0.20	(0.14)	0.19	(0.13)	0.16	(0.11)
Quadratic trend	0.06	(0.05)	0.06	(0.05)	0.08	(0.05)	0.09	(0.05)	0.10	(0.04)a
Linear tr.*Adolescent					0.47	(0.22)a	0.48	(0.22)a	0.32	(0.19)
Trends within days										
Linear trend	0.22	(0.03)f	0.22	(0.04)f	0.23	(0.04)f	0.15	(0.05)b	0.14	(0.04)c
Quadratic trend	-0.02	(0.03)	-0.03	(0.03)	0.10	(0.04)a	0.08	(0.05)	0.05	(0.05)
Cubic trend	0.06	(0.02)c	0.06	(0.02)c	0.06	(0.02)c	0.06	(0.02)b	0.05	(0.02)b
Linear trend * Friday	0.26	(0.09)b	0.21	(0.10)a	0.21	(0.09)a	0.16	(0.09)	0.10	(0.09)
Linear trend * Sunday	-0.38	(0.09)d	-0.42	(0.10)d	-0.43	(0.10)e	-0.39	(0.10)c	-0.33	(0.09)c
Quadr. trend * Sunday	-0.30	(0.08)c	-0.30	(0.08)c	-0.32	(0.08)d	-0.22	(0.08)b	-0.19	(0.07)b
Quadr. trend * females					-0.23	(0.06)c	-0.20	(0.06)c	-0.19	(0.06)c
Local setting (0=home)										
At work or school							-1.12	(0.44)a	-1.13	(0.41)b
At another place							1.11	(0.36)b	0.91	(0.34)b
Social contact (0=fam.)										
Alone							-0.09	(0.27)	0.16	(0.26)
Other people							1.99	(0.40)f	1.70	(0.38)e
Other people + family							1.99	(0.44)e	1.48	(0.42)c
Activities (0=leisure)										
Working for job/school							-2.38	(0.41)f	0.00	(0.40)
Working for the family							-2.24	(0.42)f	1.00	(0.41)b
Taking a meal							-0.26	(0.42)	-0.66	(0.39)
Regeneration							-1.04	(0.36)b	-1.94	(0.35)f
Other activities							-1.07	(0.34)b	-0.09	(0.33)
Valuation of activities									4.61	(0.15)f
Valuation of act * Ado									-1.04	(0.22)e
Outlier code: 11513									-77.96	(6.86)f

Notes: param. = fixed parameter estimates; SE = standard error. After the standard errors the significance level of the Wald-Test (parameter estimates /standard error) is indicated by letters: a < .05, b < .01, c < .001, d < .0001, e < .00001, f < .000001, two tailed.

most people weekend begins Friday afternoon and is associated with a substantially better emotional state. On Sunday the within day pattern deviates from that of the other days, because in the afternoon the emotional state turns down and decreases until evening. This can be interpreted as the mental and emotional anticipation to work- or school-demands.

Interpretation of the random effects

The random part of model-7 was elaborated to fit the within-subject error structure better to the data, but the variance and covariance components can also be interpreted and give interesting information that is not available from usual analysis (see Table 2).

The *variance of the intercept at level four* (families) shows us, how much the emotional climate might differ between families. A family with a typically high emotional state during weekdays (top 2.5 percent) will have a value of about two standard deviations above the mean ($76.4 + 2 * \sqrt{43} = 89.5$) and a family with a typically low emotional state (bottom 2.5 percent) will be two standard deviations below and has a value of about 63.3.

The *variance of the intercept at level three* (individuals) tells us, how much the members of one family might differ from each other in their average emotional state over the weekdays from Monday to Friday (because the variance at the weekend is allowed to be different). For 95 percent of the family members their emotional state will be less than $2 * \sqrt{95} = 19.5$ units apart from the family mean. This is a substantial amount of potential diversity within families. The level three random part contains

Table 2: Random parameter estimates of model-5, model-7, model-11

	Model-5	Model-7						Model-11					
Level 4 (families)													
f1 Intercept	47.1e	43.0e						44.1e					
Level 3 (persons)		p1	p2	p3	p4	p5	p6	p1	p2	p3	p4	p5	p6
p1 Intercept	85.0f	95.1f						93.7f					
p2 Weekend		-.36c	15.9d					-.37c	17.8e				
p3 Reactivity linear trend		.18a		2.39f				.16a		2.25f			
p4 Reactivity quadrat. tr.		-.26a		-.28a	0.22d			-.29a		-.35a	0.17c		
p5 Within day linear tr.				.41b		0.11b				.39b		0.11c	
p6 Within day quadr. tr.						-.97d	0.08c					-.85c	0.07b
Level 2 (days)		d1	d5	d6	d7			d1	d5	d6	d7		
d1 Intercept	33.8f	20.8f						15.6f					
d5 Within day linear tr.		.13a	1.06f					.15a	0.95f				
d6 Within day quadr. tr.		-.61f	.55f	0.42f				-.69f	.55f	0.35f			
d7 Within day cubic tr.			-.66f		0.10e				-.67f		0.10e		
d*COV* Intercept-female								5.3c					
Level 1 (observations)													
o1 Intercept	123.4f	95.0f						71.6f					
o*COV* Intercept-adolesc.								19.6f					
o*COV* Intercept-female								10.6f					

Notes: Bold figures in the diagonal are the variance parameters, below the diagonal are the correlation-coefficients. *COV* = covariance-term. After the parameter estimates the significance level of the Wald-Test is indicated by letters: a < .05, b < .01, c < .001, d < .0001, e < .00001, f < .000001, one tailed for variance estimates, two tailed for covariance estimates and correlation coefficients. Empty cells have been constricted to zero.

contains also random slope parameters and their covariances (for reasons of simplicity, only the correlations are reported in Table 2). The variation between individuals is therefore not constant over all the observations, but is a function of the variance and covariance of the other variables allowed to vary. At the weekend, for example, the variance between family members is substantially lower than during the weekdays and takes the value of 83 instead of 95 (variance of the intercept (95.1) + 2 * covariance between intercept and slope variance (2 * - 14.1) + the slope variance (15.9) = 82.8).

The *slope variance estimates at level three* tell us, how large the expected individual differences of the corresponding effects are. For individuals who show a very strong positive weekend effect (top 2.5 percent), the increase in the emotional state would be expected to be 2 * √15.85, that is 8 units above the estimated fixed effects for difference between usual weekdays and Saturday or Sunday of about 3.3 to 3.5. (The estimates here are not exactly equal to the fixed effects in Table 1, because Friday has to be taken as a normal weekday and therefore the difference between weekend and weekday becomes smaller). On the other hand, individuals on the bottom 2.5 percent will be 8 units below the estimated fixed effect and show even a decrease in mood on weekends. The correlation between the intercept and slope variance is r = -.36 and gives us the information that the higher the average emotional state of an individual during weekdays, the lower is the increase at the weekend. This might reflect a ceiling effect of the emotional state scale. The other variance estimates can be interpreted in a similar way.

The *intercept variance at level two* indicates how much the emotional state within a single individual differs over the days of the self observation, when individual differences for the weekend effect, as well as the individual differences in the trend estimates of the reactivity effect are modeled at level three. Allowing the between day effects to be different for each individual, leads to the substantial reduction in the level two intercept variance between model-5 and model-7.

All the *within day trend components* vary from day to day (level two), indicating substantial day to day deviations from the idealized pattern that show up in the fixed parameter estimates (Figure 1). Looking at the interval in which 95 percent of the linear trend estimates vary around the fixed parameter (0.22 +/- 2 * √1.06 = 0.22 +/- 2.1) reveals that one day the emotional state of the same person might increase from morning to evening, whereas the next day it might decrease. The correlations between the linear and the other trends (r = .55 with the quadratic trend and r = - .66. with the cubic trend) indicate that the within day pattern is likely to change completely. The variances of the within day slopes at level three show that there are also stable individual differences for the linear and quadratic trend component. However, the intra-individual variation between days is six to ten times larger than the variation between persons.

The *intercept variation at level one* indicates how far the single observations within each day might be apart from the values predicted by the model. Compared with model-5 level one residual variance dropped more than a quarter down to 95, mainly because trend slopes were allowed to vary at level two.

Differences between fathers, mothers and adolescents

The models fitted so far assume that there are no systematic differences between parents and their adolescent children, nor between male and female family members. This is very unlikely. Therefore we added dummy coded variables for sex, generation (parent vs. adolescent), and the interaction of generation by sex to model the family roles (*model-8*). The fit of this model does not improve significantly ($\chi^2(3) = 2.0$; $p > .20$), indicating that there are no substantial differences in the *average emotional state* between the family members.

Larson and Richards (1994) could show with the ESM-method that adolescents experience extreme emotional states more often than their parents. If this is also true in our sample, adolescents should have a higher within day variability than their parents. They also might have more changes in their emotional states from day to day. To model this *different variability* for adolescents, an adolescent-intercept covariance parameter was added at level one (observations) and at level two (days). For women comparable hypotheses exist. They are supposed to be more emotionally reactive than men are and should, therefore, also have more within day variability in their emotional state and probably also more variation in the average emotional state from day to day. To model the different variability for women, a female-intercept covariance parameter was added at both levels. The new *model-9* results in a much better fit than model-8 ($\chi^2_{(4)} = 225$; $p < .000001$). The expectations were confirmed except one. According to the Wald-test criterion, variability between days was not estimated to be larger for adolescents than for their parents. This parameter was dropped in *model-10.*

The level one intercept now represents the within day variation of the fathers emotional state that can not be explained by other estimates (the parameter estimates are equal to the ones shown in table 2 for model-11). The variability of the other family members can be inferred by adding two times the corresponding covariance to the intercept of 71.6, resulting in a variance of 92.8 for the mothers, 110.8 for the sons, and 131.0 for the daughters. Differences in the day to day variability only exist between males (intercept variance estimate at level two = 15.6) and females (intercept + 2 * level two covariance = 15.6 + 2 * 5.3 = 26.2). The results show that there are large differences in the short-term fluctuations and also in the midterm variability of the emotional state between males and females, suggesting that they might have different emotional experiences in their daily lives. For adolescents, differences are much larger than for adults, but only at the level of faster changing states.

In the next step we explored if there are any differences between the family roles in the mean pattern of the emotional state over the course of the week. Therefore, we expanded the fixed part, adding interaction terms with all the parameters describing the emotional state over time (except holidays) and each of the three dummy variables containing the family role information. Of the 33 interaction parameters, only two were significant according to the Wald-test. Keeping only the two significant interaction parameters in *model-11,* results in a better fit compared to model-10 ($\chi^2_{(2)} = 18.2; p < .001$). In model-11 the linear reactivity trend remains significant only for adolescents (Table 1), due to the significant linear trend by adolescent interaction. A further change appears in the within day trends, because the quadratic trend for females is estimated to be different from the quadratic trend for males, indicating a different within day pattern for females. The interaction effects reduce corresponding slope variance at level three and two (Table 2).

Local setting, social contacts and type of activity

In the next set of analysis we asked how the local and social setting as well as the type of current activity influences the emotional state of people. Beginning with the *local setting,* two dummy coded variables were introduced in the fixed part of model-11. One indicating being at work and the other being at another place (at friends, in the public, on the way or elsewhere), where the reference category was being at home. The resulting *model-12* had a significantly better data fit ($\chi^2_{(2)} = 74; p < .000001$).

To test the effects of *social contacts* on the emotional state, three dummy variables were added. One for being alone, the second for being together with somebody who does not belong to the family (friends, colleagues, boss, or other people), the third for being at the same time together with other family-members and somebody who does not belong to the family. The reference category was being together with one or more family members, but not with any other person. The effects of the social setting were significant (*model-13*) ($\chi^2_{(3)} = 50.7; p < .000001$). The results show that being alone is not worse than being together with the family (-0.23 units, $p = .19$). But to be with other people is related to a better emotional state, than only being with family members, no matter if other family members then are present (2,03 units, $p < .0001$) or absent (1.90 units, $p < .0001$). In the first family project we found the same results using a conventional strategy to analyze the data (Wilhelm, Horner & Perrez, 2000). It is worth noting here that controlling for the effects of social contact leads to a change in the parameter estimates of the local setting of the previous model. Being at work has now a stronger negative effect (-1.87 units, $p < .0001$) and being at another place a weaker positive effect (1.19 units, $p < .001$). This happens because the local setting is interrelated with social contacts. Ignoring the interdependence between social contact and local setting, will lead to incorrect conclusions (Wilhelm et al., 2000).

The *type of activity* a person was involved in just before the recording, was entered as a set of five dummy coded variables: working for the job; working for the family; sleep/rest; taking a meal; doing something else. Leisure time activities or doing something for oneself was the reference category. The deviance of the new *model-14* improved significantly ($\chi^2_{(5)} = 55.1$; $p < .0001$). The effects show, that following a leisure activity, or taking a meal is associated with a better emotional state, than doing something else. Working something for the job or for the family is associated with the worst emotional state.

The control of setting, social contacts, and activity reduces the weekend effect as well as the amount of increase in the emotional state from morning to evening (see model-11 vs. model-14 in Table 1). This could be expected because setting and activity as well as the social contacts are structured over time. The different effects are therefore confounded. The random parameters change only slightly (Table 3).

In a further step all the possible interaction effects between family role and setting, social contacts, and type of activity were explored, but none of them were significant.

Table 3: Random parameter estimates of model-14 and model-17

	Model-14						Model-17					
Level 4 (families)												
f1 Intercept	44.5e						34.5d					
Level 3 (persons)	p1	p2	p3	p4	p5	p6	p1	p2	p3	p4	p5	p6
p1 Intercept	92.6f						76.7f					
p2 Weekend	-.37c	16.0d					-.32b	14.6e				
p3 Reactivity linear trend	.15		2.14f				.21a		1.40f			
p4 Reactivity quadrat. tr.	-.30a		-.31a	0.16c			-.32a		-.15	0.12c		
p5 Within day linear tr.			.28a		0.12c				.27		0.12c	
p6 Within day quadrat. tr.					-.89c	0.06b					-.74c	0.07c
Level 2 (days)	d1	d5	d6	d7			d1	d5	d6	d7		
d1 Intercept	15.3f						11.4f					
d5 Within day linear trend	.17b	0.91f					.18b	0.78f				
d6 Within day quadrat. tr.	-.68f	.53f	0.34f				-.69f	.47f	0.28f			
d7 Within day cubic tr.		-.69f		0.10e				-.73f		0.08d		
d*COV* Intercept-female	5.4d						5.4e					
Level 1 (observations)												
o1 Intercept	70.3f						63.5f					
o*COV* Intercept-adolescent	19.7f						18.9f					
o*COV* Intercept-female	10.6f						9.7f					

Notes: Bold figures in the diagonal are the variance parameters, below the diagonal are the correlation-coefficients. *COV* = covariance-term. After the parameter estimates the significance level of the Wald-Test is indicated by letters: a < .05, b < .01, c < .001, d < .0001, e < .00001, f < .000001, one tailed for variance estimates, two tailed for covariance estimates and correlation coefficients. Empty cells have been constricted to zero.

Looking for outliers

Checking the model assumptions reveals that the residuals at level one and level two were more extreme at the very ends of the distribution than expected. After a closer inspection of the data we decided to control the influence of the most negative residual at level two (days) with a dummy variable. The data came from an adolescent who gave very bad estimates for his emotional state in the first two days of the observation, but without indicating that something negative had happened. Because the entire family had computer problems during the first days, these data were regarded as potentially artificial. The fit of *model-15* improved substantially ($\chi^2_{(1)}$ = 100.9; $p < .000001$). Other extreme values were not excluded because there was not enough evidence that they were artificial. Sometimes people feel in a really bad mood from one moment to another. Excluding such moments because they do not fit the statistical expectation, would give us a wrong picture of the processes as they happen in real life.

Valuation of the current activity

In the last step the *subjective valuation of the current activity*, measured on a 6-point scale ranging from very uncomfortable to very comfortable, was entered. (The variable was centered around the mean). The new *model-16* had a much better data fit than model-15 ($\chi^2_{(1)}$ = 1269.9; $p < .000001$). This variable has now a remarkable effect on the emotional state. If the current activity was rated as very uncomfortable, the emotional state was 20.9 units lower than when it was rated as very comfortable. Exploring the interaction effects between valuation and the family roles revealed one significant result that improved the fit of *model-17* ($\chi^2_{(1)}$ = 22.3, with 1 df, $p < .00001$). For adolescents the effect was weaker than for their parents (3.6 vs. 4.6 units).

The results indicate that the type of activity has a less important influence on the emotional state, than it's valuation. As could be expected, most effects due to type of activity were reduced close to zero, after controlling for valuation (Table 1). One exception is the effect of housework on mood that even changes its direction. This happens because housework was rated as being the most uncomfortable activity, but has not such a strong negative effect on mood. The same argument in reverse explains why regeneration has an even stronger negative effect. Controlling for the valuation of the current activity, further reduces the effects in the time related variables (amount of within day change, weekend effects) as well as the effects of the social setting. It also reduces the variance at each level of the random part by a substantial amount (Table 3).

Discussion and summary

The last model presented could be further extended to answer additional questions about the influence of other situational or state variables, (for example, having a conflict, feeling pain, etc.) or the impact of personality traits or family variables on the emotional state of family members.

Nonetheless, the models reported so far have shown interesting features. It could be demonstrated that basic situational factors like observation time, local setting, social contact, and current activity each have an own significant effect on the emotional state, even when the effects of the other factors are statistically controlled. However, a closer look at the effect sizes reveals that they are quite small. For example, in model-14 the biggest effect was the difference in the emotional state between Sunday and weekdays of about 3.47 units. If one takes into account the total range of the scale (0 to 100) or has a look at the standardized coefficient, which has a value of .07, this effect appears to be quite small. One reason for the rather small impact of the situational variables might be the fact that they describe objective features of daily life environments. According to appraisal theories, emotions are the result of evaluation and attribution processes (Scherer, 1988). So the subjective interpretation and appraisal of situational features should influence the emotional state more than the objective situational characteristics. In the current analysis, this interpretation is supported by the fact, that the valuation of the current activity had the highest association with the emotional state (standardized coefficient = .25).

Differences between family members were rare, despite the fact that all possible interaction effects with family roles have been explored. The biggest effects were found in the variability of the emotional state that was higher for females and adolescents.

To reduce autocorrelation, which is supposed to exist in the residuals of level one and level two, we allowed the slopes of the time related variables to vary between persons and between days. Here we followed the advise of Goldstein, Healy and Rasbash (1994), that *"it would seem preferable to incorporate as much as possible of an individual-specific structure before introducing an autocorrelation structure"* (p. 1653). Nevertheless, one can criticize that we did not estimate the amount of serial dependence in the residuals. This is possible with *MLwiN*, but not within the standard software package. One has to work with special macros (Yang, Rasbash, Goldstein & Barbosa, 1999). For our data the estimation of the adequate autocorrelation functions is especially complicated because autocorrelation is expected to exist at two levels. Ignoring serial autocorrelation in the residuals, does not effect the fixed parameter estimates, but leads to an underestimation of the corresponding standard errors as well as an underestimation of the within-subject variance and an overestimation of the between subject variance (Schwartz & Stone, 1998; Suen & Ary, 1989). Because most of the fixed effects are highly significant ($p < .001$), the conclusions drawn from these results would not change substantially, even if autocorrelation had been identified and controlled for. However, for a reliable decomposition of the between and within-subject variation, serial autocorrelation should be taken into account.

Multilevel models are able to treat specific characteristics of ambulatory assessment data that are difficult or even impossible to treat with conventional statistical strategies (see introduction). With multilevel models one can handle multiple sources of dependency, just through modeling the hierarchical levels that exist in the data. Lower level variables have not to be aggregated and can be analyzed together with higher level variables. Thus all the available information is used, resulting in a high power to detect even small effects (at the least at the lower levels). It further allows the simultaneous statistical control of many variables that might have an undesired influence on the effects of interest. This is especially important for ambulatory assessment research, where the statistical control of confounding effects is often the only way to strengthen the validity of the conclusions. Multilevel models do not rely on balanced data sets. This is a big advantage over standard repeated measurement ANOVAs that usually exclude all cases that do not provide an observation in every situation compared and therefore produce subsamples, which diminish power and create problems for generalization.

The possibility to allow for variation in the intercepts and slopes, is an easy way to reduce autocorrelation and heteroscedasticity in the data. In addition, the estimated random parameters contain information about how different effects might operate at the different levels of the hierarchy. This provides a much better description and understanding of the data, than it could be obtained with other statistical approaches.

Multilevel models share disadvantages of other multivariate data analytic methods (for example, Structural Equation Modeling). The analysis is complex and, therefore, artifacts and errors are difficult to identify. This makes a careful check of the raw data as well as the model assumptions and the control for outliers necessary (Langford & Lewis, 1998; Snijders & Bosker, 1999). Another drawback of the complexity is that the results are often not easy to communicate and that there is an implicit tendency to extend, but not to simplify interpretations (Goldstein, 1995). Despite these arguments multilevel models are powerful statistical tools that are well suited to treat the richness and complexity of real life data.

Ambulatory assessment data often create problems for the statistical analysis with conventional methods. A solution for many data-analytic problems is available in the framework of multilevel analysis. To demonstrate the usefulness of multilevel modeling, the emotional state of 314 parents and their adolescent children out of 96 families was analyzed.

Emotional state data and additional information were gathered with a computer assisted self monitoring system (FASEM-C) six times a day over the course of a week. Results show that situational features like time of the observation, local setting, social contacts, and current activity each have an own significant effect on the emotional state, even if the influence of the other variables was held constant. Mean differences between family members were rare and rather small, but there were large differences in the variation of the emotional state.

References

Cohen, J. & Cohen, P. (1983). *Applied multiple regression/correlation analysis for the behavior sciences (2nd ed.)*. Hillsdale, NJ: Erlbaum.

Goldstein, H. (1995). *Multilevel Statistical Models. (2nd ed.)*. London: Edward Arnold. Since 1999 in electronic form at: h*ttp://www.arnoldpublishers.com/support/goldstein.htm*

Goldstein, H., Healy, M.J.R. & Rasbash, J. (1994). Multilevel time series models with applications to repeated measures data. *Statistics in Medicine, 13*, 1643–1655.

Gonzalez, R. & Griffin, D. (1999). The correlational analysis of dyad-level data in the distinguishable case. *Personal Relationships, 6*, 449–469.

Hedeker, D. & Gibbons, R.D. (1996). MIXREG: A computer program for mixed-effects regression analysis with autocorrelated errors. *Computer Methods and Programs in Biomedicine, 49*, 229–252.

Jones, K. (1993). Using multilevel models for survey analysis. *Journal of the Market Research Society, 35*, 249–265.

Kenny, D.A. (1996). Models of non-independence in dyadic research. *Journal of Social Relationships, 13*, 279–294.

Kenny, D.A., Kashy, D.A. & Bolger, N. (1998). Data analysis in Social Psychology. In D.T. Gilbert, S.T. Fiske & G. Lindzey (Eds.), *The Handbook of Social Psychology, Vol. 1 (4th. ed.)* (pp. 233–265). Boston: McGraw-Hill.

Langford, I.H., Bentham, G. & McDonald, A.L. (1998). Multi-level modelling of geographically aggregated health data: A case study on malignant melanoma mortality and UV exposure in the European Community. *Statistics in Medicine, 17*, 41–57.

Langford, I.H. & Lewis, T. (1998). Outliers in multilevel data. *Journal of the Royal Statistical Society, A, 161*, 121–160.

Larson, R. & Delespaul, P.A.E.G. (1992). Analyzing Experience Sampling data: A guidebook for the perplexed. In M.W. de Vries (Ed.), *The experience of psychopathology. Investigating mental disorders in their natural settings* (pp. 58–78). Cambridge: Cambridge University Press.

Larson, R. & Richards, M. (1994). *Divergent realities. The emotional lives of mothers, fathers, and adolescents.* New York: Basic Books.

Pawlik, K. & Buse, L. (1994). "Psychometeorologie": Zeitreihenanalytische Ergebnisse zum Einfluß des Wetters auf die Psyche aus methodischer Sicht. *Psychologische Rundschau, 45*, 63–78.

Perrez, M., Schoebi, D. & Wilhelm, P. (2000). How to assess social regulation of stress and emotions in daily family life? A computer assisted family self-monitoring-system (FASEM-C). *Clinical Psychology and Psychotherapy, 7*, 326–339.

Pihet, S. (2000). *Auto-observation systématique des processus quotidiens: une méthode fiable et valide?* [Systematic self-observation of daily life processes. A reliable and valid method?] Contribution fribourgeoises en psychologie, Vol. 10. Fribourg, CH: Edition Universitaires.

Raudenbush, S.W., Brennan, R.T. & Barnett, R.C. (1995). A multivariate hierarchical model for studying psychological change within married couples. *Journal of Family Psychology, 9*, 161–174.

Rasbash, J., Browne, W., Goldstein, H., Yang, M., Plewis, I., Healy, M., Woodhouse, G., Draper, D., Langford & Lewis, T. (2000). *A user's guide to MLwiN*. London: Multilevel Models Project, Institute of Education, University of London.

Reicherts, M. & Pihet, S. (in press). Job newcomers coping with stressful situations. A micro-analysis of adequate coping and well-being. *Swiss Journal of Psychology.*

Schwartz, J.E. & Stone, A.A. (1998). Strategies for analyzing ecological momentary assessment data. *Health Psychology, 17*, 6–16.

Schwartz, J.E., Warren, K. & Pickering, T.G. (1994). Mood, location and physical position as predictors of ambulatory blood pressure and heart rate: Application of a multi-level random effects model. *Annals of Behavioral Medicine, 16*, 210–220.

Scherer, K.R. (1988). Criteria for emotion-antecedent appraisal: A review. In V. Hamilton, G.H. Bower & N.H. Frijda (Eds.), *Cognitive perspective on emotion and motivation* (pp. 89–126). Dordrecht: Kluwer Academic Publishers.

Snijders, T.A.B. & Bosker, R.J. (1999). *Multilevel analysis. An introduction to basic and advanced multilevel modelling.* London: Sage.

Snijders, T.A.B. & Kenny, D.A. (1999). The social relations model for family data: A multilevel approach. *Personal Relationships, 6*, 471–486.

Suen, H.K. & Ary, D. (1989). *Analyzing quantitative behavioral observation data.* Hillsdale, N.J.: Erlbaum.

West, S.G. & Hepworth, J.T. (1991). Statistical issues in the study of temporal data: Daily experiences. *Journal of Personality, 59*, 609–662.

Wilhelm, P., Horner, M. & Perrez, M. (2000). Humeurs et gestion du stress dans les interactions familiales: Résultats à partir de la méthode FASEM (pp. 255–274). [Mood and regulation of stress during family interactions. Results of the FASEM methodology]. In J.-P. Pourtois & H. Desmet (Eds.), *Relation familiale et résilience.* Paris: L'Harmattan.

Yang, M., Rasbash, J., Goldstein, H. & Barbosa, M. (1999). *MLwiN macros for advanced multilevel modelling (Version 2).* London: Multilevel Models Project, Institute of Education, University of London.

Part II
Psychophysiological Assessment

Chapter 13
Posture and Motion Analysis by Ambulatory Accelerometry

Hans Bussmann, Rita van den Berg-Emons, and Henk Stam
Department of Rehabilitation, Erasmus University Rotterdam, the Netherlands

Introduction

Measurement of posture and motion during normal daily life is relevant in many disciplines. Three main types of application can be distinguished. First, posture and motion can be of interest in itself and be related to a primary variable. In these cases posture and motion are assumed to represent "natural behavior", "physical activity", or (disability in) "mobility". For example, the efficacy of a physical training program can be assessed by posture and motion measurement during normal daily life. Second, measurement of posture and motion can be used to study their (unknown) effects on other signals or parameters, for example, the effect of body posture and body motion on blood pressure. Third, posture and motion analysis can be applied to facilitate the interpretation of other parameters or signals. For example, in blood pressure studies, knowledge on posture and motion will be helpful in the analysis and interpretation of blood pressure data.

In 1992, our department started a research line aimed at the development, validation, and application of an Activity Monitor (AM): an ambulatory and accelerometry-based instrument to measure posture and motion during normal daily life (van den Berg-Emons, Bussmann, Balk & Stam, 2000; Bussmann, van de Laar, Neeleman & Stam, 1998; Bussmann, Reuvekamp, Veltink, Martens & Stam, 1998; Bussmann, Tulen, van Herel & Stam, 1998; Tulen, Bussmann, van Steenis, Pepplinkhuizen & Man in 't Veld, 1997; Tulen, Stronks, Bussmann, Pepplinkhuizen & Passchier, 2000). The following postures and motions were regarded to be of major interest: lying, sitting, standing, walking, running, climbing stairs, cycling, driving a wheelchair, general (non-cyclic) movements, and the transitions between different postures. In our research, we distinguish three aspects of posture and motion: *quantity* (which posture/motion is performed, when, how often and for how long), *quality* (how is the posture/motion performed), and *physical strain* (the physiological reaction of the body related to performing postures and motions).

In the first issue of this book, Jain and colleagues described the potential of accelerometry for ambulatory posture and motion analysis, with reference to the research of our group (Jain, Martens, Mutz, Weiss & Stephan, 1996). Since then, a lot of work and research has been conducted with the AM. The aim of the present paper is to provide an overview of these developments, of the current "state of the art", and of the perspectives on ambulatory activity monitoring.

Technical description

This section provides a brief description of the technical aspects of the AM. For a more detailed description we refer to the paper of Bussmann et al. (Bussmann, Martens, Tulen, Schasfoort, van den Berg-Emons, Stam, submitted). The standard configuration of the Activity Monitor consists of four ADXL202 (Analog Devices) piezo-resistive accelerometers (about 1.5 × 1.5 × 1 cm). In most of our studies we simultaneously measure ECG. One accelerometer is attached on the lateral side of each thigh, with its sensitive axis in sagittal direction while the subject is in the anatomical position. The third (bi-axial) sensor is attached on the lower part of the sternum, with sensitive axes in the sagital and longitudinal direction. Additional sensors can be applied on the sternum (transverse axis) and on both lower arms. Each accelerometer is attached by cables to a data recorder, by means of separate Lemo jackets or with a multi-connector. Before measurements are started, the accelerometers are calibrated (+1 g, -1 g).

We currently use two recorder types. The Vitaport2™ (TEMEC Instruments, Kerkrade, the Netherlands) is a digital recorder (9 × 15 × 4.5 cm, 700 g); the universal module allows the simultaneous measurement of up to 8 channels. Continuous measurement (without changing batteries or memory cards) during several days is possible. Additionally, we use several prototypes of the so-called "Rotterdam Activity Monitor" (or "RAM") (TEMEC Instruments, Kerkrade, the Netherlands): a recorder based on Vitaport™ technology, but more dedicated to activity monitoring, and which is smaller and lighter (9 × 15 × 3.5 cm, 500 g). Acceleration signals are standardly sampled by 32 Hz and 12-bits resolution, and 30 Hz low-pass filtered. ECG signals are sampled by 64 or 128 Hz. After the measurements are completed, the data are downloaded onto a PC for analysis.

Analysis takes place after the measurements by means of the Signal Processing and Inferencing Language (S.P.I.L.) (Jain, Martens, Mutz, Weiss& Stephan, 1996). In the analysis, three parts can be distinguished: (1) feature processing, that is, new signals with specific characteristics are derived from each measured signal; (2) posture/motion detection, that is, based on the feature channels, postures and motions are determined; and (3) post-processing, that is, output signals of the posture/motion detection are processed in such a way that readable and relevant information is provided.

For posture/motion detection, three feature signals are derived from each measured accelerometer signal: the LP/angular signal, the motility signal, and the frequency signal (Figure 1). The LP/angular signals are created after low-pass filtering (Finite Impulse Response filter, cut-off frequency 0.3 Hz). The signal is subsequently converted to 1 Hz and to angles via an arcsine transformation (range: -90 to +90 degrees). The motility signals are created after subsequent high-pass filtering at 0.3 Hz, rectifying, and averaging. The frequency signal is based upon a band-pass filtered derivative (0.3–2 Hz for the legs; 0.6–4 Hz for the trunk). This band-passed signal is the input of the Fast Time Frequency Transform (FTFT) procedure, which consists of a kind of instantaneous frequency analysis (Martens, 1992). The eventual output is the (main) frequency of the measurement signal, if present. All feature signals have a time resolution of 1 Hz.

Based on the feature signals, the detection of a posture/motion (sub)category takes place. In the analysis more than 20 posture and motion (sub)categories are distinguished. For each subcategory and for each feature, a minimum and maximum value is pre-set in an Activity Detection Knowledge Base (ADKB). For consecutive moments in time (1 second), for each subcategory and for each feature, the "distance" is calculated from the actual feature signal value to the pre-set range. The calculated distances of the features are scaled and added for each subcategory. The posture/motion with the shortest distance at the end of the calculations will be selected (Figure 2).

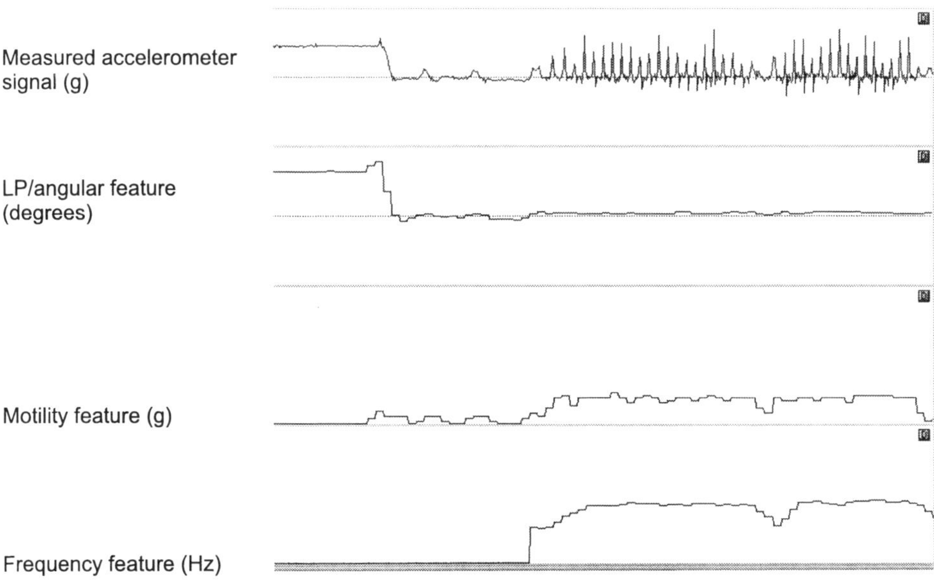

Figure 1. Measured accelerometer signal and the three feature signals derived from it.

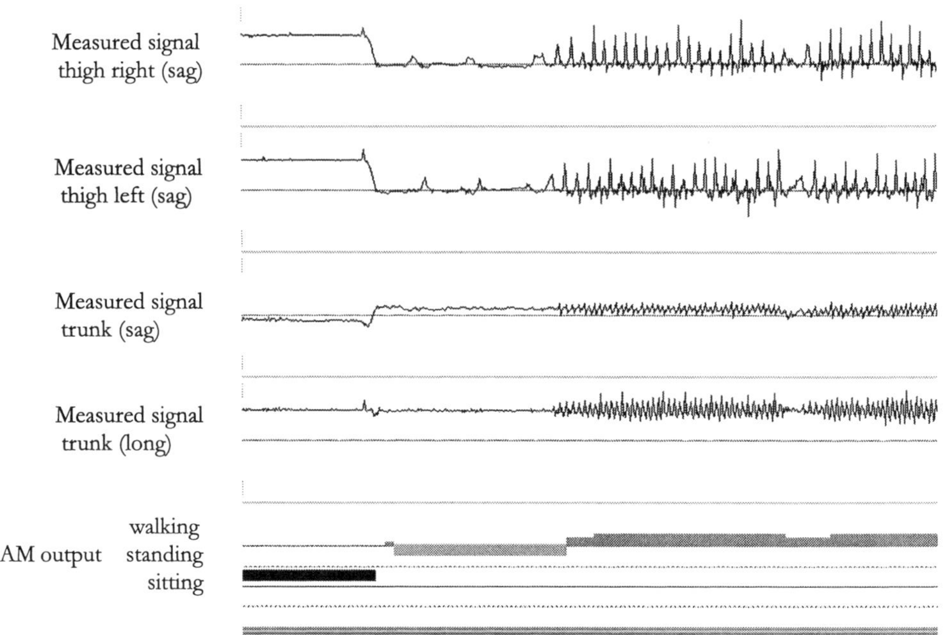

Figure 2. Four measured signals and the automatic activity detection.

After the activity detection, some (optional) post-processing procedures take place. First, posture/motion *sub*categories are reduced to a more limited number of posture/motion *main* categories. Second, a post-processing procedure is included by which activities below a certain duration are "deleted". In our studies, we apply a threshold of 5 seconds. Third, in case of postures/motions not included in the set or in case of postures/motions not correctly detected, manual editing of the AM output can take place. Fourth, the four motility signals from thighs and trunk are averaged and assigned to a body motility signal. Optionally, the ECG signal is translated into a heart rate signal. Eventually, the AM output is statistically analysed and presented in reports.

AM output variables

The output of the AM analysis can be graphically expressed and as relevant values in a spreadsheet file. Results are provided over the complete measurement period, or over selected parts of the measurement sequence. For each posture/motion category the duration – in absolute time or as percentage of the analysis period – is provided. The number of transitions is calculated for each transition category, for example, sit-to-stand, stand-to-sit, sit-to-lie. Furthermore, the number of walking periods is expressed, as required in duration categories (for example, number of walking periods < 10 seconds, number of walking periods > 10 and < 30 seconds, etc.).

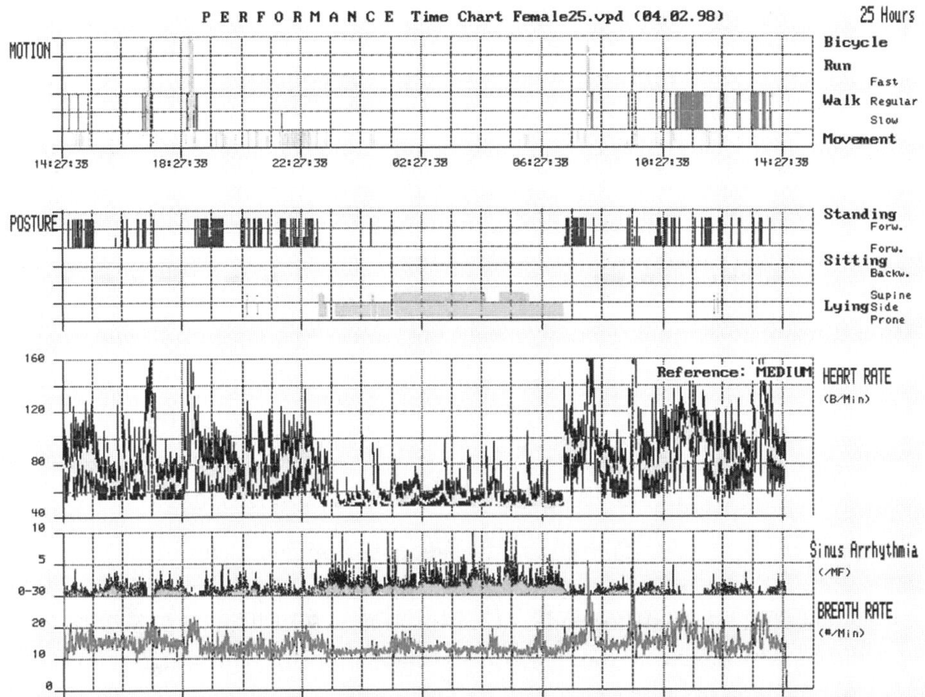

Figure 3. Example of an AM report of a 25-hour measurement. The two upper graphs show the posture and motion detection, the two lower graphs show the output of simultaneously measured physiological signals (heart rate, breathing rate, sinus arrhythmia).

The motility signals express the intensity of body segment movements, measured with accelerometry. Thus, the motility signals represent, in one way or another, the level of physical activity. The motility signals are analysed, in particular the body motility signal. Mean (body) motility is calculated over the complete analysis period, but also for each posture/motion category. For example, a high (body) motility level during sitting represents an "active" form of sitting. In the same way the (body) motility level during walking represents the "intensity" of walking, that is, walking speed. Similar to motility, heart rate data can be analysed: that is, mean heart rate over the analysis period(s), as well as for each posture/motion category (Figure 3)

Validity studies

The validity of the AM for detecting postures and motions has been reported in five papers (van den Berg et al., 2000; Bussmann, Tulen et al., 1998; Bussmann, Reuvekamp et al., 1998; Bussmann, van de Laar et al. 1998; Bussmann, Martens et al., submitted). In these studies able-bodied subjects, amputees, students participating in a psychophysiological study, failed back surgery patients, and heart failure patients were involved. Subjects generally performed a large number of functional activities in their own manner and pace. In these latter studies – with the exception of the study of van den Berg et al. (2000) and one study of Bussmann et al. (Bussmann, Martens et al., submitted) – a first and more simple version of the AM was used. In this first version of the AM – identical in sensor configuration, but different in analysis program – different motions could not be distinguished, the analysis scheme was more hierarchical, and part of the analysis (posture-motion detection) was not distance-based but Boolean. Because both AM versions were based on the same input signals, the data obtained during the three validity studies previously published could also be used to examine the validity of measurements with the current version of the AM. Validity was assessed by calculating agreement scores (sensitivity, predictive value [PV]) between AM output and video output, and by comparing the number of walking periods, and the duration of activities determined by both methods.

The overall agreement between AM output and videotape analysis for the four studies was 89%, 93%, 81%, and 90%, respectively. The overall sensitivity percentages for standing ranged from 84 to 97% and the PV percentages from 80 to 92%. For sitting these ranges were 86–94% and 92–99%, and for lying 91–98% and 71–97%, respectively. For walking the range of sensitivity percentages was 79–86%, the range of PV percentages 79–87%. These percentages were 92–97% and 83–91% for cycling, and 24–76% and 91–100% for climbing stairs. Thus, generally the agreement percentages were high; only the sensitivity percentages for climbing stairs were clearly lower, generally due to the misdetection as walking. The duration of walking was slightly underestimated (–0.8%, –0.8% and –4.1%). The number of walking periods was well determined (total number AM versus video: 169 vs. 170, 255 vs. 240, 110 vs. 94). The number of transitions according to AM and videotape analysis was 230 vs. 214, 86 vs. 94, 228 vs. 205, and 153 vs. 149.

It can be concluded that the current version of the AM allows valid measurement of most postures and motions. The validity is even stronger than the results suggest: the agreement percentages were significantly lowered by "grey area" postures and motions. For example, the detection of shuffling as standing (walking according to videotape analysis), the detection of cycling with periods without moving the legs as sitting (still cycling according to videotape analysis criteria), and the detection of sitting with the trunk strongly backwards as lying on the back (still sitting according to videotape analysis criteria). Postures were generally well determined, as were walking and cycling. The ability to distinguish climbing stairs was less powerful, although improvement may be gained by the more stable accelerometers we currently use and the correction for angular attachment deviations. A recent study showed that a configuration with additional accelerometers attached at the lower arms allows a valid detection of driving a wheelchair (unpublished data).

Applications

The AM has been used in several explorative and evaluative studies. The results of some studies are already published or in the pipeline, whereas others are still in progress.

The AM has been used to study the activity level of chronic heart failure (CHF) patients compared to healthy controls (van den Berg, Bussmann, Balk & Stam, accepted). Everyday physical activity in patients with chronic CHF was measured with a novel Activity Monitor; measurements were performed during two consecutive days. The results showed significant differences in percentage of the measurement period that subjects were active (CHF 3.9%, controls 11.3%), in number of transitions (90 vs. 133), in number of walking periods (63 vs. 181) and in motility (0.06 vs. 0.15). A similar study was performed in patients with meningomyelocele (MMC) (Berg van den-Emons, Bussmann, Brobbel, Roebroeck, van Meeteren & Stam, submitted) and in patients with cerebral palsy (CP). As in CHF patients, MMC patients were less active (6.5% vs. 12.7%), and performed less transitions (84 vs. 151), and the number of walking/wheelchair driving periods was lower (122 vs. 185) compared with controls. In CP patients, however, preliminary data show no significant differences in percentage of the day being active (9.8% vs. 10.7%); other measures were also not significantly different between the groups.

A number of projects is currently ongoing:

- following the descriptive study in CHF patients, an evaluative study investigating the effect of an aerobic training program on daily activity in these patients;
- another study (Free University Amsterdam) is evaluating the effects of pyridostigmine on fatigue and activity pattern in post-polio patients;
- in patients with amputation of a lower leg, the effect of a novel prosthesis socket on gait pattern and daily physical activity – measured with the AM – is being studied;
- the AM is clinically used in the evaluation of a multidisciplinary program for patients with chronic pain.

Future research projects will focus on:

- the effect of exercise training on daily physical activity in Guillain-Barré patients;
- the extent of hypoactivity in MMC and CP patients, and its relation with physical fitness, disability and quality of life;
- the potential of ambulatory techniques to measure pain (behavior) in young children after major surgery;
- the recovery of physical activity in spinal cord injury patients.

In other departments of our university hospital, activity monitoring is applied in a psychopharmacological study (Tulen, Bussmann et al., 1997), in a drug study in migraine patients (Tulen, Stronks et al. 2000), and in a study on ambulatory blood pressure measurement. These studies are described in more detail in the chapter by Tulen et al., this Volume.

Measurement of arm-hand use

An important extension of the standard AM configuration is due to the relevance of measuring arm-hand use in specific patient groups. For example, Uswatte et al. (Uswatte, Miltner, Foo, Varma, Moran & Taub, 2000) studied the validity of ambulatory measurement of arm-hand use in stroke patients. In our department research is aimed at patients with reflex sympathetic dystrophy, but also in other patient groups and in other disciplines (for example, ergonomics) measurement of arm-hand use will be relevant. Studies performed so far indicate that with the use of two additional accelerometers attached to the lower arm, most types of arm-hand use can be accurately determined. The measurement of arm-hand use is based on the motility signals derived from the lower-arm accelerometer signals. The added value of the AM is mainly determined by the combination of these motility signals and the standard AM output (postures and motions). For example, using only accelerometers on the lower arms should lead to the classification arm-hand use when the subject is walking. Due to the simultaneous posture/motion classification, this type of arm-hand use can be distinguished from arm-hand use during sitting or standing.

Quality and physical strain

Although the signal of piezo-resistive accelerometers is difficult to interpret – because the signal is a combination of a component of the gravitational acceleration and a component of the inertial acceleration – it contains a lot of information about quality of postures and motions, that is, movement pattern, co-ordination, speed, etc. In our research, walking and the sit-to-stand transition receive special interest. In walking, parameters such as stride frequency, walking speed, symmetry, and stability can be derived from the acceleration signals. In a study on the acceleration signal during walking, we found that the signal of the thigh sensor is highly reproducible in able-bodied subjects (Bussmann, Damen & Stam, 2000). In another study, we found that the acceleration signals of thighs and trunk can be used to assess stability of movement in elderly subjects (Slagter, Bussmann, Wagenaar, van der Cammen & Stam, 1998). With respect to the sit-to-stand transition, parameters such as movement time, movement pattern, and phasing of leg and trunk movements are considered important and are automatically determined.

In literature, acceleration signal-based parameters are used in the long-term measurement of energy or oxygen consumption. As mentioned earlier in this paper, AM motility signals express the intensity of body segment movements, measured with accelerometry. Body motility appeared to have a close relationship with oxygen uptake and heart rate during walking (Bussmann, Hartgerink, van der Woude & Stam, 2000). Although recent studies show a more complex picture when motility is used as physical strain measure in persons with different economies (Bussmann, van den Berg-Emons, Angulo, Stijnen & Stam, submitted) and in activities other than walking, the use of motility may increase the validity of ambulatory long-term measurement of physical strain.

Comparison with other instruments

The AM is not the only instrument aimed at the measurement of postures and motions or physical activity during normal daily life. In the measurement of these constructs, two major categories can be distinguished.

Accelerometry-based instruments have been developed for and applied in research on the *level of physical activity*. These instruments do not provide specific information about postures and motions, but do give general data on activity level. The output of these instruments can be compared with the motility feature of the AM. For example, data express when a subject was active and how active he was, but do not represent the type of activity performed. In these instruments, the level of physical activity measured with accelerometry is frequently related or translated to energy expenditure. Examples of this type of instruments are the Caltrac, CSA, Tracmor, TriTrac, AMS, and Actigraph. Instruments such as these have the advantages of practical feasibility (unobstrusiveness) and prolonged measurement periods, but are – as mentioned – restricted in their potential to give detailed information. However, it has to be noted that for many research and clinical questions detailed data are not necessary.

Other instruments are more similar to the AM, in the sense that some (or more) *postures and motions* are automatically detected. The background and applications are generally very different, as are the methods used and the set of postures/motions that are distinguished. For example, Anastadiades and Johnston (1990) used EMG to distinguish static and dynamic activities. Walker et al. used a mercury switch and an accelerometer for the measurement of postures and number of steps (Walker, Heslop, Plummer, Essex & Chandler, 1997). Tuomisto et al. used accelerometers, a hydrostatic tube, EMG and heart rate in a validation study on posture and motion detection (Tuomisto, Johnston & Schmidt, 1996). In other studies – as in the studies with the AM – also piezo-resistive accelerometers are used, and especially for their potential to measure both postures and motions. Examples of these instruments are the DynaPort system as reported by Busser and Uiterwaal et al. (Busser, Ott, Uiterwaal, Lummel van, Blank, 1997; Uiterwaal, Glerum, Busser & van Lummel, 1998), the instrument developed and used by Fahrenberg and Foerster et al. (Fahrenberg, Foerster, Mueller & Smeja, 1997; Foerster, Smeja & Fahrenberg, 1999), the activity monitor used by Dunnewold and colleagues (Dunnewold, Hoff, van Pelt, Fredrikze, Wagemans & van Hilten, 1998), the instrument of Ma and Barbenel (Ma & Barbenel, 1997), and the AMMA system developed by Kiani et al. (Kiani, Snijders & Gelsema, 1997, 1998). The AM as described in this paper is also applied by Tulen et al. (Tulen, Bussmann et al., 1997; Tulen, Stronks et al., 2000). Generally, qualitative comparison of the AM with the other systems is difficult. Instruments discriminate different activity categories, are used for different aims, or validity is determined following a different or unknown method.

Potential and restrictions of activity monitoring

Fahrenberg (1996) has provided an overview of the advantages and disadvantages of ambulatory measurements. Here, we briefly discuss some of the points that are specifically of interest for activity monitoring.

The major advantage of ambulatory activity monitoring is the ecological validity: natural, spontaneous behavior is objectively measured in a natural setting. In rehabilitation medicine, and increasingly in other disciplines, the consequences of diseases for daily functioning are considered of upmost importance. Furthermore, long-term measurement increases the chance of "catching"events (for example, ticks, tremors). Additionally, activity monitoring provides data about what a person actually does, and not about what a person can, thinks he does, or says he does. And last, the simultaneous measurement of different physical and physiological signals (for example, accelerometry, EMG, ECG, blood pressure, temperature) can and will reveal new knowledge.

Nevertheless, it can not be stated that ambulatory activity monitoring is the only relevant way of measurement of a subject's behavior during normal daily life. Some important limitations, however, have to be mentioned. In ambulatory (activity) monitoring there is no or only limited control on confounding factors. For example, in research on changes over time in the sit-to-stand transition during normal daily life the way of performance will be influenced by type of chair and chair height; differences found may be due to chair-related factors and not to subject-related factors. Another point of interest is the natural between-measurement variance. For example, the activity pattern of a person during day 1 may and will be different from the activity pattern on another day. These factors – the lack of control within and between measurements and the natural variability – will have their effect on the reliability of measurements. The search for instruments that are as unobtrusive as possible is an inherent characteristic of ambulatory research. Instruments, however, and the knowledge of the subject about the instrument and measurement, may influence the behavior of subjects (reactivity effect). Other critical factors are the load on patients/subjects and researchers/clinicians, the time and efforts required for ambulatory measurements, non-acceptance of ambulatory techniques, and the costs of the instrument and measurements. For example, due to production in small batches, the cost of a complete AM system currently is about US$ 11,000.

Ambulatory activity monitoring is a relatively novel technique, and the "acceptance" and widespread use of a technique depends on a number of factors. Brand and Crowninshield (Brand & Crowninshield, 1981) described six criteria a patient evaluation tool has to meet when it is to be used outside of a few research institutions: 1) correlation with functional capacity; 2) measured parameter must not be directly observable and semiquantifiable; 3) parameters must clearly distinguish between normal and abnormal; 4) no significant alteration of the performance; 5) the measurement must be accurate and reproducible; and 6) results in a form readily identifiable in a physical or physiological analog. None of these criteria is inherently unsolvable for activity monitoring and some (points 1, 2, 4, 6) are related to specific advantages of ambulatory activity monitoring. Point 5 stresses the relevance of reliability and validity studies. Therefore, we started our AM research with accurate and extensive validity studies, followed by studies aimed at sensitivity and evaluation. Some additional remarks can, however, be made. First, we have experienced that clinicians may not be directly aware of the added value of activity monitoring; they think that they can get the information in another, more simple way (point 2). This fact necessitates action from two sides: clinicians should "open" their minds for new initiatives, and researchers should be able to make clear the benefits of a new technique. A researcher will be mainly interested in values, clinicians will expect a clear and professional report with relevant and easy to interpret results. Being critical about, and making clear the real added value of ambulatory activity monitoring will be important issues for current advocates of this technique. Other relevant topics concern the ongoing search for more user- and patient-friendly and less obstrusive instruments.

Future developments

Expected developments can be classified into four categories: instrument, measurement, costs, and applicability. Technical and instrumental developments may include smaller sensors, wire-less sensors, smaller and lighter data recorders, faster and real-time analysis, feedback applications, and developments within the field of data transport and telecommunication. Methodological and measurement-related developments may involve the (further application of) combined measurement of several physiological, physical and other signals. As mentioned above, the costs of detailed activity monitoring – as provided with the AM – are still relatively high. A current economic dilemma is the investment associated with large-scale production to substantially lower this price. In the previous paragraph we mentioned some factors influencing the widespread use of ambulatory techniques. Although not all factors have been addressed, these are the type of factors which will largely determine the success of ambulatory activity monitoring, and ambulatory techniques in general, in the future.

References

Anastasiades, P. & Johnston, D.W. (1990). A simple activity measure for use with ambulatory subjects. *Psychophysiology, 27*, 87–93.

Berg van den-Emons, H. J.G., Bussmann, J.B.J., Balk, A.H.M.M. & Stam, H. (2000). Validity of ambulatory accelerometry to quantify physical activity in heart failure. *Scandinavian Journal of Rehabilitation Medicine, 32*, 187–192.

Berg van den, R., Bussmann, H., Balk, A. & Stam, H. (accepted) Everyday physical activity in patients with chronic congestive heart failure as measured with a novel Activity Monitor. *Physical Therapy.*

Berg van den-Emons, H.J., Bussmann,. J.B., Brobbel, A.S., Roebroeck M.E., Meeteren van, J., Stam, H.J. (submitted). Everyday physical activity in adolescents and young adults with meningomyelocele as measured with a novel activity monitor.

Brand, R.. & Crowninshield, R.D. (1981). Comment on criteria for patient evaluation tools. *Journal of Biomechanics, 14* ,655

Busser, H.J., Ott, J., Uiterwaal, M., Lummel van, R.C. & Blank, R. (1997). Ambulatory monitoring of children's activity. *Medical Engineering & Physics, 19*, 440–445.

Bussmann, J.B.J. & Stam, H.J. (1998). Techniques for measurement and assessment of mobility in rehabilitation: a theoretical approach. *Clinical Rehabilitation, 12*, 455–464.

Bussmann, J.B.J., Tulen, J.H.M., Herel van, E.C.G. & Stam, H.J. (1998). Quantification of physical activities by means of accelerometry: a validation study. *Psychophysiology, 35*, 488–496.

Bussmann, J.B.J., Laar van de, Y.M., Neeleman, M.P. & Stam, H.J. (1998). Ambulatory accelerometry to quantify motor behavior in patients after failed back surgery. *Pain, 74*, 153–161.

Bussmann, H.B.J., Reuvekamp, P.J., Veltink, P.H., Martens, W.L.J. & Stam H.J. (1998). Validity and reliability of measurements obtained with an "Activity Monitor" in people with and without a transtibial amputation. *Physical Therapy, 78*, 989–998.

Bussmann, J.B.J., Hartgerink, I., Woude van der, L.H.V. & Stam, H.J. (2000). Measuring physical strain during ambulation with accelerometry. *Medicine & Science in Sports & Exercise, 32*, 1462–1471.

Bussmann, J.B.J. (1998). Ambulatory monitoring of mobility-related activities in rehabilitation medicine. PhD thesis. Delft: Eburon.

Bussmann, J.B.J., Damen, L. & Stam, H.J. (2000). Analysis and decomposition of signals obtained by thigh-fixed accelerometry during walking. *Medical & Biological Engineering & Computing, 38*, 632–638.

Bussmann, J.B.J., Martens, W.L.J., Tulen, J.H.M., Schasfoort, F.C., van den Berg-Emons, H.J.G. & Stam, H.J. (submitted). Measuring daily behavior using ambulatory accelerometry: the Activity Monitor.

Bussmann, J.B.J., van den Berg-Emons, H.J.G., Angulo, S.M., Stijnen, Th. & Stam, H.J. (submitted). Measurement of physical strain during prosthetic gait by accelerometry.

Dunnewold, R.J., Hoff, J.J., van Pelt, H.C., Fredrikze, P.Q., Wagemans, E.A. & van Hilten, B.J. (1998). Ambulatory quantitative assessment of body position, bradykinesia, and hypokinesia in Parkinson's disease. *Journal of Clinical Neurophysiology, 15*, 235–242.

Fahrenberg, J., Foerster, F., Mueller, W. & Smeja, M. (1997). Assessment of posture and motion by multi-channel piezoresistive accelerometer recordings. *Psychophysiology, 34,* 607–612.

Fahrenberg, J. (1996) Ambulatory assessment: issues and perspectives. In: J. Fahrenberg & M. Myrtek (Eds.), *Ambulatory assessment; computer-assisted psychological and psychophysiological methods in monitoring and field studies* (pp. 3–20). Seatle: Hogrefe & Huber Publishers.

Foerster, F., Smeja, M. & Fahrenberg J. (1999). Detection of posture and motion by accelerometry: a validation study in ambulatory monitoring. *Computers in Human Behavior, 15*, 571–583

Jain, A., Martens, W.L.J., Mutz, G., Weiss, R.K. & Stephan, E. (1996). Towards a comprehensive technology for recording and analysis of multiple physiological parameters within their behavioral and environmental context. In: J. Fahrenberg & M. Myrtek (Eds.), *Ambulatory assessment; computer-assisted psychological and psychophysiological methods in monitoring and field studies* (pp. 215–236). Seatle: Hogrefe & Huber Publishers.

Kiani, K., Snijders, C.J. & Gelsema, E.S. (1997). Computerized analysis of daily life motor activity for ambulatory monitoring. *Technology & Health Care, 5*, 307–318.

Kiani, K., Snijders, C.J. & Gelsema, E.S. (1998). Recognition of daily motor activity classes using an artificial neural network. *Archives of Physical Medicine and Rehabilitation, 79*, 147–154.

Ma, J. & Barbenel, J.C. (1997). A new ambulatory monitoring instrument of posture and mobility related activities. *Biomedical Sciences Instrumentation, 33*, 88–93.

Martens, W.L.J. (1992). The Fast Time Frequency Transform (F.T.F.T.): a novel approach to the Instantaneous Spectrum. In: *Proceedings IEEE Engineering in Medicine & Biology Society.*

Slagter, A.H., Bussmann, J.B.J., Wagenaar, R.C., Cammen van der, T.J., Stam, H.J. (1998). Quantifying quality of moving in the elderly based on ambulatory accelerometry. *Student Health Technology Information, 48*, 249–253.

Tulen, J.H.M., Bussmann, J.B.J., Steenis van, H.G., Pepplinkhuizen, L. & Man in 't Veld, A.J. (1997). A novel tool to quantify physical activities: ambulatory accelerometry in psychopharmacology. *Journal of Clinical Psychopharmacology, 17*, 202–207.

Tulen, J.H.M., Stronks, D., Bussmann, J.B.J., Pepplinkhuizen, L. & Passchier, J. (2000) Towards an objective quantitative assessment of daily functioning in migraine; feasibility study. *Pain, 86*, 139–149.

Tuomisto, M.T., Johnston, D.W. & Schmidt, T.F.H. (1996). The ambulatory measurement of posture, thigh acceleration and muscle tension and their relationship to heart rate. *Psychophysiology, 33*, 409–415.

Uiterwaal, M., Glerum, E.B., Busser, H.J. & van Lummel, R.C. (1998). Ambulatory monitoring of physical activity in working situations, a validation study. *Journal of Medical Engineering & Technology, 22*, 168–172.

Uswatte, G., Miltner, W.H.R., Foo, B., Varma, M., Moran, S. & Taub, S. (2000). Objective measurement of functional upper extremity movement using accelerometer recordings transformed with a threshold filter. *Stroke, 31*, 662–667.

Walker, D.J., Heslop, P.S., Plummer, C.J., Essex, T. & Chandler, S. (1997) A continuous patient activity monitor: validation and relation to disability. *Physiological Measurement, 18*, 49–59.

Chapter 14
Accelerometry in Clinical Psychophysiology

Joke Tulen[1], Anita Volkers[1,2], Dirk Stronks[1,2],
Marinel Cavelaars[3], and Wim Groeneveld[4]
[1]Departments of Psychiatry, [2]Medical Psychology and Psychotherapy,
[3]Internal Medicine, and [4]Biomedical Physics and Technology,
Erasmus Medical Center Rotterdam, The Netherlands

Introduction

Behavior and cardiovascular psychophysiology

Cardiovascular variability is determined by a complex interaction of both extrinsic (for example, light-dark cycle, sleep, posture, locomotor activity, mental activity, emotions, feeding, temperature, sensory input) and endogenous factors (for example, respiration, pulsatility of flow, baroreflex sensitivity, intrinsic circadian rhythm) (Pickering, 1991). For research as well as for clinical purposes it is relevant to determine the contribution of each of these factors to overall hemodynamic variability, because this may have consequences for diagnosis and treatment in a variety of disease states. Delineation of the effects of the behavioral factors (body posture, physical activities) becomes especially relevant in prolonged (24-hr) ambulatory cardiovascular measurements: a situation in which control for (extrinsic) confounding factors usually is reduced or absent.

To quantify behavior, research in clinical psychophysiology can benefit much from accelerometry. Questions related to situational, psychosocial, and emotional factors involved in cardiovascular functioning under ambulatory conditions can be addressed more reliably when correcting for overt behavior (body postures, locomotor activity, motility, (in)voluntary movements, (non)specific movements) as quantified by means of accelerometers (for example, Clarck, Denby, Pregibon, Harshfield, Pickering, Blank & Laragh, 1987; Fahrenberg & Myrtek, 1996; Kario, Schwartz & Pickering, 1999; Sherwood & Turner, 1993; Tulen, Boomsma, Man in 't Veld, 1999). An accurate description of the interaction between overt behavior and psychophysiological functioning has relevance for a variety of disease states. In some disorders, the focus of interest lies on the abnormalities observed in cardiovascular regulation, with physical activity as a major confounding factor. In other disorders, abnormalities in behavioral processes predominate with cardiovascular regulation as a dependent variable. Apart from clarifying pathophysiological processes in certain disease states, a detailed quantification of physical activities offers the opportunity to study the efficacy and possible side-effects of (non)pharmacological treatments on behavioral processes in interaction with psychophysiological functioning. This chapter focuses on possibilities to measure, or control for, overt behavior when interpreting psychophysiological functioning of psychiatric, neurological, and cardiovascular disorders under ambulatory conditions. The instruments and data presented are based on our studies performed with a variety of patient categories (depression, Gilles de la Tourette syndrome, migraine, hypertension) and a psychopharmacological study performed with healthy volunteers (effects of benzodiazepines). The findings of the migraine study and benzodiazepine study have been published before (Tulen, Bussmann, van Steenis, Pepplinkhuizen & Man in 't Veld, 1997; Tulen, Stronks, Bussmann, Pepplinkhuizen & Passchier, 2000).

Methodology

Wrist-actigraphy: assessment of 24-hr motor activity patterns

Wrist-actigraphy can be used as an easy-to-use objective method to quantify spontaneous motor activity for a continuous period of several days in the habitual environment of subjects. When measured from the non-dominant wrist, several studies have demonstrated the validity and reliability of the method (Middelkoop, van Dam, Smilde-van den Doel & van Dijk, 1997; Patterson, Krantz, Montgomery, Deuster, Hedges & Nebel, 1993; Tryon, 1991); it can be used to discriminate rest- from activity-periods and to provide motor activity parameters related to diurnal sleep/wake patterns.

Equipment, sensor, and parameters: The actigraph used for our experiments (Geahwiler Electronic; size: 51 x 36.5 x 21 mm) contains a monoaxial piezoelectric acceleration sensor which counts the number of supra-threshold movements (accelerations > 0.1 g) per 30 sec epochs. The analogue signal of the sensor was sampled at a frequency of 8 Hz and subsequently band-pass filtered (0.25–3.0 Hz). The summed number of motor activity counts of each epoch was stored as a 1-byte value in a 32 Kbyte solid state memory. After completion of the measurement period, the data were uploaded to a personal computer for further analysis. The raw data files were screened visually and in reference to the daily log that the subjects kept, for quality of the recording, moments of actigraph removal, the occurrences of special activities, and to indicate bed-in and bed-out times (to define the sleep period). For each sleep-wake period, the following parameters were computed: motor activity level during wake and sleep (number of counts per epoch as percentage of the maximum number of counts possible, 253), fragmentation index of motor activity during wake and sleep (number of groups of consecutive zero count epochs divided by the total number of zero count epochs), immobility index during sleep (number of zero count epochs divided by the total number of zero count epochs), and, on the basis of the daily log total sleep time and sleep latency time. In addition, a clock-time based analysis was applied to compute half-hour activity counts from 06:00 hrs in the morning till 06:00 hrs the next morning.

In our studies, the subjects wore a wrist-actigraph continuously for a period of four days and nights, either from Monday till Friday morning or from Tuesday till Saturday morning, in their habitual environment (in the case of healthy subjects) or on the psychiatric ward (in the case of depressed patients). The subjects were asked to perform their normal activities at home or at the ward and to remove the actigraph only during bathing. The first day and night of the recording were considered as habituation period. The wrist-actigraphy data of the last three days and nights were used for analyses.

Daily physical activities: the Activity Monitor

Objective quantification of daily physical activities such as body postures (lying, sitting, standing) and dynamic activities (that is, walking, cycling, climbing stairs, postural transitions) can be realised by means of body-mounted accelerometers. Based on accelerometry, an Activity Monitor has been developed comprising four accelerometers, a portable digital recorder, and additional computer analysis software (see chapter 13 of Bussmann, van den Berg-Emons & Stam for a detailed description and examples). Validation studies in healthy subjects, amputees, and patients after failed back surgery showed high percentages of agreement (85–90%) between the automatic computer classification of the accelerometry signals and the visual analysis of simultaneously recorded videotapes (Bussmann, 1998; Bussmann, Reuvekamp, Veltink & Martens, 1998; Bussmann, Tulen, van Herel & Stam, 1998; Bussmann, van de Laar, Neeleman & Stam, 1998).

Equipment, sensors, and parameters: The Activity Monitor uses a portable digital recorder (Vitaport2™ System; TEMEC Instruments, Kerkrade, The Netherlands) for data-acquisition, that is carried on a belt around the waist. Definition of the sample rate and preprocessing settings of the acceleration signals and transfer of the Vitaport data to Personal Computer occurred by means of Vitagraph™ software (TEMEC Instruments). Four IC-3031 uni-axial piezo-resistive accelerometers were employed to quantify activities. The accelerometer signals are a combination of a component of the gravitational force (giving absolute angle information) and a component of the acceleration of the sensor (Veltink, Bussmann, de Vries, Martens & van Lummel, 1996). Two sensors were attached to the skin over the sternum: in the upright standing position, one sensor being sensitive parallel to the field of gravity (the longitudinal- or Y-axis) and one sensor attached perpendicular to the Y-axis sensor, sensitive along the sagittal- or X-axis. The two sensors on the upper legs were sensitive along the sagittal- or X-axis (according to Bussmann, 1998;

Bussmann, Veltink, Koelma, van Lummel & Stam, 1995). The accelerometer signals were stored digitally on the flashdisk of the recorder at a sample frequency of 32 Hz (description of signal processing procedures: chapter 13). The output signal of the computerized activity detection was processed to obtain the following parameters over a selected period of time: the total time spent in each posture (lying, sitting, standing) or as movement (summation of time spent as walking, cycling, climbing stairs, or as unspecified movements), the total number of transitions between lying, sitting and standing, and a total body motility index. For each analysis period, the time spent in the different body postures or as movement was expressed in minutes; total body motility was expressed in arbitrary units per sec, whereas the number of transitions during the periods were counted.

The Activity Monitor was used in a 'semi'-ambulatory setting during which healthy subjects were measured on four occassions for several hours in the laboratory as part of a pharmacological study, and in an ambulatory setting during which measurements were obtained from migraine patients before, during, and after a migraine attack in the habitual environment of the patients. Attachment of sensors and equipment required about 30 min, including testing of the signals and a brief calibration procedure of the signals in the sitting and standing posture. Instructions were provided regarding use of the equipment, checking the equipment's functional state, including practical advice for handling the recorder and sensors during a sleep period. The healthy subjects of the pharmacological study could move about freely in a room where they could relax, study, walk around or sleep; no specific instructions regarding type of activities were provided. The migraine subjects were instructed to perform their normal daily activities during the 48-hr headache-free measurement period, to keep a regular sleep-wake pattern and to avoid abnormal physical and mental exertions. The first 24-hrs of recording were considered to be a habituation period; data of the second day were used for analysis. When measured during their migraine and recovery period (about 72 hrs), no specific instructions were provided.

Accelerometry to quantify head movements

Accelerometers also can be used to quantify specific types of abnormal behavior, such as obsessive compulsive behaviors, involuntary movements, or tics. Sensor position is a relevant issue here, since these behaviors show high variability regarding body localisation and high intersubject variation. Recurrent and involuntary motor and vocal tics constitute the typical characteristics of patients with the syndrome of Gilles de la Tourette (Shapiro, Shapiro, Young & Feinberg, 1988). An increase in head tics is a frequently reported initial symptom of Tourette patients, therefore, we initiated experiments to quantify head movements and tics in Tourette patients by means of accelerometry.

Equipment, sensors, and parameters: Registration of the head movements occurred by means of 3 uni-axial 5g piezo-resistive accelerometers (IC-sensors 3031) that were attached to an elastic band, placed around the head, just above the eyebrows of the subject. These accelerometers provide signals that are a combination of a component of the gravitational force (absolute angle information) and a component of the acceleration of the sensor (Veltink, Bussmann, de Vries, Martens & van Lummel, 1996). Sensor1, placed above the left ear, measured the position and movements of the head in the lateral plane (that is, towards the left or right shoulder); sensor2, placed on the forehead, measured the position and movements of the head in the sagittal plane (that is, forwards or backwards); and sensor3, also placed on the forehead, measured the position and movements of the head also in the lateral plane (that is, rotation of the head to the left or to the right). The accelerometer signals were stored at a sample frequency of 64 Hz on a portable digital recorder. The datafiles were uploaded to a Personal Computer and analyzed using the program Windaq-ex™ (version 1.38; Dataq Instruments) and custom software (written in LabView™ 5.1). Our quantification was based on the signals of sensor1 (lateral), sensor2 (sagittal), and the difference signal of the signals of sensor3 and sensor1 (sensor3–sensor1; transversal plane) (example recording: see Figure 1). Videotapes were compared with the corresponding accelerometer signals in search for specific types of tics. Fast head movements could be recognised, primarily corresponding to isolated or bursts of motor tics of the patients (head jerking); the number of isolated fast head movements with typical features and a total duration of less than or equal to 0.22 sec were counted visually. Countings were checked with reference to the videotapes and a clinical expert. A head motility index was computed for each plane (lateral, sagittal, transversal) in order to obtain a general motility measure, reflecting changes both in frequency and intensity of movements: each of the three signals was high-pass filtered (0.5 Hz) and rectified; the resulting signals were integrated over 1 min intervals.

As a first approach we applied our method to Tourette patients and healthy controls in a controlled situation and looked for task-specific effects on head movements and head tics, in order to optimise recording procedures and develop signal processing tools. In subsequent studies we plan ambulatory recordings of head movements in both Tourette and ADHD patients.

Multichannel recording of accelerometry and cardiovascular signals

When combining accelerometry with physiology, a digital recorder is advisable that allows multichannel storage of signals with varying sample frequencies and preprocessing options, and with sufficient capacity to monitor for prolonged periods of time. If a combination with other recording devices is made (for instance a non-invasive blood pressure monitor), synchronization of measurements is a relevant issue.

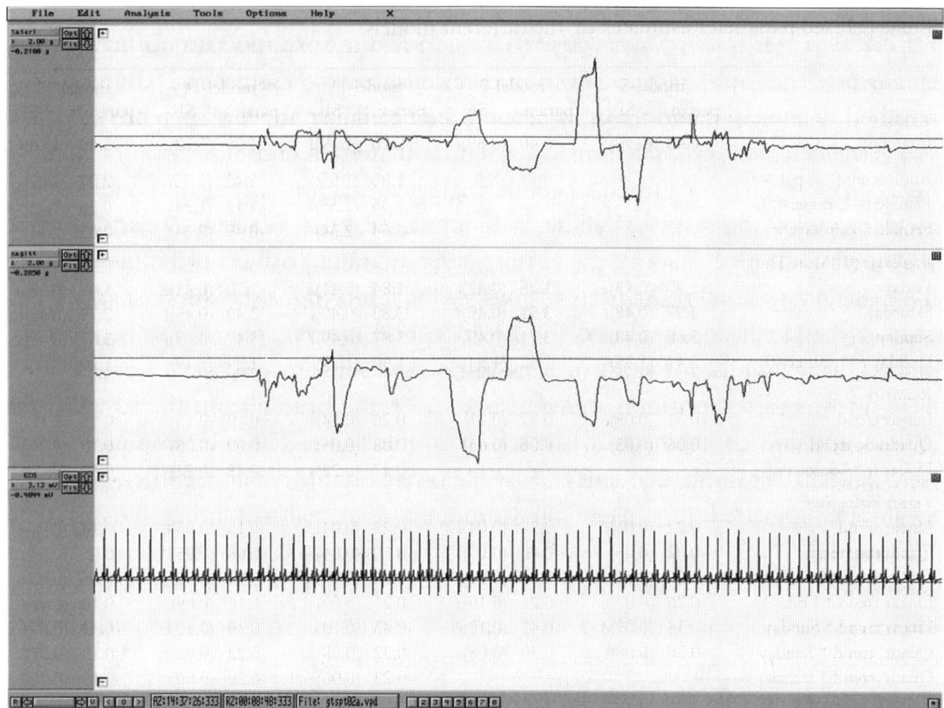

Figure 1. Illustration of head movements in the lateral (upper curve) and sagittal (middle curve) plane of a Tourette patient during calibration procedures (moving the head forward and backward, followed by moving the head to the right and to the left). The lower curve depicts the ECG. Time scale: 70 sec.

Heart rate recordings: Heart rate (bpm) was derived from a precordial ECG lead by means of adhesive disposable Ag/AgCl electrodes. The ECG signal was preprocessed and digitised at a sample frequency of 128 Hz on the Vitaport2 recorder. Transfer of the data file to Personal Computer occurred by means of Vitagraph™ software; analysis of the ECG signal was performed by means of a Signal Processing and Inferencing Language (S.P.I.L.™), which operates within the Vitagraph™ software. R-waves were dectected with a 2 ms accuracy, R-R intervals were transposed to heart rate time series, and stored at a sample frequency of 4 Hz. Within Vitagraph™, this heart rate time series was scrutinised visually for movement artifacts, R-wave dectection failures, and technical quality of the recordings; a linear interpolation procedures was applied to correct the heart rate time series where necessary. S.P.I.L. software routines were used to link the heart rate time series to the different classes of static and dynamic activities. For each selected analysis period, mean heart rate (bpm), standard deviation, and maximum and minimum values of heart rate were computed per static and dynamic activity category.

Blood pressure recordings: Non-invasive blood pressure was recorded by means of a Spacelabs 90207 BP monitor which was connected to the Vitaport2 recorder by means of a pressure transducer in order to synchronize the blood pressure and activity recordings. Blood pressure measurements were obtained at 15 min intervals during daytime and at 20 min intervals during the night. The daytime parts of the measurements were defined on the basis of the activity monitor. Average daytime and nocturnal systolic blood pressure, diastolic blood pressure, and heart rate values were calculated for each subject. Furthermore, mean total body motility (see chapter by Bussmann for a description of motility) was calculated over each 15 min period preceding each blood pressure measurement. Mean daytime total motility values were divided into three levels based on the pooled daytime total motility values of all subjects: low (lowest 0.333 part of the pooled data), moderate (middle 0.333 part), and high (upper 0.333 part). Blood pressure and heart rate values were studied in relation to the three defined motility levels.

Combined assessments of heart rate and accelerometry occurred in the studies with migraine, Tourette, and hypertensive patients, and also during the psychopharmacological study with healthy volunteers. Blood pressure recordings were obtained only from the hypertensive subjects, who were monitored in combination with accelerometry for a 24-hr period in their habitual environment.

Daily logs

In ambulatory research, daily logs are essential to document relevant events (for example, time point of medication intake), specific or unusual physical or psychological activities, leisure time activities, means of transportation, work or weekend day, and to obtain repeated assessments of self-rating questionnaires focused, for instance, on sleep quality and mood. Within the log used for the studies with depressed and migraine patients, the following brief self-rating questionnaires were filled in by the subjects: 1) the *Subjective Sleep Quality Scale* (SSQ; version: De Diana, 1976): at breakfast; 2) the *Profile Of Mood States* (POMS; validated Dutch version: Wald & Mellenbergh, 1990): at breakfast, lunch, dinner, and before sleep; and 3) the *Stanford Sleepiness Scale* (SSS; Hoddes, Zarcone, Smythe, Phillips & Dement, 1973). Subjective Sleepiness was assessed by means of a Dutch translation of the SSS, at similar time points as the POMS. These questionnaires are short and only take a few minutes to fill in.

Clinical applications

Psychomotor function and sleep in depression

Background: Psychomotor alterations (retardation and agitation) and sleep disturbances are two important clinical features of depression. In hospitalised severely depressed patients it is problematic to obtain ambulatory recordings of multiple signals to assess behavioral and psychophysiological functioning in relation to these clinical features: the equipment and sensors induce too great a burden for the patient. However, wrist-actigraphy has succesfully been applied to measure 24-hr spontaneous motor activity patterns in depressed patients; in combination with sleep logs it can provide additional information about changes in sleep/wake schedules or sleep quality. Thusfar, equivocal findings have been reported regarding the relationships between severity of depression and motor activity levels during wake and sleep in depressed patients (for example, Raoux, Benoit, Dantchev, Denise, Franc, Allilaire & Widlocher, 1994; Royant-Parola, Borbely, Tobler, Benoit & Widlocher, 1986; Sobin & Sackheim, 1997), which may have been due to differences in study population (bipolar versus unipolar depressed patients) and treatment status (medicated versus unmedicated). Relationships between severity of depression and self-reported sleep disturbances have seldom been studied. We evaluated 24-hr motor activity patterns and sleep characteristics in a group of unmedicated unipolar depressed patients and a group of healthy controls in order to clarify differences between patients and controls regarding diurnal motor activity patterns and sleep characteristics. Furthermore, within the patient group, we investigated relationships between severity of depression and motor activity patterns and between severity of depression and self-reported sleep characteristics.

Subjects and procedures: Fifty-eight hospitalised depressed patients (18 males, 40 females; mean age: 52.1 years, SD: 8.9), who met the DSM-IV criteria for major depressive disorder, subtype unipolar, participated in the study (DSM-IV, APA, 1994). The patients had an initial score of >17 on the 17-item version of the Hamilton Rating Scale of Depression (HRSD; Hamilton, 1960) and were studied after a psychotropic drug-free period of at least 7 days. Specific exclusion criteria were severe motor disabilities, and diseases (for example, Parkinson disease, arthritis), and drugs interfering with the motor activity pattern. Sixty-four healthy subjects (33 males, 31 females; mean age: 48.5 years, SD: 9.9) with no personal history of mental illness, sleep disorders, current medical illness or medication use formed the control group. It could not be excluded that the difference in study environment between patients and controls (hospital versus home) was a potential confounding factor in this study.

Depression, motor activity, and sleep characteristics: Depressed patients showed a significantly lower motor activity level during wake, less fragmentation of activity during wake, a reduced immobility level during sleep, a reduced total sleep time and a lower subjective sleep quality than controls, whereas motor activity level during sleep and sleep latency time were significantly increased in patients versus controls (Table 1). The alterations in diurnal motor activity pattern in the depressed patients are illustrated in Figure 2. No significant correlations were observed between the severity of depression and motor activity levels during wake and sleep, the fragmentation index during wake and sleep, and the immobility index during sleep. However, total sleep time and subjective sleep quality showed a significant inverse correlation with the severity of depression, whereas sleep latency time was significantly positively correlated with the severity of depression (Table 1).

Table 1. Mean (SD) motor activity and sleep parameters (based on the averaged values of the 3 recording days and nights) for depressed patients and controls.

	Patients	Controls	T-test p-values	Patients: partial corr coeff. with HRDS
HRSD score	27.2 (4.6)			
MW	6.9 (3.5)	11.6 (5.4)	<.001	0.01 (ns)
FragW	0.4 (0.1)	0.5 (0.08)	<.001	-0.05 (ns)
MS	0.8 (0.6)	0.6 (0.3)	<.001	-0.07 (ns)
FragS	0.05 (0.03)	0.05 (0.02)	ns	-0.02 (ns)
Imm	0.91 (0.06)	0.93 (0.03)	<.05	-0.05 (ns)
TST (min)	373.8 (96)	414.9 (52)	<.01	-0.31 (p<.05)
SLT (min)	73.4 (44)	22.4 (22)	<.001	0.34 (p<.05)
SSQ score	2.6 (2)	8.4 (2)	<.001	-0.50 (p<.001)

HRSD: Hamilton Rating Scale for Depression; MW, motor activity during wake; MS, motor activity during sleep; FragW, fragmentation index during wake; FragS, fragmentation index during sleep; Imm, immobility index during sleep; TST, total sleep time; SLT, sleep latency time; SSQ, subjective sleep quality; ns: non-significant

Evaluation: Our findings underline the presence of disturbances in motor activity level during daytime and sleep in depressed patients. Although we observed no significant relationships between severity of depression and motor activity patterns during wake or sleep, more severely depressed patients were found to have a shorter sleep period length, a longer sleep latency, and a worse sleep quality. Actigraphy has been suggested to be a suitable method to differentiate between subtypes of depression (for example, bipolar vs unipolar; Teicher, 1995). Our data show that self-reported sleep characteristics, rather than characteristics of motor activity pattern, correlate with severity of depression within unipolar depression. Maybe severity of depression is not related to interindividual variations in motor activity level within this patient group but clinical symptoms such as anxiety, agitation and psychotic features are (Parker, 2000). It will be interesting to study diurnal motor activity patterns and sleep characteristics in relation to these features and to explore their potential to predict treatment response, to evaluate mood, sleep, and psychomotor improvement after treatment, and to quantify side-effects of antidepressants.

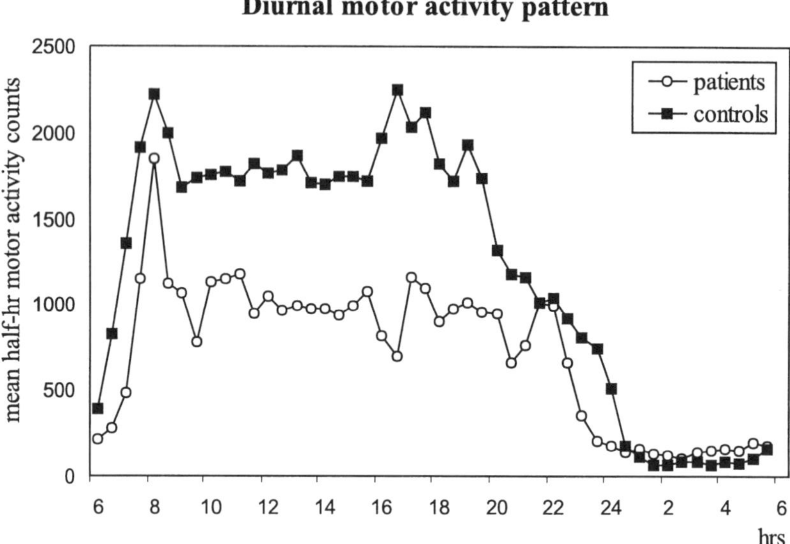

Figure 2. Mean half-hr motor activity counts, averaged for the three 24-hour periods, for the controls and the depressed patients separately.

(In)voluntary movements and tics in the syndrome of Gilles de la Tourette

Background: The syndrome of Gilles de la Tourette is a chronic neuropsychiatric disorder characterized by recurrent and involuntary motor and vocal tics and complex behavioral symptoms (for example, Shapiro, Shapiro, Young & Feinberg, 1988). Objective quantification of the frequency and intensity of tics in patients with the syndrome of Gilles de la Tourette is essential for diagnostic purposes, for evaluation of therapy efficacy, and to increase our understanding of the pathophysiology of the disease. The difficulty of developing reliable methods for objective assessment of tic severity relates to the variable presentation of tic symptoms, comprising aspects of body localisation, frequency, intensity, complexity, and noticeability, in addition to time- and situation-specific variations within and across subjects (Kurlan & McDermott, 1992; Peterson & Leckman, 1998; Shapiro, Shapiro, Young & Feinberg, 1988). Ambulatory accelerometry can be used as a tool to objectively quantify (in)voluntary movements and tics in GTS and to study these movements in relation to the psychophysiological condition of the patient. As a first approach, we quantified head movements and head tics in Tourette patients.

Subjects, procedures, and measurements: Nine patients (7 males, 2 females; mean age: 37.6 years, SD: 12.9) with current symptoms of Tourette's syndrome were diagnosed by a senior psychiatrist (DSM-IV criteria, APA, 1994). All patients suffered from multiple and single motor and vocal tics, as well as obsessive compulsive behaviors, and scored mild to moderate on severity of the syndrome (Yale Global Tic Severity Scale: Leckman, Riddle, Hardin, Ort, Swartz, Stevenson & Cohen, 1989). The control group consisted of 14 healthy volunteers (7 males, 7 females; mean age: 31.8 years, SD: 14.3). Each subject participated in an 1-hr session in which a videocamera as well as accelerometers recorded the movements of the head during: a) a 10 min period of rest (Rest1), b) a conversation of 5 min during which the subject talked with the researcher about his/her hobbies, c) a 5 min period of rest (Rest2), and d) watching a 15-min video of an entertaining program. The first 4 min of each rest or task period were analysed for number of fast head tics and intensity of head motility. Only head motility data of the lateral plane are presented, because the results for the other 2 planes were similar.

Isolated fast head movements and head motility: The fast head movements always corresponded to isolated or complex bursts of motor tics in the Tourette patients (head jerking). Figure 3 depicts the occurrence of bursts of fast head movements and changes in heart rate. Isolated fast motor tics were characterized by one sharp peak, not related or influenced by other head movements. Tourette patients showed a significantly higher number of isolated fast head movements during both rest periods and during video watching in comparison with controls (Table 2). Furthermore, the number of isolated fast head movements increased significantly from Rest2 to video watching, but not from Rest1 to conversation. Conversation induced a significant increase in head motility levels in both controls and patients in the lateral plane, whereas video watching did not. The patients showed significantly higher head motility levels during rest and task periods than controls (Table 2; all periods: $p<.05$).

Evaluation: Head motility levels during periods of rest and tasks were higher in Tourette patients than in controls. This suggests a chronic hyperactivity in the patients, although increased motility reflects both increased (non-)specific head movements and head tics. As expected, our countings of the isolated fast head movements (tics) revealed a significantly higher number of tics in patients versus controls during periods of rest, but also a very large inter-individual variability. Although watching a videotape did not significantly affect head motility in controls and patients, the number of isolated fast head movements showed a significant increase in the patients. This increase of head tics corresponds with our finding of an increase in number of eye tics in these patients during the same task (Tulen, Azzolini, de Vries, Groeneveld, Passchier & van de Wetering, 1999). In about 90% of the tics, premonitory sensations appear to precede the tic (Leckman, Walker, Goodman, Pauls & Cohen, 1993). In the near future, combined recordings of tics and heart rate or other physiological signals will allow us to study whether the concept of 'premonitory sensations' in Tourette has a physiological basis: Figure 3 sugg-

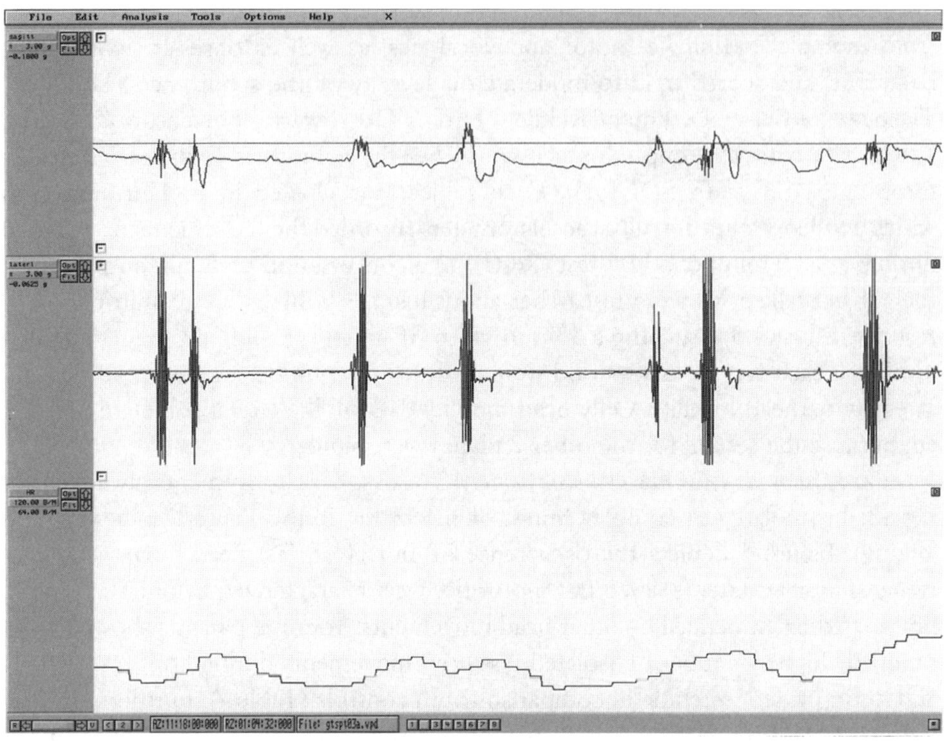

Figure 3: Head movements in the sagittal (upper curve) and lateral (middle curve) plane of a Tourette patient, illustrating the occurrence of bursts of fast head movements. The correspon-ding heart rate changes are depicted in the lower curve. Time scale: 60 sec.

Table 2. Mean (range) number of fast head movements as well as mean (SD) head motility levels (int/min) during rest and task periods, for the controls and the Tourette patients separately.

	Fast head movements		M-W test	Head motility lateral plane		M-W-test
	Controls	Patients	p-values	Controls	Patients	p-values
Rest1	0.0 (0-0)	17.0 (0-60)	.002	8820 (3632)	24904 (18313)	.007
Conv.	0.6 (0-3)*	19.4 (0-114)	ns	32959 (11756)*	48684 (2000)*	.039
Rest2	0.0 (0-0)	18.4 (0-81)	.002	11516 (7181)	29791 (15588)	.001
Video	0.1 (0-1)	34.9 (0-111)*	.004	11159 (5283)	22993 (18262)	.033

Conv.: conversation; M-W test: Mann-Whitney U test; ns: non-significant

*:p<.05; **: p<.01: Wilcoxon test; significant within-group increase from rest1 to conversation, or from rest2 to video watching

gests that there might be a relationship between the occurrence of tics and changes in heart rate. Both in standardized and ambulatory settings, accelerometry may contribute to a more objective description of the severity and temporal dynamics of tics or (non)-specific movements in relation to psychophysiological processes.

Effects of psychopharmaca on daily functioning

Background: Investigation of drug-induced psychophysiological effects in relation to daily behavioral patterns can provide useful information regarding treatment evaluation for both acute and chronic disease states. We explored whether the anxiolytic and sedative properties of benzodiazepines influence the postural and locomotor activities of normal daily life as well as postural-related heart rate changes. Effects of two oral doses of alprazolam (0.5 and 1.0 mg) were compared with one oral dose of lorazepam (2 mg) in a placebo-controlled design in healthy males. Alprazolam was chosen because it specifically may attenuate adrenomedullary activity (Breier, Davis, Buchanan, Listwak, Holmes, Pickar & Goldstein, 1992), but does not appear to influence cardiac vagal (parasympathetic) tone (McLeod, Hoehn-Saric, Porges & Zimmerli, 1992). In addition, it has been suggested that alprazolam may induce less sedation in comparison with clinically equivalent anxiolytic doses of other benzodiazepines (Dawson, Jue & Brodgen, 1984). Lorazepam was used as an active control: lorazepam may attenuate sympathetic nervous system activity and influence cardiac vagal tone (Tulen, Mulder, Pepplinkhuizen, Man in 't Veld, van Steenis & Moleman, 1994), and at an oral dose of 2 mg, lorazepam clearly induces sedation (Preston, Ward, Broks, Traub & Stahl, 1989). Furthermore, responses to the high dose of alprazolam (1 mg) may be compared with responses to the (approximately) clinically equivalent oral dose of 2 mg lorazepam (for example, Ellinwood, Heatherly, Nikaido, Bjornsson & Kilts, 1985; Huybrechts, 1991). Our measurements were obtained during a 4-hr ambulatory recording period, between 5 to 9 hrs after oral dose administration.

Subjects, procedures, and measurements: In a double-blind randomized cross-over study, 12 healthy male volunteers (mean age: 22 years, range 19–25) received either an oral dose of 2 mg lorazepam, or 0.5 mg alprazolam, or 1 mg alprazolam, or a placebo, on four different days, which were separated by at least five days. At 8:15 hrs, the subjects received the oral dose of alprazolam, lorazepam or placebo. During the morning part of the experiment, details of cardiovascular and catecholaminergic responses were studied during a standardized laboratory schedule of supine rest, active standing (orthostatic challenge), and mental load (Van den Berg, Tulen, Boomsma, Noten, Moleman & Pepplinkhuizen, 1996). The afternoon part of the study (from 13.00 till 17.00 hrs) comprised ambulatory measurements of heart rate and accelerometry in a living room in the hospital where the subjects could move around freely, study, relax, or sleep. Changes in sleepiness were assessed by means of the Stanford Sleepiness Scale at 13.00, 15.00, and 17.00 hrs.

Effects of benzodiazepines on physical activities, heart rate, and sedation: After benzodiazepine administration, the subjects spent significantly more time in the lying position (MANOVA: $p<.01$; lorazepam highest: 35%, placebo lowest: 11%), and significantly less time in the sitting position ($p<.01$; lorazepam lowest: 53%, placebo highest: 76%) (Table 3). Lorazepam and alprazolam had no effect on the time spent in static standing or general dynamic activities. After benzodiazepine administration, total body motility during static activities reduced significantly ($p<.025$), with motility after lorazepam administration being lowest. Mean heart rate showed a significant increase from supine to sitting, to standing, and to dynamic body movements ($p<0.001$) (Table 3). Lorazepam induced an overall increase in mean heart rate of about 6% and alprazolam a minor decrease of 2%, versus placebo ($p<0.003$); the effects were not posture-dependent. Sleepiness was significantly increased after alprazolam (0.5 and 1 mg) and lorazepam administration, in comparison with placebo ($p<.001$); the effect appeared strongest at 13.00 hrs and showed a significant time-dependent decline from 13.00 to 17.00 hrs ($p<.001$; Table 3).

Evaluation: This study illustrates the potential advantages of combining physiological measurements with accelerometry in pharmacological research. Apart from studying the effects of anxiolytics or hypnotics in ambulatory situations, details of spontaneous dynamic activities and postural transitions may be informative to analyse after acute and chronic administration of drugs that are known to induce postural hypotension or tachycardia (antidepressants; neuroleptics; mao-inhibitors). More than a mere quantification and inventarisation of potential side-effects, the study of these processes may provide objective indices of the patient's actual behavior before and after therapeutic interventions. As such, relationships between mobility and acute or chronic disease states (cardiovascular, psychopathological, movement disorders) (for example, Tyron, 1991) or behavioral processes (Montoye & Taylor, 1984) may be quantified objectively in order to evaluate the effects of (pharmaco)therapeutic interventions in relation to normal daily functioning more reliably.

Migraine attacks and daily functioning

Background: Migraine is a paroxysmal disorder, with attacks of unilateral, pulsating headache associated with nausea, vomiting, photophobia, and phonophobia (Headache Classification Committee of the International Headache Society, 1988). The repeated recurrence of migraine attacks significantly reduces quality of life and leads to impaired functioning (physically, emotionally, and socially) both at home and at work (Kryst & Scherl, 1994; Passchier, de Boo, Quaak & Brienen, 1996). Dependent on the severity of the attack, migraine can necessitate bed rest and/or reduced activity, and it can induce mood disturbance and physiological arousal. The research done on daily functioning during an actual migraine attack is limited and mostly based on self-report measures (for example, Stewart, Lipton, Kolodner,

Table 3. Effects of benzodiazepines on physical activities, mean heart rate, and sedation (from: Tulen, Bussmann, van Steenis, Pepplinkhuizen, & Man in 't Veld: Journal of Clinical Psychopharmacology, 17, 202-207, 1997)

mean (SD)		Placebo	Alprazolam (0.5 mg)	Alprazolam (1 mg)	Lorazepam (2 mg)
Activities					
Static	lying (%)	11 (15)	26 (20)	26 (20)	35 (19)
	sitting (%)	76 (15)	62 (21)	60 (19)	53 (19)
	standing (%)	6 (3)	6 (3)	6 (2)	5 (2)
Dyn. movement (%)		7 (3)	6 (2)	7 (3)	6 (2)
Motility (au)		2.26 (1.25)	1.88 (0.96)	1.90 (0.70)	1.61 (0.75)
Activity periods (n)		25.7 (7.3)	27.1 (10.7)	33.2 (11.7)	29.1 (8.2)
Heart Rate (bpm)					
Static	lying	66.4 (8.3)	63.5 (7.4)	64.9 (8.7)	69.6 (7.3)
	sitting	72.8 (8.4)	71.9 (10.5)	72.8 (7.2)	78.1 (7.8)
	standing	86.3 (12.2)	83.7 (12.9)	84.2 (8.2)	91.6 (8.8)
Dyn. movement		92.0 (9.9)	90.4 (10.8)	90.0 (6.3)	96.4 (7.9)
Sedation (SSS)					
13.00 hrs		1.8 (0.9)	2.7 (1.1)	3.0 (1.0)	3.2 (1.5)
15.00 hrs		1.3 (0.7)	1.9 (0.8)	2.5 (0.9)	2.5 (1.4)
17.00 hrs		1.1 (0.3)	1.4 (0.5)	1.5 (0.7)	1.8 (1.0)

SSS: Stanford Sleepiness Scale; %: percentage of time spent in activity category versus total recording time; dyn.: dynamic; n: number; au: arbitrary units

Liberman & Sawyer, 1999). We do not know how the subjective reports of migraine-induced disability relate to the behavioral and psychophysiological aspects of daily functioning. Yet, quantification of the patient's behavior in relation to their subjective perspective of level of functioning and psychophysiological condition during a migraine attack can provide an improved understanding of the relationships between diurnal mobility patterns, migraine, and effectiveness of therapeutic interventions.

Subjects, procedures, and measurements: Six migraine patients (all females; mean age: 39.8 years, range: 29 – 49) with the diagnosis 'migraine' (criteria: IHS, 1988) were studied. Patients with a positive history of drug abuse, psychiatric illness, or current medical illness other than migraine, were excluded from the study. The patients used their habitual medication for the acute treatment of migraine (2 patients used no medication), but did not use prophylactic anti-headache medication during the study.

Severity and duration of migraine attacks: Patient 1 used no anti-migraine medication; the patient reported a significant improvement (that is, a reduction in the severity of the attack, as a result of which at least some daily activities could be resumed) of her relatively mild headache after 4 hrs (Table 4). An untreated severe attack (patient 3) lasted 10 hrs before a significant improvement was observed; treatment of a severe attack with sumatriptan (injection; patient 5) resulted in a significant improvement after 1 hr; treatment of a moderate attack with sumatriptan (nasal spray; patient 4) reduced migraine complaints after 2 hrs, whereas treatment of moderate or severe attacks with ibuprofen or ergotamine (preceded by paracetamol) (patients 2 and 6) resulted in improvements after 4 or 5 hrs. In patient 4, the migraine attack developed in the late evening at a time point when she usually went to bed ('migraine period' between 23:00 hrs p.m. till 01:00 hrs a.m.); all other migraine attacks developed and were monitored during daytime.

Migraine and daily activities: example: Patient 3 (29 years) suffered from a severe, menstruation associated, migraine attack (with severe nausea and vomiting, photophobia, and phonophobia) that lasted 2 days. She used no medication for the treatment of her migraine attack. A significant improvement was reported after 10 hrs of recording. However, a substantial part of the first recovery day was also spent in bed, still with complaints of vomiting and photophobia and phonophobia.

Quantitative comparisons between migraine and the headache free period (Table 4): Patient 1 and 2 required no bed rest during their relatively light attacks: no change in time spent 'lying down' was observed versus the headache free period. In these patients, the changes in number of postural transitions, or the changes in number of min spent sitting, standing, or moving, versus the headache free period were variable. Patients 3, 5 and 6 required bed rest during their attacks and responded in an

Table 4. Per patient, for each migraine attack, the difference in time spent in different body positions and dynamic activities as well as in the number of postural transitions between the migraine period and the corresponding time period of the baseline day (in absolute number of min and as % of the duration of the migraine period) (based on Tulen, Stronks, Bussmann, Pepplinkhuizen, & Passchier: Pain, 86, 139-149, 2000).

Pat.	MP Min	Lying min	(%)	Sitting min	(%)	Standing min	(%)	Movements min	(%)	Trans. n	Motility % vs bsl
1	240	-0	(-0)	+32	(+13)	-21	(-9)	-11	(-5)	+1	-30
2	240	+1	(+0)	-43	(-18)	+24	(+10)	+19	(+8)	-5	-16
3	600	+584	(+97)	-441	(-74)	-63	(-11)	-91	(-15)	-55	-94
4	120	+11	(+9)	-6	(-5)	-4	(-3)	-2	(-2)	0	-75
5	60	+49	(+82)	-23	(-38)	-16	(-27)	-9	(-15)	-12	-90
6	240	+21	(+9)	+48	(+20)	-37	(-15)	-33	(-14)	-16	-51

Pat: patients; MP: migraine period in min; Trans.: transitions; motility, % vs bsl: motility, percentrage of change versus baseline; a positive value implies more time spent in that position/activity during migraine, a minus sign implies less time spent in that position/activity during migraine, in correspondence with the baseline day.

unequivocal manner to migraine, compared with the headache free period: the number of postural transitions decreased, the time spent in the lying position increased, and the time spent in the standing position or moving decreased. The time spent in the sitting position revealed variable changes versus the headache free period. Patient 3 (severe untreated attack, migraine period: 10 hrs) showed the largest behavioral changes (in absolute number of min) versus the headache free period, patient 5 (severe attack, sumatriptan injection, migraine period: 1 hr) the smallest. The migraine attack of patient 6 showed an intermediate pattern between patients 3 and 5 (possibly due to the slower effectivity of paracetamol and ergotamine in comparison with a sumatriptan injection). Patient 4 only showed minor changes versus the baseline period because of the late occurrence of her 'migraine period': although the migraine attack was sufficiently severe to require bed rest, during the comparable time period of the headache free recording she already slept for a large part of the time. In terms of percentage, the reduction in total body motility versus the baseline period was much larger in the patients who required bed rest (patients 3, 4, 5, 6: between 50 and 95% reduction) than in those who did not (patients 1 and 2: 30 and 16% reduction, respectively). During daytime migraine, supine heart rate was higher (mean: 78.0, SD: 13.6 bpm) than heart rate during the baseline sleep period (mean: 73.6, SD: 9.0 bpm).

Evaluation: With the restriction of the time required to travel to the patient and attach the sensors (about 1 hr), the migraine attacks and recovery periods were monitored. Overall, our findings indicate that migraine always influences behavior by reducing total body motility and that, dependent upon the severity of the attack, effectiveness of acute treatment, and the time of day, the time spent in various body positions, activities, and number of postural transitions are affected. Because a migraine attack is unpredictable in its occurrence, with our approach the patients will always suffer from headache for a certain period of time before measurements can take place. However, ambulatory accelerometry can be used as a valid and objective tool to quantify the daily activities in relation to heart rate changes during interictal periods. This may, for instance, help to clarify issues regarding chronobiological and autonomic nervous system disturbances in migraine. Furthermore, when using ambulatory accelerometry during migraine episodes, the main advantage is the possibility to evaluate the behavioral changes from headache till full recovery; this provides an opportunity to monitor the time-dependent effects of acute treatments of migraine on diurnal mobility patterns in relation to variations in severity of the illness and psychophysiological functioning.

Physical activity and ambulatory blood pressure in hypertension

Background: The diurnal variation of blood pressure is to a large extent determined by the sleep-wake cycle. This variation in blood pressure is considered to have prognostic value: several studies demonstrated that individuals who do not exhibit a nocturnal decline in blood pressure (nondippers) have an increased risk of cardiovascular morbidity and mortality compared to individuals who experience a normal nocturnal decline (dippers) (for example, Rizzoni, Muiesan, Montani, Zulli & Calebich, 1992; Verdecchia, Schillaci, Guerrieri, Gatteschi, Benemio, Boldrini & Porcellati, 1990). It is unclear to what extent the type and intensity of daily physical activities are of relevance in this issue, yet these are important determinants of the momentary fluctuations of blood pressure which can induce their effect independent of psychosocial or emotional factors (Gellman, Spitzer, Ironson, Llabre, Saab, DeCarlo Pasin, Weidler & Schneiderman, 1990). In order to clarify relationships between diurnal physical activities and blood pressure variation, we assessed the effect of total body motility (degree of physical activity) on daytime blood pressure during ambulatory measurements.

Subjects, procedures, and measurements: Sixteen subjects (13 hypertensives, 3 normotensives; 8 males, 8 females; mean age: 49.5 years, SD: 12.5) were studied for 24 hrs during which ambulatory measurements of non-invasive blood pressure (Spacelabs 90207 BP monitor) and body postures and physical activities by means of accelerometry were performed in their habitual environment.

Motility, blood pressure, heart rate, and body posture: Daytime and nighttime values of systolic and diastolic blood pressure and heart rate showed, on group level, a clear diurnal variation: during daytime systolic and diastolic blood pressure and heart rate were higher than during nighttime (systolic blood pressure, day: 138.6 (SD: 15) mmHg, night: 117.8 (16); diastolic blood pressure, day: 86.3 (12), night: 68.8 (13); heart rate, day: 79.1 (9) bpm, night: 66.4 (9)). Figure 4 illustrates that total body motility values are related to body posture; the highest values being observed when the subject is in the upright position (reflecting motility due to activities such as walking or climbing stairs). Systolic and diastolic blood pressure responses as well as heart rate responses increased significantly with increasing motility levels (Figure 5; ANOVAs with post-hoc comparisons between level1 [low] and level2 [moderate], and between level2 [moderate] and level3 [high]: all p-values $<.05$), the proportional increase being similar for systolic and diastolic blood pressure.

Evaluation: Sofar, relationships between physical activity and diurnal blood pressure variability have primarily been investigated by means of wrist actigraphy (for example, Kario, Schwartz & Pickering, 1999; Gretler, Carlson, Montano & Murphy, 1993). These studies found that it is essential to interpret ambulatory blood pressure data in the light of concomitant activity data. In this study, we calculated total body motility under ambulatory conditions based on the activity monitor. In contrast to

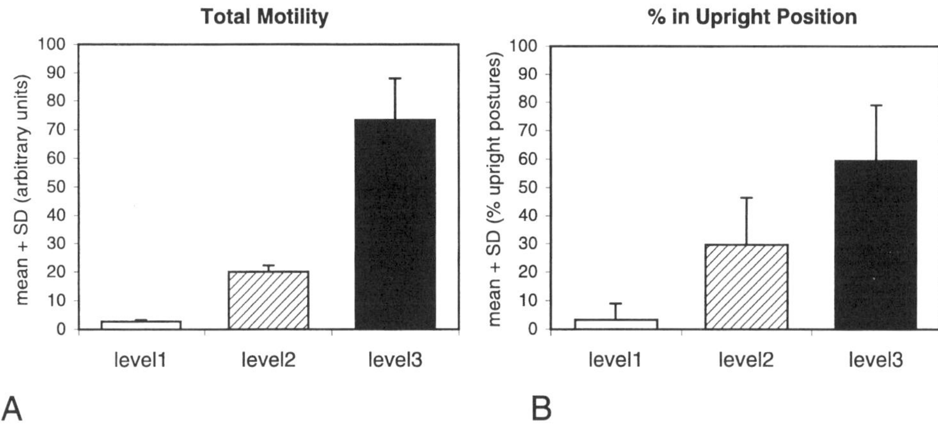

Figure 4. Mean + SD values of total motility perceding each blood pressure measurement (A) and mean + SD percentages of upright position (B) related to the 3 defined levels of motility: level1 (low), level2 (moderate), and level3 (high).

wrist actigraphy, the total motility index provides us with a global measure of body activity based on intensity of trunk and leg movements. During normal daily activities, blood pressure and heart rate increased with increasing levels of body motility. Postural changes are relevant to monitor in these processes, because they appeared to have a large effect on body motility and may independently affect heart rate and blood pressure (for example, Tulen, Boomsma & Man in 't Veld, 1999). Therefore, when unraveling diurnal blood pressure variability in order to determine which components have clinical relevance for hypertension, combined assessments of physical activity and cardiovascular signals are necessary. The findings obtained with these analyses can subsequently be used to evaluate more reliably the situational, psychosocial and emotional factors involved in blood pressure variability in the habitual environment of (hypertensive) subjects.

Discussion

Benefits and limitations of our methods to quantify overt behavior

Wrist-actigraphy to quantify 24-hr motor activity patterns: A major advantage of the wrist-actigraph is that it is small-sized and easy-to-use. As an unobtrusive device it can be used to obtain reliable information of 24-hr motor activity patterns in situations where more complex measurements (with more sensors and larger recorders) are undesired. Patterns and levels of motor activity during wake and sleep can be studied in relation to clinical, emotional, and subjective sleep indices to evaluate global aspects of psychomotor (dys)functions in neuropsychiatric and neurological disorders. As a global measure of physical activity, actigraphy has also been used in car-

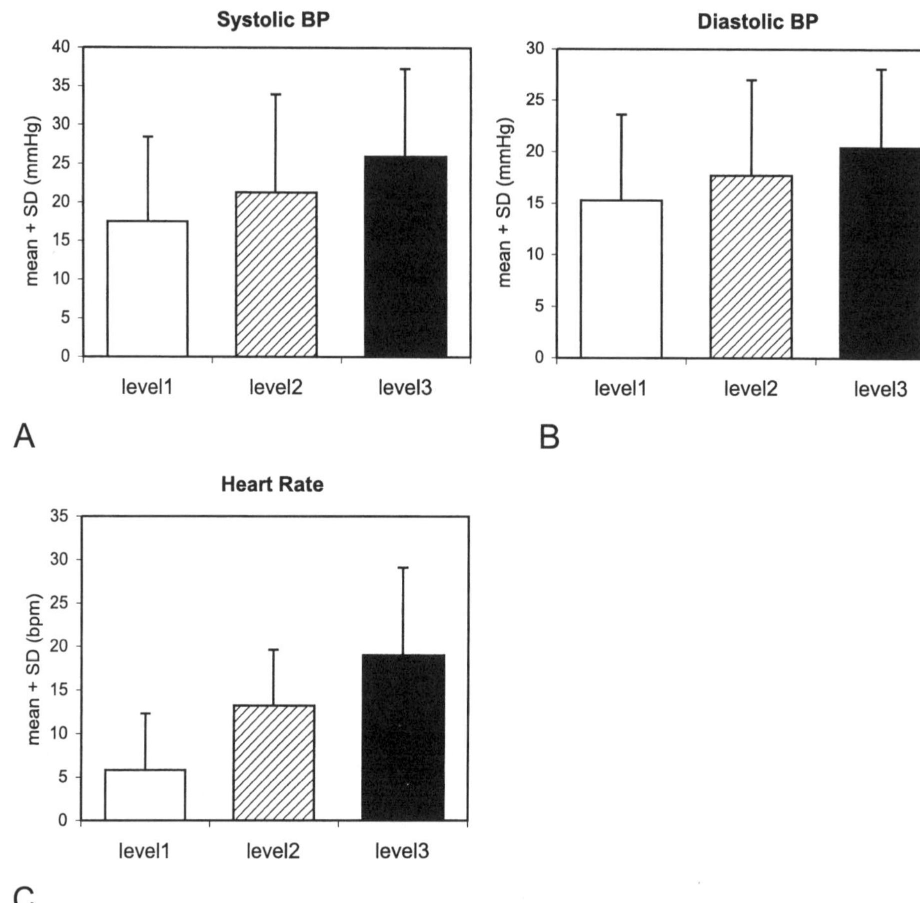

Figure 5. Mean + SD values of systolic (A), diastolic (B) blood pressure and heart rate (C) responses to the 3 levels of total motility. For each level, the mean differences with nighttime values are presented.

diovascular studies (for example, Kario, Schwartz & Pickering, 1999). However, when it is relevant to study the morphology of (non)specific movements and/or focus on particular behavioral patterns, whether or not in relation to physiological processes, other sensors, measuring devices and high resolution processing techniques need to be used. Contemporary activity monitors that measure bodily accelerations in various planes (for example, Leenders, Sherman & Nagaraja, 2000; Welk, Blair, Wood, Jones & Thompson, 2000) offer some extra possibilities, but still can not fully capture the morphological features of (non)specific movements.

The Activity Monitor to quantify daily physical activities: This method has several advantages over current subjective and objective methods to assess aspects of daily physical activities: a) in comparison with the use of daily logs and/or questionnaires it has the advantage of being more objective and accurate (Patterson, Krantz, Montgomery, Deuster, Hedges & Nebel, 1993), b) in comparison with quantification of overall 24-hr motor activity patterns by means of wrist-actigraphy, it has the advantage of enabling to study details of posture-related behavioral activities, and c) the Vitaport2 recorder allows combined measurements of multiple signals with varying sample frequencies; therefore, the method can be used to quantify posture- and activity-related cardiovascular changes under ambulatory conditions, which results in a more reliable interpretation of ambulatory recorded cardiovascular measurements. The present limitations of the method relate to the fact that a) body-mounted sensors are used, which do not allow bathing, swimming or intensive sports involving a lot of sweating, and b) the size and weight of the recorder (dimensions: 15x9x4.5 cm, 700 gr.).

Accelerometry to quantify head movements and tics: Similar sensors were used as for the Activity Monitor, therefore the same advantages apply. The use of these accelerometers made it possible to obtain objective quantitative data regarding spontaneous head movements and tics. The experience we obtained with this experiment can now be used to explore other movement dysfunctions in neuropsychiatric or neurological disorders. In combination with the use of a multichannel digital recorder, quantification of these spontaneous movements in relation to cardiovascular parameters is possible. The limitations of our method to quantify head movements are restricted to 1) sensor position: because of the oval characteristics of the head, the sensors could not be placed entirely perpendicular to the direction of the gravitational field; therefore, some 'cross-talk' between the 3 planes (lateral, sagittal, transversal) occurred, and 2) attachment of sensors on a head band is somewhat inconvenient and needs to be replaced with something more practical and less noticeable before ambulatory measurements in daily life situations can be made.

Future developments

Combined monitoring of psychophysiological and behavioral parameters is essential for research purposes in a variety of psychological and medical disciplines. Our studies illustrate the potential advantages of this research strategy. Developments in the near future should, among others, focus on the following aspects:

Feature extraction, automatic signal processing, validation, and multisignal analysis:

a) implementation and validation of signal features related to fast head movements/tics or other simple tics and dystonic or tonic tics in automatic signal processing procedures may facilitate the quantification of the severity and temporal dynamics of the tics. At first instance this will require controlled studies in which computerized output needs to be validated against visually analysed videotapes. Once the validity of the automatic procedures has been established, it is possible to move from controlled to ambulatory studies.

b) spectral analyses of the accelerometer signals (for instance by means of Joint Time-Frequency Analysis) may be explored for its potential to reflect intensity and periodicity of (in)voluntary movements and tics.

c) further exploration and validation of locomotor activities, (in)voluntary movements, (non)specific movements, and tics in a variety of ambulatory situations, but particularly in the habitual environment of subjects.

d) a detailed quantification of relationships between cardiovascular time-series and activity parameters, for example, heart rate and blood pressure responses to postural changes, motility, various dynamic activities, and (non)specific movements or tics.

e) synchronizing the behavioral and cardiovascular measurements with the assessments of subjective mood and sedation, in order to improve an accurate description of the interaction between these parameters.

Instrumentation:

f) optimization of sensor position, size, configuration, and manner in which the sensors are attached to the body is something that requires attention in the future, also when other types of tics or behavioral abnormalities are studied under ambulatory conditions.

g) when using digital recorders for multisignal measurements in ambulatory research, development of smaller and lighter recorders with high storage capacity remains a relevant issue; only when the patients are not hampered by the equipment and sensors, can reliable information be obtained about normal behavioral patterns or spontaneous (non)specific movements.

Conclusion

Monitoring of behavioral activities by means of accelerometry is a promising and original method which deserves a special place in clinical psychophysiological research. Our studies illustrate that accelerometry by means of body-mounted piezo-resistive sensors forms an objective approach to quantify daily physical activities (body posture, physical and locomotor activity) or behavioral dysfunctions (psychomotor retardation, (in)voluntary movements, tics) in relation to psychophysiological functioning in a variety of diseases. As such, accelerometry may contribute to an increase of our understanding of pathophysiological processes; furthermore, it may be used for diagnostic purposes and for evaluation of therapy efficacy.

Acknowledgements

The benzodiazepine study was performed with financial support from the Dutch Ministery of Economic Affairs and Pharmacia & UpJohn BV; the migraine study was supported by a research grant from Glaxo Wellcome BV. The authors are grateful to the following persons who contributed to individual experiments: Walter van den Broek, Jan Bruijn, Marlies Wegewijs-de Jong, Marieke Gieteling, Hans Bussmann, Judith Romers, Sander de Vries, Ben van de Wetering, Frans van den Berg, Ton van den Meiracker, Arie Man in 't Veld, Hugo van Steenis, Jan Passchier, and Lolke Pepplinkhuizen (University Hospital Rotterdam – Dijkzigt and Erasmus University Rotterdam).

References

American Psychiatric Association. (1994). *Diagnostic and statistical manual of mental disorders.* (4th ed.) Washington, DC: Author.

Breier, A., Davis, O., Buchanan, R., Listwak, G.J., Holmes, C., Pickar, D. & Goldstein, D.S. (1992). Effects of alprazolam on pituitary-adrenal and catecholaminergic responses tometabolic stress in humans. *Biological Psychiatry, 32*, 880–890.

Bussmann, J.B.J. (1998). *Ambulatory monitoring of mobility-related activities in rehabilitation medicine.* PhD thesis, Erasmus University Rotterdam, Eburon.

Bussmann, J.B.J., Laar van de, Y.M., Neeleman, M.P. & Stam, H.J. (1998). Ambulatory accelerometry to quantify motor behavior in patients after failed back surgery: a validation study. *Pain, 74*, 153–161.

Bussmann, J.B.J., Reuvekamp, P.J., Veltink, P.H. & Martens, W.L.J. (1998). Validity and reliability of measurements obtained with an 'Activity Monitor' in people with and without a transtibial amputation. *Physical Therapy, 78*, 989–998.

Bussmann, J.B.J., Tulen, J.H.M., Herel van, E.C.G. & Stam, H.J. (1998). Quantification of physical activities by means of ambulatory accelerometry: a validation study. *Psychophysiology, 35*, 488–496.

Bussmann, J.B.J., Veltink, P.H., Koelma, F., Lummel van, R.C. Stam, H.J. (1995). Ambulatory monitoring of mobility-related activities; the initial phase of the development of an Activity Monitor. *European Journal of Physical Medicine and Rehabilitation, 5*, 2–7.

Clark, L.A., Denby, L., Pregibon, D., Harshfield, G.A., Pickering, T.G., Blank, S. & Laragh, J.H. (1987). A quantitative analysis of the effects of activity and time of day on the diurnal variations of blood pressure. *Journal of Chronic Disease, 40*, 671–681.

Dawson, E.D., Jue, S.G. & Brodgen, R.N. (1984). Alprazolam, a review of its pharmacological-properties and efficacy in the treatment of anxiety and depression. *Drugs, 27*, 132–147.

De Diana, I.P.F. (1976). Two stochastic sleep quality scales for self-rating subject's sleep. *SleepResearch, 5*, 101.

Ellinwood, E.H., Heatherly, D.G., Nikaido, A.M., Bjornsson, T.D. & Kilts, C. (1985). Comparative pharmacokinetics and pharmacodynamics of lorazepam, alprazolam and diazepam. *Psychopharmacology, 86*, 392–399.

Fahrenberg, J. & Myrtek, M. (1996). *Ambulatory assessment. Computer-assisted psychological and psychophysiological methods in monitoring and field studies.* Seattle WA: Hogrefe & Huber Publishers.

Gellman, M., Spitzer, S., Ironson, G., Llabre, M., Saab, P., DeCarlo Pasin, R., Weidler, D.J. & Schneiderman, N. (1990). Posture, place, and mood effects on ambulatory blood pressure. *Psychophysiology, 27*, 554–551.

Gretler, D.D., Carlson, G.F., Montano, A.V. & Murphy, M.B. (1993). Diurnal blood pressure variability and physical activity measured electronically and by diary. *American Journal of Hypertension, 6*, 127–133.

Hamilton, M. (1960). A rating scale for depression (HRS). *Journal of Neurology Neurosurgery & Psychiatry, 23*, 56–61.

Headache Classification Committee of the International Headache Society (1988). Classification and diagnostic criteria for headache disorders, cranial neuralgias and facial pain. *Cephalalgia 8* (suppl 7),10–73.

Hoddes, E., Zarcone, V., Smythe, H., Phillips, R. & Dement, W. (1973). Quantification ofsleepiness: a new approach. *Psychophysiology, 10*, 431–436.

Huybrechts, I. (1991). The pharmacology of alprazolam: a review. *Clinical Therapeutics, 13*, 100–117.

Kario, K., Schwartz, J.E. & Pickering, T.G. (1999). Ambulatory physical activity as a determinant of diurnal blood pressure variation. *Hypertension, 34*, 685–691.

Kryst, S. & Scherl, E. (1994). A population-based survey of the social and personal impact of headache. *Headache, 34*, 344–350.

Kurlan, R. & McDermott, M.P. (1992). Rating tic severity. In: R. Kurlan (Ed.). *Handbook of Tourette's syndrome and related tic and behavioral disorders* (pp 199–220). New York: Marcel Dekker..

Leckman, J.F., Riddle, M.A., Hardin, M.T., Ort, S.I., Swartz, K.L., Stevenson, J. & Cohen, D.J. (1989). The Yale Global Tic Severity Scale: initial testing of a clinician-rated scale of tic severity. *Journal of the American Academy of Child and Adolescence Psychiatry, 28*, 566–573.

Leckman, J.F., Walker, D.E., Goodman, W.K., Pauls, D.L. & Cohen, D.J. (1993). Premonitory urges in Tourette's syndrome. *American Journal of Psychiatry, 150*, 98–102.

Leenders, N.Y.J.M., Sherman, W.M. & Nagaraja, H.N. (2000). Comparisons of four methods of estimating physical activity in adult women. *Medicine and Science in Sports and Exercise, 32*, 1320–1326.

McLeod, D.R., Hoehn-Saric, R., Porges, S.W. & Zimmerli, W.D. (1992). Effects of alprazolamand imipramine on parasympathetic cardiac control in patients with generalized anxietydisorder. *Psychopharmacology, 107*, 535–540.

Middelkoop, H.A.M., van Dam, E.M., Smilde-van den Doel, D.A. & van Dijk, G. (1997). 45-hour continuous quintuple-site actimetry: relations between trunk and limb movement and effects of circadian sleep-wake rhythmicity. *Psychophysiology, 34*, 199–203.

Montoye, H.J. & Taylor, H.L. (1984). Measurement of physical activity in population studies: areview. *Human Biology, 56*, 195–216.

Parker, G. (2000). Classifying depression: should paradigms lost be regained? *American Journal of Psychiatry, 157*, 1195–1203.

Passchier, J., Boo de, M., Quaak, H.Z.A. & Brienen, J.A. (1996). Health-related quality of lifeof chronic headache patients is predicted by the emotional component of their pain. *Headache, 36*, 556–560.

Patterson, S.M., Krantz, D.S., Montgomery, L.C., Deuster, P.A., Hedges, S.M. & Nebel, L.E. (1993). Automated physical activity monitoring: validation and comparison with physiological and self-report measures. *Psychophysiology, 30*, 296–305.

Peterson, B.S. & Leckman, J.F. (1998). The temporal dynamics of tics in Gilles de la Tourettesyndrome. *Biological Psychiatry, 44*, 1337–1348.

Preston, G.C., Ward, C.E., Broks, P., Traub, M. & Stahl, S.M. (1989). Effects of lorazepam onmemory, attention, and sedation in man: antagonism by Ro 15–1788. *Psychopharmacology, 97*, 222–227.

Pickering, T.G. (1991). *Ambulatory monitoring and blood pressure variability*. London: SciencePress Ltd.

Raoux, N., Benoit, O., Dantchev, N., Denise, P., Franc, B., Allilaire, J.F. & Widlocher, D. (1994). Circadian pattern of motor activity in major depressed patients undergoingantidepressant therapy: relationship between actigraphic measures and clinical course. *Psychiatry Research, 52*, 85–98.

Rizzoni, D., Muiesan, M.L., Montani, G., Zulli, R., Calebich, S. & Agabiti-Rosei, E. (1992). Relationship between initial cardiovascular structural changes and daytime and night-time blood pressure monitoring. *American Journal of Hypertension*, *5*, 180–186.

Royant-Parola, S., Borbely, A.A., Tobler, I., Benoit, O. & Widlocher, D. (1986). Monitoring oflong-term motor activity in depressed patients. *British Journal of Psychiatry*, *149*, 288–293.

Shapiro, A.K., Shapiro, E.S., Young, J.G. & Feinberg, T.E. (1988). *Gilles de la Tourette syndrome.* New York: Raven Press.

Sherwood, A. & Turner, J.R. (1993). Postural stability of hemodynamic responses duringmental challenge. *Psychophysiology*, 30, 237–244.

Sobin, C. & Sackeim, H.A. (1997). Psychomotor symptoms of depression. *American Journal of Psychiatry*, *154*, 4–17.

Stewart, W.F., Lipton, R.B., Kolodner, K., Liberman, J. & Sawyer, J. (1999). Reliability of the migraine disability assessment score in a population-based sample of headache sufferers. *Cephalalgia*, *19*, 107–114.

Teicher, M.H. (1995). Actigraphy and motion analysis: new tools for psychiatry. *Harvard Review of Psychiatry,* 3, 18-35.

Tryon, W.W. (1991). Activity measurement in psychology and medicine. New York: Plenum Press.

Tulen, J.H.M., Azzolini, M., de Vries, J.A., Groeneveld, W.H., Passchier, J. & van denWetering, B.J.M. (1999). Quantitative study of spontaneous eye blinks and eye tics in Gilles de la Tourette's syndrome. *Journal of Neurology Neurosurgery* & *Psychiatry*, *67*, 800–802.

Tulen, J.H.M., Boomsma, F. & Man in 't Veld, A.J. (1999). Cardiovascular control and plasma catecholamines during rest and mental stress: effects of posture. *Clinical Science*, *96*, 567–576.

Tulen, J.H.M., Bussmann, J.B.J., van Steenis, H.G., Pepplinkhuizen, L., Man in 't Veld, A.J. (1997). A novel tool to quantify physical activities: ambulatory accelerometry in psychopharmacology. *Journal of Clinical Psychopharmacology*, 17, 202-207.

Tulen, J.H.M., Mulder, G., Pepplinkhuizen, L., Man in 't Veld, A.J., van Steenis, H.G., & Moleman, P. (1994). Effects of lorazepam on cardiac vagal tone during rest and mental stress: assessment by means of spectral analysis. *Psychopharmacology*, 114, 81-89.

Tulen, J.H.M., Stronks, D.L., Bussmann, J.B.J., Pepplinkhuizen, L. & Passchier, J. (2000). Towards an objective quantitative assessment of daily functioning in migraine: a feasibility study. *Pain*, *86*, 139–149.

Tyron, W.W. (1991). Activity measurement in psychology and medicine. New York: Plenum Press.

Van den Berg, F., Tulen, J.H.M., Boomsma, F., Noten, J.B.G.M., Moleman, P. & Pepplinkhuizen, L. (1996). Effects of alprazolam and lorazepam on catecholaminergic and cardiovascular activity during supine rest, mental load, and orthostatic challenge. *Psychopharmacology*, *128*, 21–30.

Veltink, P.H., Bussmann, J.B.J., Vries de, W., Martens, W.L.J. & Lummel van, R.C. (1996). Detection of static and dynamic activities using uniaxial accelerometers. *IEEE RehabEng*, *4*, 375–385.

Verdecchia, P., Schillaci, G., Guerrieri, M., Gatteschi, C., Benemio, G., Boldrini, F. & Porcellati, C. (1990). Circadian blood pressure changes and left vertricular hypertrophy in essential hypertension. *Circulation*, *81*, 528–536.

Wald, F.D.M., Mellenbergh, G.J. (1990). De verkorte versie van de nederlandse vertaling van de Profile Of Mood States (POMS). *Nederlands Tijdschrift voor de Psychologie*, *45*, 86–90.

Welk, G.J., Blair, S.N., Wood, K., Jones, S. & Thompson, R.W. (2000). A comparative evaluation of three accelerometry-based physical activity monitors. *Medicine and Science in Sports and Exercise*, *32*, S489–S497.

Chapter 15
Assessment of Posture, Motion, and Hand Tremor by Calibrated Accelerometry

Friedrich Foerster
Forschungsgruppe Psychophysiologie, Department of Psychology, University of Freiburg, Germany

Introduction

The assessment of physical activity is a basic issue in psychophysiological ambulatory monitoring. However, diary-type records of activity are of questionable reliability and validity, and, in any case, lack resolution in time. The objective measurement of movement and posture, and the kinematic analysis of behavior in general, has greatly profited from the progress made in sensor technology and advanced methods in signal analysis. This is evident from a number of recent publications (see also the Book Chapters by Bussmann et al. and Tulen et al.).

Physical activity is defined here as gross body movement that usually involves, in varying degrees, the upper and lower extremities and the movement of the neck (head) and trunk. This activity is apparent in changing body position (lying supine, sitting, standing), in walking and climbing stairs, and in many kinds of motor performance. In the psychophysiological laboratory, subjects are usually instructed not to move in order that the recording artifacts can be avoided. In ambulatory monitoring studies, however, physical activity is as much an essential aspect of psychophysiological activation as is a source of unwanted variance.

The design of the assessment of physical activity will depend on the specific aims of a given study. Among these are:

- measurement of over-all physical activity to assess energy expenditure or the subject's activity level for the 24-hour period;
- detection of change in body position (for example, lying supine, sitting, standing), body rotation (for example, during sleep), and often occurring movement behaviors (for example, walking, climbing stairs);
- kinematic analysis, that is, detection of more specific movements (for example, using a tool, typing a keyboard), individual features of gait, and, moreover, diagnosis of movement disorders (for example, hand tremor in Parkinson's disease,

restless legs syndrome), and the clinical use of kinematic analysis for the evaluation of treatment and rehabilitation programs in patients with movement pathologies.

Methodology

The conventional methodology made use of wrist-worn actometers, tilt-switch transducers, mechanical pedometer, piezo-ceramic sensors, and other electronic devices to register movements. Actometer devices are suitable for many applications and they are less expensive than the infrared-light methodology of kinematic analysis, easier to apply than recordings of the electromyogram, and more convenient than video tape analysis. The measurement of activity in psychology, psychophysiology, and medicine was reviewed by Tryon (1991; see also Bussmann, 1998; Fahrenberg & Myrtek, 2001; Patterson et al., 1993).

The progress in the assessment of movement and posture resulted from three developments: First, the wide bandwidth of new piezoresistive (for example, ICSensor Model 3031, Analog Devices ADXL202) and piezocapacitive sensors paved the way for the development of a new methodology with calibrated accelerometers. The DC signal output (that is, signal output < 0.5 Hz) allows the assessment of change in position in relation to the gravitational axis (that is, inclination in degrees), and the AC signal output > 0.5 Hz is used to represent acceleration in terms of the gravitation, that is, g (or milli-g), along the sensitive axis of the device; second, the development of pocket-sized digital data recorders has especially facilitated multi-channel ambulatory monitoring and 24-hour recording of activity in daily life; and, third, the increase in computer capacity that enabled advanced methods of signal analysis, in particular, joint time (amplitude) – frequency analysis and specific methods of filtering (for example, Qian & Chen, 1996), benefited behavior analysis, too. Software has been developed for automatic detection of motion patterns in multi-channel recordings.

Multi-channel (multi-site) accelerometry with calibrated sensors is thus a very promising methodology, and researchers are becoming increasingly aware of the many advantages this approach has to offer and of its potential fields of application in psychology and medicine (see Bussmann, 1998; Jain, Martens, Mutz, Weiß & Stephan, 1996; Veltink & van Lummel, 1994). The actual posture and the pattern of motion (beyond the measurement of physical activity) basically provide a frame of reference for the evaluation of many behaviors, symptoms, and physiological changes. For example, the assessment of resting condition vs. walking or climbing stairs appears to be an essential aspect in the psychophysiological investigation of cardiovascular change and energy expenditure under naturalistic conditions.

Ambulatory blood pressure monitoring is a good example that both, an index of the over-all physical activity and the detection of motion patterns (including change of posture), are essential aspects of any thorough evaluation of BP variability in daily life, that is, BP responses to certain activities or events and BP recovery in leisure time and sleep. It should be noted that the ambulatory monitoring equipment commonly used for 24-hour ECG or blood pressure recordings does not permit measurement of physical activity. The patients are required instead to indicate change of body position, exercise, etc., by entries in a diary. However, concurrent recordings of physical activity appear to be superior to this method in terms of a precisely timed evaluation of cardiovascular reactivity in a psychophysiological context. Such recordings could indicate whether a sudden rise in blood pressure is caused by standing up, that is, by hydrostatic effects and compensatory regulation, by physical exercise, that is, by metabolic requirements; or whether this change was possibly caused by an emotional response or mental effort. For obvious reasons, an actimeter worn on the wrist (for example, Van Egeren, 1992), would not be the best choice to indicate the amount of physical exercise relevant for change in cardiovascular measures.

Body position, is certainly, an important aspect, too. In recent research on BP recovery and BP decrease during sleep (dipper and non-dipper), many authors seem to neglect body position during sleep. Unnoticed body rotation from the left to the right side may introduce an arbitrary BP change in the order up to 20 mmHg (caused by height differences concerning arm cuff/level of the heart and hydrostatic effects), that is, in the order of the assumed recovery effects (Fahrenberg, 2000; Pickering, 1991; Schwan & Pavek, 1989).

In the literature, various strategies were suggested to account for physical activity in psychophysiological recordings of cardiovascular changes: regression models (Anastasiades & Johnston, 1990; Tuomisto, Johnston & Schmidt, 1996), cross-correlation techniques (Fahrenberg, Heger, Foerster & Müller, 1991), a segmentation of recordings to separate data periods with/without physical activity (Käppler, Becker & Fahrenberg, 1993), and a real-time algorithm for partialling out heart rate variance due to physical activity in order to retain psychologically relevant components (Myrtek et al., 1988, see, also the Book Chapter by Myrtek & Foerster, this Volume).

In the following, an account of the developments and refinements of accelerometry in this laboratory, based on four method studies, will be given. Initially, motion was predominantly seen as unwanted variance that should be controlled by appropriate recordings to detect changes in posture and motion. In due course, it became evident that a one-channel recording of physical activity would not suffice. In the process of developing accelerometry for such applications, the kinematic analyses became a research issue in itself. Furthermore, the assessment of one particular movement disorder, the hand tremor in Parkinson's disease, emerged as an interesting clinical application of this methodology. Two 24-hour monitoring studies in PD patients have been completed so far.

Detection of posture and motion

Basic issues

Multi-channel accelerometry was recently evaluated in a number of ambulatory monitoring studies. The evaluation indicated the importance of the following questions raised: Which algorithms are suitable for the *detection of motion patterns and posture*, and which *sensor placements* would provide a minimal configuration to assess a broad spectrum of functional activities? (Busser, 1994; Busser, Ott, van Lummel, Uiterwaal & Blank, 1997; Bussmann, 1998; Bussmann, Tulen, van Herel & Stam, 1998; Bussmann, Veltink, Martens & Stam, 1994; Fahrenberg, Foerster, Müller & Smeja, 1997; Fahrenberg, Müller, Foerster & Smeja, 1996; Foerster, Smeja & Fahrenberg, 1999; Kiani, Snijders & Gelsema, 1997; van de Weijer, Smits, de Haan & van Lummel, 1994; see also Veltink, Bussmann, de Vries, Martens & van Lummel, 1996). A third issue was the choice of a sensor placement or a sensor configuration for a *valid prediction of general physical activity and energy expenditure* (Bouten, Verboektet-van de Venne, Westerterp, Verduin & Janssen, 1996; Middelkoop, van Dam, Smilde-van den Doel & van Dijk, 1997; Myrtek, Brügner & Müller, 1996; Patterson et al., 1993; Richardson, Leon, Jacobs, Ainsworth & Serfass, 1995; Sherman et al., 1998; Tuomisto et al., 1996; Walker, Heslop, Plummer, Essex & Chandler, 1997).

With a few exceptions, the aforementioned studies refer only to a small number of motion patterns. It is clear that in addition to standing, sitting, lying, walking, climbing stairs, further behaviors should be included (Bussmann et al., 1998; Foerster et al., 1999): Subtypes of lying, that is, lying on the right or left side, supine or with back supported, and a preferred position at sleep onset, are necessary to monitor bed rest and nightly body rotation; samples of walking at normal and fast pace are preferable to test the discrimination between walking and climbing of stairs. Indeed, the majority of investigations have only used a few sensors, and several studies have not explicitly referred to the DC-component as an indication of posture (inclination): they seemed to be content with just the analysis of movement. In addition, the subject samples studied were always small. Posture and motion patterns do exhibit a remarkable inter-individual variability. Therefore, a larger number of subjects is required to investigate such patterns. The selection of a minimal configuration would be of practical interest in this context.

Calibrated accelerometry for the detection of posture and motion

Calibration refers here, firstly, to the calibration procedure regarding each piezoresistive sensor and recorder channel, and, secondly, to the standard protocol which provides the basic reference patterns (see below). Four method studies from this laboratory were concerned with the development and refinement of multi-channel accelerometry (see, Table 1 for an overview).

Table 1. Detection of posture and motion: Summary of four method studies.

	First Study	Second Study	Third Study	Fourth Study
Design	Lab Building Pilot study evaluation of Sensors	Lab Building Cross validation	Lab Building/ Field Validation against participant observer	Lab Building Conditions 4X repeated (permutation)
Student Participants	N=26 male Age: 20-33 years	N=26 male Age: 21-33 years	N=24 male Age: 21-34 years	N=31 male Age: 20-32 years
Sensors	ZAK tri-axial, VITAPORT uni-axial, PAR tri-axial, 2-channel EMG, VITAPORT body-position transducer	ICS 3031, medNatic, VITAPORT body-position transducer	ICS 3031	ICS 3031, ADXL 202
Placement	Forearm, Lower leg, Recorder	Regio infraclavicularis, Wrist, Thigh, Lower leg	Sternum, Wrist, Thigh, Lower leg	Sternum, Thigh
Conditions	Sitting, Standing, Supine rest, Motor performance (key-board), Stairs up, Stairs down	Sitting, Standing, Supine rest, Motor performance (key-board), Walking, Stairs up, Stairs down, Cycling	Sitting, Standing, Supine rest, Sitting and talking, Motor performance (keyboard), Walking, Stairs up, Stairs down, Cycling	Sitting (upright, forward, backward), Standing, Lying (supine, left, right), Walking (normal, fast), Stairs up, Stairs down, Cycling
Analysis	Discrimance analysis	DC-AC-decom-position, fixed threshold, dis-criminance analysis	DC-AC-decom-position, reference-pattern based classification	DC-AC-decom-position, reference-pattern based hierar-chical classification
Specific Issues	Evaluation of accelerometers, EMG, body position sensor	Discrimination between conditions, detection of static and dynamic behaviors	Validation of accelerometric against behavior observation	Distinguishing of subtypes of moving behavior and posture (esp. walking-stairs-discrimination)
Reference	Fahrenberg, Müller, Foerster & Smeja, 1996	Fahrenberg, Foerster, Smeja & Müller, 1997	Foerster, Smeja & Fahrenberg, 1999	Foerster & Fahrenberg, 2000

The first investigation was designed to evaluate accelerometry (comparing different sensor types) and the EMG in the discrimination of seven conditions, and within-subject correlation between sensor types, between recording sites. The correlation between measures of activity and heart rate changes were also investigated (Fahrenberg et al., 1996).

The second study used only piezoresistive sensors in the development of calibrated accelerometry, which comprises the decomposition of position (the degree of inclination) and motion (acceleration). Recordings were made under eight conditions (as previously, and including cycling). A classification based on four parameters was correct in almost 100 % of patterns when subsequently applied to a second trial (recorded in reversed order). The findings indicated a noteworthy between-subject variation in behaviors, for example, walking or climbing stairs (Fahrenberg et al., 1997). Such variability makes the classification of motion patterns by stepwise discriminant analysis or the use of a set of normative data difficult. Instead, the recording of a standard protocol proved to be a superior method for detecting the essential motions and postures. This standard protocol consists of a fixed sequence of behaviors, recorded for at least 30 s each, allowing for individual differences of movement and some deviations in positioning of the sensitive axes due to individual morphology. The recorded patterns were subsequently employed as a reference.

The third study comprised nine conditions. The recordings were continued outside the laboratory building and a participant observer classified the various postures and motions. The findings indicated a high agreement between automatic detection and observation. Some participants, however, showed discrepancies in specific motions or they exhibited mixed patterns. Generally, the discrimination between walking and climbing stairs was less satisfactory (Foerster et al., 1999).

The fourth method study aimed at a further refinement of calibrated accelerometry. The new investigation was to evaluate the hierarchical classification of patterns, especially with regard to the difficult discrimination between walking and climbing stairs (Foerster et al., 1999). An extended standard protocol contained static and dynamic behaviors which were not accounted for previously: subsets of sitting posture (leaning forward and backward), and lying (body rotation and a lying position, back supported and knees slightly bent). The measurement of body rotation required an additional sensor placed on the sternum, sensitive in y-direction (transversal). A sensor for the z-direction (vertical) indicates lying independently of body rotation and should be useful for distinguishing between climbing stairs and walking.

The increase in the number of sensors and axial representations of movements raised the question about the choice of sensor configuration sufficient to detect the major classes of posture and motion correctly. The answer will depend partly on the actual selection of movements and functional activities, although the main classes of posture and a set of basic motion patterns may be regarded as core patterns. Which sensor placement gives the minimal configuration for detection of these core patterns? An extended configuration using a larger number of sensors may be able to detect, for example, essential subtypes of moving or lying in bed, and may therefore be preferable for a full 24-hour recording.

Sensor placement

The sensors (IC Sensor Model 3031) were piezoresistive. They have wide bandwidth (i.e., DC and AC response), high sensitivity ~ 1 mV/g (standard range ± 2 g), and a typical accuracy of ± 0.2 %. The frequency response is practically linear up to the kHz range. The sensors (supplied by Vitaport, Becker Meditec, Karlsruhe,

Germany) were mounted, 20 x 20 x 2 mm, and weigh 4 g. In more recent studies, also two-axial ICS 3031 and ADXL 202 sensors, housing 20 x 20 x 4. The flat design of today's accelerometers permits the placement of sensors on many parts of the body, even on the distal phalanx of the finger. The terminology is inconsistent across laboratories (Table 1). We suggest the descriptive terms sagittal (x-direction), transversal (y-direction), and vertical (z-direction) instead of the anatomical terminology referring to the anterioposterior, mediolateral, and craniocaudal axes.

Table 2. Axes and planes

	Terms		Direction with reference to gravitational axis (Sternum vertical)
1	*Sagittal*		*x*
		anterioposterior ventral–dorsal (pointing forward)	
2	*Transversal*		*y*
		mediolateral lateral horizontal (pointing sideways)	
3	*Vertical*		*z*
		craniocaudal longitudinal (pointing up)	

Note: Positive direction means that a positive signal is obtained when, for example, a three-axial sensor placed on the sternum of the standing subject indicates movement forward, sideways, and up.

Each sensor was calibrated for a specific Vitaport2 amplifier channel by measuring the signal under controlled inclination, that is, by rotating the sensor providing a signal output corresponding to + 1 g and - 1 g (the gravitational constant) or 0 respectively 180 degrees to the gravitational axis. The DC output is zero when the sensitive axis is perpendicular to the gravitational axis. The recordings were obtained with a 32 Hz sampling rate and low pass filtering at 20 Hz.

The sensors were used as follows:
Sternum. Three uni-axial sensors were placed adjacently at the sternum about 5 cm below the jugulum, the sensitive axes pointing in a vertical (1), sagittal (2), and transversal (3) direction, that is, in the z-, x- and y-direction, respectively.

Thigh. Frontal aspect of right (4) and left (5) thigh, distal from m. rectus femoris, about 5 cm above the patella, the sensitive axis of the sensors was roughly perpendicular to the surface, that is, to the frontal aspect of the sternum and the frontal aspect of the thigh.
The sensors were attached with adhesive medical tape (Fixomull® Stretch, Beiersdorf AG, Hamburg).

The Vitaport 2 (Becker Meditec, Karlsruhe, Germany) was used for the multichannel recording. Vitaport 2 is a general purpose digital recorder/analyzer (32 bit microprocessor, 16 MHz). It weighs 700 g. More recently, the Varioport Recorder was used with smaller dimensions, reduced weight (170 g), and low power consumption designed for prolonged ambulatory recording.

Hierarchical classification of posture and motion patterns

Pre-processing

The DC and AC components of the raw signal were separated by means of a first order FIR digital filter with a cut-off frequency at 0.5 Hz (3 dB). Raw signal, DC-values, and rectified AC-values were averaged across data points for each condition and monitoring segment. Walk frequency was calculated by means of short-time Fourier transform within the frequency band of 0.5 to 4 Hz using the z- (vertical) axis of the sternum sensor (Fahrenberg et al., 1997; Foerster et al., 1999; Qian & Cheng, 1996).

Classification

Data segments were classified by referring to the standard protocol variable profiles. Similarity is determined by the so called L distances (see, for example, Halmos, 1950). The L distance between two conditions j and k with the variables i=1...nv is defined as

(1) $dist_{jk} = \Sigma_{i=1...nv} | x_{ij} - x_{ik} |$

Unlike the L distance (Euclidian Distance) $\sqrt{\Sigma_{i=1...nv}(x_{ij} - x_{ik})^2}$, which makes an adjustment for the risk of variables with large differences, the large and small diffferences are treated equally in the L distance.

The variables have to be standardized whenever they have different scaling (for example, AC and DC variables). The most common standardization factor is the standard deviation as used, for example, for the z-transformation. In our investigation, however, we used a standardization factor suitable for the L distance, namely the average absolute differences between the ns standard protocol conditions: for variable i we formulate:

(2) $s_i = \Sigma_{j=1...ns}\Sigma_{k<j} | x_{ij} - x_{ik} | / [ns(ns-1)/2]$

This factor is a measure of discrimination of variable i between the ns standard protocol conditions (or a respective subset of them). Hence, the standardized L distance is given by

(3) $d_{jk} = \Sigma_{i=1...nv} | x_{ij} - x_{ik} | / s_i$

Each of the standard protocol conditions represents a point in the nv-dimensional space given by the nv variables. A certain data segment m was labeled according to the standard protocol condition j to which it was nearest, that is, whose L_1 distance d_{jm} was the smallest under the ns standard protocol conditions.

Hierarchical classification was conducted with a SAS© datastep macro using subsequent subsets of variables to discriminate subsets of conditions. Table 3 summarizes the steps denoting variables and standard protocol situations used. After determining posture (lying, sitting, standing) and motion (yes/no) on the basis of discrimation (1) and (2), lying was categorized in detail by (4), and, if the subject was in supine position, by (5); sitting by (6); walking on the level and up stairs by (3), and, if walking was selected, by (7); and, finally, bicycle by (8). This classification procedure was applied to the three sets of repeated behaviors, that is, 39 (3 x 13) conditions.

Table 3. Hierarchical classification

Step	Specification	Discrimination between Conditions (number of conditions)	Variables/Sensors used	Standardization necessary
1	Posture	lying (4), sitting (3), standing	DC of 3 sternum, 2 thigh	no
2	Motion	all	AC of 3 sternum, 2 thigh	no
3	Stairs	walking (2), stairs (2)	AC and raw signal of 2 sternum (sagittal, vertical), 2 thigh, walk frequency	yes
4	Lying	lying (4)	DC of sternum lateral	no
5	Supine	lying on back, supine	DC of sternum sagittal and vertical	no
6	Sitting	sitting (3)	DC of sternum sagittal and vertical	no
7	Walking	walking (2)	walk frequency	no
8	Bicycle	sitting forward, bicycle	AC of sternum sagittal, 2 thigh	no

Five-sensor configuration

An almost perfect concordance was found between the behavior protocol in the laboratory and the classification based on calibrated accelerometry with a five-sensor configuration. The overall agreement was impaired only by 38 (3.2 %) misclassifications, most of which concerned the discrimination between sitting upright/leaning backward and the discrimination between dynamic activities, that is, walking, and climbing stairs (Foerster & Fahrenberg, 2000).

Two-sensor configuration

With this configuration, that is, z-direction of the sternum sensor and x-direction of the right thigh, the agreement for classes of lying, standing, moving, and sitting, was almost perfect indicating only 1.3 % misclassifications. Since the sternum sensor x-direction (sagittal) and the y-direction (transversal) were disregarded here, subtypes of walking, of sitting, and of lying could not be distinguished.

Standard configuration

A minimum set of sensors can be used for a given application, for example, a two-sensor configuration would clearly suffice to differentiate between four basic classes (sitting, standing, lying, moving) in ambulatory monitoring. Thus, a sensor configuration for standard accelerometric detection of frequently occurring posture and motion patterns is proposed (see Table 4). The methodology developed here can be easily adopted to account for further motion patterns on condition that appropriate variation regarding the sensitive axes of sensors exist and such motions were included in the standard protocol.

Table 4. Proposed sensor configuration for standard accelerometric detection of posture and motion patterns.

Number of sensors	Placement	Direction of axis	Suited for detection of
2	Sternum right Thigh	z x	Basic classes: Sitting, Standing Lying, and Moving (pace and vigor of stride)
4*	as above, and Sternum left Thigh	 x x	Subtypes of Sitting and Moving (Walking, Climbing stairs, Cycling)
5	as above, and Sternum	 y	Body rotation in bed

Note: * Recommended for optimal discrimination

Pace and vigor of stride

The quantification of gait, that is, rate and vigor of walking, was examined. However, the vigor of stride was not included in the classification procedure. Rate and amplitude were calculated by means of short-time Fourier transform (STFT; see Qian & Chen, 1996; Foerster & Smeja, 1999) within the frequency band of 0.5 to 4 Hz using the vertical axis of the sensor placed on the sternum. The sternum sensor proved to be superior in estimating pace; using a thigh sensor would only indicate every second step. The signal amplitude of walking represents, however, the vigor of stride.

Conclusions

The findings from this series of four method studies basically correspond with the findings reported by the Rotterdam Group (see, Chapters by Bussmann et. al; Tulen et al.; this Volume). They show that a large variety of static and dynamic motion behaviors can be correctly detected by multi-channel accelerometry, appropriate signal processing, and statistical analysis. The reliability of the software detection of motions and postures was established in repeated measurement designs and the validity of the classification procedure was successfully evaluated against behavior observation in the laboratory (videotaped in some instances) and in daily life (ambulatory monitoring and participant observation). Of course, further agreement studies between automatic classification procedures and observation may be useful for a further refinement and extension of the methodology. One might expect that under naturalistic conditions a number of mixed patterns, unusual or idiosyncratic behaviors may occur which challenge the present strategies. In particular, the investigation of movement disorders appears to be a rewarding research orientation.

The algorithm for the detection of posture and motion patterns is still an issue in the refinement of accelerometry. Several suggestions have been made as to how to achieve an adequate data reduction and to differentiate between a variety of dynamic activities under investigation. The development of pattern recognition systems based on different strategies was proposed. Such classifier systems could be designed by using statistical algorithms, conventional or fuzzy logic, or artificial neural networks (Kiani et al., 1997; Martens, 1994). However, only two approaches have been used to a greater extent (Bussmann et al., 1998; Fahrenberg et al., 1997; Foerster et al., 1999):

Fixed-threshold classification. Motion patterns, for example, walking, climbing stairs, and cycling, can be differentiated by applying a threshold to the signal of the thigh accelerometer. The threshold is derived from empirical studies and is used for all subjects. The discrimination between more classes of motion patterns requires a greater number of threshold values and appropriate normative studies. Substantial interindividual differences in static and dynamic behaviors clearly lead to misclassifications.

Reference-pattern based classification. The detection of motion patterns can be improved if individual reference patterns for each postural and activity condition were obtained by an initial recording of the essential patterns under investigation. In the case of such a standard protocol, multivariate analyses and pattern similarity coefficients can be used for the detection and labeling of an actual segment, that is, motion pattern with reference to the standard protocol (Foerster et al., 1999).

In view of these considerations, the use of a reference-pattern based classification, rather than a fixed threshold classification, is suggested whenever possible. The standard protocol takes less than a minute of recording time for every posture and motion. The protocol can be easily adapted to specific subsets of behaviors and the strategy is highly flexible since certain reference patterns may be included later, if necessary, after the conclusion of the monitoring. Further refinement of the reference pattern based classification was achieved by a hierarchical strategy which classifies postures and, subsequently, uses reference patterns for the discrimination between subsets of dynamic activities.

Measurement of Tremor

Tremor is a significant symptom of Parkinson's disease. This low frequency tremor, with a frequency range of about 3 to 7 Hertz, is usually manifest in one or both hands; the face, legs, and other regions may also be affected. In clinical practice, the severity of tremor is usually assessed during the neurological examination. The Unified Parkinson's Disease Rating Scale UPDRS (Fahn et al., 1987) contains several items concerning the localization and occurrence of tremor during rest and movement, whereby occurrence and amplitude are rated together on five-point scales. In addition to symptom ratings, clinical studies often include EMG recordings of hand tremor. These measurements are mostly conducted for only a brief period of time during rest and postural tremor test. However, short-term recordings of tremor may not reflect a patient's disability since the tremor activity exhibits significant fluctuations and diurnal changes (Cleeves & Findley, 1987; Elble & Koller, 1991). Patients with moderate tremor amplitude may be significantly disabled if their tremor is constant, whereas other patients may be disabled because of intermittently severe tremor.

24-hour assessment of tremor activity

Clinical studies on the course of tremor and appropriate medication, necessitate repeated measurement designs that may include, besides standardized rest and postural tremor tests, long-term recordings. Furthermore, 24 hour ambulatory monitoring would facilitate the investigation of how tremor activity is affected by change of posture, by time of day and night and, possibly, by emotional and behavioral events.

The quantification of tremor amplitude changes appears to be of particular interest in long-term assessments, whereas tremor frequency shows little intrasubject variation. The current view is that there are few diagnostic situations in which such amplitude values are helpful (Deuschl, Krack, Lauk & Timmer, 1996). The assessment of this view would be easier if more long-term studies about tremor amplitude change were available. The quantification of tremor amplitude is, of course, the basis of reliable detection of tremor occurrence, that is, the discrimination of tremor and non-tremor segments according to an objective cut-off value.

Ambulatory recordings of wrist activity and day-to-day variability in patients with Parkinson's disease have been reported (van Hilten, Hoff & Roos, 1993; van Hilten, Middelkoop, Kerkhof & Roos, 1991), and the use of accelerometry has been suggested as a valid means to assessing tremor, posture, and motion (van Hilten et al., 1993; van Someren et al., 1993, van Someren et al., 1998; Zimmermann et al., 1994). For recording tremor in the longterm, a method was developed, based on the EMG and the use of portable analog recorder devices (Bacher, Scholz & Diener, 1989; Spieker, Boose, Jentgens & Dichgans, 1995; cf. Tremor Analyzer, CSM, Filderstadt, Germany).

Advantages in accelerometry

Compared to EMG recordings, accelerometry has some practical advantages. EMG recordings usually require abrasion of the skin and application of an electrolyte. Properties of the skin-electrode system exhibit systematic and time-dependent changes. Such limitations may become especially evident in clinical investigations that involve repeated measurement designs and long-term recordings, for example, 24 hour ambulatory recordings. The processing of the EMG raw signal requires certain assumptions such as those concerning stationarity and filter settings. Although EMG recordings can be calibrated, that is, in micro Volts, this does not ensure a reliable comparison of the severity of tremor activity in between and within-subject designs. Accelerometry appears to have major advantages: the ease in application of sensors, the quantification of the amplitude of tremor activity, and moreover, the availability of an objective decision rule as to whether tremor is present or not.

The aim of the present work was to develop a practical method of assessing the tremor activity in patients with Parkinson's disease during standardized tasks and under conditions of daily life. Important tremor parameters were amplitude, frequency, and occurrence in percent of time. It should be noted that amplitude refers here to the actometer raw signal and, therefore, signifies acceleration (milli-g) which equals the second derivative of the amplitude of movement (mm). However, movement amplitude can be calculated from acceleration amplitude by integrating it twice, assuming, the tremor signal is sinusoidal. Joint amplitude-frequency analysis was used to quantify these parameters (Foerster & Smeja, 1999). Furthermore, the recently developed methodology of kinematic analysis for detecting posture and motion based on multi-channel accelerometry (see above) was applied.

Tremor analysis using Short Time Fourier Transform STFT (TREMOR Program)

In order to determine frequency and amplitude of the acceleration signal an analysis was done by a variant of the Joint Time-Frequency Analysis JTFA, that is, the Short Time Fourier Transform STFT (Qian & Chen, 1996). STFT calculates for

Table 5. Parameters for the STFT: Criteria for depicting tremor activity.

Parameter	Description	Value	
		Study 1	Study 2
Frequency band	Tremor frequency is searched within this band	2-7 Hz	3-7 Hz
Step frequency	Step frequency of the spectrum is related to the length of the FFT: length (seconds) = 1/step frequency (Hz)	0.5 Hz	0.5 Hz
Power ratio	Ratio = power of peak frequency / total power (Has tremor frequency sufficient power?)	0.5	a
Between ratio	Ratio = power within the band / total power (Has tremor band sufficient power?)	a	0.5
Within ratio	Ratio = power of peak frequency / power of band (sharpness of the frequency peak)	a	0.05
Peak estimation	by searching the greatest peak within the band with quadratic interpolation (peak) or by estimating the "expected value", that is, the weighted mean	peak	expected value
Windowing	FFT using rectangle or Hanning window	Hanning	Hanning
Amplitude threshold	Peak amplitudes below the threshold are missing data	0.005 g	0.01 g
Amplitude output	Acceleration (g) or movement (cm)	accel.	accel.
Episode length	Tremor episodes must be longer than this threshold	1 second	1 second

Note: [a] Ratio criteria modified.

each data point of a raw signal a complete Fourier spectrum. Based on the power spectrum, the method transforms the raw signal into two new signals with the same sampling rate, namely the peak frequency within a predefined band and the amplitude of this frequency. In the present form, STFT uses 10 parameters (Table 5).

Primary data analysis was done with program TREMOR implemented under Windows (95 or 98). Besides tremor analysis, the program prepares the accelerometer signals for classification of posture and motion (decomposition of AC and DC by a first-order FIR digital filter with cutoff frequency of 0.5 Hz at 3 dB as well as the walk frequency and vigor, using STFT in 0.5 to 4 Hz, no missing data criteria used). Furthermore, heart rate and the mean squared successive difference MSSD are derived from the ECG using a special filter ("canonical filter") which compares each QRS complex with an individual averaged QRS). The essential results of this analysis can be controlled on the screen. Data analysis of a 24 hr recording of tremor activity in one channel required about six minutes computer time on a Pentium PC.

Figure 1 shows an example of the steps in STFT. In Figure 1a, a typical accelerometer signal is depicted. The signal has values between 0.4 g and 1.4 g and a DC-level of about 0.9 g. The DC-level is due to the rest position of the hand: episodes of high amplitude and short tremor intervals. Before STFT was applied the DC-component was removed by a first order FIR digital filter with cutoff frequency of 3 Hz. The STFT now produces the time series of the tremor frequency (Figure 1b)

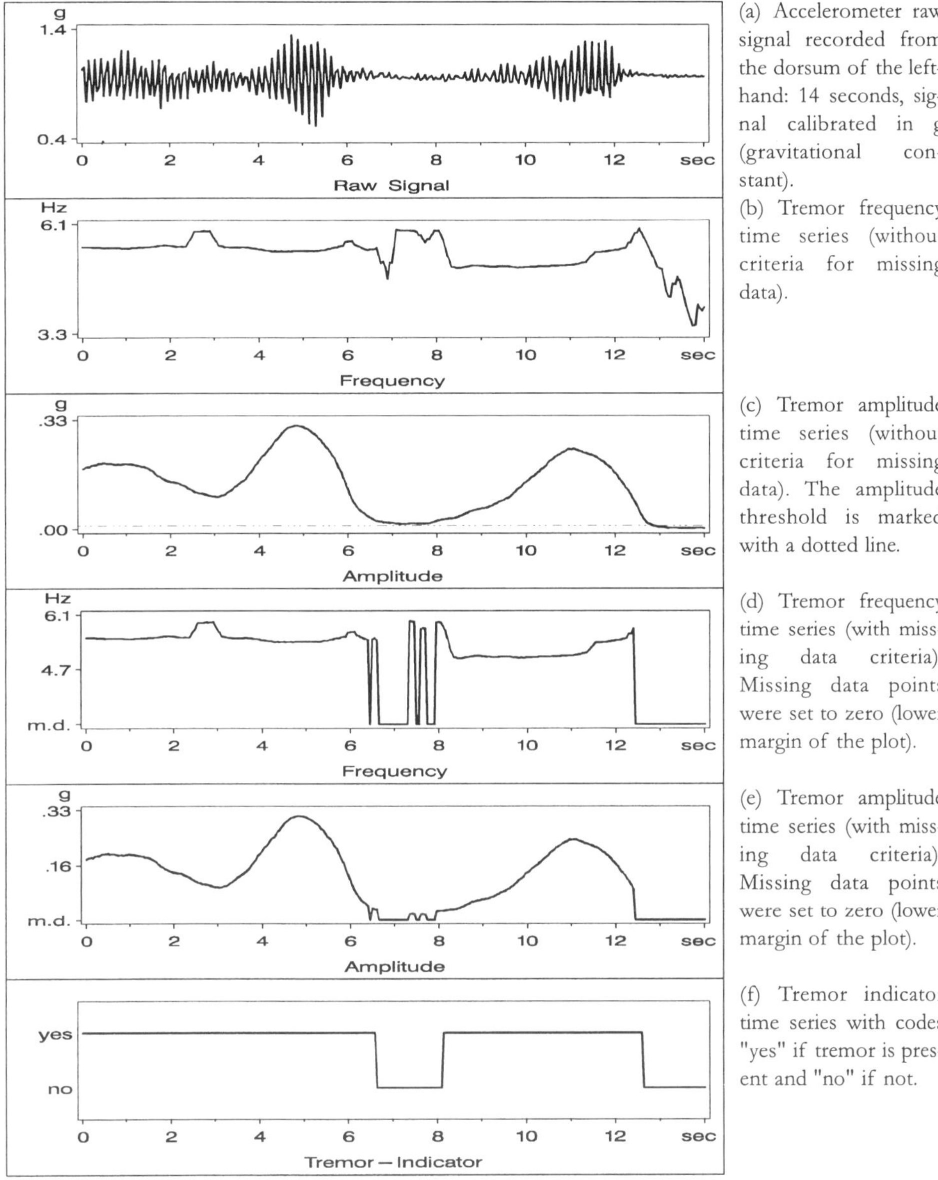

(a) Accelerometer raw signal recorded from the dorsum of the left-hand: 14 seconds, signal calibrated in g (gravitational constant).

(b) Tremor frequency time series (without criteria for missing data).

(c) Tremor amplitude time series (without criteria for missing data). The amplitude threshold is marked with a dotted line.

(d) Tremor frequency time series (with missing data criteria). Missing data points were set to zero (lower margin of the plot).

(e) Tremor amplitude time series (with missing data criteria). Missing data points were set to zero (lower margin of the plot).

(f) Tremor indicator time series with codes "yes" if tremor is present and "no" if not.

Figure 1. An example for the STFT-analysis

and amplitude (Figure 1c) and (with the criteria, Table 5) the same time series with missing data during intervals in which the criteria are not fulfilled (Figure 1d and 1e). Finally, in Figure 1f the tremor index is shown.

Data points of the tremor signals, which meet the criteria given in Table 5, are defined "tremor points". The ratio between the number of "tremor points" in an interval and the total length of the interval is defined as "tremor occurrence" (%). The other tremor variables are frequency (Hz) and amplitude (gravitational constant g or cm). The output of the TREMOR program is stored in an ASCII file which can be directly read into SAS. SAS programs were used for the hierarchical classification (see above) and statistical analyses.

Selected findings from two studies

First study

In the first study, 25 right-handed patients with Parkinson's disease were recorded in a rest condition, in a postural tremor test (both tasks repeated once under conditions of distraction), and during 24 hour ambulatory monitoring. A repeated measurement MANOVA was used to test the effects of posture and night-day differences in tremor activity. Further issues included consistencies of amplitude measurements across hands, between tasks, and between segments of recordings.

Individual differences in tremor frequency were not correlated to amplitude or occurrence time, however, moderate correlations did exist between amplitude and occurrence time (cut-off value 0.005 g) in the order of .50. Findings indicated an increase between resting tremor and postural tremor in the three tremor parameters, an increase under distraction, and enhanced activity in sitting compared to standing/walking. Individual recordings revealed in some instances that changes in tremor activity occurred when a patient was emotionally upset or strained. Such descriptive evidence would favor further development of more precise psychophysiological methods in ambulatory monitoring of tremor in PD patients. This methodology appeared to be appropriate for the detection of diurnal changes in tremor activity, especially amplitude changes, and for the psychophysiological investigation of enhanced tremor caused by task demands and emotional reactions (Foerster & Smeja, 1999; Smeja, Foerster, Fuchs, Emmans, Hornig & Fahrenberg, 1999).

Second Study

The second investigation dealt with the relationship between rest and postural tremor tasks and tremor during monitoring and investigated the changes during the course of treatment, that is, the rehabilitation program provided by the clinic (Foerster, Thielgen, Fuchs, Hornig & Fahrenberg, 2001). In the Parkinson-Klinik Wolfach, 30 patients with Parkinson's disease (age M = 64.8, SD = 8.9) with Hoehn and Yahr scores between 1 and 3 (M = 2.3, SD = 0.7, 17 F, 13 M) participated in the 24-hour monitoring. Clinically, all patients were selected because they had exhibited tremor. In 20 patients, a second recording was obtained toward the end of the in-patient rehabilitation program (mean interval 18 days, SD = 2.8). In this study, treatment components and medication varied between patients and was not controlled in this study. Besides the accelerometer devices on both hands, three sensors were also placed at the sternum and one sensor at the thigh of the dominant leg. An electrocardiogram (modified Nehb anterior) was also recorded in order to obtain heart rate data.

The initial recordings took place during the first week in which the patients were admitted to the rehabilitation center. The standard protocol included (1) a sequence of static and dynamic behaviors (recordings 30 s each) to obtain reference patterns for the detection of posture and motion in the subsequent monitoring, and (2) assessment of rest tremor, postural tremor, and hand tremor without and with distraction by counting numbers backward (recordings 120 s each). Subsequently, the 24 hour monitoring began. The patients could move unrestricted within the premise and vicinity of the rehabilitation center and they were instructed to adopt their usual course of daily life.

The correlations between tremor parameters occurrence (% of time), amplitude (g) and frequency (Hz) were computed for the two tasks and the tremor-dominant hand (in 16 patients the right hand). During rest and postural tremor, occurrence and amplitude correlated r =.57, frequency and occurrence .07, and frequency -.25 with amplitude. However, under conditions of distraction a somewhat different relationship emerged: occurrence and amplitude r = .43, frequency and occurrence -.28 and -.31 with amplitude. In certain segments of the monitoring, the relationship between amplitude and occurrence was even higher: during sitting .70, during meals .85, during the night .66. The recordings allowed for the investigation of the relationship between tremor activity and heart rate. A within-subject correlation coefficient .36 for the dominant hand (pooled across 30 patients, 260 time points) indicated a small, however noteworthy, relationship between tremor variability and a cardiovascular measure of activation. When a coefficient of "systemic correlation", which, in this case, is a more appropriate statistic for estimating the functional covariation (Stemmler & Fahrenberg, 1989), was computed, the coefficients shrank to .14 for tremor occurrence and heart rate and .10 for amplitude and heart rate.

Once again, the distraction condition caused a significant and substantial increase in tremor occurrence and tremor amplitude. During the monitoring, segments like "sitting (without meals)", "meals", "standing" and "day" versus "night" differed in occurrence time and amplitude whereas frequency was rather stable. The most pronounced tremor activity was noted during the initial tasks for assessment of rest and postural tremor under distraction, and the lowest during the night segment (Figure 2).

During the monitoring, tremor occurrence was predicted best by the postural tremor test under distraction. Coefficients of correlation ranged between .64 to .56 for the daytime segments (Table 6). The corresponding coefficients for tremor amplitude were generally lower, however, with the exception of night-time tremor

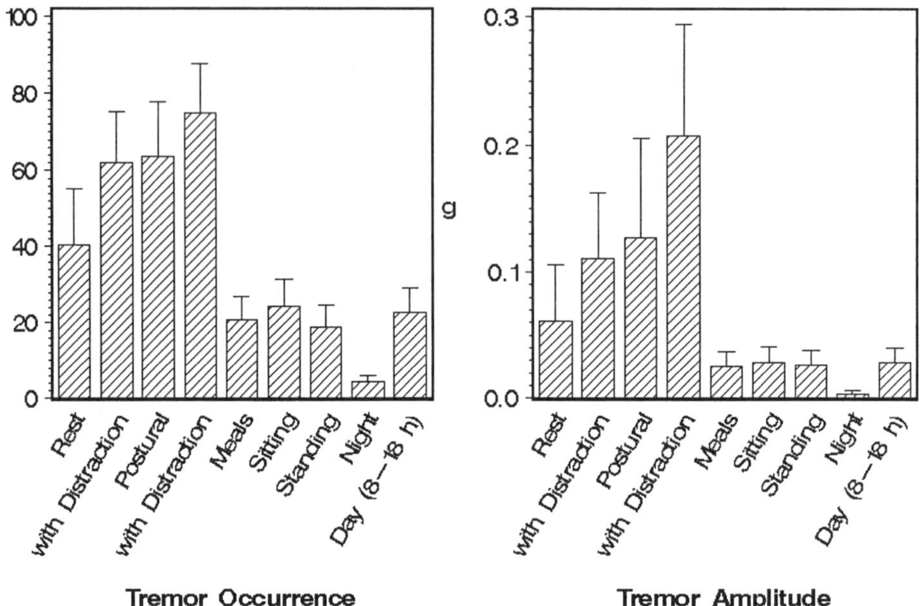

Figure 2. Means and 2SE of tremor occurrence and amplitude for specific segments
Note: Sitting Segment (without "Meal" Segment)

amplitudes which were predicted fairly well by the standard protocol (.73). For tremor frequency, which exhibited only low variability, likewise, substantial coefficients were found. The regression analyses indicated generally a moderate to high "laboratory-field" relationship, whereby the measures taken from the postural tremor test under distraction exceeded the other measures.

Figure 3 depicts the diurnal changes in tremor and heart rate and the changes from the first to the second recording. There was little hand tremor during the night and during the rest periods after lunch (12–13 h). The peaks of the tremor occurrence and amplitude in the late afternoon may indicate initial effects, that is, a reactivity caused by the recording which usually began at this time.

ANOVA with two repeated measurement factors "hours" and "recordings" showed a significant hour effect for tremor occurrence ($p<.001$; hours 8–18, $p=.016$), amplitude ($p=.001$; hours 8–18, $p=.014$), and heart rate ($p<.001$; hours 8–18, $p<.001$). Significant changes from first to second recording were found for daytime only (8–18) regarding tremor occurrence ($p=.009$), tremor frequency ($p=.002$), and heart rate ($p=.017$). A reduction of tremor frequency from first to second recording was evident only during the monitoring, whereas during laboratory tasks an increase in frequency was noted. The pattern of change varied between patients, and in some cases, also between tremor parameters occurrence and amplitude. It is noteworthy that in a few patients there was an increase instead decrease

Table 6. Laboratory-field prediction: The best predictor variables based on a stepwise multiple regression

Meals		Sitting		Standing		Night		Day	
Best Predictor		Best Predictor		Best Predictor		Best Predictor		Best Predictor	
R	p	R	p	R	p	R	p	R	p
Tremor Occurrence									
Postural under distraction		Postural under distraction		Postural under distraction		Standard Protocol		Postural under distraction	
.62	<.001	.62	<.001	.56	<.001	.48	.008	.64	<.001
Tremor Amplitude									
Postural under distraction		Mean of two Distraction		Mean of two Distraction		Standard Protocol		Mean of two Distraction	
.52	.003	.52	.004	.43	.017	.73	<.001	.51	.004
Tremor Frequency									
Mean of Resting and Postural		Mean of two Distraction		Postural under distraction		Postural under distraction		Mean of two Distraction	
.68	<.001	.65	.002	.75	<.001	.60	.004	.74	<.001

Notes: The predictor variables were: resting tremor and postural tremor test (both without and with distraction), likewise the mean of resting and mean of postural tremor test, and the mean of the eight conditions of the standard protocol used as reference for the detection of posture and motion. Criterion variables were the five segments from the first 24-hour-monitoring (Meals, Sitting without meals, Standing, Night, Day 8-18 h). Data from first recording. Due to missing data: N=29 for tremor occurrence and amplitude, N=20 for tremor frequency.

in tremor from first to second recording. On average, however, tremor decreased from the beginning to the end of the rehabilitation program.

The over-all effect in tremor reduction shown in Figure 3, however, appears to be rather small. A general trend to reduced symptoms was evident, however, the t-tests for distinct monitoring segments and, likewise, rest and postural tremor tasks, were not significant. The significant increase in heart rate during the treatment, especially during the night, was probably caused by the anti-parkinson medication.

Distinct psychophysiological episodes where the tremor was obviously enhanced by emotional activation or mental effort were even less frequent than had been cautiously expected on the basis of the first investigation. At present, this finding is open to scrutiny, because the assessment of psychologically meaningful events by diary, kept by the patients for hourly entries, was not very effective. There were, however, several findings which underline the role of emotional states in the attenuation and aggravation of tremor activity in these patients. Distraction during rest and postural tremor tasks enhanced the occurrence and amplitude of tremor. The clear increase in tremor activity at the beginning of the monitoring (usually 4 p.m.) can be attributed to emotional and situative conditions. The assessment of tremor activity under distraction provides the best predictor variable in laboratory-field comparisons. The ambulatory monitoring is a suitable method to further investigate such relationships and to objectively assess the external validity (generalizability) of

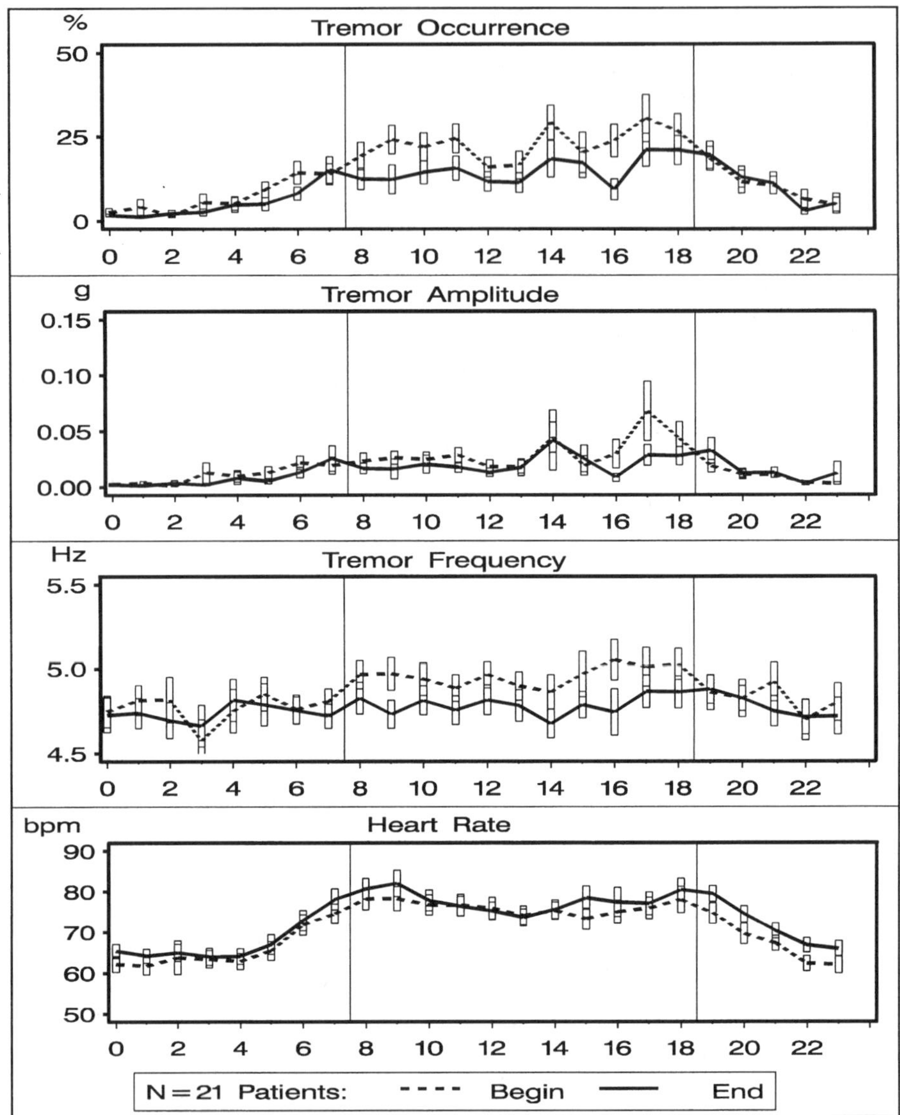

Figure 3. Reduction of tremor during the rehabilitation program: Means and SE of one-hour segments from the 24-hour-monitoring.

Conclusions and perspectives

Kinematic analysis based on accelerometry is a valuable methodology appropriate for many research and applied fields. One-channel uncalibrated actimetry may still be useful in behavior analysis, however, the accelerometry using calibrated sensors and refined strategies in signal analysis and pattern classification clearly has many advantages. These developments are reflected in the related Chapters in this volume, as compared to the previous volume (Fahrenberg & Myrtek, 1996).

Progress in the methodology of kinematic analysis will include, for example, the assessment of gait, of limb or head movements, of stability of posture, of tremor activity, and the detection of other movement disorders by specific filtering techniques. The tentative use of certain parameters or motion patterns, detected on-line, for feedback and control of behavior, for example, in rehabilitation of patients with movement disorders, and applications of this kind appear to be within the scope of this methodology.

The multi-channel accelerometry and classification of static and dynamic motion behaviors is used to date only in a few institutions. A serious drawback is the apparent number of requirements regarding data recorder and software.

Issues in methodology

Some of the prevailing issues in methodology were pointed out in the preceding sections regarding the detection of posture and motion. However, several issues exist which are common to all applications of accelerometry. There are some aspects of this methodology which need further attention: technical features of the sensors in terms of intra-sensor and inter-sensor variation, temperature drift of sensors, and the optimal housing for multi-axial sensors. The available accelerometer differ in axial sensitivity (change in mV/degree of inclination), frequency range, resonant frequency, damping, and temperature drift. In many instances, such specifications are not given by manufacturers. The directional sensitivity is not an all-or-none characteristic but has to be measured by relating signal amplitude and angle of inclination. The available sensors, furthermore, differ in size and mass, hardiness, and price. Substantial differences can exist among such IC sensors in sensitivity and offset which may affect reproducibility of measurements.

It should be noted that the flat design of most sensors suggest that such sensors are attached to the body surface so that the axial orientation becomes defined. The positioning must be designed with care, especially for uni-axial sensors, because the response characteristics depend on the degrees of inclination between axis and direction of movement (acceleration). At present, it appears appropriate to provide regular checks of the + 1 to – 1 range of all sensors, channel by channel, at least at the start and end of a particular study. If large temperature differences occur in the order of 20 degrees Celsius, for example, in monitoring studies during the cold season, the temperature drift of sensors may lead to unwanted variance.

At present, the sensor electronics and housings for biomedical applications are manufactured in rather small numbers by a few companies and the applications are far from achieving a standardization of technical features. This state of affairs precludes general statements concerning the selection of sensors. Desirable features would include: housings small and flat as possible, directions (sensitive axes) as required in such applications and flexible connections. The advantages in multi-site recordings will make multi-connectors and, eventually, multiplex amplifier technology desirable to save recorder channels for other signals in ambulatory monitoring of physiological and behavioral changes.

Basically, the time has come for the cross-laboratory standardization of accelerometry and guidelines, concerning algorithms and the optimal sensor configurations, like the standard ECG leads in cardiology.

Acknowledgements

This research was supported by the Deutsche Forschungsgemeinschaft. Marcus Cheetham helped to improve the English version of this chapter.

References

Anastasiades, P. & Johnston, D.W. (1990). A simple measure of activity for use with ambulatory subjects. *Psychophysiology, 27,* 87–93.

Bacher, M., Scholz, E. & Diener, H.C. (1989). 24 hour tremor quantification based on EMG recording. *Electroencephalography and Clinical Neurophysiology, 72,* 176–183.

Bouten, C.V.C., Verboeket-van de Venne, W.P.G., Westerterp, K.R., Verduin, M. & Janssen, J.D. (1996). Daily physical activity assessment: comparison between movement registration and doubly labeled water. *Journal of Applied Physiology, 81,* 1019–1026.

Busser, H.J. (1994). Using the piezoresistive accelerometer in posture and motion monitoring. In P.H. Veltink & R.C. van Lummel (Eds.), *Dynamic analysis using body fixed sensors. Second World Congress of Biomechanics. Amsterdam 1994* (pp. 107–109). The Hague, The Netherlands: McRoberts.

Busser, H.J., Ott, J., van Lummel, R.C., Uiterwaal, M. & Blank, R. (1997). Ambulatory monitoring of children's activity. *Medical Engineering and Physics, 19,* 440–445.

Bussmann, H. (1998). *Ambulatory monitoring of mobility-related activities in rehabilitation medicine.* Delft, The Netherlands: Eburon.

Bussmann, J.B.J., Tulen, J.H.M., van Herel, E.C.G. & Stam, H.J. (1998). Quantification of physical activities by means of ambulatory accelerometry: A validation study. *Psychophysiology, 35,* 488–496.

Bussmann, J.B.J., Veltink, P.H., Martens, W.L.J. & Stam, H.J. (1994). Activity monitoring with accelerometers. In P.H. Veltink & R.C. van Lummel (Eds.), *Dynamic analysis using body fixed sensors. Second World Congress of Biomechanics. Amsterdam 1994* (pp. 13–17). The Hague, The Netherlands: McRoberts.

Cleeves, L. & Findley, L. (1987). Variability in amplitude of untreated essential tremor. *Journal of Neurology, Neurosurgery and Psychiatry, 50,* 704–708.

Deuschl, G., Krack, P., Lauk, M. & Timmer, J. (1996). Clinical neurophysiology of tremor. *Journal of Clinical Neurophysiology, 13,* 110–121.

Elble, R.J. & Koller, W.C. (1991). *Tremor.* Baltimore: Johns Hopkins University Press.

Fahn, S., Elton, R. L. and Members of the UPDRS Development Committee (1987). Unified Parkinson's disease rating scale. In S. Fahn, C.D. Marsden, D. Calne & M. Goldstein (Eds.), *Recent developments in Parkinson's disease* (pp. 153–164). Florham Park, NJ: Mac Millan.

Fahrenberg, J. (2000). *Die Messung des Finger-Blutdrucks. Eine Methodenstudie mit zwei Geräten.* Research Report No. 150. University of Freiburg, Germany: Institute of Psychology.

Fahrenberg, J., Foerster, F., Müller, W. & Smeja, M. (1997). Assessment of posture and motion by multi-channel piezoresistive accelerometer recordings. *Psychophysiology, 34,* 607–612.

Fahrenberg, J., Heger, R., Foerster, F. & Müller, W. (1991). Differentielle Psychophysiologie von Befinden, Blutdruck und Herzfrequenz im Labor-Feld-Vergleich. *Zeitschrift für Differentielle und Diagnostische Psychologie, 12,* 1–25.

Fahrenberg, J., Müller, W., Foerster, F. & Smeja, M. (1996). A multi-channel investigation of physical activity. *Journal of Psychophysiology, 10,* 209–217.

Fahrenberg, J. & Myrtek, M. (Eds.) (1996). *Ambulatory Assessment: computer-assisted psychological and psychophysiological methods in monitoring and field studies.* Seattle, WA: Hogrefe & Huber.

Fahrenberg, J. & Myrtek, M. (2001). Monitoring und Assessment. In F. Rösler (Ed.), *Enzyklopädie der Psychologie. Serie Biologische Psychologie. Band 4: Grundlagen und Methoden der Psychophysiologie* (S. 657–798). Göttingen: Hogrefe.

Foerster, F. & Fahrenberg, J. (2000). Motion pattern and posture: Correctly assessed by calibrated accelerometers. Behavior Research Methods, Instruments & Computers, 32, 450–457.

Foerster, F. & Smeja, M. (1999): Joint amplitude and frequency analysis of tremor activity. *Electromyography Clinical Neurophysiology, 39,* 11–19.

Foerster, F., Smeja, M. & Fahrenberg, J. (1999). Detection of posture and motion by accelerometry: A validation study in ambulatory monitoring. *Computers and Human Behavior, 15,* 571–583.

Foerster, F., Thielgen, T., Fuchs, G., Hornig, A. & Fahrenberg, J. (2001). *24-stündige Tremor-Untersuchungen an Parkinson-Patienten.* Research Report No. 151. University of Freiburg, Germany: Institute of Psychology.

Halmos, P.R. (1950): *Measure Theory.* Princetown, NJ, Van Nostrand.

Jain, A., Martens, W.L.J., Mutz, G., Weiß, R.K. & Stephan, E. (1996). Towards a comprehensive technology for recording and analysis of multiple physiological parameters within their behavioral and environmental context. In J. Fahrenberg & M. Myrtek (Eds.), *Ambulatory assessment. Computer-assisted psychological and psychophysiological methods in monitoring and field studies* (pp. 215–235). Seattle, WA: Hogrefe & Huber.

Käppler, C., Becker, H.-U. & Fahrenberg, J. (1993). Ambulantes 24-Stunden-Monitoring als psychophysiologische Assessmentstrategie: Reproduzierbarkeit, Reaktivität, Retrospektionseffekt und Bewegungskonfundierung. *Zeitschrift für Differentielle und Diagnostische Psychologie, 14,* 235–251.

Kiani, K., Snijders, C.J. & Gelsema, E.S. (1997). Computerized analysis of daily life motor activity for ambulatory monitoring. *Technology & Health Care, 5,* 307–318.

Martens, W.L.J. (1994). Exploring the information content and some applications of body mounted piezoresistive accelerometers. In P.H. Veltink & R.C. van Lummel (Eds.), *Dynamic analysis using body fixed sensors. Second World Congress of Biomechanics. Amsterdam 1994* (pp. 9–12). The Hague, The Netherlands: McRoberts.

Middelkoop, H.A.M., van Dam, E.M., Smilde-van den Doel, D.A. & van Dijk, G. (1997). 45-hour continuous quintuple-site actimetry: Relations between trunk and limb movements and effects of circadian sleep-wake rhythmicity. *Psychophysiology, 34,* 199–203.

Myrtek, M., Brügner, G., Fichtler, A., König, K., Müller, W., Foerster, F. & Höppner, V. (1988). Detection of emotionally induced ECG changes and their behavioral correlates: A new method for ambulatory monitoring. *European Heart Journal, 9 (Supplement N),* 55–60.

Myrtek, M., Brügner, G. & Müller, W. (1996). Interactive monitoring and contingency analysis of emotionally induced ECG changes: Methodology and applications. In J. Fahrenberg & M. Myrtek (Eds.). *Ambulatory Assessment: computer-assisted psychological and psychophysiological methods in monitoring and field studies* (pp. 115–127). Seattle, WA: Hogrefe & Huber.

Patterson, S.M., Krantz, D.S., Montgomery, L.C., Deuster, P.A., Hedges, S.M. & Nebel, L.E. (1993). Automated physical activity monitoring: Validation and comparison with physiological and self-report measures. *Psychophysiology, 30,* 296–305.

Pickering, T.G. (1991). *Ambulatory monitoring and blood pressure variability.* London: Science Press.

Qian, S. & Chen, D. (1996): *Joint Time-Frequency Analysis. Methods and Applications.* Upper Saddle River, NJ: Prentice Hall PTR.

Richardson, M.T., Leon, A.S., Jacobs, D.R., Ainsworth, B.E. & Serfass, R. (1995). Ability of the Caltrac accelerometer to assess daily physical activity levels. *Journal of Cardiopulmonary*

Rehabilitation, 15, 107–113.

Schwan, A. & Pavek, K. (1989). Change in posture during sleep causes errors in non-invasive automatic blood pressure recordings. *Journal of Hypertension, 7* (suppl 6), S62–S63.

Sherman, W.M., Morris, D.M., Kirby, T.E., Petosa, R.A. Smith, B.A., Frid, D.J. & Leenders, N. (1998). Evaluation of a commercial accelerometer (Tritrac) to measure energy expenditure during ambulation. *International Journal of Sports Medicine, 19*, 43–47.

Smeja, M., Foerster, F., Fuchs, G., Emmans, D., Hornig, A. & Fahrenberg, J. (1999). 24 hr assessment of tremor activity and posture in Parkinson's disease by multi-channel accelerometry. *Journal of Psychophysiology, 13*, 245–256.

Spieker, S., Boose, A., Jentgens, Ch. & Dichgans. J. (1995). Long-term tremor recordings in parkinsonian and essential tremor. *Journal of Neural Transmission, 46 (Suppl.),* 339–349.

Stemmler, G. & Fahrenberg, J. (1989). Psychophysiological assessment: Conceptual, psychometric, and statistical issues. In G. Turpin (Ed.), *Handbook of clinical psychophysiology* (pp. 71–104). Chichester: Wiley.

Tryon, W.W. (1991). *Activity measurement in psychology and medicine.* New York: Plenum Press.

Tuomisto, M.T., Johnston, D.W. & Schmidt, T.F.H. (1996). The ambulatory measurement of posture, thigh acceleration, and muscle tension and their relationship to heart rate. *Psychophysiology, 33*, 409–415.

van de Weijer, J.G.W., Smits, M.G., de Haan, A.F. & van Lummel, R.C. (1994). Detecting sleeping postures by accelerometry. The development of a bedrest monitor. In P.H. Veltink & R.C. van Lummel (Eds.), *Dynamic analysis using body fixed sensors. Second World Congress of Biomechanics. Amsterdam 1994* (pp. 23–25). The Hague, The Netherlands: McRoberts.

van Egeren, L.F. (1992). The relationship between job strain and blood pressure at work, at home, and during sleep. *Psychosomatic Medicine, 54,* 337–343.

van Hilten, J.J., Hoff, J.I. & Roos, R.A.C. (1993). Ambulatory activity monitoring: an evaluation of day-to-day variability in patients with Parkinson's disease and healthy elderly. *Journal of Ambulatory Monitoring, 6,* 219–223.

van Hilten, J.J., Hoogland, G., van der Velde E.A., van Dijk, J.G., Kerkhof, G.A. & Roos, R.A.C. (1993). Quantitative assessment of Parkinsonian patients by continuous wrist activity monitoring. *Clinical Neuropharmacology, 16,* 36–45.

van Hilten, J.J., Middelkoop, H.A.M., Kerkhof, G.A. & Roos, R.A.C. (1991). A new approach in the assessment of motor activity in Parkinson's disease. *Journal of Neurology, Neurosurgery and Psychiatry, 54,* 976–979.

van Someren, E.J., van Gool, W.A., Vonk, B.F., Mirmiran, M., Speelman, J.D., Bosch, D.A. & Swaab, D. F. (1993). Ambulatory monitoring of tremor and other movements before and after thalamotomy: a new quantitative technique. *Journal of the Neurological Sciences, 117*, 16–23.

van Someren, E.J., Vonk, B.F., Thijssen, W.A., Speelman, J.D., Schuurman, P.R., Mirmiran, M. & Swaab, D. F. (1998). A new actigraph for long-term registration of the duration and intensity of tremor and movement. *IEEE Transactions on Biomedical Engineering, 45,* 386–395.

Veltink, P.H., Bussmann, H.B.J., de Vries, W., Martens, W.L.C. & van Lummel, R.C. (1996). Detection of postures and movements using uni-axial accelerometers. *IEEE Rehabilitation Engineering, 4,* 375–385.

Veltink, P.H. & van Lummel, R.C. (Eds.) (1994). *Dynamic analysis using body fixed sensors. Second World Congress of Biomechanics. Amsterdam 1994.* The Hague, The Netherlands: McRoberts.

Walker, D.J., Heslop, P.S., Plummer, C.J., Essex, T. & Chandler, S. (1997). A continuous patient activity monitor: validation and relation to disability. *Physiological Measurement, 18*, 49–59.

Zimmermann, R., Deuschl, G., Hornig, A., Schulte-Mönting, J., Fuchs, G. & Lücking C.H. (1994). Tremors in Parkinson's disease: Symptom analysis and rating. *Clinical Neuropharmacology, 17,* 303–314.

Chapter 16
Ambulatory Monitoring of Blood Pressure in Daily Life: A Tool for Investigating Psychosocial Processes

Andrew Steptoe
Psychobiology Group, Department of Epidemiology and Public Health
University College London, UK

Introduction

One of the most striking developments in clinical and experimental psychophysiology over the past two decades has been the advance in ambulatory assessment techniques. No longer are studies confined to the laboratory or clinical setting, and to the investigation of acute physiological responses to laboratory stimuli. The progress in technology has permitted measurement of many variables to be made in naturalistic settings, allowing the covariation of physiological function, behavior and emotion state to be studied under everyday life conditions.

The techniques of ambulatory monitoring can be used for many purposes, from exploring theoretical issues in psychophysiology to diagnosis and the evaluation of therapy. The present chapter will describe recent research on the use of ambulatory methods in the investigation of psychosocial processes related to cardiovascular disease risk. I will describe how ambulatory techniques are not only valuable for assessing the everyday physiological activity of individuals at varying risk of cardiovascular disease, but also for exploring the precise ways in which psychosocial factors may influence cardiovascular function. The focus will be on ambulatory monitoring of blood pressure, accompanied by accelerometer measures of physical activity. However, before discussing these topics, I will briefly outline some important aspects of current assessment methods that are not widely appreciated, but place significant limitations on the interpretation of ambulatory monitoring studies.

The impact of ambulatory monitoring on everyday activities

A major advantage of ambulatory monitoring in psychophysiology is that behavioral and emotional influences on cardiovascular function can be assessed under everyday conditions. Interest in ambulatory monitoring evolved from dissatisfaction with laboratory methods in cardiovascular psychophysiology, and in particular with the inferences that were drawn about cardiovascular disease etiology from acute physiological stress reactivity studies (Parati et al., 1991). Critics of acute stress testing have argued that laboratory testing evaluates short-term physiological adjustments to arbitrary behavioral stimuli, and has limited reliability and ecological validity (Pickering & Gerin, 1990). By contrast, since ambulatory monitoring is carried out in "real life", it does not have these limitations. Of course, a problem with interpreting ambulatory data is that posture and physical activity also vary across the day, and have profound effects on blood pressure and heart rate (Gellman et al., 1990; Kario, Schwartz & Pickering, 1999). But developments in the objective measurement of physical activity and posture described elsewhere in this volume now allow these factors to be assessed and to be taken into account statistically.

The virtue of ambulatory monitoring therefore lies in part in its representativeness of physiological function in everyday life. However, just because measures are taken from freely moving individuals does not mean that the situation is typical of normal life. In fact, there are a number of aspects of ambulatory monitoring that may disrupt the participant's normal activities. Firstly, the apparatus itself may be bulky and uncomfortable, with electrodes, sensors, and storage devices restricting the person's movement. Ambulatory blood pressure monitoring devices are improving in this respect, and are now lighter and less obtrusive. Nevertheless, the standard measurement technique for blood pressure still requires periodic squeezing of the arm during inflation of the cuff, and this is itself uncomfortable. It has been reported, for example, that hypertensives are more physically active in the night than normotensives during ambulatory monitoring, and that this pattern is associated with greater sleep disturbance (Leary & Murphy, 1998). This difference may be due to the greater cuff inflation pressure for hypertensives, leading to more pain that may in turn produce smaller nocturnal blood pressure dipping.

Secondly, people may be embarrassed by ambulatory monitoring and therefore curtail their activities. The presence of cables and the periodic noise of cuff inflation may lead participants to avoid social or physical activities during the monitoring period. A participant may choose to postpone a shopping trip or visit to the theatre on the days of ambulatory monitoring, so as not to be exposed to unwarranted enquiries or ridicule.

Another aspect of ambulatory monitoring that may disrupt normal activity is the need to be immobile during arm cuff inflation and deflation, so as to ensure more reliable recordings. In psychophysiological studies, blood pressure readings are often accompanied by diary assessments in which people register their mood, activities and social situation. Some electronic or pencil and paper diaries are extremely elaborate and take several minutes to complete. This has the effect of further disrupting ongoing activity.

Finally, there is a more subtle influence of ambulatory monitoring on participants, particularly those involved in clinical studies. People with hypertension and other cardiovascular conditions may limit their physical activities in order to reduce the likelihood of having too many high readings. They may believe that their blood pressures will be elevated by certain situations, and want to minimise such exposures so as to give the impression that their blood pressure is under good control. All these factors may serve to reduce the representativeness of periods of ambulatory blood pressure monitoring.

A test of the influence of ambulatory monitoring on physical activity

It has previously been shown with self-report diaries that everyday activities appear to be disrupted by ambulatory blood pressure monitoring (Blanchard, Cornish, Wittrock & Jaccard, 1990). We have investigated the influence of ambulatory monitoring on objective measures of everyday activities in a study of 24 men and women assessed over the working day (Costa, Steptoe, Cropley & Griffith, 1999). Blood pressure was recorded every 20 minutes from 8.00 am to 6.00 pm using SpaceLabs 90217 ambulatory monitors, and then every 30 minutes in the evening. Participants were instructed to carry on as normal, but to keep their arms still during cuff inflation and deflation. Blood pressure readings were accompanied by completion of a diary, in which location, posture, and activity were recorded. Physical activity was assessed with triaxial accelerometers (TriTrac-R3D). These solid state monitors contain accelerometers that assess movements in three planes and use the integrated vector magnitude to calculate estimated energy expenditure (Sherman et al., 1998). In addition, participants wore the accelerometers on a separate working day and evening, during which no blood pressure monitoring or diary completion was required. By comparing the energy expenditure on the two days, it was possible to evaluate the impact of the ambulatory blood pressure monitoring protocol.

The energy expenditure results are summarised in Figure 1. Accelerometer data were collected in one minute epochs, and these were averaged to produce the hourly means illustrated. It can be seen that physical activity was reduced on the day of ambulatory blood pressure monitoring, compared with the day on which activity alone was measured. The participants did indeed appear to limit their physical activity during the monitoring day, even though the work demands and requirements were the same on the two days. We also found that physical activity was not only lower during the minutes surrrounding each blood pressure reading (due to keeping still and then filling in the diary), but also during the periods between blood pressure readings.

These findings are relevant primarily to blood pressure monitoring with standard arm cuff systems, and not to cardiovascular measures with continuous assessments of the electrocardiogram or the Portapres. However, there may be some restrictions of everyday activities with all devices, particularly when self-report assessments are included. Thus although ambulatory monitoring has many advantages, limitations of generalizability must still be recognised.

Ambulatory monitoring and psychosocial factors

One of the main uses of ambulatory monitoring in health-related cardiovascular psychophysiology is to investigate psychosocial influences on biological function.

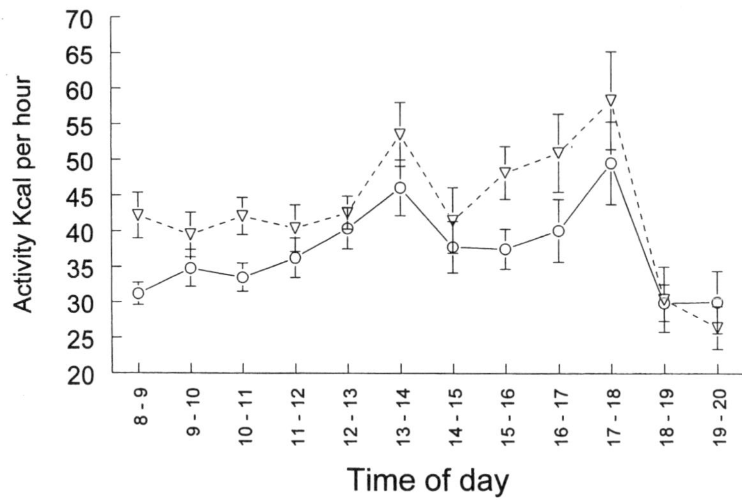

Figure 1. Mean activity calories per hour between 8.00 am and 8.00 pm, recorded on a day of ambulatory blood pressure monitoring (solid line), and a day of activity monitoring alone (dotted line). Error bars indicate S.E.M. From Costa et al (1999).

Many types of psychosocial factor are studied. For example, much research is directed towards delineating the impact of work stress on blood pressure and heart rate (Belkic et al., 2000). The cardiovascular correlates of social isolation are also of considerable interest (Horsten, Ericson, Perski & al., 1999), and ambulatory methods have also been extended to explore the influence of marital status and family structure on blood pressure (Brisson et al., 1999; Steptoe, Lundwall & Cropley, 2000). Psychological factors such as hostility and coping style are also studied using ambulatory blood pressure techniques (Carels, Sherwood & Blumenthal, 1998). In all these instances, the main approach has been to study between-subject effects, by comparing the blood pressure and heart rate of individuals with high and low levels on the psychosocial characteristic in question.

However, ambulatory methods can also be used to investigate the impact of psychosocial factors on cardiovascular function in more detail. I will illustrate these possibilities with two recent analyses we have conducted with blood pressures recorded from a sample of schoolteachers. The first example concerns the interaction between stress and social support.

Ambulatory blood pressure, stress, and social support

Social support is an important influence on cardiovascular function and well-being. A number of epidemiological studies have documented the association between cardiovascular disease risk and both low social support and limited social networks (Hemingway & Marmot, 1999; Uchino, Cacioppo & Kiecolt-Glaser, 1996). The question arises of what psychobiological mechanisms mediate this link. Blood pressures recorded under clinical conditions have been found to be inversely associated with social support in a number of studies. But the evidence relating social support with blood pressure recorded in naturalistic conditions is surprisingly limited. A Swedish research group has established that low work social support is associated with raised heart rate during sleep, work and leisure (Unden, Orth-Gomér & Elofsson, 1991). More recently, it was reported that low social support as assessed with the Interpersonal Support Evaluation List (ISEL) was related to reduced heart rate variability in healthy middle-aged women (Horsten et al., 1999). This finding is interesting, since reduced heart rate variability predicts poor outcome following myocardial infarction (La Rovere et al., 1998). However, Linden et al (1993) found that systolic blood pressure over the day was inversely associated with social support only among female and not male university students, implying a gender difference in response. Another recent study demonstrated in an adult population that support rated on the ISEL was positively associated with the amount of systolic blood pressure dipping at night rather than with levels in the day (Ituarte, Kamarck, Thompson & Bacanu, 1999), while Brownley et al (1996) found that support was associated with reduced blood pressure only in adults with high hostility scores.

It is apparent that several factors may moderate the impact of social support on ambulatory cardiovascular activity. Another factor that is relevant is whether social support has direct effects on health outcomes, or buffers the impact of life stress (Cohen & Wills, 1985). There is evidence to support both points of view. For example, Rosengren et al. (1993) observed that mortality in middle-aged men over a seven year period increased with the number of stressful life events they experienced, but only in those with low emotional support, illustrating the buffering effect of support. Social support at work has also been found to buffer the impact of chronic work stress on cardiovascular disease (Johnson & Hall, 1994). By contrast, much of the research on social networks has shown that social isolation is associated with increased risk irrespective of life stress (Berkman, Vaccarino & Seeman, 1993). In this analysis, we set out to discover whether ambulatory cardiovascular data could throw light on the issue.

Data were analyzed from 62 schoolteachers who were part of a larger study of work stress and cardiovascular risk (Steptoe, 2000). One year before ambulatory monitoring, participants had completed the ISEL (Cohen, Mermelstein, Kamarck & Hoberman, 1985). This questionnaire consists of 40 items designed to assess perceived availability of four separate types of support: tangible support or the perceived availability of practical aid, appraisal support or the availability of people to talk to and to provide advice, self-esteem support measuring self-confidence and positive social comparisons, and belonging support or the perceived availability of social contacts with whom one can do things. Responses to the items were scored in a binary format and summed to generate a total support score. The sample was divided by median split into high support and low support groups (mean scores 37.5

versus 28.7). Blood pressure and heart rate were recorded every 20 minutes between 9.00 am and 5.40 pm on a working day. Readings were accompanied by ratings of subjective pressure or stress, scored on a 7-point scale. As in the study described earlier, energy expenditure was recorded in 1-minute epochs using TriTrac research ergometers. The energy expenditure for the 5 minutes preceding each blood pressure reading was used to estimate concurrent physical activity.

We reasoned that if social support has a main effect on blood pressure and heart rate, then levels during the day should be lower in the high than low support groups. If, on the other hand, social support has a buffering effect, then interactions with the level of stress at the time of readings might emerge. The blood pressure, heart rate and energy expenditure values associated with ratings of high stress were therefore averaged for each individual, and compared with values associated with low stress. Energy expenditure was significantly greater during high than low stress periods, indicating that subjective ratings of stress were associated with increased physical activity. Energy expenditure was therefore treated as a covariate, along with body mass index, in the analysis of cardiovascular activity.

The results for systolic and diastolic pressure are shown in Figure 2, the main effect of stress was significant in both analyses, with higher systolic and diastolic pressure at times when participants were experiencing greater stress. However, this effect interacted with social support. Blood pressure was raised during high stress periods only among participants in the low social support group. For both systolic and diastolic pressure, the effect of stress was significant in the low support ($P < 0.01$) but not in the high support group.

These data are an illustration of the stress buffering role of social support. There was no main effect of support, so social support was only influential under conditions of high momentary perceived stress. This finding may account for the discrepancies in the literature linking support with cardiovascular activity. The impact of social support on cardiovascular activity may be more pronounced when people experience stress in their lives.

Psychosocial influences on ambulatory function: exposure or reactivity

Another way in which ambulatory cardiovascular data can be used is to help us try and understand the processes through which psychosocial factors stimulate differences in cardiovascular activity. The demonstration that psychosocial factors such as social isolation or work stress are associated with differences in cardiovascular activity in every day life is only the first step: within-subject techniques are required to identify the intervening pathways. A number of models of the influence of psychosocial factors can be proposed, and ambulatory techniques are beginning to be used to disentangle these.

Take the case of job strain, a psychosocial factor that is strongly related to cardiovascular disease risk. It has been demonstrated in several investigations that ambulatory blood pressure is elevated in people who work in jobs characterised by high demands and low control, when these are defined both by self-report and by independent assessments (Belkic et al., 2000; Schnall, Landsbergis & Baker, 1994). The association between job strain and blood pressure is more robust in men than women, among whom other factors appear to be influential (Brisson, 2000). A question that emerges is what processes mediate the association between blood pressure and job strain. One possibility is that differences are due to variations in body weight or in health behavior such as alcohol consumption and cigarette smoking, with a greater prevalence of these risk factors among people in high strain jobs. However, this explanation has been discounted in many studies, since they have shown that associations persist after controlling for these factors (Schnall et al., 1994). Psychophysiological processes may therefore be involved.

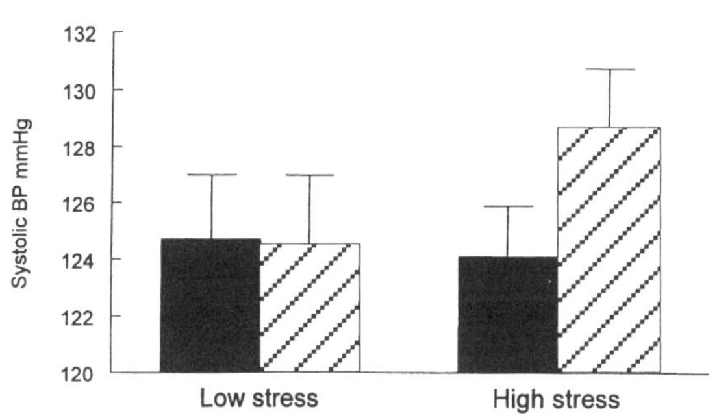

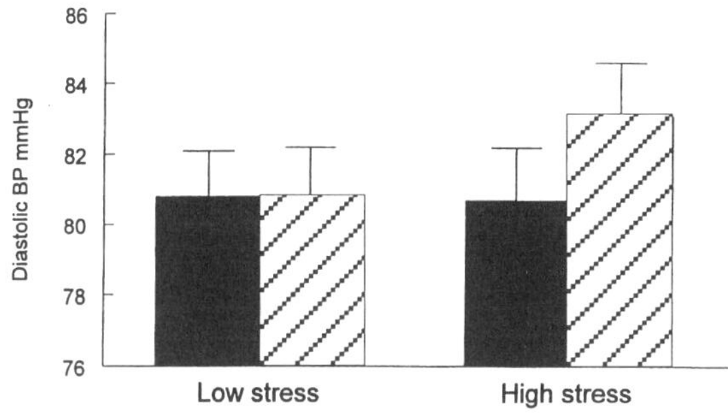

Figure 2. Mean systolic pressure (upper panel) and diastolic pressure (lower panel), adjusted for concurrent energy expenditure and body mass, during periods of high stress and low stress over the working day. The high social support group is depicted in the solid bars, and the low support group in the hatched bars. Error bars indicate S.E.M. From Steptoe (in press).

But what is the psychophysiological mechanism? There are at least three possibilities, and these are illustrated in Figure 3. Model 1 is that people in high strain jobs are more physiologically responsive than those in low strain jobs to stimuli that are encountered during the working day. Responsivity is taken here to include both heightened reactivity to events, and delayed recovery following stressors. It is known that ambulatory blood pressure is affected by episodes of negative affect and conflictual social interaction (Brondolo, Karlin, Alexander, Bobrow & Schwartz, 1999; Kamarck et al., 1998). It has also been found in experimental studies that people who rate their jobs as high demand and low control show exaggerated cardiovascular reactions to uncontrollable stressors (Steptoe, Cropley & Joekes, 1999). It is plausible therefore that the differences in blood pressure observed with high and low job strain may arise from differences in reactivity to daily stressors.

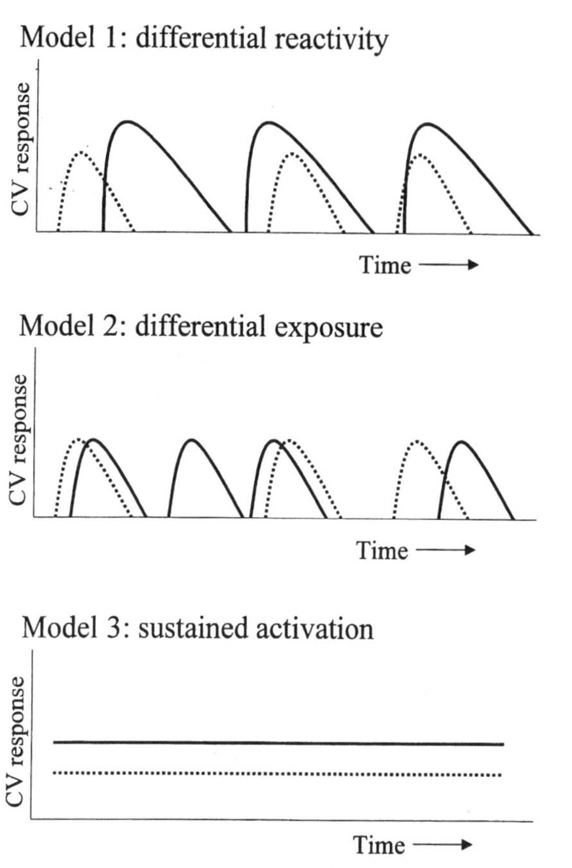

Figure 3. Three hypothetical models of the association between job strain and cardiovascular activity under naturalistic conditions. The solid lines represent high job strain, while the dotted lines represent low job strain. For details, see text.

Heightened stress reactivity may translate into higher levels over the working day.

The second possibility is that effects arise from variations in exposure to stimuli that provoke cardiovascular responses (model 2). People working in high strain jobs may experience adverse events more often in their working lives than do low strain groups. If they encounter more events during a typical day that are uncontrollable or highly demanding, this may lead to more frequent cardiovascular activation. A general elevation of blood pressure may then arise from more frequent stress-induced responses. If model 2 operates, then job strain might not be associated with heightened responsivity, but with differential exposure.

The third model is that the elevated blood pressure of people in high strain jobs is not related to responsivity on a day-to-day basis at all. It may instead arise from pervasive chronic strain leading to heightened autonomic and neuroendocrine activation. Such a mechanism is less interesting from the psychophysiological point of view, since ambulatory monitoring is not needed to detect the pattern; rather, it could be identified with conventional clinical measures, without using special apparatus to investigate physiology in everyday life. However, an argument against model 3 is that in many studies, blood pressures have been shown to be different only during ambulatory monitoring, and not with conventional clinical measurements (Light, Turner & Hinderliter, 1992; Steptoe et al., 1999). This suggests that the mediating processes are stimulated by the conditions of everyday life.

I have illustrated these alternative mechanisms in relation to work stress, although similar distinctions may be drawn for other psychosocial factors as well. The interesting issue in the present context is whether we can use ambulatory data to try and tease out these competing models of the processes linking psychosocial factors with cardiovascular risk.

An investigation of competing models

We have recently conducted an analysis of ambulatory blood pressure, heart rate and activity recorded from 122 male and female school teachers that set out to test the models of psychophysiological processes described above (for details see Steptoe, in press). The findings are statistically independent of the effects described in the section on stress and social support. The analysis focussed on job control, since a number of clinical and epidemiological studies have demonstrated that lack of control in the work environment is a determinant of cardiovascular disease risk (Bosma et al., 1997; Schnall et al., 1990). As before, we analyzed blood pressure and heart rate recorded every 20 minutes over the working day. Every blood pressure reading was accompanied by ratings of how much control participants felt at the time. The control ratings could range from 1 = *no control* to 7 = *complete control.*

An average of 24.9 ± 2.2 blood pressure readings out of a maximum possible 26 was obtained from each participant over the working day. Scrutiny of the ratings of control indicated that episodes of low perceived control were relatively infrequent. For example, only 22 of the 122 participants gave ratings of 1 or 2 on the 7-point scale at any point over the working day. Blood pressure, heart rate, and energy expenditure readings that accompanied ratings 1 – 4 on the control scale were therefore aggregated to estimate the cardiovascular adjuncts of low perceived control. These averages were contrasted with the blood pressure, heart rate, and energy expenditure readings that accompanied ratings of 6 or 7 (high perceived control) on the rating scale.

The purpose of this analysis was to contrast the differential reactivity and differential exposure models linking work characteristics and cardiovascular function. Before the ambulatory monitoring session, participants had completed a standard assessment of job control derived from Karasek and Theorell (1990). Based on the extent of agreement with statements such as "I have control over how I do my job", the cohort were divided into high job control (n = 71) and low job control (n = 51) groups. The uneven size of the two groups was due to ties in the scores. Altogether, there were 25 men and 46 women in the high job control group, compared with 20 men and 31 women in the low job control group. The two groups did not differ in age distribution, occupational status, body mass index, or in the proportion of cigarette smokers.

It was hypothezised that within-subjects, episodes of low perceived control would be associated with higher blood pressure and heart rate than episodes of high perceived control. We reasoned that if differential reactivity (model 1) underlies the influence of job control, then the low job control group should be more reactive to episodes of low perceived control over the working day. That is, the difference in blood pressure and heart rate between high and low perceived control episodes

Table 1. Cardiovascular activity associated with high and low perceived control over the working day

	High perceived control	Low perceived control	Significance
Systolic pressure (mmHg)	124.9 (12.2)	128.3 (15.4)	.007
Diastolic pressure (mmHg)	80.4 (6.9)	82.1 (8.7)	.028
Heart rate (bpm)	77.9 (8.5)	80.2 (10.8)	.023
Energy expenditure (kcal/5min)	8.57 (2.8)	8.48 (2.59)	.15

Note: Means with standard deviations in parentheses

should be greater in the low job control group. If, on the hand, the critical pathway is differential exposure, then reactivity to episodes of low perceived control might not differ between groups. Rather, the low job control group should experience more frequent episodes of low perceived control over the working day.

The average blood pressure, heart rate and energy expenditure values recorded during episodes of high and low perceived control are summarised in Table 1. These are within-subject effects, so the analysis is limited to the 57 participants who recorded periods of both high and low perceived control over the day. It can be seen from Table 1 that low perceived control was associated with significant increases in systolic pressure, diastolic pressure and heart rate. Energy expenditure levels did not differ in the high and low perceived control conditions, so the cardiovascular effects are unlikely to be secondary to differences in physical activity. The blood pressure and heart rate responses to low control are relatively small. This is not too surprising, given the many other influences over cardiovascular activity during ambulatory monitoring. Nevertheless, the result is important, since it corroborates the findings of laboratory studies that have demonstrated heightened cardiovascular activity in response to conditions of low control (for example, Steptoe, Fieldman, Evans & Perry, 1993). These data indicate the influence of low perceived control can be observed under naturalistic conditions in spontaneous everyday life situations. However, there was no difference between job control groups in the effects. Thus no evidence was found to support the differential reactivity model.

What about the differential exposure model? This was investigated in two ways. Firstly, the number of people in the high and low job control groups who experienced any episodes of low perceived control over the day was compared. Significantly more teachers in the low job control group (58.8%) than in the high job control group (38.0%) reported at least some episodes of low perceived control ($P = 0.28$). Secondly, across the complete sample (n = 122), the proportion of blood pressure readings associated with low perceived control was compared in the high and low job control groups. Again, effects were significant, with a greater proportion of blood pressure readings being associated with low perceived control in the low job control than high job control groups (14.6% versus 7.2%), ($P = 0.016$). Both these findings support the exposure hypothesis, in demonstrating that low job control is associated with more frequent experience of low perceived control over the working day.

Conclusion

The analyses of cardiovascular activity, social support, and job control detailed above have been presented for illustrative purposes only. The purpose of these illustrations was to demonstrate that ambulatory data provide powerful investigative tools for psychosocial research. Instead of limiting analyses to between-subject comparisons of ambulatory activity, it is possible to use repeated measure data to explore the relevance of theoretical models in naturalistic situations. As ambulatory methods become more widely available, it may become possible to investigate phenomena of major public health interest, such as the socio-economic gradient in cardiovascular risk, as well (Matthews et al., 2000). I am confident that the use of ambulatory techniques for investigating broader psychosocial influences on cardiovascular regulation and disease risk will be of increasing importance over the next decade.

Acknowledgement

The research described here was supported by the Medical Research Council, UK. I am grateful to a number of colleagues for their contributions, including Mark Cropley, Marco Costa, Katherine Joekes and Jayne Griffith.

References

Belkic, K., Landsbergis, P., Schnall, P., Baker, D., Theorell, T., Siegrist, J., Peter, R. & Karasek, R. (2000). Psychosocial factors: review of the empirical data among men. In P. L. Schnall, K. Belkic, P. Landsbergis& D. Baker (Eds.), *The Workplace and Cardiovascular Diseases (Occupational Medicine* Vol. 15, Number 1, pp. 24–46). Philadelphia: Hanley and Belfus.

Berkman, L. F., Vaccarino, V. & Seeman, T. (1993). Gender differences in cardiovascular morbidity and mortality: The contribution of social networks and support. *Annals of Behavioral Medicine, 15*, 112–118.

Blanchard, E. B., Cornish, P. J., Wittrock, D. A. & Jaccard, J. (1990). Effects of 24-hour ambulatory blood pressure monitoring on daily activities. *Health Psychology, 9*, 647–652.

Bosma, H., Marmot, M. G., Hemingway, H., Nicholson, A. C., Brunner, E. & Stansfeld, S. A. (1997). Low job control and risk of coronary heart disease in Whitehall II (prospective cohort) study. *British Medical Journal, 314*, 558–565.

Brisson, C. (2000). Women, work, and CVD. In P. L. Schnall, K. Belkic, P. Landsbergis& D. Baker (Eds.), *The Workplace and Cardiovascular Diseases* (*Occupational Medicine* Vol. 15, Number 1, pp. 49–57). Philadelphia: Hanley and Belfus.

Brisson, C., Laflamme, N., Moisan, J., Milot, A., Masse, B. & Vezina, M. (1999). Effect of family responsibilities and job strain on ambulatory blood pressure among white-collar women. *Psychosomatic Medicine, 61*, 205–13.

Brondolo, E., Karlin, W., Alexander, K., Bobrow, A. & Schwartz, J. (1999). Workday communication and ambulatory blood pressure: implications for the reactivity hypothesis. *Psychophysiology, 36*, 86–94.

Brownley, K. A., Light, K. C. & Anderson, N. B. (1996). Social support and hostility interact to influence clinic, work, and home blood pressure in black and white men and women. *Psychophysiology, 33*, 434–445.

Carels, R. A., Sherwood, A. & Blumenthal, J. A. (1998). Psychosocial influences on blood pressure during daily life. *International Journal of Psychophysiology, 28*, 117–129.

Cohen, S., Mermelstein, R., Kamarck, T. & Hoberman, H. M. (1985). Measuring the functional components of social support. In I. G. Sarason & B. R. Sarason (Eds.), *Social Support: Theory, Research and Applications* (pp. 73–94). Dordrecht: Martinus Nijhoff.

Cohen, S. & Wills, T. A. (1985). Stress, social support, and the buffering hypothesis. *Psychological Bulletin, 98*, 310–357.

Costa, M., Steptoe, A., Cropley, M. & Griffith, J. (1999). Ambulatory blood pressure monitoring is associated with reduced physical activity during everyday life. *Psychosomatic Medicine, 61*, 806–811.

Gellman, M., Spitzer, S., Ironson, G., Llabre, M., Saab, P., Pasin, R., Weidler, D. J. & Schneiderman, N. (1990). Posture, place and mood effects on ambulatory blood pressure. *Psychophysiology, 27*, 544–551.

Hemingway, H. & Marmot, M. (1999). Evidence based cardiology: psychosocial factors in the aetiology and prognosis of coronary heart disease: systematic review of prospective cohort studies. *British Medical Journal, 318*, 1460–1467.

Horsten, M., Ericson, M., Perski, A., Wamala, S.P., Schenck-Gustafsson, K. & Orth-Gomér, K. (1999). Psychosocial factors and heart rate variability in healthy women. *Psychosomatic Medicine, 61*, 49–57.

Ituarte, P. H., Kamarck, T. W., Thompson, H. S. & Bacanu, S. (1999). Psychosocial mediators of racial differences in nighttime blood pressure dipping among normotensive adults. *Health Psychology, 18*, 393–402.

Johnson, J. V. & Hall, E. M. (1994). Social support in the work environment and cardiovascular disease. In S. A. Shumaker & S. M. Czajkowski (Eds.), *Social Support and Cardiovascular Disease* (pp. 145–166). New York: Plenum Press.

Kamarck, T. W., Shiffman, S., Smithline, L., Goodie, J. L., Paty, J. A., Gnys, M. & Yi-Kuan Jong, J. (1998). Effects of task strain, social conflict, and emotional activation on ambulatory cardiovascular activity: daily life consequences of recurring stress in a multiethnic adult sample. *Health Psychology, 17*, 17–29.

Karasek, R. A. & Theorell, T. (1990). *Healthy Work*. New York: Basic Books.

Kario, K., Schwartz, J. E. & Pickering, T. G. (1999). Ambulatory physical activity as a determinant of diurnal blood pressure variation. *Hypertension, 34*, 685–691.

La Rovere, M. T. & al. (1998). Baroreflex senstivity and heart-rate variability in prediction of total cardiac mortality after myocardial infarction. *Lancet, 351*, 478–484.

Leary, A. C. & Murphy, M. B. (1998). Sleep disturbance during ambulatory blood pressure monitoring of hypertensive patients. *Blood Pressure Monitoring, 3*, 11–15.

Light, K. C., Turner, J. R. & Hinderliter, A. L. (1992). Job strain and ambulatory work blood presssure in healthy young men and women. *Hypertension, 20*, 214–8.

Linden, W., Chambers, L., Maurice, J. & Lenz, J. W. (1993). Sex differences in social support, self-deception, hostility, and ambulatory cardiovascular activity. *Health Psychology, 12*, 376–80.

Matthews, K. A., Raikkonen, K., Everson, S. A., Flory, J. D., Marco, C. A., Owens, J. F. & Lloyd,

C. E. (2000). Do the daily experiences of healthy men and women vary according to occupational prestige and work strain? *Psychosomatic Medicine, 62*, 346–353.

Parati, G., Trazzi, S., Ravogli, A., Casadei, R., Omboni, S. & Mancia, G. (1991). Methodological problems in evaluation of cardiovascular effects of stress in humans. *Hypertension, 17(Suppl)*, III50–III55.

Pickering, T. G. & Gerin, W. (1990). Cardiovascular reactivity in the laboratory and the role of behavioral factors in hypertension: a critical review. *Annals of Behavioral Medicine, 12*, 3–16.

Rosengren, A., Orth-Gomer, K., Wedel, H. & Wilhelmsen, L. (1993). Stressful life events, social support, and mortality in men born in 1933. *British Medical Journal, 307*, 1102–1105.

Schnall, P. L., Landsbergis, P. A. & Baker, D. (1994). Job strain and cardiovascular disease. *Annual Review of Public Health, 15*, 381–411.

Schnall, P. L., Pieper, C., Schwartz, J. E., Karasek, R. A., Schlussel, Y., Devereux, R. B., Ganau, A., Alderman, M., Warren, K. & Pickering, T. G. (1990). The relationship between 'job strain,' workplace diastolic blood pressure, and left ventricular mass index. Results of a case-control study. *Journal of the American Medical Association, 263*, 1929–35.

Sherman, W. M., Morris, D. M., Kirby, T. E., Petosa, R. A., Smith, B. A., Frid, D. J. & Leenders, N. (1998). Evaluation of a commercial accelerometer (Tritrac-R3 D) to measure energy expenditure during ambulation. *International Journal of Sports Medicine, 19*, 43–47.

Steptoe, A. (2000). Stress, social support and cardiovascular activity over the working day. *International Journal of Psychophysiology, 37*, 299–308.

Steptoe, A. (in press). Job control, perceptions of control, and cardiovascular activity: an analysis of ambulatory measures collected over the working day. *Journal of Psychosomatic Research.*

Steptoe, A., Cropley, M. & Joekes, K. (1999). Job strain, blood pressure, and responsivity to uncontrollable stress. *Journal of Hypertension, 17*, 193–200.

Steptoe, A., Fieldman, G., Evans, O. & Perry, L. (1993). Control over work pace, job strain and cardiovascular responses in middle-aged men. *Journal of Hypertension, 11*, 751–759.

Steptoe, A., Lundwall, K. & Cropley, M. (2000). Gender, family structure and cardiovascular activity during the working day and evening. *Social Science and Medicine, 50*, 231–239.

Uchino, B. N., Cacioppo, J. T. & Kiecolt-Glaser, J. K. (1996). The relationship between social support and physiological processes: a review with emphasis on underlying mechanisms and implications for health. *Psychological Bulletin, 119*, 488–531.

Unden, A. L., Orth-Gomér, K. & Elofsson, S. (1991). Cardiovascular effects of social support in the work place: twenty-four-hour ECG monitoring of men and women. *Psychosomatic Medicine, 53*, 50–60.

Chapter 17
The Assessment of Blood Pressure Variability in Behavior Modification: The Identification of Relevant Situation and Mood Factors

Lutz Mussgay[1], Frithjof Niegot[1], and Heinz Rüddel[1,2]
[1]*Psychosomatic Hospital St.-Franziska-Stift, Bad Kreuznach, Germany, and*
[1,2]*Department of Behavioral Medicine and Rehabilitation, Center for Psychobiological and Psychosomatic Research, University of Trier*

Introduction

Moods and emotional states affect body processes. With regard to the cardiovascular system, negative affective states and perceived stress in general have shown the best correlation with heart rate and blood pressure (Franck, Herrmann & Fahrenberg, 1996; James & Pickering, 1991; James, Yee, Harshfield, Blank & Pickering, 1986; Langewitz, Rüddel & Von Eiff, 1987; Shapiro, Goldstein & Jamner, 1990; Southard et al., 1986). A sustained elevation of blood pressure is likely to induce vascular alterations with various consequences such as strokes and myocardial infarctions. Elevations of blood pressure level have received much more attention than blood pressure changes that occur in everyday life in response to varying situational and emotional requirements. Blood pressure changes are more or less seen as error variance that should be avoided. Even 24–hours ambulatory blood pressure monitoring mainly has a focus on blood pressure level throughout the day and the night and cancels out unwanted fluctuations. Our approach, on the contrary, tries to make use of the "unwanted" variance. We used blood pressure changes during 24–hour ambulatory blood pressure monitoring for the identification of relevant situation and mood factors. The accumulated evidence was to be used in the individual therapeutic setting for the tailoring of treatment strategies for patients suffering from essential hypertension or being at high risk to develop hypertension (borderline hypertensives). The rationale dates back to the work of Luborsky and Auerbach (1969) and has since been applied in a much refined fashion by other researchers (Franck et al., 1996; Heger, 1990; Jacob et al., 1999; Kamarck et al., 1998; Käppler, 1994; Rau, 1993; Shapiro et al., 1993; Shapiro, Jamner & Goldstein, 1997; Shapiro, Jamner, Goldstein & Delfino, in press). It makes use of the observation that the given individual will exhibit blood pressure elevation in situations that put strain on the processing and coping resources. It is known that the amount of activity, of mood changes, and of various challenging situations during everyday life, all affect blood pressure (Fahrenberg, 1996). Research up to now, however, has not led to a common understanding about the effects of certain situation and mood factors and their relation to blood pressure changes. The only generally accepted exception is the influence of negative affect on blood pressure elevations (Shapiro et al., in press; Shapiro, et al., 1997). Apart from this finding, the search for a specific response pattern, that is valid across subjects has proven to be unsuccessful. Psychotherapy, however, focuses on a given individual. The quest for conditions affecting blood pressure has to be individual in nature and, therefore, need not be concerned with interindividual response patterns. Its potential lies in the analysis of individually different response tendencies.

Table 1, extracted from Fahrenberg (1996, page 168), lists principal sources of blood pressure variations. Some variables like seasonal components or periodic changes and high frequency ones like Mayer-Waves can be discarded for the intended purpose. Others have to be excluded because their registration is difficult or unreliable on a repeated basis throughout 24 hours or is not possible with the measuring devices currently available. This applies to noise, moisture and temperature as well as to salt intake. Nevertheless, an approach which sets out to combine 24–hour blood pressure monitoring with the assessment of psychological and situational factors has to include the major remaining sources of variation in order to distinguish therapeutically relevant from irrelevant factors. Of prime importance are

Table 1. Principal sources of blood pressure variation (except specific clinical conditions, e.g., pheochromocytoma, autonomic neurophathia) (extracted from Fahrenberg, 1996, p. 168).

Periodic components
Respiration; Mayer waves; ultradian,
circadian (diurnal), and seasonal components
Physical activity
Posture, changing from supine to upright position
Dynamic and static (isometric) exercise
Ingestion of food and drink
Micturation and defaecation
Smoking, alcohol, caffeine, salt
Behavioral, mental and emotional activity
Anticipation of tasks or events
Mental effort, emotional activation
Social interaction, talking, sexual intercourse
Behavioral/ emotional challenge (stress-strain)
Ambient conditions
Temperature, moisture
Noise

parameters like activity level and heart rate in order to identify blood pressure rises that are exercise related. Even posture has known effects on mood (Gellman et al., 1990). A description of prevailing situational characteristics, the number of persons present, an estimate of familiarity, aspects of coping with the situations and ratings of emotion and mood states are necessary to extract a sufficiently detailed picture of possible influences on blood pressure. The final interpretation will also have to consider influences of medication, especially if their presumed effects cover the antihypertensive spectrum. Antihypertensive medication, however, does not typically affect situational reactivity. Its main consequences are attenuation of the general blood pressure level (Mills & Dimsdale, 1991). Thus, the conclusions regarding individually relevant effects of situation context is reliably possible. On the other hand, the interpretation of blood pressure peaks can never be more than a hypothesis about contributing influences. In single case designs the accumulated data base is not sufficient to reliably quantify the relative contribution of all major influences. Also, normative data are not available which would help to clarify individual response tendencies.

A further necessary prerequisite for the inclusion of a given patient into the diagnostic procedure has to consider the issue of individual response patterns. Only patients that are likely to react primarily with their cardiovascular, or more specifically, with their blood pressure system to challenging and stressful situations can be included. In clinical practice testing this would be too time consuming, so tentatively the fact of a moderately or severely elevated blood pressure at clinical measurements can be taken as an index of response specificity of the blood pressure system. Our approach collects data in the field, not in the laboratory. Ideally, the recording should be done in the natural environment of the patient. Individual vulnerabilities would then be challenged most realistically. In this respect, an assessment during inpatient rehabilitation can best be a substitute with limited representativity compared to assessments in everyday life. Still a lot of potentially relevant challenges can be expected to be encountered. This applies mainly to existing vulnerabilities in all types of social contact. A promising way out of this dilemma is the inclusion of standard provocation challenges like mental arithmetic or public speaking. Pioneering work of Fahrenberg and others (for an overview see Fahrenberg, 1996) has shown the advantage of electronic diaries as tools to collect on the spot ratings on a regular basis over a prolonged length of time. Their use offers the best chances to register unbiased judgments pertaining to the actual situation. In contrast to a typical interview session where the subjective evaluations of the patient prevail, the inclusion of cardiovascular and blood pressure data in relation to situation and mood ratings allows a rather objective analysis of influencing factors. Due to the limiting factors addressed above, the ensuing hypotheses should be verified together with the patient.

Methodology

The following chapter describes operative and procedural details of our approach, lists the range of parameter assessed and presents the analytical strategies summarized in the report sheet.

For 24–hour blood pressure measurement a standard ambulatory device is used (Tonoport, ParMed/Hellige) and run on oscillatory or auscultatory mode as required to achieve maximal accuracy. Although the output of an actometer can be registered by this device to yield objective data on activity levels, the approach as it is presented here did not use this option, however, but relied on subjective ratings of the patient. This has several reasons: Firstly, the application of an actometer at calve-level would hinder the patient unduly, as it requires to cope with the wiring for the total of 24 hours which, beside having to undress while attaching the transducer, is rather awkward during night hours. We expected quite a few patients to refuse assessment or at least to discontinue it. Secondly, the device we used has to run on auscultatory mode in order to register activity. This, however, would not have been reliably possible in all patients. Especially, overweight patients are difficult to measure in this mode.

Blood pressure was assessed every 20 minutes during the day (7:00 h – 22:00 h) and every 30 minutes during night hours. Additionally, patients could start a measurement by pressing a predesigned button. Patients were not informed about their resulting blood pressure values. The LCD-display of the device was covered by sticky tape to avoid feedback and possible confoundation. A second set of parameters was gathered with a palm–top–computer (HP 200 LX) providing a LCD–display of 80 x 54 signs and a keyboard. For presentation of the questions, an interactive Turbo-Pascal program was written. Patients were instructed to switch on the electronic diary and answer the set of items at each cuff inflation during the day. From a main menu the user could skip into four subbranches by typing in No. 1–4, respectively. The first branch provided the patient with a detailed description of the purpose of the assessment as well as of the way how to handle the electronic diary and how and when to type in the required situation and mood ratings. The second branch was to be activated at each blood pressure measurement. A fixed set of questions had to be answered. Table 2 lists all items together with the type of response required. The items were chosen on the basis of reports by the groups of Fahrenberg (Fahrenberg, 1996), Schwenkmezger (Hank & Schwenkmezger, 1996) and Perrez (Perrez & Reicherts, 1996; Perrez & Reicherts, 1989). Economy considerations, however, dictated some alterations and abbreviations without limiting the scope of the items unnecessarily.

The third branch asked for some final estimates regarding the acceptance of important aspects of the assessment procedure. Table 3 lists these items (translated) together with the mean ratings of 13 test patients. The fourth branch, finally,

Table 2. Items of branch 2 that have to be answered at each automatically started or self induced blood pressure measurement (translated from German). Either a code had to be typed in or a rating had to be indicated ranging from 0 = total disagreement to 6 = total agreement/very much.

Situation categories: What are you engaged with at the moment ?			
		What exactly are you doing ?	
1	Therapy/diagnostic procedure	1	Individual therapy session or examination
		2	Group therapy
		3	Sport therapy
		4	Relaxation/Feldenkrais session
		5	Other
2	Leisure time activities	1	Conversation
		2	Sports
		3	Relaxation/reading
		4	Contemplating
		5	Religious activity
		6	TV/radio
		7	Shopping
		8	Promenating
		9	Other
3	Meals		
4	Grooming/hygiene, dressing or undressing		
5	one of the compulsory activities	1	Mental arithmetic
		2	Climbing stairs
		3	Resting
		4	Publicly speaking
6	Other		

Persons present: What persons are present at the moment ?	Code
I am alone	1
a familiar person	2
an unfamiliar person	3
several familiar persons	4
several unfamiliar persons	5
A larger group of persons	6
Coping ratings	Rating
The persons present put me under strain	0-1-2-3-4-5-6
The present situation needs a lot of effort	0-1-2-3-4-5-6
The present situation is familiar to me	0-1-2-3-4-5-6
I am able to cope with the situation effectively	0-1-2-3-4-5-6
Activity estimate: How strongly did you exert yourself ?	0-1-2-3-4-5-6
Posture: In what posture was the measurement taken ?	Code
Standing	1
Sitting	2
Lying	3
Walking	4
Mood ratings	Rating
I'm feeling anxious	0-1-2-3-4-5-6
I'm sad	0-1-2-3-4-5-6
I'm excited	0-1-2-3-4-5-6
I'm happy	0-1-2-3-4-5-6
I'm feeling tense	0-1-2-3-4-5-6
I'm angry	0-1-2-3-4-5-6
I'm suppressing my anger	0-1-2-3-4-5-6
I'm feeling irritable	0-1-2-3-4-5-6
I'm feeling exhausted	0-1-2-3-4-5-6

had to be activated by the patient, whenever he or she was asked to respond by the start of a blood pressure measurement, but was not able to answer the items of branch 2 immediately because he was currently engaged in other important activi-

Table 3. Items to assess acceptance of electronic diary and mean ratings of 13 test-persons (translated from German).

Nr.	Item	Mean	SD
1	I slept well	2.8	1.9
2	I was disturbed during sleep by cuff inflations	3.2	2.4
3	I was disturbed in my sleep by other causes	1.7	1.9
4	I was disturbed during the day by cuff inflations	4.0	1.0
5	I liked the blood pressure measurement very much	2.5	2.2
6	Handling the blood pressure device was no problem	4.0	2.0
7	Answering the electronic diary disturbed me very much	2.2	2.2
8	I very much liked answering computer questions	3.8	1.9
9	Handling the palm-top computer was very easy	4.4	1.7
10	The instructions on the computer-monitor were very helpful	5.2	0.6
11	The additional written instruction was very helpful	5.4	0.8
Ratings: 0 = I do not agree; 6 = I agree fully			

ties. Skipping to this option required no further response. Just after the delay patients were supposed to switch on the computer again and to indicate the reason for the delay. Alternatives were: therapy session, medical examination or other reasons. The patient could then start manually a blood pressure recording and answer the questions of branch 2 as usual. For each patient the completion of a set of four standard situations was scheduled at some time throughout the recording period. These situations were included to confront the patient with challenges he or she would otherwise have tended to avoid. One situation asked for physical exercise. Patients had to climb up four flights of stairs as fast as possible and then to start a blood pressure measurement and giving the additional ratings. A further situation induced a mental challenge. Arithmetic calculations had to be repeated for 15 minutes. We used the Konzentrations-Leistungs-Test (KLT, Düker & Lienert, 1959). A third stressful experience asked the patients to present themselves in public in a staged application for a vacant post. After five minutes of preparation they had eight minutes to convince two opposing unfamiliar staff members of their qualification for this particular job. The set of challenges were very similar to the Trierer Social Stress Test (TSST) (Kirschbaum, Pirke & Hellhammer, 1993). A fourth situation explicitly did not ask for any kind of activity, instead patients had to relax in a quiet room, preferably the clinic chapel, and spend there 30 minutes at rest with a self–induced measurement at the end. This situation was supposed to serve as a baseline measure. Due to the standardized implementation of the four situations, they provided the additional advantage to compare baseline values as well as reactivity indices between patients. Compliance to undergo these situations, however, was not good in some patients; particularly public speaking was most often avoided.

Report preparation

Figure 1 gives the schematic overview of the subsequent analytical stages. First, the two data sets had to be combined. This was done with a PC–based SAS–system. Tonoport data (blood pressure, heart rate) were aligned with electronic diary data (activity estimate, situation characteristics, posture, and mood ratings) according to the respective time stamps of each measurement. A time lag of maximal three minutes before and 13 minutes after each blood pressure measurement was allowed. A file resulted, that contained a varying number of complete data sets covering the waking hours of a 24–hour period. The actual number depended largely on the diligence and reliability of the part-taking patient.

Data were analyzed further using two strategies. The first approach looked at the data in a way to highlight the impact of mood ratings and aspects of situational coping on blood pressure. The second approach recombined the data in order to pronounce the impact of situation characteristics on blood pressure.

Since exercise has known effects on blood pressure, in a first step its influence was removed by regression analysis separately from systolic and diastolic blood pressure. The corresponding sequence of activity ratings and pressure values throughout the 24–hour registration period entered into the calculation process. The activity corrected blood pressure was used for the further steps. Each 24–hour set of mood ratings was regressed on the corrected systolic and diastolic blood pressure values separately. The resulting regression coefficients are then expressing the contribution of each situation or mood dimension to the systolic or diastolic blood pressure course. These coefficients were supposed to be of prime importance for therapeutic purposes, since they highlight the relative importance of certain situational and mood factors as regards blood pressure changes. More specifically, they describe the individual vulnerability pattern of a patient in response to the encountered challenging situations.

The second analytical strategy sums up blood pressure and heart rate values as well as coping and mood ratings separately for the different situation characteristics. For all categories of situations, persons present, standard situations, and posture (see Table 2) the respective mean values were calculated. Finally, the maximal systolic and diastolic blood pressure, the respective time of occurrence, situation category, coping, and mood ratings were extracted.

All results were combined and entered into a report. Figure 2 presents an example.

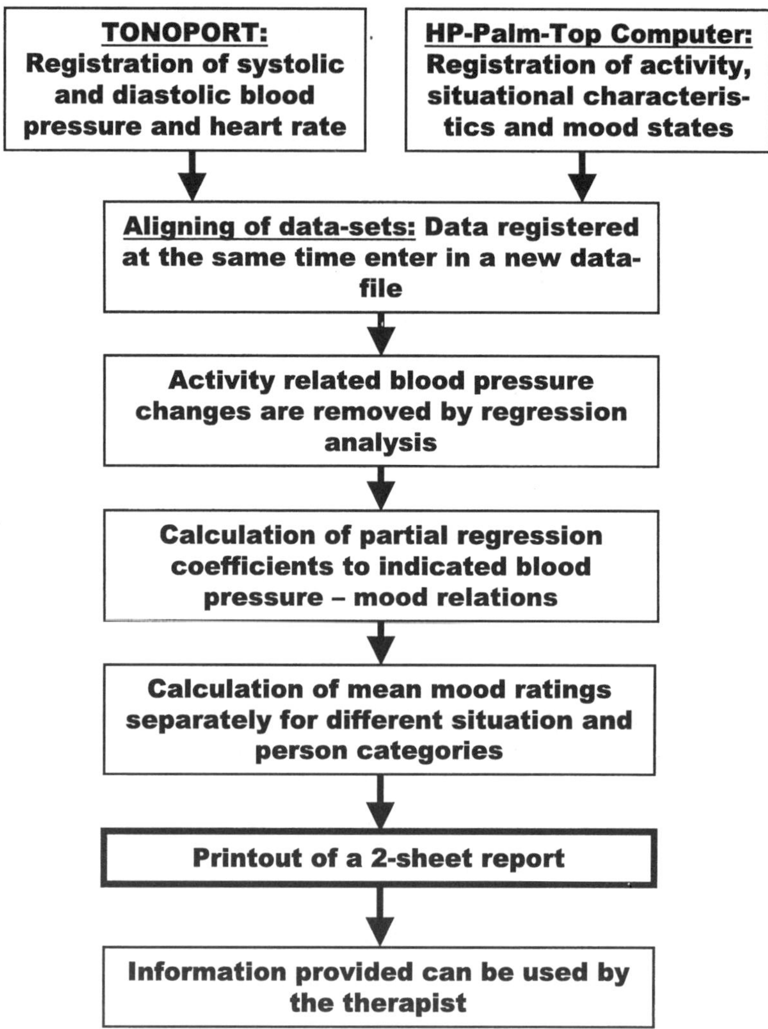

Figure 1. Data sampling and subsequent analytical steps leading to the report

The report is supposed to provide the therapist with all information he or she may need to evaluate the patient's response pattern and to provide a sufficient basis for a thorough exploration of the patient.

Acceptance

In clinical routine acceptance was sufficiently good. Most patients could handle the equipment after a short introduction. The frequency of typing in the required ratings depended strongly on the discipline and motivation of the patient. In some

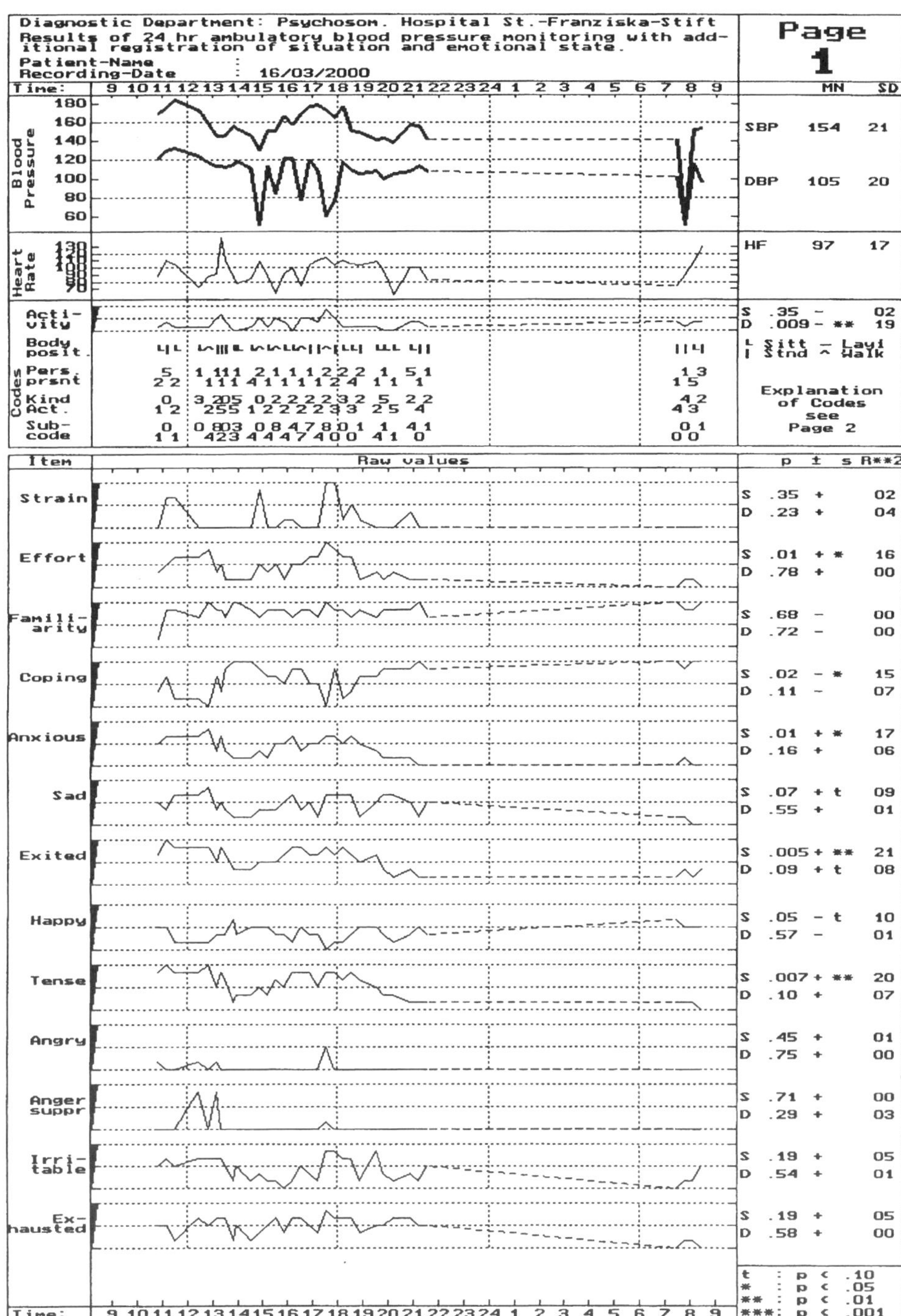
Diagnostic Department: Psychosom. Hospital St.-Franziska-Stift
Results of 24 hr ambulatory blood pressure monitoring with additional registration of situation and emotional state.
Patient-Name :
Recording-Date : 16/03/2000
Page 1
Time: 9 10 11 12 13 14 15 16 17 18 19 20 21 22 23 24 1 2 3 4 5 6 7 8 9
MN SD
Blood Pressure
SBP 154 21
DBP 105 20
Heart Rate
HF 97 17
Acti-vity
S .35 - 02
D .009 - ** 19
Body posit.
Sitt Stnd Layi Walk
Codes
Pers. prsnt
Kind Act.
Sub-code
Explanation of Codes see Page 2
Item
Raw values
p ± s R**2
Strain
S .35 + 02
D .23 + 04
Effort
S .01 + * 16
D .78 + 00
Famili-arity
S .68 - 00
D .72 - 00
Coping
S .02 - * 15
D .11 - 07
Anxious
S .01 + * 17
D .16 + 06
Sad
S .07 + t 09
D .55 + 01
Exited
S .005 + ** 21
D .09 + t 08
Happy
S .05 - t 10
D .57 - 01
Tense
S .007 + ** 20
D .10 + 07
Angry
S .45 + 01
D .75 + 00
Anger suppr
S .71 + 00
D .29 + 03
Irri-table
S .19 + 05
D .54 + 01
Ex-hausted
S .19 + 05
D .58 + 00
t : p < .10
* : p < .05
** : p < .01
***: p < .001
Time: 9 10 11 12 13 14 15 16 17 18 19 20 21 22 23 24 1 2 3 4 5 6 7 8 9

Page 2

Blood Pressure and Heart Rate: Mean Values for Activities, Persons and Body Positions.

Valid Entries: 34

	Activity		Sub-Class	N	SBP	DBP	HR	Evaluation: Strain	Effort	Familiarity	Coping	Emot. State: Anxious	Sad	Excited	Happy	Tense	Angry	Anger suppr.	Irritable	Exhausted
1	Therapy	1	One-to-one	1	169	121	88	0	2	1	2	3	3	4	3	5	1	0	3	3
		2	Group	0	.	.	.	.	.	.	.	.	.	.	.	.	.	.	.	.
		3	Exercise	0	.	.	.	.	.	.	.	.	.	.	.	.	.	.	.	.
		4	Relax/Feldkr	1	145	111	85	0	1	5	6	1	1	2	3	2	0	0	1	1
		5	Other	0	.	.	.	.	.	.	.	.	.	.	.	.	.	.	.	.
2	Leisure Time	1	Conversat.	4	157	110	105	1	2	5	4	2	2	3	2	2	0	0	2	2
		2	Exercise	0	.	.	.	.	.	.	.	.	.	.	.	.	.	.	.	.
		3	Relax/Read	0	.	.	.	.	.	.	.	.	.	.	.	.	.	.	.	.
		4	Contemplat.	7	159	114	98	1	3	5	3	3	3	4	2	3	0	0	2	3
		5	Religious	0	.	.	.	.	.	.	.	.	.	.	.	.	.	.	.	.
		6	TV/Radio	0	.	.	.	.	.	.	.	.	.	.	.	.	.	.	.	.
		7	Shopping	2	173	98	89	0	4	5	4	2	2	4	2	5	0	0	2	4
		8	Promenade	3	156	86	90	2	4	5	3	3	3	4	1	4	1	2	3	4
		9	Other	0	.	.	.	.	.	.	.	.	.	.	.	.	.	.	.	.
3	Meals			5	164	108	100	2	4	5	3	3	3	4	2	4	0	1	4	3
4	Hygiene/Dressing			3	118	89	88	0	1	6	6	0	1	1	3	1	0	0	1	1
5	Standardsit.	1	Calculation	2	141	103	78	0	2	5	5	1	4	2	2	2	0	0	2	4
		2	Clmb. Stairs	1	146	113	142	0	3	5	2	4	3	5	2	5	0	0	4	4
		3	Rest	2	154	117	82	0	1	6	6	1	1	2	3	2	0	0	2	2
		4	Speach	0	.	.	.	.	.	.	.	.	.	.	.	.	.	.	.	.
0	Other			3	150	98	110	3	2	4	5	3	2	4	3	4	0	0	3	3
	PERSONS PRESENT																			
1	Alone			21	150	107	91	0	2	5	4	2	2	3	2	3	0	0	2	3
2	One familiar person			7	164	95	105	3	4	4	3	3	3	4	2	4	1	0	3	3
3	One unfamiliar person			1	153	96	130	0	0	6	6	0	0	2	3	0	0	0	3	0
4	Several familiar persons			2	148	110	95	2	2	4	4	2	2	3	2	4	0	0	2	2
5	Several unfamiliar persons			3	162	118	106	2	2	5	5	2	2	3	3	3	0	0	2	3
6	Large group of persons			0	.	.	.	.	.	.	.	.	.	.	.	.	.	.	.	.
	BODY-POSITION																			
1	Standing			13	149	104	104	1	2	5	4	2	2	3	2	3	0	0	2	3
2	Sitting			16	157	115	93	1	2	5	4	2	3	3	2	3	0	0	2	3
3	Laying			0	.	.	.	.	.	.	.	.	.	.	.	.	.	.	.	.
4	Walking			5	156	78	90	2	4	5	3	3	3	4	2	5	1	0	3	4
	BLOOD PRESSURE: MAXIMUM																			
S	Systolic at		11 hr 29	Sit 2/1		Per 2	BP 2	4	4	5	1	4	4	5	1	5	0	0	3	1
D	Diastolic at		11 hr 29	Sit 2/1		Per 2	BP 2	4	4	5	1	4	4	5	1	5	0	0	3	1

Report:

Date: Signature:

Figure 2. Page 1 displays blood pressure, heart rate, activity level, posture (sitting, laying, standing, walking), situation and person codes, coping and mood ratings on a 24-hour basis. Dashed lines denote breaks in responding of more than one hour duration. The column on the right gives either mean values and standard deviations (blood pressure, heart rate) or, in the lower part of the page, the results of the regression analyses separately for systolic (S) and diastolic (D) blood pressure. The p-column gives probability estimates of the regression coefficients. The direction of the duration can either be positive (+) or negative (-). In case of significance (right column, bottom) the appropriate sign occurs to highlight the relevance. The explained variance (in %) appears in the right column.
Page 2 presents averaged blood pressure, heart rate, coping, and mood ratings separately for all situations (inclusive standard situations), persons present, and posture (see Table 2). Column N indicates the number of occurrences. The total number of valid data sets is given in a box near the top of the page. The last two lines contain maximum values of systolic and diastolic blood pressure and relevant information regarding the respective situation, persons, posture, and ratings.

cases the instructions were met rather compulsively, while other patients delivered not enough data to warrant analysis. Complaints about feeling disturbed by the regular pump operation, especially at night, were quite frequent. The additional rating task with the electronic diary, however, was very rarely found obtrusive or troublesome. There were compliance problems with the standard stress situations, especially with public speaking.

In order to familiarize therapists with the newly established approach, introductory courses were held in regular intervals. After some time of experience with the procedure it was proposed to reduce the complexity of the report sheets. Some therapists found it difficult to extract the most relevant information from the summarized data. A further reduction of data, however, seems unjustified, as the complexity with which blood pressure is related to environment and mood factors has to be considered an unchangeable reality. Therapists therefore will have to be trained more extensively to handle the host of information Taken together, the approach was successfully implemented and provides valuable information on many patients.

Results

Pooling the individually oriented analytical approaches to use psychophysiological monitoring for behavior modification, leads to a valuable data pool that offers the chance to gain deeper insight into concomitants of blood pressure regulation. However, we have to deal with an apparent dilemma. Stimulus specific response patterns have not turned up yet or concern only very broad concepts like negative affect. So any statistical analysis will have to apply strategies that leave sufficient room for differentiation between patients or subgroups of patients instead of focusing on the blood pressure behavior of the entire group. This part of the experimental variance will then cover individual response patterns. In order to solve this dilemma we have pursued a strategy to establish regularities that apply to the entire group in a uniform sense and then to search for response patterns that are valid only for subgroups of patients.

129 patients had completed the assessment. 18 had to be excluded, because their compliance was too poor and led to less than 20 valid pairings of blood pressure, heart rate, and emotional ratings, leaving 111 patients to be considered in the analysis. 54 (48,6 %) were females, 58 (51,4 %) males. Their mean age was 47.8 (±9.9) years. When classified according to their main diagnoses, 44.9 % of the patients had mood (affective) disorders (ICD10: F3), another 44.1 % suffered from neurotic, stress related and somatoforme disorders (ICD10: F4), 3.1 % were classified as disorders of adult personality and behavior (ICD10: F6), and 7.1 % showed behavioral syndromes associated with physiological disturbances and physical factors (ICD10: F5). All together the 111 patients completed 3.616 concurrent data sets (yielding a mean answer rate of 32.6, with a maximal rate of 50). Mean blood pressure was 137/93 mmHg (137/91 for males; 138/95 for females), mean heart rate was 88.1 bpm (88.7 for males, 87.5 for females).

Figure 3 shows mean ratings for activity, coping, and mood. In general, the level of activity was rather low. Most situations were conceived of requiring a lot of effort, on the other hand the feeling of being familiar with the situation prevailed. As regards mood, in accordance with the perception of situations being strenuous, the emotional experience was rated as a feeling of tension, albeit not in the extreme. Exhaustion was indicated to a comparable degree. As regards positive mood states feelings of happiness were indicated to a slightly lower degree. A tendency to per-

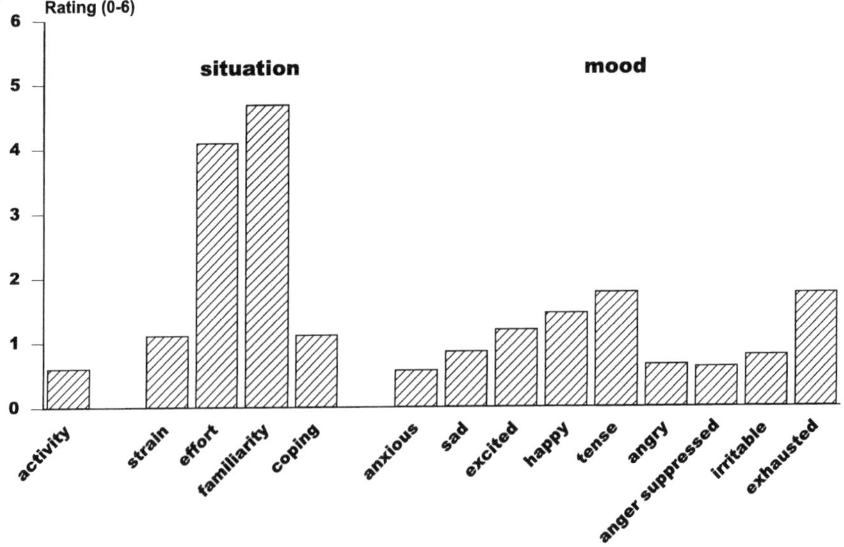

Figure 3. Mean ratings of 111 assessments yielding a total of 3616 data sets

ceive most situations as stressful and strenuous may be related to a predominance of affective and somatoforme disorders in our sample of patients.

Some literature reports center around the importance of negative affect in relation to high blood pressure (Carels et al., 2000; Shapiro et al., 1997; Shapiro et al., in press). We therefore compared blood pressure and heart rate for positive and negative affect, while taking the intensity of the respective ratings into account. Feelings of happiness as well as familiarity and effective coping with a situation were taken to indicate positive affect, whereas feelings of sadness, anger, suppression of anger, and tension were considered indicative of negative affect. For each intensity (0–5) of the ratings (because of very few ratings with the extreme value of 6 this intensity was left out) the respective mean blood pressure and heart rate were calculated (Figure 4).

It is obvious, that heart rate and blood pressure differed considerably between positive and negative affect. However, the difference was not affected by the respective intensity. Systolic blood pressure behaved somewhat differently. There was only a slight tendency to higher values for negative affect at high intensities, however, the difference got more accentuated without leading to higher absolute values of systolic blood pressure. Our findings, although supporting the notion of a stronger impact of negative affect on cardiovascular activity is not in accord with the litera-

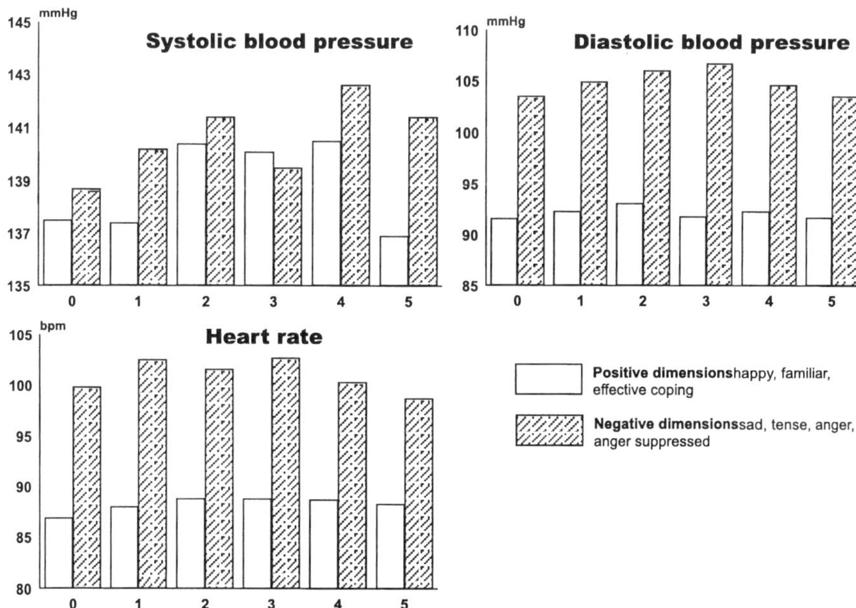

Figure 4. Systolic, diastolic blood pressure and heart rate for positive and negative situation and mood dimensions separated for different rating intensities (rating 6 is left out due to very few occurrences).

ture (Shapiro et al., in press) as regards the dependency on rating intensity.

A further analytical approach to describe the impact of coping and mood factors on physiological parameters was offered by the comparison of subgroups with extreme ratings in either of the coping and mood dimensions. Two groups were formed, one comprising the upper third of the sample, the other the lower third of the distribution. The midsection had been discarded for this purpose. These groups were then compared by t–tests on each of the physiological parameters (systolic blood pressure, diastolic blood pressure, heart rate).

Figure 5 exhibits the resulting p–values. It turned out that the extreme groups differed significantly in some mood dimensions in physiological parameters. Systolic blood pressure was significantly related to differences in sadness, excitement, tension and marginally to anxiety and exhaustion; diastolic values went along with differences in tension and exhaustion. Heart rate was significantly related to differences in exhaustion and marginally to sadness. Here again, a preponderance of negative affects emerges from this analysis. Carels et al. (2000) make a point in relating the variability of emotional states to blood pressure. Their approach is based on the assumption that "more emotionally responsive persons are responding to a greater number of stressful events during daily life, while another (explanation) is, that people who evidence considerable emotional responsivity perceive daily events as more

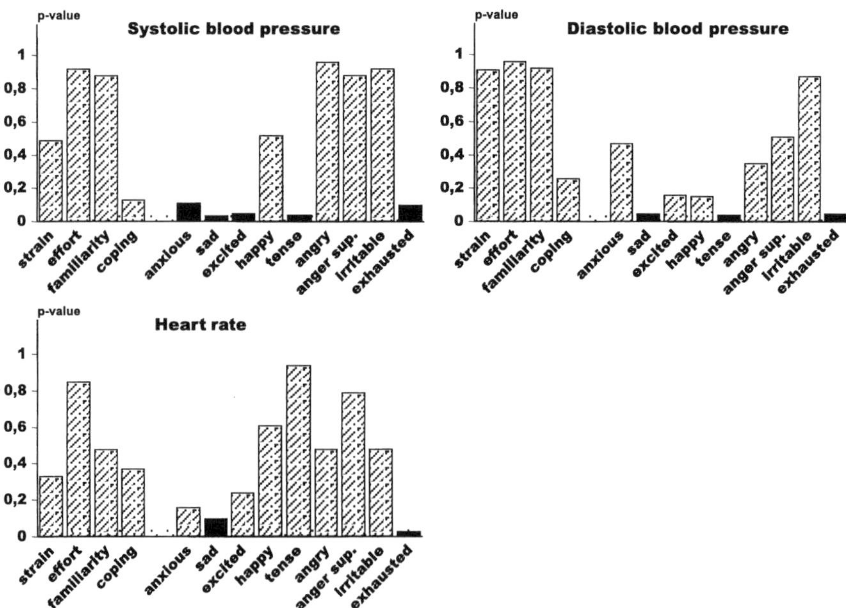

Figure 5. P-values of the t-test-comparison on ratings for situation coping and mood for the two extreme rating groups (upper and lower third) seperately for systolic, diastolic blood pressure and heart rate. Significant (< .05%) and marginally (<.10%) significant differences are presented as black bars, the 5% area is indicated by the dotted pattern.

stressful than those who are not responsive". Accordingly, emotional responsivity is operationalized by the standard deviations of different emotional ratings. The registered ambulatory blood pressure and heart rate values are seen as dependent variables. We chose the same approach. Standard deviations of all separate coping and mood ratings were calculated for each individual patient. Again extreme groups (upper versus lower third) were formed and the physiological parameters compared by t–test (see Figure 6).

A high variance in perceived strain, familiarity and feelings of effective coping, excitement and exhaustion was related to systolic blood pressure differences. Variance of excitement and exhaustion and marginally of familiarity brought about differences in diastolic blood pressure. Differences in heart rate finally were related to variability in effective coping and marginally in perceived strain, excitement, tension, and exhaustion. All results by and large confirm the report of Carels et al. (2000) in highlighting a pronounced influence of the variability of negative affect on blood pressure and heart rate. In comparison, the influence of positive affect is limited.

Group oriented analyses of these data sets do not consider the individual deviations from a general pattern of responsivity. The direction of the relatedness between the two data sets is one such example that can offer valuable additional information by highlighting the disparity within the data. With increasing intensity of ratings, the

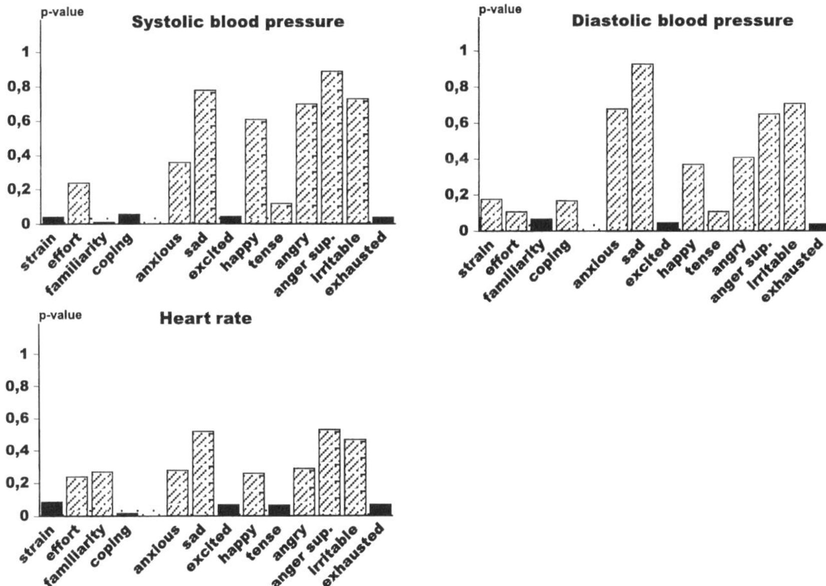

Figure 6. P-values of the t-test-comparison on the ratings for situation coping and mood for the two extreme standard deviation groups (upper and lower third) seperately for systolic, diastolic blood pressure, and heart rate. Significant (< .05%) and marginally (< .10%) significant differences are presented as black bars, the 5% area is indicated by the dotted pattern.

physiological parameters can either increase or decrease. In order to answer this question, the results of all the regression analyses that had been calculated between each individual data set of subsequent mood and coping ratings on one hand and blood pressure and heart rate on the other were considered in this respect.

Table 4 presents the results of this survey. As it turns out, there were very few significant coefficients for systolic blood pressure for positive relationships. In the average only 8.8 % of the regression analyses exceeded the significance level of 5 %, about 10.5 % exceed the level of 10 %. In the average 30.5 % yielded coefficients that are negative, indexing inverse relationships with physiological parameters. Roughly, the same applied for diastolic blood pressure. Here, however, even more negative relationships turned out to be significant as in systolic blood pressure. Obviously, there is no uniform relationship pattern present. This finding again hints into the direction of individual response patterns.

In order to follow up this line of reasoning, a cluster analytic approach was pursued. Mean positive and negative emotional ratings (positive emotions containing familiarity with the situation, happiness, and the feeling of effective coping, negative emotions were sadness, anger, suppression of anger, and anxiety) were separated into four clusters, explaining 76 % of the variance.

Table 5 depicts the resulting pattern together with the respective blood pressure and heart rate values. Cluster 1 described 9 patients with a tendency to medium ratings of both positive and negative emotions. Their blood pressure occupied an intermediate range with 139/92 mmHg. The same applied for the heart rate. A second cluster comprised 34 patients with medium ratings for positive and very low ratings for negative emotions. Blood pressure and heart rate were slightly lower than before. A third cluster (n = 25) described patients with high positive and medium negative ratings. Their blood pressure and heart rate were highest. The last cluster comprised 38 patients with the highest positive ratings and very low negative ones. Their systolic blood pressure was the lowest. Diastolic pressure and heart rate tended to the lower end of the spectrum, but were slightly above the value of cluster 2. It is somewhat surprising that also high positive ratings like in cluster 3 obviously went along with heightened blood pressure and faster heart rate. This effect was marginally significant for systolic blood pressure relative to clusters 2 and 4. All other effects were not significant. Obviously not only negative mood states are activating the sympathetic nervous system and hence leading to increases in blood pressure and heart rate. This finding points more in the direction of patterns of negative and positive affect having specific effects on the cardiovascular system depending on the particular combination. This finding is in line with the recent, yet unpublished, results of Shapiro et al. (in press).

Table 4. Direction of relationship between blood pressure (systolic and diastolic) and coping and mood ratings in 111 patients. The table contains the percentage of significant regression coefficients for either negative or positive relations on a 10% or 5% level as well as the percentage of relations with coefficients lower than zero.

Ratings for	Systolic blood pressure					Diastolic blood pressure				
	(-)		< 0%	(+)		(-)		< 0%	(+)	
	5%	10%		10%	5%	5%	10%		10%	5%
Coping										
strain	0	0	25.0	5.2	2.1	1.0	2.1	24.0	5.2	3.1
effort	0	0	23.0	6.7	4.8	1.9	1.9	22.9	4.8	4.8
Familiarity	0	0	33.6	7.5	4.7	0	1.9	33.0	7.5	2.8
effective coping	0	0	31.4	5.7	3.8	1.9	3.8	30.0	4.8	2.9
Mood										
anxious	0	0	26.0	3.9	3.9	1.3	2.6	27.3	3.9	2.6
sad	0	0	32.1	3.8	3.8	0	2.6	30.0	5.1	2.6
excited	0	0	19.8	6.9	5.0	0	1.0	18.8	5.0	1.0
happy	0	0	25.2	6.8	3.9	0	1.0	26.0	5.8	2.9
tense	0	0	26.6	3.7	1.8	0.9	1.8	25.0	6.4	2.8
angry	0	0	25.6	7.0	4.7	1.2	2.3	25.0	3.5	2.3
anger suppressed	0	0	25.3	7.0	2.4	1.2	2.4	25.0	6.0	2.4
irritable	0	0	33.7	5.6	3.4	2.2	4.5	33.7	3.4	2.2
exhausted	0	0	29.3	5.1	4.0	2.0	3.0	30.0	7.1	5.1
Mean	0	0	30.6	10.5	8.8	3.5	6.5	28.8	9.1	7.4

Table 5. Results of a cluster analysis on positive and negative mood states and respective systolic and diastolic blood pressure and heart rate means.

Cluster	Positive	Negative	N	Syst. BP	Diast. BP	Heart rate
1	2.1	2.7	9	139	92	88
2	1.9	0.3	34	137	92	87
3	2.4	1.2	25	144	95	90
4	2.9	0.2	38	134	94	88

Discussion

The issue of stimulus specificity remains unsolved. Obviously, the kind of analytical approach determines, at least to some part, the resulting patterns. When looking at the entire sample like other literature reports (Carels et al., 2000; Käppler, 1994; Franck et al., 1996; Shapiro et al., 1997; Shapiro et al., in press; Steptoe, Roy & Evans, 1996), effects of negative affect on blood pressure and heart rate are verified. Approaches that try to identify subgroups with different response tendencies on the other hand come up with the somewhat contradictory finding that positive affect in addition to negative affect also has blood pressure and heart rate rising qualities. Kamarck et al. (1998) points to the substantial heterogeneity regarding the effects of psychosocial influences on ambulatory cardiovascular activity. This notion can be seen as further support for analytical strategies basing on subgroup differentiation.

In this sense it is somewhat awkward that Shapiro et al. (1997) did not include positive affect into their assessment. Consequently they were only able to show the impact of negative affect on blood pressure. Similarly, Kamarck et al. (1998) asked only for negative emotional qualities and, not surprisingly, came up with the finding of elevated blood pressure and heart rate during periods of emotional (high negative or high arousal) activation. In the new study of Shapiro et al. (in press) positive affect ratings were included. In the analysis, however, the analytical approach again concentrated on the whole sample and did not distinguish subgroups. They look at the combination of different moods and their differential effects on blood pressure. Feeling happy, however, was the only positive mood dimension included, thus their results cannot be readily compared with our findings. The surface contour plots they are presenting, however, also indicate that interactions between positive and negative affect have to be considered. Franck et al. (1996) report results that point into the same direction as our findings. In their study systolic blood pressure was elevated when patients felt well, compared to the lack of such a feeling. The main effects reported, however, centre around negative mood dimensions. Jacob et al. (1999)

present a likely explanation that is able to reconcile the apparently contradictory findings. Their data show, that the degree of engagement of a mood rather than the degree of unpleasantness is the relevant factor for blood pressure rises. Again, they did not distinguish subgroups. There may be the danger of circularity when in further studies only negative affective qualities are included and when these qualities then are only studied on the whole sample.

On the other hand our results should be regarded with some reservation. The intensity of negative and/or positive emotions differs between patients. This way patients with high intensity emotion ratings have a stronger impact and therefore dominate the resulting pattern. Although data have been gathered in the field, they are not typical for the every day life of the patients. Specific individual challenges do not occur, also the overall level of activity is different from a typical workday outside the hospital.

We consider our approach promising for clinical practice, since the inclusion of physiological data into the therapeutic process greatly enlarges the validity of any behavior modification in patients with elevated blood pressure. Factors responsible for physiological reaction like blood pressure rises are typically not known by the patients. So instead of relying on subjective evaluations, the therapist has access to objective evidence. The individual response pattern is a valuable basis for the formulation of hypotheses about major sources of vulnerability in a given patient. Additionally, the report sheet is likely to prompt a fruitful exchange about individual ways of coping with every day life stressors. The demonstration of physiological changes in response to typical challenges may be a further motivating factor for behavioral changes. Quite often patients are naive in regard to their bodily reactions to stress. Highlighting the physiological effects of moderate challenges, therefore, provides new insights into the damaging properties of long-term stress exposition. Taken together, there is no doubt as to the clinical relevance, provided the therapist is ready to invest some time for a thorough analysis of the report provided. In addition the resulting data sets offer promising ways into the analysis of concomitants of blood pressure behavior.

Summary

An approach was presented that related blood pressure changes throughout a 24–hour ambulatory blood pressure monitoring to concurrent changes in environmental and mood factors by use of a computerized assessment procedure. The resulting data are analyzed and presented on a two-sheet report to be used by the therapist for the generation of hypotheses about an individual vulnerability pattern in response to daily challenges for the planning of therapeutic strategies. The data set of 111 patients that have yet completed the assessment procedure was analyzed to yield group specific information regarding the relatedness of blood pressure and heart rate to coping and mood factors. In accordance with literature reports, a prominent influence of negative affect could be verified. A second cluster analytic approach tried to differentiate subgroups of patients with different response tendencies. These results demonstrate nicely that in contrast to the analysis concerning the total sample the more differentiated approach also highlights the fact of blood pressure rising qualities of positive emotions at least in subgroups of patients.

References

Carels, R.A., Blumenthal, J.A. & Sherwood, A. (2000). Emotional responsivity during daily life: relationship to psychosocial functioning and ambulatory blood pressure. *International Journal of Psychophysiology, 36*, 25–33.

Düker, H. & Lienert, G. (1959). *Der Konzentrations-Leistungs-Test (KLT)*. Göttingen: Hogrefe.

Fahrenberg, J. (1996). Concurrent assessment of blood pressure, physical activity, and emotional state in natural settings. In J. Fahrenberg & M. Myrtek (Eds.), *Ambulatory Assessment. Computer assisted psychological and psychophysiological methods in monitoring and field studies* (pp. 165–187). Seattle: Hogrefe & Huber.

Franck, M., Herrmann, J.M. & Fahrenberg, J. (1996). Psychophysiologisches Blutdruck-Monitoring. *Nieren- und Hochdruckkrankheiten, 5*, 1995–201.

Gellmann, M., Spitzer, S., Ironson, G., Llabre, M., Saab, P., DeCarlo Pasin, R., Weidler, D. J. & Schneiderman, N. (1990). Posture, place, and mood effects on ambulatory blood pressure. *Psychophysiology, 27*, 544–551.

Hank, P. & Schwenkmezger, P. (1996). Computer-assisted versus paper-and-pencil-based self-monitoring: an analysis of experimental and psychometric equivalence. In J. Fahrenberg & M. Myrtek (Eds.), *Ambulatory Assessment. Computer assisted psychological and psychophysiological methods in monitoring and field studies* (pp. 85–100). Seattle: Hogrefe & Huber.

Heger, R. (1991). *Psychophysiologisches 24-Stunden-Monitoring: Methodenentwicklung und erste Ergebnisse eines multimodalen Untersuchungsansatzes bei 62 normotonen und blutdrucklabilen Studenten*. Frankfurt a.M.: Peter Lang.

Jacob, R.G., Thayer, J.F., Manuck, S.B., Muldoon, M.F., Tamres, L.K., Williams, D.M., Ding, Y. & Gatsonis, C. (1999). Ambulatory blood pressure responses and he circumplex model of mood: a 4-day study. *Psychosomatic Medicine, 61*, 319–333.

James, G.D., Yee, L.S., Harshfield, G.A., Blank, S.G. & Pickering, T.G. (1986). The influence of happiness, anger, and anxiety on the blood pressure of borderline hypertensives. *Psychosomatic Medicine, 48*, 502–508.

James, G.D. & Pickering, T.G. (1991). Ambulatory blood pressure monitoring: Assessing the diurnal variation of blood pressure. *American Journal of Physical Anthropology, 84*, 343–349.

Kamarck, T.W., Shiffman, S.M., Smithline, L., Goodie, J.L., Paty, J.A., Gnys, M. & Yi-Kuan Jong, J. (1998). Effects of task strain, social conflict, and emotional activation on ambulatory cardiovascular activity: daily life consequences of recurring stress in a multiethnic adult sample. *Health Psychology, 17*, 17–29.

Käppler, C. (1994). *Psychophysiologische Bedingungsanalyse von Blutdruckveränderungen im alltäglichen Lebenskontext*. Dissertation, University of Freiburg. Frankfurt a. M.: Lang.

Käppler, C., Becker, H.-U. & Fahrenberg, J. (1993). Ambulantes 24-Stunden-Monitoring als psychophysiologische Assessmentstrategie: Reproduzierbarkeit, Reaktivität, Retrospektionseffekt und Bewegungskonfundierung. *Zeitschrift für Differentielle und Diagnostische Psychologie, 14(4)*, 235–251.

Kirschbaum, C., Pirke, K.-M. & Hellhammer, D. (1993). The ‚Trier Social Stress Test' – a tool for investigating psychobiological stress response in a laboratory setting. *Neuropsychobiology, 28*, 76–81.

Luborsky, L. & Auerbach, A.H. (1969). The Symptom-Context Method. Quantitative studies of symptom formation in psychotherapy. *Journal of the American Psychoanalytic Association, 17,* 68–99.

Mills, P.J. & Dimsdale, J.E. (1991). Cardiovascular reactivity to psychosocial stressors. A review of the effects of beta-blockade. *Psychosomatics, 32(2),* 209–220.

Mussgay, L. & Rüddel, H. (1996). Ambulatory blood pressure monitoring: Promises and limitations in behavioral medicine. In J. Fahrenberg & M. Myrtek (Eds.), *Ambulatory Assessment. Computer assisted psychological and psychophysiological methods in monitoring and field studies* (pp. 365–374). Seattle: Hogrefe & Huber.

Parati, G., Ravogli, A. & Mancia, G. (1994). Clinical use of ambulatory blood pressure monitoring: a critical appraisal. *Journal of Cardiovascular Risk, 1(2),* 108–119.

Perrez, M. & Reicherts, M. (1996). A computer-assisted self-monitoring procedure for assessing stress-related behavior under real life conditions. In J. Fahrenberg & M. Myrtek (Eds.), *Ambulatory Assessment. Computer assisted psychological and psychophysiological methods in monitoring and field studies* (pp. 51–68). Seattle: Hogrefe & Huber.

Perrez, M. & Reicherts, M. (1989). Belastungsverarbeitung: Computerunterstützte Selbstbeobachtung im Feld. *Zeitschrift für Differentielle und Diagnostische Psychologie, 2*, 129–139.

Langewitz, W., Rüddel, H. & Von Eiff, A.W. (1987). Influence of perceived level of stress upon ambulatory blood pressure, heart rate, and respiratory frequency. *Journal of Clinical Hypertension. 3*, 743-748.

Rau, R. (1993). *Handlungssicherheit bei der Dispatchertätigkeit im Elektroenergieversorgungssystem. Eine psychophysiologische Untersuchung.* Dissertation, University of Dresden.

Shapiro, D., Goldstein, I.B. & Jammer, L.D. (1990). Relative contributions of trait characteristics and moods to daytime ambulatory blood pressure and heart rate. *Journal of Psychophysiology, 4*, 347–356.

Shapiro, D., Jammer, L.D. & Goldstein, I.B. (1993). Ambulatory stress psychophysiology: the study of ‚compensatory and defensive counterforces' and conflict in a natural setting. *Psychosomatic Medicine, 55*, 309–323.

Shapiro, D., Jammer, L.D., Goldstein, I.B. & Delfino, R.J. (in press). Striking a chord: moods, blood pressure, and heart rate in everyday life. *Psychophysiology.*

Southard, D.R., Coates, T.J., Kolodner, K., Parker, F.C., Padgett, N.E. & Kennedy, H.L. (1986). Relationship between mood and blood pressure in the natural environment: An adolescent population. *Health Psychology, 5*, 469–480.

Steptoe, A., Roy, M. & Evans, O. (1996). Psychosocial influences on ambulatory blood pressure over working and non-working days. *Journal of Psychophysiology, 10*, 218–227.

Chapter 18
Ambulatory 24-Hour Monitoring of Brachial and Finger Blood Pressure in Normotensive and Hypertensive Males

Reingard Seibt, André Berndt, Dieter Knöpfel, and Klaus Scheuch
Department of Work and Organizational Psychology, University of Technology Dresden, Germany

Introduction

The contemporary occupational situation is characterized by increasing dynamics and flexibility of work. Therefore, it is necessary to develop adequate innovative techniques to assess work-related strain and its consequences. In this context occupational physiology is faced with the need for appropriate non-invasive techniques for the reliable assessment of strain.

In the field of occupational physiology, arterial blood pressure and heart rate are the most frequently used strain measures. These parameters reflect the activation of the cardiovascular system in a work environment. Raised blood pressure proved to be an epidemiologic risk factor for cardiovascular diseases (Schnall & Landsbergis, 1994; Blumenthal et al., 1995; Johnson et al., 1996). The possible impact of occupational strain on the pathogenesis of hypertension has been discussed in several studies (Pickering, 1993; Seibt et al. 1998b; Siegrist et al., 1992; Theorell et al., 1993; van Egeren, 1992).

The development of new non-invasive methods for the long-term monitoring of cardiovascular parameters changed the profile of stress-strain research (Seibt & Scheuch, 1999). Beyond 24-hour ECG, many psychophysiological and work physiological studies have used the technique of ambulatory 24-hour blood pressure monitoring (ABPM). This technique provides to examine a wide spectrum of everyday blood pressure (Mancia et al., 1997; Parati et al., 1998; Rau, 1998; Schrader, 1995; Seibt et al, 1998b).

In the literature there are several hints of a so-called *carry-over-effect* of cardiovascular activation from the work place to leisure time and sleep (James et al., 1993; Pickering et al., 1991, 1993; van Egeren, 1992). There is also much uncertainty regarding the prognostic validity of single blood pressure peaks and blood pressure variability (Floras et al., 1988; Frattola et al., 1993; Gosse et al., 1989; Mancia et al., 1997; Parati et al., 1998; Pickering, 1997). Moreover, it was observed that the blood pressure variability in hypertensives was higher than the variability in normotensives (Krönig, 1993; Pickering, 1998). The diurnal rhythm is important for the evaluation of blood pressure variability (Baumgart & Rahn, 1990; Krönig, 1993; Siegel et al., 1992). In this context the increased blood pressure rise in the morning is of special diagnostic interest. In this period a high frequency of cardiovascular events was obtainted (Baumgart & Rahn, 1990; Mansoor, 1999; Pasqualetti et al., 1990; Siegel et al., 1992).

In stress-strain research, most of the 24-hour blood pressure examinations utilize the method of Riva-Rocci (brachial blood pressure, measured on the upper arm). The measurement principle is either oscillometric or auscultatoric. Advantages and disadvantages of these methods are discussed in Schrader (1995). Using the Riva-Rocci method, blood pressure can be registered only discontinuously, which does not allow the detection of single blood pressure peaks and short-term situation-related blood pressure changes (Mallion et al., 1999; Parati, 2000; Seibt & Scheuch, 1999). It is therefore questionable whether this blood pressure variability is a sufficient indicator for the evaluation of the total spectrum of variability.

Since 1982, a continuous arterial finger blood pressure measurement technique has been available (finger blood pressure) with the *Finapres* device (Ohmeda 2300; Englewood, U.S.A). A crucial advantage of the *Finapres* method (Peňáz technique) compared with the traditional Riva-Rocci method is that rapid blood pressure changes can be registered. At the end of the eighties, the new device *Portapres* was developed which for the first time can register long-term blood pressure under everyday conditions continuously (Imholz et al., 1990, 1993, 1998; Langewouters et al., 1993). However, until now neither *Finapres* nor *Portapres* have been widely used in clinical practice, and both systems are insufficiently validated for assessments in occupational physiology (Seibt & Scheuch, 1999).

Objectives

The aim of this study was to examine the validity of discontinuously (brachial blood pressure) and continuously (finger blood pressures) measured 24-hour blood pressure in normotensives and hypertensives. In particular, it should be investigated whether the blood pressure behavior is different between both groups. Advantages and disadvantages of both measurement principles should be critically considered, too.

Since the level and the variability of blood pressure do not only depend on the diurnal dynamic but also on type and intensity of activity, the 24 hour period had to be separated into the following time periods: *work, leisure time, sleep,* and *morning.* These following questions should be cleared:

- whether brachial and finger blood pressure show a similar 'circadian' rhythm,

- whether the postulated wider blood pressure variability in hypertensives could be confirmed,
- whether there are differences between brachial and finger blood pressure concerning level and variability during *work, leisure time, sleep, and morning,*
- whether 'work stress' influences blood pressure during *leisure time* and *sleep* (*carry-over-effect*),
- what relations exist between brachial and finger blood pressure?

Methods

Subjects

In order to recruit well-defined blood pressure groups 20 normotensives and 20 hypertensives were selected from a sample of 51 males (aged 22 to 55 years) according to the results of a 3-day self-measurement of the brachial BP (Seibt et al., 1996). Each group contained 10 younger and 10 older males with mean ages of 27.7 ± 4.7 and 50 ± 5.3 years, respectively. All subjects were right-handed. The group of the younger normotensives consisted of students, all other subjects were members of faculties in scientific institutes. All participants were untreated and showed no signs of hypertension-related organ damages. This was ascertained by medical history and by a clinical classification program (e. g., echo cardiography, duplex sonography, clinical parameters). There were no differences between mean blood pressure (BP) values of the left and the right arm.

There were no age differences between the diagnostic groups (see Table 1). However, the hypertensives showed a significantly ($p = .006$) higher body mass index. Within each group there were no significant blood pressure differences between the younger and the older males. Therefore these age groups were not considered separately in the following.

The self-measurements (6 per day) were taken under resting conditions (device: *Visomat 20*; company: Hestia, Mannheim / Germany). The criterion for the diagnosis of normotension or hypertension was based on the mean values of systolic blood pressure (SBP) and diastolic blood pressure (DBP). Hypertension was diagnosed when the mean value was above 135 mmHg SBP and/or 85 mmHg DBP (Seibt et al., 1996; Mengden et al., 2000). According to this diagnostic criterion, normotensives differed from hypertensives by significantly ($p = .000$) lower SBP and DBP (see Table 1). In sum, both groups can be assumed to be comparable.

Ambulatory 24-hour monitoring

According to the diagnostic criterion of the self-measurement, normotensives differed from hypertensives by significantly higher SBP and DBP Body Mass Index (see Table 1).

In order to assess the impact of the occupational load on the cardiovascular system a 24-hour monitoring was performed during a typical working day. Arterial BP was registered simultaneously at two different parts of the body. The first position was the arteria brachialis of the right upper arm (brachial BP), and the second position was the middle or ring finger of the left hand (finger BP). The subjects were asked to fill in a detailled diary (all quarter hours) with a description of their activities (e. g., physical or mental stress), and to note carefully the times at which they started their work, went to bed and awoke.

Brachial blood pressure

Brachial BP was registered with the automatic long-term measurement device *TM 2420* (company: Bosch + Sohn GmbH, Jungingen / Germany), which works according to the Riva-Rocci auscultatory (sphygmomanometric) technique. The Korotkov sounds are received with a microphone which is placed optimally above the arteria brachialis. In order to omit artifacts (e. g., environmental sounds or muscle contractions) a dual microphone technique was adopted. The measuring interval during the 24 hours was 15 minutes (96 values per day).

Finger blood pressure

Finger BP was registered continuously with the *Portapres 2* (in the following described as *Portapres*) device (company: TNO Biomedical Instrumentation, Amsterdam / The Netherlands), which is a further development of the systems *Portapres 1* and *Finapres*. It is characterized by an automatic height correction and a two finger switching system (Langewouters, 1993). The blood pressure measurement is based on the volume clamp technique of Peñáz et al. (1973) and a physiological calibration (Physiocal system) according to Wesseling et al. (1986, 1995).

Table 1. Characterization of normotensives (n = 20) and hypertensives (n = 20)

Parameter	Normotensive	Hypertensive	t-value	p-value
Age [years]	36.6 ± 13.5	41.7 ± 11.3	t = 1.29	.204
BMI [kg/m²]	23.8 ± 3.0	26.3 ± 2.2	t = 2.94	.006
	Blood pressure self-measurement			
SBP [mmHg]	123.8 ± 5.9	138.9 ± 13.5	t = 4.59	.000
DBP [mmHg]	76.6 ± 6.2	87.7 ± 6.8	t = 5.40	.000

Note: BMI: body mass index; SBP: systolic blood pressure; DBP: diastolic blood pressure

The reliability of the BP measurement depends on the proper size of the finger cuff and its proper fitting. In order to avoid measurement errors due to decreased blood flow and its consequences (for example, numb feeling in the finger tip), the measurement switched between the two fingers every 15 minutes (Langewouters, 1993). After each finger switching, the physiological calibration was performed automatically to observe the finger circulation. The values we used were outside of the calibration interval.

Data analysis

The strain of the cardiovascular system was investigated for the following time periods: *work*, *leisure time*, *sleep*, and *morning*. For these time periods the arithmetic mean values and the standard deviations (as measure of the blood pressure variability) were calculated. The analysis of the finger BP began with the aggregation of the beat-to-beat values for each minute and with the calculation of their standard deviation. In order to compare the measurements of both blood pressure recording techniques, the mean scores and the standard deviations of the minutes were selected when the brachial measurements were carried out.

The 24-hour monitoring began between 7 a.m. and 9 a.m. (before the beginning of the work). While the "Deutsche Liga zur Bekämpfung des Bluthochdrucks" recommends to use standardized day (6 a.m. to 10 p.m.) and night (10 p.m. to 6 a.m.) periods (German Hypertension League, 1995; Krönig, 1993), in our study the real individual *waking* and *sleeping* periods were calculated. The individual evaluation based on the diary and the changes of the cardiovascular data (Seibt et al., 1996; van Ittersum et al., 1995). In addition, the changes of the height correction system were considered.

Definition of time periods: *Work* comprises the time between beginning and finishing of the work at the work place. After leaving the work place, *leisure time* begins, which includes all indoor and outdoor activities. *Sleep* lasts from going to bed till getting up. The time between waking up and the end of the 24-hour measurement (before the beginning of work) is defined as the *morning* period. The *waking* period contains all time periods except for *sleep*. The recovery process of the cardiovascular system after *work* is assessed by means of *leisure time* and *sleep* (*carry-over-effect*).

The most important sources for variability of BP are the diurnal changes associated with the *wake-sleep-cycle*. That's why the dynamics over 24 hours are to be mapped firstly. By using the *waking* versus *sleeping* periods the so called "dippers" and "non-dippers" should be identified by both measurement techniques. According to the diagnostic criteria of the German Hypertension League (1995) "non-dippers" are defined by a reduction from *wake* (initial value: 100 %) to *sleep* of less than 10 % in SBP and 15 % in DBP, respectively, and the remaining subjects are classified as "dippers".

Statistics

The statistical calculations of the data were performed with the program SPSS (version 9.0). Each calculation considered age and body mass index as covariates. The significance level for the statistical tests was $\alpha = 5$ %. The Kolmogoroff-Smirnov-test was performed to test the normality of the distributions. Differences between mean values were tested with t-tests for dependent or independent samples whenever the data were normally distributed and the variances were homogeneous. Changes in the time courses of BP were investigated with multivariate ANOVAs with repeated measurements (saturated model). The statistical relations between different BP scores were calculated with the Pearson-Bravais correlation coefficient. Correlation coefficients were interpreted in the following way: $0 < r \leq 0.2$: very low; $0.2 < r \leq 0.5$: low; $0.5 < r \leq 0.7$: medium; $0.7 < r \leq 0.9$: high; $0.9 < r \leq 1$: very high (Brosius & Brosius, 1995).

Results

Course of brachial and finger blood pressure over 24 hours

Figure 1 shows group mean values of the 24-hour courses for brachial and finger BP in both groups. All scores were synchronized so that the beginning was 8 a.m. (first record). For brachial BP the 15-minute intervals are depicted, while for finger BP the mean values over one minute are shown.

Both, brachial and finger BP decrease over night (more than 20 %) and increase in the *morning* (SBP: $F = 317.76$; $p = .000$; DBP: $F = 181.25$; $p = .000$). In the *waking* periods no systematic blood pressure changes can be obtained (SBP: $F = 3.06$; $p = .060$; DBP: $F = 1.90$; $p = .164$). It is remarkable that sometimes brachial and finger BP behave in different ways.

The circadian change can be found in normotensives and hypertensives, but the level of BP is significantly higher ($F = 17.10$; $p = .000$) in hypertensives. The nocturnal fall of BP is significantly ($t = 2.25$ to 3.24; $p = .037$ to $.004$) lower in brachial than in finger BP (see Table 2). However, there are no significant differences between both groups in the nocturnal fall of BP. Hypertensives only show a trend to have a smaller reduction of finger BP in the night (SBP: 22 %; DBP: 24 %) than normotensives (SBP: 26 %; DBP: 29 %). The relatively flat transitions between *waking* and *sleeping* periods in the evening and in the *morning* are due to different times of going to bed (9:30 p.m. to 1:30 a.m.) and getting up (4:00 a.m. to 9:30 a.m.). The sleeping duration was similar for both groups (normotensives: 7:12 ± 0:52 h; hypertensives: 7:27 ± 0:28 h).

According to the diagnostic criteria of the German Hypertension League (1995), among the hypertensives the number of "non-dippers" is twice as high (40 %) as for normotensives. When the finger BP is considered, only 10 % of the normoten-

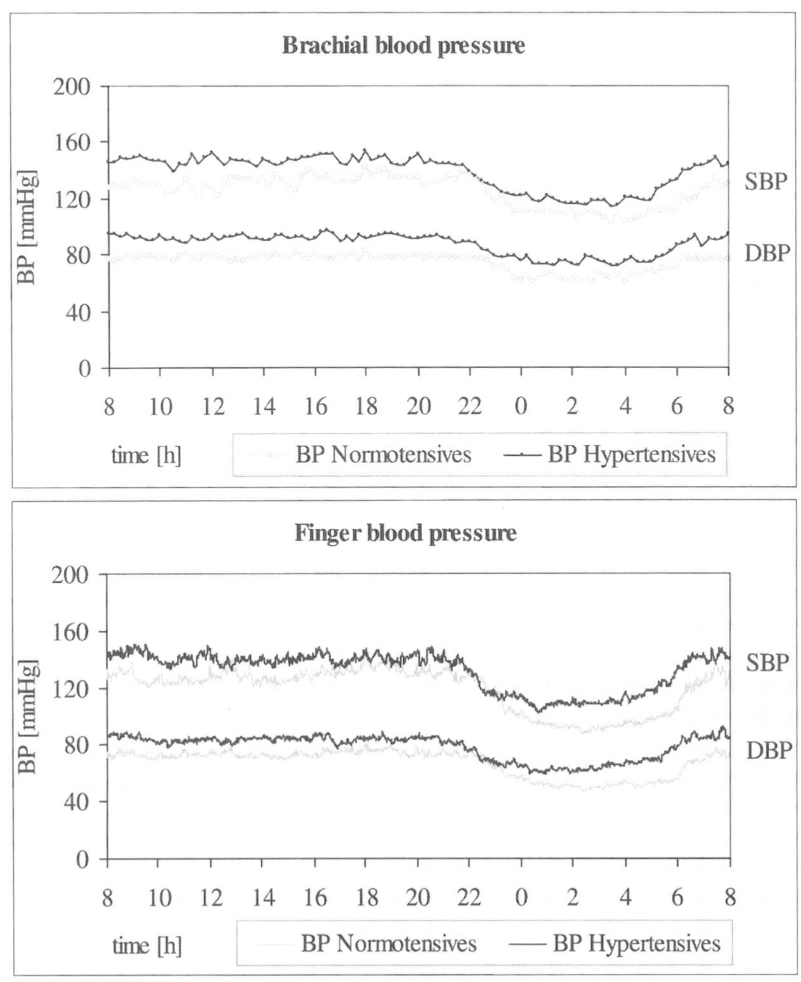

Figure 1. Means of 24-hour courses of brachial and finger systolic (SBP) and diastolic (DBP) blood pressure (BP) in normotensives (n = 20) and hypertensives (n = 20)

Table 2. Nocturnal fall of brachial and finger systolic (SBP) and diastolic (DBP) blood pressure (BP) in normotensives (n = 20) and hypertensives (n = 20) (M and SD)

	Normotensive		Hypertensive	
Method	SBP	DBP	SBP	DBP
Brachial BP [mmHg]	25.3 ± 6.4	15.5 ± 5.3	26.2 ± 7.0	17.0 ± 5.7
Finger BP [mmHg]	33.7 ± 8.2	21.4 ± 6.8	30.6 ± 9.7	20.1 ± 7.4

sives and 5 % of the hypertensives would be characterized as "non-dippers". This indicates differences in the sleep behavior between the groups.

Brachial and finger BP in normotensives and hypertensives

In order to assess the influence of work on the cardiovascular system for normotensives and hypertensives, the behavior of brachial and finger BP during *work, leisure time, sleep, and morning* was compared between the two groups with t-tests for independent samples. Furthermore, these time periods were analyzed separately for each group with t-tests for dependent samples (see Figures 2 and 3).

Mean values

Hypertensives compared to normotensives have significantly higher mean values in the brachial (t = 3.32 to 6.25; p = .002 to .000) and finger (t = 2.16 to 4.91; p = .037 to .000) BP during the four time periods (see Figure 2). The differences are more obvious for the DBP (t = 3.38 to 6.26; p = .002 to .000) than for the SBP (t = 2.16 to 4.66; p = .037 to .000). The group differences are minimal in the finger SBP (t = 2.16 to 3.45; p = .037 to .002) and maximal in the brachial DBP (t = 5.00 to 6.26; p = .000).

During all time periods, the brachial BP is higher than the corresponding finger BP (see Figure 2). In normotensives these differences for the SBP are significant only during *sleep* (t = 6.00; p = .000), while for the DBP significant (t = 2.36 to 5.71; p = .029 to .000) differences were found for *work*, *leisure* time and *sleep*. For these time periods the hypertensive group shows significant differences in SBP (t = 3.31 to 4.39; p = .004 to .000) and in DBP (t = 7.32 to 8.37; p = .000). In the *morning* period there are no significant differences between the mean values of brachial and finger BP in both groups. But, the brachial BP tends towards higher values.

As expected, *sleep* differs from *work*, *leisure time* and *morning* by significantly lower brachial (t = 10.11 to 18.72; p = .000) and finger (t = 10.64 to 18.46; p = .000) BP mean values. This is true for SBP and DBP, and for normotensives as well as for hypertensives. This means that both groups show a distinct sleeping-waking rhythm which can be found not only for brachial but also for finger BP.

Comparing the *waking* periods one with another, there are significantly lower values for *work* than for *leisure time* in the brachial (t = 3.95; p = .001) and finger (t = 2.13; p = .047) SBP in normotensives. There are also no differences in the DBP between *work*, *leisure time* and *morning* for both measurement techniques. Hypertensives, however, show significantly higher means for finger DBP in the *morning* compared with *work* (t = 3.08; p = .006) and *leisure time* (t = 3.24; p = .004), while all other BP mean values do not differ significantly between *work*, *leisure time* and *morning*.

From a diagnostic point of view, the mean values of the normotensives in the brachial SBP during *leisure time* (135 ± 8 mmHg) already touch the hypertensive

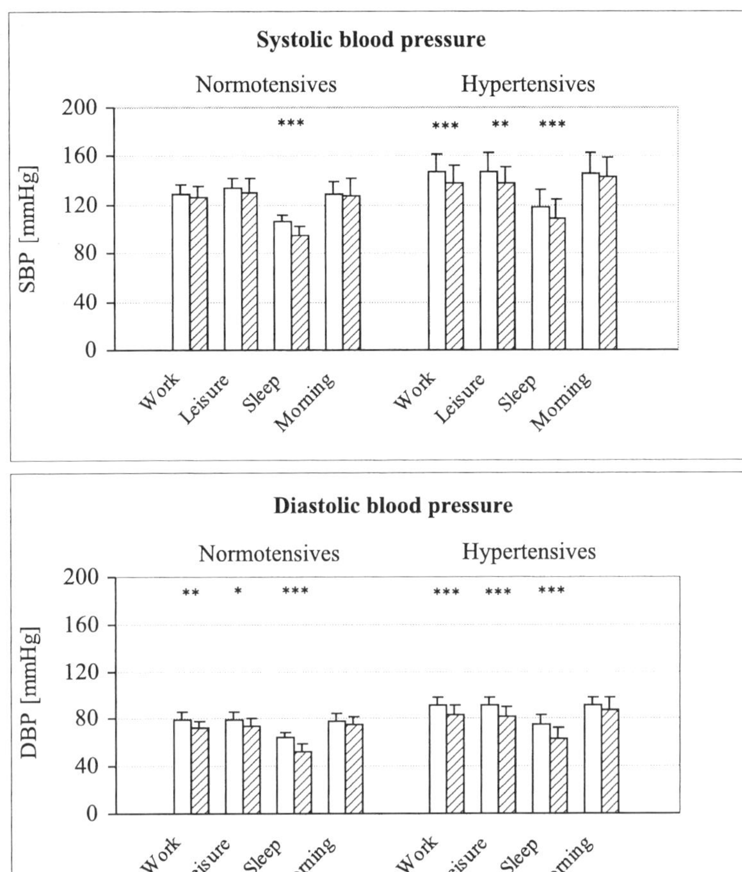

Figure 2. Level of brachial and finger systolic (SBP) and diastolic (DBP) blood pressure (BP) for different time periods in normotensives (n = 20) and hypertensives (n = 20) (M and SD)

range (defined by waking mean: SBP: >135 mmHg; DBP: >85 mmHg). All brachial mean values of the hypertensive group are clearly in the hypertensive range during the *waking* periods (*work*: 147/92 mmHg; *leisure time*: 148/92 mmHg; *morning* 146/91 mmHg). In both groups *work* does not indicate an increased strain of the cardio-vascular system.

Variability

The variability of the data is depicted with mean standard deviations for the four time periods in Figure 3. The hypertensive group shows a slightly higher variability of BP values than the normotensive group. This is especially true for the *sleeping* and

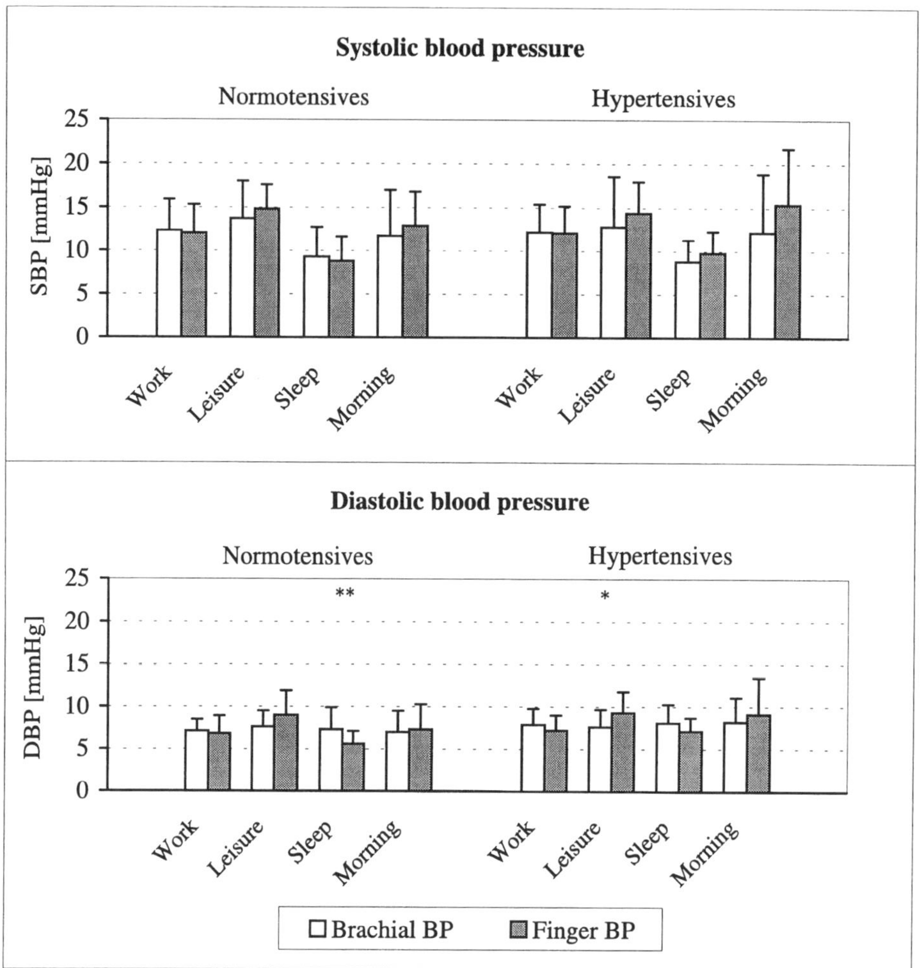

Figure 3. Variability of brachial and finger systolic (SBP) and diastolic (DBP) blood pressure (BP) for different time periods in normotensives (n = 20) and hypertensives (n = 20) (M and SD)

morning periods, independent from the measurement technique. However, this difference is significant ($t = 3.05$; $p = .004$) only for finger DBP during *sleep*.

The mean standard deviations of both BP measurement techniques change from one time period to the next one in a different way, e. g., the variability of brachial BP is not generally lower than that of finger BP. While the standard deviation of the brachial SBP and DBP during the *leisure time* and *morning* is always lower than the corresponding variability of the finger BP, *sleep* shows an opposite trend, which is, however, only significant ($t = 2.86$; $p = .010$) for the DBP in normotensives.

In general, the variability of the SBP (range: 9 to 27 mmHg) is much higher than the variability of the DBP (range: 5 to 19 mmHg). The lowest variability is found for the DBP during *sleep* (normotensives: 5.6 ± 1.5 mmHg; hypertensives: 7.1 ± 1.6

mmHg). Compared with *waking* periods, during *sleep* the brachial (t = 2.22 to 4.02; p = .039 to .001) and finger (t = 3.62 to 7.20; p = .002 to .000) SBP demonstrate a significantly lower variability in both groups. The corresponding comparisons in DBP can only be found for finger BP (t = 2.19 to 4.15; p = .041 to .001).

When only the *waking* periods are compared one with another, there are no significant variability differences in brachial BP. Generally, the brachial DBP shows a relative homogeneous variability (range: 4.8 to 10.8 mmHg). The highest variability is noticed for the finger SBP during *leisure time* in normotensives (14.8 ± 2.8 mmHg) and during *morning* in hypertensives (15.4 ± 6.4 mmHg). Compared with the *work* the *leisure time* variability is higher for finger SBP (normotensives: t = 3.13; p = .006; hypertensives: t = 2.66; p = .015) and DBP (normotensives: t = 2.83; p = .011; hypertensives: t = 3.84; p = .001). But, there are no significant variability differences between the *leisure time* and *morning*. Generally speaking, the variability during *work* indicates a relative homogeneous profile of activity, while for the *leisure time* there is a much wider variability.

Correlations

The relations between brachial and finger BP were investigated with (Pearson-Bravais) correlation coefficients (see Table 3).

Brachial and finger BP behave in different ways under *waking* and *sleeping* condition in normotensives and hypertensives. In the normotensive group the very low correlations (especially those of DBP: r = -.26 to .34) in all time periods indicate that brachial and finger BP are relatively independent from one another. Contrary to the expectations even during *sleep* (SBP: r = .23; DBP: r = -.26) there is no statistical association between the BP recording techniques; only for *leisure time* (r = .53) and *morning* (r = .50) the correlations of the SBP are in an intermediate range. By contrast the hypertensive group shows higher correlations in all time periods for the SBP (r = .63 to .81) and DBP as well (r = .55 to .76).

Table 3. Correlation coefficients between brachial and finger systolic (SBP) and diastolic (DBP) blood pressure in normotensives (n = 20) and hypertensives (n = 20)

	Normotensive		Hypertensive	
Time period	SBP	DBP	SBP	DBP
Work	.19	.25	.79 ***	.71 ***
Leisure time	.53 *	.34	.63 **	.74 ***
Sleep	.23	-.26	.81 ***	.76 ***
Morning	.50 *	.08	.75 ***	.55 *

Note: Significance levels: * p < .05 ** p < .01 *** p < .001.

Discussion

Measurement of brachial and finger blood pressure

One central aim of this study was to test the applicability of continuously recorded BP as a new parameter for long-term investigations in occupational physiology. It should be cleared whether such investigations can be assumed to be representative for typical daily behavior. The subjects were asked not to change their usual behavior during the recording day. However, there are some restrictions due to the special technique. The recording devices make certain activities difficult to perform, and the course of the behavior is interrupted every 15 minutes because of the need to fill in the diary. Some usually performed activities might be omitted at all because every activity had to be written down in the diary. Because of the finger cuffs, the use of the hand connected with the *Portapres* is limited (for example, heavy physical load, rapid movements, driving a car). That means, using the Portapres is rather recommendable in professional groups with predominantly mental stress. Furthermore, the conspicious application of the devices, the disturbing sounds during the night and restrictions concerning personal hygiene might cause an unusual situation for the participants and for their social environment (Jain, 1995; Schmidt et al., 1992).

The individual blood pressure scores were not uniform, especially among the normotensives. In some cases *Portapres* and *TM 2420* yielded very similar values, while in other cases there were great differences, sometimes more than 20 mmHg. Fahrenberg et al. (1997) reported similar findings from a methodological study which was designed to compare *Portapres* data with those obtained from brachial BP within a 2-hour period. Neither finger switching nor influences of the temperature could explain these blood pressure differences. The validity of finger blood pressure is restricted because comparable intraarterial measurings (gold standard) are missing, too. Several authors found a good correspondence between this finger blood pressure and intraarterial blood pressure (Idema et al., 1989; Imholz et al., 1993, 1998; Langewouters et al., 1998; Parati et al., 1989; Staessen et al., 1995). However, recent studies reported higher degrees of systolic blood pressure variability with the *Finapres* method (Omboni et al., 1998; Parati, 2000).

In a 24-hour examination recording conditions cannot be kept constant. Changes of the environmental temperature (e. g., indoor and outdoor temperature) can have an impact on the blood flow in the finger and therefore on the finger BP. The fixing of the finger cuffs and of the height correction system cannot be controlled throughout the 24-hour measurement, which can also cause errors. In this study a good correspondence between the blood pressure values of the two fingers could be achieved in nearly all subjects by multiple switching and repositioning the cuffs at the beginning of the investigation. In some cases there were differences between the blood pressure values of the third and fourth finger which presumably were caused by certain anatomic-morphological properties of the fingers (Meurer et al., 1992; Veerman et al., 1994).

The height correction system (which controls the height difference between finger and heart) can also be assumed as a potential cause for the deviations. Since the fingers which contain the cuffs are outside the hydrostatic interference level (ca. 5 to10 cm below the diaphragm) most of the time, BP is often influenced by a hydrostatic effect. When arm and hand are rapidly moved, hydrostatic pressure differences will probably not be accurately corrected, which can cause an overestimation or underestimation of the BP. The main source of measurement errors, however, lies in muscle contractions and movements of the measured finger.

The reliability of *Portapres* investigations depends on the degree of hand movements, a careful application of the cuffs and optimal blood flow of the fingers (Fahrenberg et al., 1997; Imholz et al., 1993, 1998; Jones et al., 1993; Langewouters et al., 1998; Schmidt et al., 1992). But then again, this cannot be guaranteed under everyday conditions. The blood pressure recording with *TM 2420* is less vulnerable to individual behavior or environmental influences than the *Portapres*. The percentage of measurement errors was about 3 % with the *TM 2420* and 5 % with the *Portapres* (for example, BP values outside the physiological range).

40 % of the people reported that finger blood pressure recording was more uncomfortable than brachial recording. Schmidt et al. (1992) found that about 50 % of the subjects felt to be handicapped by the *Portapres*, especially by the cuffs. In accordance with our results, *sleep* was only marginally disturbed for the majority of the subjects.

In summary it may be said that the reliability of the both blood pressure measuring methods is influenced by different conditions. Primarily, the control of body position and physical activity is necessary (Fahrenberg et al., 1997; Seibt & Scheuch, 1999).

Reliability of brachial and finger blood pressure measurement under everyday conditions

Brachial BP was significantly higher than finger one in both groups and all time periods. For hypertensives this difference (average: 8 mmHg) was about twice as high as for normotensives. Under "ideal conditions", both measurement techniques should yield identical results according to Staessen et al. (1995). The difference found in our study can be caused by different regulatory mechanisms (Seibt et al., 1998a), special anatomic-physiological properties (Meurer et al., 1992; Veerman et al., 1994), and several measuring principles (Bos et al., 1996, Imholz et al., 1998; Scheuch et al. 1998).

It is supposed that the regulatory mechanisms of arterial BP are embedded in a very complex system which includes parts of the central and autonomic nervous system, finger receptors, and neurohumoral factors. From the aorta to the finger arteries, muscular elements of the vessel wall are increasing and elastic elements are decreasing. During early stages of hypertension a media hypertrophy probably occurs which causes an adaptation disturbance of the finger vessels. Already minor diameter changes in the arterioles can evoke great changes in resistance, which change BP (Meurer et al., 1992; Veerman et al., 1994).

Among normotensives there were no prognostically significant correlations between brachial and finger BP, that is, brachial and finger BP are nearly independent under everyday conditions. Among hypertensives, though, there were moderate correlations with an explained variance of about 50 %. This difference between normotensives and hypertensives can have physiological reasons. But, in small samples a low interindividual variability can cause coincidental effects. In the investigations of Jain (1995), activity (accelerometry, EMG) explained about one third of the variability of finger SBP and about one fourth of the variability of finger DBP. Generally speaking, the analyses point out unstable regulatory mechanisms in normotensives, whereas these mechanisms are more stable in the hypertensive group.

Some studies postulate a characteristic biphasic blood pressure profile for 24 hours called "circadian rhythm" (Baumgart & Rahn, 1990; Krönig, 1993; Siegel et al., 1992; Schrader, 1995). The highest values should occur in the first hours after getting up and in the early evening, while the mean values decrease slightly around noon and significantly during night. However, Mancia et al. (1983) concluded that the classic form of the 24-hour "circadian rhythm" does not exist. This is also confirmed by our results. Here, the brachial and finger blood pressure profiles were only characterized by a marked decrease in the night and an increase in the *morning*. This was especially true for diastolic finger blood pressure. Normotensives as well as hypertensives showed these changes, but in hypertensives the general BP level was higher. There were no differences between hypertensives and normotensives regarding to the nocturnal fall. We believe that the endogenously controlled rhythm is overruled by exogenous factors, especially by different physical and mental activities. From this view the reduction of blood pressure during the night is a result from a lower sympathetic nervous system activity (Grassi & Esler, 1999) that appears to be the principal determinant of the nocturnal fall in blood pressure. Several scientists postulate a *carry-over-effect* (Pickering, 1993; Pickering et al., 1991; Rau, 1998; van Egeren, 1992). In our investigation there were no significant differences in the mean values of BP between *work* and *leisure time*. Both time periods are influenced by a lot of different activities. Therefore a *carry-over-effect* during *leisure time* is not provable. The wide variability (especially of finger blood pressure) and the elevated blood pressure mean values during *leisure time* indicate rather a stressful than a recovery period in this case.

More reliable, statements about recovery can be derived from the blood pressure reduction during *sleep*. This decrease can be interpreted as a cardiovascular recovery in comparison to the *waking* period (Seibt et al., 1998a). BP during *sleep* was significantly lower than during *waking* periods. *Sleep* values of brachial BP were clearly in the normotensive range for the normotensive group (limits: 120/70 mmHg), while in the hypertensive group the mean values were in the borderline region (SBP: 118 ± 14 mmHg; DBP: 75 ± 8 mmHg). For finger BP these values were even lower in both groups. The relatively wide range of BP during *sleep* indicates differences in sleep quality, which can vary between normal sleep, mild disturbed sleep and sleep loss. 40 % of the hypertensives have a less than 15 % reduction in brachial blood pressure from *waking* values. However, light sleep disturbances are assumed to have only minor influence on BP (Schrader, 1995). A recent study of Mansoor (2000) in which physical activity was monitored demonstrated greater levels of sleep activity in "non-dippers" than in "dippers".

The variability of BP is influenced by several endogenous (for example, age, level of BP) and exogenous (e. g., posture, physical or mental stress) factors, but also by features of the recording technique and analysis (Krönig, 1993). Blood pressure variability cannot be completely registered by using of the discontinuous measurement. The standard deviation (which is often used as a measure of variability) does not take into account the temporal dependencies of blood pressure changes.

Blood pressure variability was higher in hypertensives than in normotensives, especially in DBP. In both groups brachial blood pressure variability was lower than finger blood pressure variability in *leisure time* and *morning*, while during *sleep* the opposite relationship was true. This result can be influenced by the body position during the *sleep* (for example, compressed arteria brachialis, hydrostatic effects). In our study this variance source was not examined more detailed. Generally, the variability during *sleep* was much lower than during the *waking* period. Here the hypertensive group showed the higher blood pressure variability. In the *waking* period there was no systematic difference. Mancia et al. (1983) reported similar results. The reason for the higher variability in hypertensives might be the lower baroreceptor sensitivity due to a loss of elasticity of the vascular walls. Already among mild hypertensives the different regulatory mechanisms are partially disturbed (Grassi & Esler, 1999). An increased blood pressure variability could indicate premature changes of vessel walls (Asmar et al., 1988; Veerman et al., 1994). Special analyses of brachial and finger blood pressure should help to discover regulatory mechanisms which are involved in maladaptation processes and which contribute to the development of hypertension.

The spectrum of blood pressure variability and the dynamics of BP are reflected better by the minute average values of the beat-to-beat measurement than by the 15-minute measurements. However, the gigantic amount of beat-to-beat data often does not correspond with the relatively rough protocol and the vague statements about the activities. So, the scores obtained by continuous blood pressure measurement often cannot be assigned to the different activities.

Summary and conclusions

Brachial blood pressure (intermittently measured) and finger blood pressure (continuously measured) represent original and specific parameters for the cardiovascular responses to everyday stress. The crucial advantage of both methods lies in the non-invasive, mobile long-term measurement and, therefore, in the applicability for occupational physiological field investigations. However, the blood pressure measurement with *Portapres* under everyday conditions is more subject to disturbances and requires a higher degree of compliance. Therefore in the near future, our main concern should be to clarify the impact of possible sources of error. Until now, we also do not know much about the prognostic relevance of finger blood pressure.

Both measurement techniques reflect the "circadian rhythm" of the blood pressure with sufficient accuracy. Normotensives as well as hypertensives showed a clear decrease of blood pressure in the *sleeping* period, the hypertensives being characterized by a lower reduction, especially in the finger blood pressure. The lack of this rhythm can be a hint for disturbed cardiovascular regulation (e. g., secondary hypertension).

A clear disadvantage of the intermittent measuring techniques is the low temporal accuracy. Compared with finger blood pressure, discontinuous measurement of brachial blood pressure does not permit a sufficient analysis of blood pressure peaks and short-term, situation-specific blood pressure responses (Seibt & Scheuch, 1999). This is also true for blood pressure variability over 24 hours as a whole. In order to evaluate work-related cardiovascular strain responses and the corresponding recovery processes, the discontinuous measurement is economic and expressive. With the beat-to-beat measurement valuable additional statements can be won only by a differentiated analysis with a high temporal resolution. This is of special importance for temporal periods with clinical relevance (for example, blood pressure rise in the morning, sleep apnoe).

The discrepancy between continuously recorded blood pressure values and relatively rough activity protocol information is a limitation of the expressiveness. In order to utilize the many data obtained with continuous measurement, it is necessary to aggregate the data, but this restricts the depiction of the dynamics and the spectrum of blood pressure variability. Nevertheless, hypertensives, compared with normotensives, showed a trend towards a higher variability in both measurement techniques. Moreover, hypertensives had significantly higher mean values in all time periods.

The postulated *carry-over-effect* could not be confirmed. Until now, there is not so much knowledge about the assessment of cardiovascular strain during *work*. A scaled evaluation (scoring system) of the daily total strain in general and of special *work* and *leisure time* activities in particular can help to assess the magnitude of strain more reliably (Rau, 1998; Seibt et al., 1996, 1998b). Here the type and duration of physical activity and emotional strain have to be considered but also beginning and duration of *work* and *sleep*. The additional registration of bodily activity and position could enhance the diagnostic expressiveness (Jain, 1995; Schmidt et al., 1992).

The low number of subjects limits the generalizability of the results obtained in this study. The results should therefore be doublechecked again in further studies. Nevertheless, they may stimulate further research on strain under everyday conditions. Since each technique has specific advantages and disadvantages, it is necessary to choose the appropriate technique for each objective. But, the introduction of new diagnostic technique often raises as many questions as answers.

References

Asmar, R.G., Brunel, P.C., Pannier, B.M., Lacolley, P.J. & Safar, M.E. (1988). Arterial distensibility and ambulatory blood pressure monitoring in essential hypertension. *American Journal of Cardiology*, *61*, 1066–1070.

Baumgart, P. & Rahn, K.H. (1990). Morgendlicher Blutdruckanstieg: vor oder nach dem Aufwachen? *Klinische Wochenschrift*, *68*, 320–323.

Blumenthal, J.A., Thyrum, E.T. & Siegel, W.C. (1995). Contribution of job strain, job status and marital status to laboratory and ambulatory blood pressure in patients with mild hypertension. *Journal of Psychosomatic Research*, *39*,133–144.

Bos, W.J.W., van Goudoever, J., van Montfrans, G.A., van den Meiracker, A.H. & Wesseling, K.H. (1996). Reconstruction of brachial artery pressure from noninvasive finger pressure measurements. *Circulation*, *94*, 1870–1875.

Brosius, G. & Brosius, F. (1995). *SPSS. Base System und Professional Statistics.* Bonn: International Thomson Publishing.

Fahrenberg, J., Herrmann, J., & Lutz, B (1997). *Kontinuierliche Blutdruckmessung am Finger (Portapres 2) im Vergleich zu oszillometrischer (SpaceLabs 90207) und auskultatorischer (Boucke Tensiomat FIB 4/6) Technik.* Forschungsbericht No. 129, Albert-Ludwigs-Universität Freiburg, Psychologisches Institut.

Floras, J.S., Hassan, M.O., van Jones, J., Osikowska, B.A., Sever, P.S. & Sleight, P. (1988). Factors of influencing blood pressure and heart rate variability in hypertensive humans. *Hypertension*, *11*, 273–281.

Frattola, A., Parati, G., Cuspidi, C., Albini, S. & Mancia, G. (1993). Prognostic value of 24-hour blood pressure variability. *Journal of Hypertension*, *11*, 1133–1137.

German Hypertension League (1995). Statement on ambulatory blood pressure monitoring by the German Hypertension League. *Journal of Human Hypertension*, *9*, 777–779.

Gosse, P., Roudant, R., Reynaud, P., Julien, E. & Dallocchio, M. (1989). Relationship between left ventricular mass and noninvasive monitoring of blood pressure. *American Journal of Hypertension*, *2*, 631–633.

Grassi, G. & Esler, M. (1999). How to assess sympathetic activity in humans. *Journal of Hypertension*, *17*, 719–734.

Idema, R.N., van den Meiracker, A.H., Imholz, B.P.M., Man in't Veld, A.J., Settels, J.J., van Eck, H.J.R. & Schalekamp, M.A.D.H. (1989). Comparison of Finapres non-invasive beat-to-beat finger blood pressure with intrabrachial artery pressures during and after bicycle ergometry. *Journal of Hypertension*, *7*, 58–59.

Imholz, B.P.M., Langewouters, G.J., van Montfrans, G.A., Parati, G., van Goudoever, J., Wesseling, K.H., Wieling, W. & Mancia, G. (1993). Feasibility of ambulatory, continuous 24-hour finger arterial pressure recording. *Hypertension*, *21*, 65–73.

Imholz, B.P.M., van Montfrans, G.A., Parati, G., Villani, A., Gropelli, A., Langewouters, G.J., Wesseling, K.H., Mancia, G., Wieling, W. (1990). First experience with Portapres. *Journal of Hypertension, 8* (Suppl. 3), 87.

Imholz, B.P.M., Wieling, W., van Montfrans, G.A. & Wesseling, K.H. (1998). Fifteen years experience with finger arterial pressure monitoring: Assessment of the technology. *Cardiovascular research, 38*, 605–616.

Jain, A., Martens, W.L.J., Mutz, G., Weiß, R.K. & Stephan, E. (1995). Towards a comprehensive technology for recording and analysis of multiple physiological parameters within their behavioral and environmental context. In J. Fahrenberg & M. Myrtek (Eds.), *Ambulatory assessment: computer-assisted psychological and psychophysiological methods in monitoring and field studies.* (pp. 215–235). Seattle: Hogrefe & Huber.

James, G.D.,Cates, E.M., Pickering, T.G. & Laragh, J.H. (1993). Parity and perceived job stress elevate blood pressure in young normotensive working woman. *American Journal of Hypertension, 2*, 637–639.

Johnson, J.V., Stewart, W., Hall, E.M., Fredlund, P. & Theorell, T. (1996). Long-term physiosocial work environment and cardiovascular mortality among swedish men. *American Journal of Public Health, 86*, 324–331.

Jones, R.D.M., Kornberg, J.P., Roulson, C.J., Visram, A.R. & Irwin, M.G. (1993). The Finapres 2300e finger cuff. The influence of cuff application on the accuracy of blood pressure measurement. *Anaesthesia, 48*, 611–615.

Krönig, B. (1993). Blutdruckvariabilität – ein diagnostisches Dilemma. In I.W. Franz (Ed.), *Belastungsblutdruck bei Hochdruckkranken. Diagnostische, prognostische und therapeutische Aspekte.* (pp. 3–14). Berlin: Springer.

Langewouters, G.J. (1993). *Portapres^{TM} Model 2.0. User Manual.* Amsterdam: TNO Biomedical Instrumentation Research Unit.

Langewouters, G.J., Settels, J.J., Roelandt, R. & Wesseling, K.H. (1998). Why use Finapres or Portapres rather than intraarterial or intermittent non-invasive techniques of blood pressure measurement ? *Journal of Medical Engineering & Technology, 22*, 37–43.

Mallion, J.M., Baguet, J.P., Siché, J.P., Tremel, F., de Gaudemaris, R. (1999). Clinical value of ambulatory blood pressure monitoring. *Journal of Hypertension, 17*, 585–595.

Mancia, G., Ferrari, A., Gregorini, L., Parati, G., Pomidossi, G., Bertinieri, G., Grassi, G., Di Rienzo, M., Pedotti, A. & Zanchetti, A. (1983). Blood pressure and heart rate variabilities in normotensive and hypertensive human beings. *Circulation Research, 53*, 96–104.

Mancia, G., Parati, G., Di Rienzo, M. & Zanchetti, A. (1997). Blood pressure variability. In A. Zanchetti & G. Mancia (Eds.), *Handbook of Hypertension. Pathophysiology of Hypertension*, (Vol. 17, pp. 117–169). Amsterdam: Elsevier.

Mansoor, G.A. (1999). Patterns of ambulatory blood pressure monitoring: linkage of data analysis to the diseases process. *Blood pressure monitoring, 4*, 149–154.

Mengden, T., Weisser, B., Uen, S. & Vetter, H. (2000). Blutdruckselbstmessung – gestern, heute, morgen. *Nieren- und Hochdruckkrankheiten, 29*, 263–276.

Meurer, K.A., Saborowski, F. & Hossmann, V. (1992). Kreislauf. In W. Kaufmann & G.W. Löhr (Eds.), Pathophysiologie. *Ein kurzgefasstes Lehrbuch.* (pp. 443–474). Stuttgart: Thieme.

Omboni, S., Parati, G., Castiglioni, P., Di Rienzo, M., Imholz, B.P.M., Langewouters, G.J., Wesseling, K. H. & Mancia G. (1998). Estimation of blood pressure variability from 24-hour ambulatory finger blood pressure. *Hypertension, 32*, 52–58.

Parati, G. (2000). Continuous finger monitoring of blood pressure: advantages, problems and perspectives. *Blood Pressure Monitoring, 5*, 47–49.

Parati, G., Casadei, R., Gropelli, A., Di Rienzo, M. & Mancia, G. (1989). Comparison of finger and intra-arterial blood pressure monitoring at rest and during laboratoring testing. *Hypertension, 13*, 647–655.

Parati, G., Di Rienzo, M., Ulian, L., Santucciu, C., Girard, A., Elghozi, J.L. & Mancia, G. (1998). Clinical relevance of blood pressure variability. *Journal of Hypertension*, 16 (Suppl. 3), 25–33.

Pasqualetti, P., Natali, G., Casale, R. & Colantonio, D. (1990). Epidemiological chronorisk of stroke. *Acta Neurologica Scandinavica*, *81*, 71–74.

Peñáz, J. (1973). Photoelectric measurement of blood pressure, volume and flow in the finger. In R. Albert, W. Vogt & W. Helbig (Eds.), *Digest of the X. International Conference on Medical and Biological Engineering, Dresden*, 104.

Pickering, T.G. (1993). Applications of ambulatory blood pressure monitoring in behavioral medicine. *Annals of Behavioral Medicine*, *15*, 26–32.

Pickering, T.G. (1998). Variability of blood pressure. *Blood Pressure Monitoring*, *3*, 141–145.

Pickering, T.G., Schnall, P.L., Schwartz, J.E. & Pieper, C.F. (1991). Can behavioral factors produce a sustained elevation of blood pressure? Some observations and a hypothesis. *Journal of Hypertension, 9* (Suppl. 8), 566–568.

Rau, R. (1998). Ambulantes psychophysiologisches Monitoring zur Bewertung von Arbeit und Erholung. *Zeitschrift für Arbeits- und Organisationspsychologie*, *42*, 185–196.

Scheuch, K., Berndt, A., Knöpfel, D. & Seibt, R. (1998). Brachialer und peripherer Blutdruck über 24 Stunden – eine vergleichende Studie. *Zeitschrift für Arbeits- und Organisationspsychologie*, *42*, 219–233.

Schmidt, T.F.H. (1992). A new dimension of blood pressure measurement in man: 24-h ambulatory continuous noninvasive recording with Portapres. In T.F.H. Schmidt, B.T. Engel & G. Blümchen (Eds.), *Temporal variations of the cardiovascular system*. (pp. 181–221). Berlin: Springer.

Schnall, P.L. & Landsbergis, P.A. (1994). Job strain and cardiovascular disease. *Annual Review of Public Health*, *15*, 381–411.

Schrader, J. (1995). *Blutdruck-Langzeitmessung*. München: Medikon.

Seibt, R., Boucsein, W. & Scheuch, K. (1998a). Effects of different stress settings on cardiovascular parameters and their relationship to daily life blood pressure in normotensives, borderline hypertensives and hypertensives. *Ergonomics*, *41*, 634–648.

Seibt, R., Naumann, H.J. & Hinz, A. (1996). Bewertungskriterien der Blutdruckselbstmessung und der 24-Stunden-Blutdruckmessung. *Nieren- und Hochdruckkrankheiten*, *25*, 337–340.

Seibt, R., Naumann, H.J., Scheuch, K. & Misterek, M. (1998b). Influence of workload on cardiovascular system in normotensives and hypertensives using the 24-hour ambulatory blood pressure monitoring. *Journal of Psychophysiology*, *12*, 325.

Seibt, R. & Scheuch, K. (1999). Blutdruckmessung und –bewertung in der Arbeitsmedizin. *Arbeitsmedizin Sozialmedizin Umweltmedizin*, *34*, 363–367.

Siegel, D., Black, D.M., Seeley, D.G. & Hulley, S.B. (1992). Circadian variation in ventricular arrhythmias in hypertensive man. *American Journal of Cardiology*, *69*, 344–347.

Siegrist, J., Peter, R., Motz, W. & Strauer, B.E. (1992). The role of hypertension, left ventricular hypertrophy and psychosocial risks in cardiovascular disease: prospective evidence from blue-collar men. *European Heart Journal*, *13* (Suppl. D), 89–95.

Staessen, J.A., Fagard, R., Thijs, L., Amery, A. & the paricipants in the fourth international consensus conference on 24-hour ambulatory blood pressure monitoring. (1995). A consensus view on the technique of ambulatory blood pressure monitoring. *Hypertension*, *26*, 912–918.

Theorell, T., Ahlberg-Hulten, G., Jodko, M., Sigala, F. & de la Torre, B. (1993). Influence of job strain and emotion on blood pressure in female hospital personnel during workhours. *Scandinavian Journal of Work, Environment and Health*, *19*, 313–318.

Van Egeren, L. (1992). The relationship between job strain and blood pressure at work, at home, and during sleep. *Psychosomatic Medicine*, *54*, 337–343.

Van Ittersum, F.J., Ijzerman, R.G., Stehouwer, C.D.A. & Donker, A.J.M. (1995). Analysis of twenty-four-hour ambulatory blood pressure monitoring: what time period to assess blood pressures during waking and sleeping? *Journal of Hypertension*, *13*, 1053–1058.

Veerman, D.P., Imholz, B.P.M., Wieling, W., Karemaker, J.M. & van Montfrans, G.A. (1994). Effects of aging on blood pressure variability in resting conditions. *Hypertension*, *24*, 120–130.

Wesseling, K.H., de Witt, B., van der Hoeven, G.M.A., van Goudoever, J. & Settels, J.J. (1995). Physiocal, calibrating finger vascular physiology for Finapres. *Homeostasis*, *36*, 67–82.

Wesseling, K.H., Settels, J.J., de Wit, B. (1986). The measurement of continuous finger arterial pressure noninvasively in stationary subjects. In T. F. H. Schmidt, T.M. Dembroski, G. Blümchen (Eds.), Biological and psychological factors in cardiovascular disease. (pp. 355-375). Berlin: Springer.

Chapter 19

Respiratory Pathophysiology of Clinical Anxiety Outside the Laboratory: Assessment of End-Tidal pCO_2, Respiratory Pattern Variability, and Transfer Function RSA

Frank H. Wilhelm[1], Georg W. Alpers[1], Alicia E. Meuret[1], and Walton T. Roth[2]
[1]*Department of Psychiatry and Behavioral Sciences, Stanford University,*
[2]*VA Palo Alto Health Care System Palo Alto, CA, USA*

Introduction

Anxiety disorders are common in the general population and often debilitating. The diagnostic criteria, as laid out in the current 4th edition of the Diagnostic and Statistical Manual for Mental Disorders (DSM-IV)(American Psychiatric Association, 1994), include various symptoms that indicate autonomic or respiratory dysregulation. One line of anxiety research is engaged in finding physiological correlates of patient self-reports of physical symptoms that could either help in understanding the mechanisms involved in the disorder or aid in the diagnostic decision process.

In this chapter we will describe new methods of ambulatory physiological monitoring that can help detect activation disturbances concomitant with anxiety. Ambulatory monitoring is an important, expanding new technological development that up till now has been applied mainly to cardiovascular problems (electrocardiographic and blood pressure abnormalities) and epilepsy. The time is ripe for psychiatry to also benefit from this method. We envision a time when new patients complaining of anxiety and stress will routinely be monitored to complement their self-report in determining the severity and nature of their symptoms and what treatment is appropriate, and then will be monitored again during and after treatment to complement self-report data in evaluating its success. In the future, success of treatments could also be judged in terms of their ability to reverse abnormal physiological patterns.

We think that ambulatory assessment is important and can complement laboratory studies of anxiety for two main reasons: First, it allows assessment of anxiety when and where it happens. Panic attacks, which can occur in panic disorder (PD), social phobia, or specific phobia, often take place in situations that are not easily reproducible inside a laboratory. In addition, they sometimes happen unexpectedly, seemingly "out of the blue", and the limited laboratory window of observation may easily miss such attacks. Furthermore, the most widely used behavioral treatment of anxiety is exposure to anxiety provoking stimuli and situations, which is often conducted outside the laboratory. For example, height phobia is typically treated by asking patients to remain on top of a high building until the anxiety starts to subside. Agoraphobia is treated by helping patients to expose themselves to many situations, such as elevators, shopping malls, or riding on a train. Ambulatory assessment methodologies can help evaluate experiential and physiological changes during this kind of therapy. Second, ambulatory assessment allows to estimate to what extent abnormalities represent a "state" anxiety effect or a persisting "trait" characteristic of anxiety patients. In other words, ambulatory measurement outside the laboratory can help determine to what extent a physiological characteristic is a trait feature persisting over 24 hours, or a shorter-term state induced by the laboratory or testing situation itself. Patients with anxiety disorders are often particularly anxious in the laboratory, and as a consequence, a supposed laboratory baseline hardly represents a basal state. Laboratory baseline assessment is influenced by at least three acute factors: what went on before it (clinical tests, challenge procedures), the conditions of the baseline measurements (such as the invasiveness of the measurement apparatus, the confining quality of the testing room), and what the subject anticipates will happen after it.

Of course, laboratory studies still must be an integral part of comprehensive anxiety research since they allow tight control and experimental variation of stimulus conditions. Many recent studies of our group have been conducted in the laboratory: CO_2 inhalation (Roth et al., 1992), repeated breath holding (Roth et al., 1998b), prolonged quiet sitting (Wilhelm et al., in press-c; Wilhelm et al., in press-d), hyperventilation (Wilhelm et al., in press-a), giving a speech in front of others (Gerlach et al., in press; Hofmann et al., 1995), being touched (Wilhelm et al., 2000a), and approaching a phobic stimulus (Roth et al., 1994). But we also have been long aware of the shortcomings of an exclusive focus on laboratory studies and have complemented with studies in ambulatory situations: flying in an airplane (Wilhelm & Roth, 1998a), driving a car on the freeway or over bridges (Alpers & Wilhelm, 2000), walking through a shopping mall (Whittal et al., 1996), and 24-hr monitoring (Margraf et al., 1987; Wilhelm et al., 2000c).

How ambulatory studies have profoundly changed the way we think about PD today were outlined in our previous chapter in this book series (Wilhelm & Roth, 1996). The first part of the chapter focussed on the empirical data on ambulatory PD assessment. We concluded that panic attacks are usually of only moderate intensity (at least as measured by heart rate changes), hyperventilation plays only a small role in the symptomatology of panic attacks (based on transcutaneous pCO_2 monitoring studies), and cognitions contribute to the severity of attacks. Here we will provide an update of these conclusions based on results from our recent studies. In the previous chapter we outlined some principal methodological complications in ambulatory anxiety research and presented a recent study of flying phobics to highlight our advances. These included long-term recording of electrodermal activity and calibrated respiration, development of computer programs to eliminate artifacts in these channels, control for speech activation, and the development and application of a new method to derive additional heart rate in the field (Wilhelm & Roth, 1998c). In the current book chapter we will describe some of our recent advancements in ambulatory methodology by describing how we measure several physiological parameters that have not been measured outside the laboratory in freely moving subjects for extended periods before. Here we will outline a new approach for establishing standardized baselines in unsupervised subjects outside the laboratory and other strategies for dealing with factors interfering with ambulatory assessment. This will be followed by the presentation of the protocols and preliminary data from two ongoing ambulatory projects examining psychophysiological changes in driving phobia during exposure treatment and in PD during 24–hr assessment.

Methodological Innovations

Novel Physiological Measures Outside the Laboratory

Our current focus in research with anxiety disorder patients is the respiratory system. Abnormalities in respiration have been postulated as central in anxiety disorders for several decades. The "hyperventilation syndrome" was believed to lie at the root of a variety of "psychosomatic" complaints and mood disturbances, and since the establishment of PD as a diagnostic category, episodes of hyperventilation have been particularly associated with panic attacks (Ley, 1985). A hypothesis of cognitive-behavioral theory has been that small increases in anxiety initiate hyperventilation and result in hypocapnea (decreased pCO_2) with its attendant symptoms, and that perception of those symptoms causes anxiety and hypocapnea to spiral upward in a positive feedback loop. On the other hand, the suffocation false alarm hypothesis (Klein, 1992) considers PD patients to be particularly sensitive to hypercapnea (increased pCO_2), and to react to it secondarily with acute or subacute hyperventilation, which lowers pCO_2 below levels that will trigger an alarm. To evaluate the empirical basis for the different theories about respiratory abnormalities in anxious patients, we have extended measurements that only used to be made within the laboratory into ambulatory settings. We will present two novel ambulatory respiratory measures here: end-tidal pCO_2 and respiratory pattern variability. In addition, we will present a novel approach to measure changes in cardiac vagal control in the field, because respiratory influences play an important role in this assessment.

Ambulatory recording is rare for the measurement of respiratory variables in anxiety. A notable exception is a 24-hr ambulatory study from the Columbia group (Martinez et al., 1996) using a portable respiratory monitor. Tidal volume averaged for 2-min periods showed larger variability in PD patients than in matched controls. Unfortunately, the monitor did not allow recording and analysis of breath-by-breath values. Tidal volume, rather than respiratory rate increases characterized the periods of anxiety and limited symptom attacks. These results indicate that PD patients experience large fluctuations in anxiety during everyday life that are accompanied by changes in tidal volume over periods of minutes.

End-tidal PCO2

Shortness of breath is a common complaint among anxious patients and it ranks high among symptoms reported during panic attacks. In view of the fact that voluntary hyperventilation can lead to a pattern of physical and psychological symptoms in healthy individuals resembling anxiety symptoms, it has been hypothesized that hyperventilation plays a major role in the symptomatology of PD (Ley, 1985). Since end-tidal pCO_2 is the hallmark of hyperventilation it has received special attention in research.

The respiratory system functions basically to supply oxygen (O_2) to the organs of the body to use in combustion of fuel and to rid the body of the "waste product" gas, carbon dioxide (CO_2), resulting from this metabolism. CO_2 plays a crucial role in maintaining the acid-base balance within the internal milieu of the body. Hyperventilation, defined as" breathing in excess of metabolic requirements" (Gardner, 1994), can occur dramatically and acutely with deep or fast breathing, or as the result of more subtle perturbation of normal breathing such as sighing. Hyperventilation lowers blood pCO_2 making blood pH slightly more alkalotic and causing a leftward shift in the oxygen-hemoglobin dissociation curve. Fried (1987) believes that this shift, combined with the constriction of the cerebral arteries produced by alkalosis, can impair O_2 delivery to the brain to the extent that its function in some regions is compromised by the resulting hypoxia. Other effects of alkalosis are to increase intracellular calcium, sympathetic neuronal catecholamines, coronary artery tone, peripheral resistance, and cardiac arrhythmias, and to decrease extracellular calcium and potassium, which affect neuronal excitability (Gilbert, 1999). These multiple, diverse effects have raised suspicion that hyperventilation is a mediator of many clinical symptoms accompanying acute anxiety or panic.

The human body has evolved several redundant systems to limit an increase in arterial pCO_2. When CO_2 builds above the normal setpoint – for example, as a result of physical exercise or of attenuated ventilation – chemoreceptors located in the arteries (aorta, carotis) and brain stem powerfully stimulate ventilation, thus reducing pCO_2 swiftly. On the other hand, when pCO_2 falls below the normal set-point, the resulting reduction in stimulation of chemoreceptors has only mild effects on a reduction of ventilation, and pCO_2 normalizes relatively slowly. Under some circumstances, for example, during extended stress or anxiety states, pCO_2 may not normalize for a long time. A typical normal level for arterial pCO_2 in healthy individuals during rest is 40 mm Hg. Inter-individual variations at baseline of ± 4 mm Hg are considered typical. The pCO_2 threshold for onset of perceptible symptoms due to overbreathing is about 20 mm Hg (Rafferty et al., 1992), but physiological regulation processes may be disturbed by less acute reductions in pCO_2. Arterial pCO_2 is difficult to measure, but it can be approximated quite accurately by end-tidal pCO_2, which is the level of pCO_2 reached at the end of a normal expiration. At this point in time, the expired gas mixture contains air from the depth of the lungs that participated in alveolar gas exchange.

PCO_2 is measured by a capnometer (also called capnograph) using gas infrared spectroscopy. A sample of expired air from the nose or mouth is continously sucked into the device by a pump, dehumidified, and analyzed for its CO_2 content (which is computed from the peak in the CO_2 dispersion spectrum). End-tidal CO_2 is the partial pressure of carbon dioxide measured in the expired air at the end of each expiration, when the CO_2 level reaches a plateau. This value is close to alveolar and arterial levels of pCO_2. Since barometric pressure and temperature can affect the measurement, many capnographs self-calibrate for these environmental changes.

Recently a small portable capnometer, the Capnocount® mini (size = 6.5 x 12.8 x 3.5 cm, weight = 320 g, Figure 1) was developed by Weinmann Co., Germany, for use in patient monitoring in emergency medicine applications outside the hospital (measurement of respiration rate and pCO_2 during intubation, reanimation, and transport). The device measures end-tidal pCO_2 and respiratory rate, and values are updated breath-by-breath on an LCD display. The accuracy of the device's measurements corresponds to the quality standards of stationary hospital equipment. It automatically recalibrates pCO_2 measurement to changing temperature and pressure. The pump flow rate can be switched between 50, 100, and 150 ml/min. At the lowest flow rate, the device produces a barely audible humming sound.

The device runs for up to 3 hr with an internal rechargeable battery (7.2 V) and can store end-tidal pCO_2 and respiratory rate every 2 sec for up to 8 hr. We use this unmodified version in a treatment study for panic patients (see section "24-hr Monitoring in panic disorder" below). Patients take the device and two charged batteries home to conduct breathing exercises twice daily for about 20 min, utilizing the pCO_2 and respiratory rate feedback from the device. The stored data from the practice sessions are downloaded to a PC at a base station when the patient returns a week later.

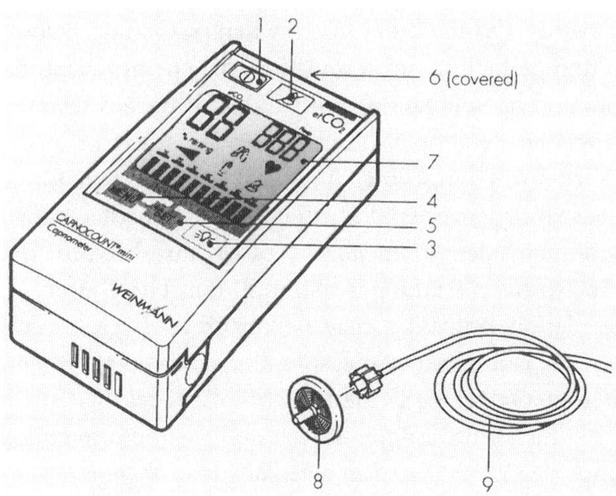

Figure 1. Portable capnometer (expired pCO_2 measurement device). Descriptors: 1 = on/off switch; 2 = alarm mute button; 3 = light switch; 4 = menu selection key; 5 = menu setting key; 6 = input for gas sampling; 7 = LCD display for pCO_2, respiratory rate, and device status; 8 = water filter; 9 = sampling tube.

We employ a custom-made modification of the device for our ambulatory research projects. The raw pCO_2 waveform is output as a digital signal, registered by the serial port input of the Vitaport 2 device, and recorded continuously with a sample rate of 25 Hz. This allows a full disclosure analysis of end-tidal pCO_2 data using our customized software described below. Given the complexities of distortions to end-tidal plateaus, reliance on online detection algorithms did not appear sufficient for research applications. The voltage for operating the device continuously for periods up to 25 hr is supplied by an external commercially available camcorder type battery (Lithium-Ion, 7.2 V, 5400 mAh).

A typical pCO_2 waveform sampled from the nostrils is depicted in Figure 2. An adequate quantification of end-tidal levels has to make sure that pCO_2 reaches a plateau. End-tidal pCO_2, which is close to alveolar and arterial values, is determined as the levels at which pCO_2 stops rising at the end of expirations. In the first phases of expiration, air from the lungs is mixed with air in anatomical dead spaces. Expirations with a low percentage of alveolar air can be recognized by the fact that the pCO_2 waveform does not reach a nearly horizontal plateau, but rather increases steeply and then breaks off suddenly (Bass & Gardner, 1985). Thus, only breaths in which pCO_2 waveforms reach a distinct plateau can be considered valid measurements of end-tidal, and therefore arterial, levels.

We (FW) have developed software for the supervised automated analysis of the expired pCO_2 waveform. The program loads the pCO_2 channel data, performs low-

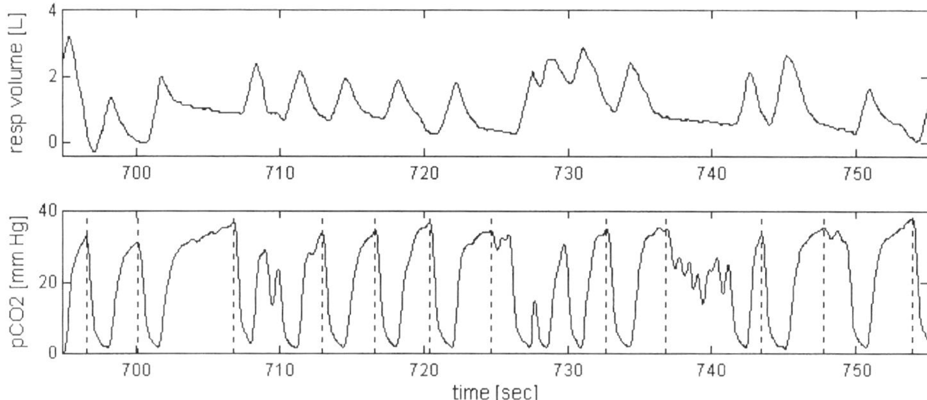

Figure 2. Software for the analysis of expired pCO_2 waveforms. One-minute display during editing of the expired pCO_2 channel (lower graph). Qualifying end-tidal pCO2 plateaus are marked. The upper graph depicts respiratory volume change (in liters).

pass filtering, and searches for local minima and maxima that fulfill certain criteria. The criterion for a valid end-tidal pCO_2 measurement is a steady slope of not more than 12 mm Hg/sec during the 0.25 sec before an end-expiratory peak. We require valid plateaus to be present in 50% of breaths in a measuring epoch for it to be considered. The program displays 1-min segments of pCO_2 data with lines indicating end-tidal plateaus, and their value in mm Hg. The operator can reset or exclude certain plateau markers with a few mouse clicks. The calibrated respiration channel (lung volume change in liters) is displayed in parallel to aid in deciding if an outlier plateau is due to measurement artifact or unusual respiratory behavior, for example, sighing or suspended breathing. This additional information has proven invaluable for accurate analysis of expired pCO_2 data. It also helps in identifying incomplete exhalations with a low percentage of alveolar air, which are indicated by lower than normal depth of breathing. Occlusion of nostrils and/or mouth breathing is a problem that sometimes occurs, especially during periods of speaking and during sleep. To assure adequate sampling even if one nostril is completely occluded, we use dual prong sample cannulas with one opening for each nostril. Tests in our laboratory have shown that even very small amounts of expired air reaching at least one nostril are sufficient to measure end-tidal pCO_2 accurately. Thus, even during periods of vocalization when most air is exhaled through the mouth typically a high percentage of exhalations can be scored for measurement of end-tidal pCO_2.

PCO_2 is unique among physiological activation measures in that exercise and emotional activation do not change it in the same way. Exercise typically does not change pCO_2 appreciably because the increased production of CO_2 by muscle metabolism is compensated for by increased ventilation even at exercise onset (as a result of corollary discharge), while intense anxiety accompanied by hyperventilation decreases pCO_2 by up to 20 mm Hg. Thus, decreases in pCO_2 during an experiment can be interpreted straightforwardly as being a result of increased ventilation accompanying emotional activation. In contrast, parameters like heart rate, skin conductance, blood pressure, respiratory rate, or tidal volume typically increase both during exercise and emotional activation, which necessitates the independent measurement of physical activity levels using accelerometry to allow unambiguous interpretation.

The empirical database regarding pCO_2 in PD patients measured in the laboratory is sizeable. Studies were largely stimulated by theories relating hyperventilation to anxiety (Clark, 1986; Klein, 1992; Ley, 1985). When examined at rest, end-tidal pCO_2 has often been noted to be lower in PD patients than in controls (for example, Hegel & Ferguson, 1997; Papp et al., 1997). Rapee (1986) found that during a rest period before hyperventilation, PD patients had lower pCO_2s and higher heart rates than patients with generalized anxiety disorder (GAD). Munjack, Brown, et al. (1993) reported that venous pCO_2 at rest (without the prospect of any stressor such as hyperventilation) was lower in PD patients than GAD patients, and that in GAD patients pCO_2 was lower than in controls. One of our recent analyses (Wilhelm et al., in press-d) confirmed that quietly sitting PD patients had lower pCO_2 than either GAD patients or controls. In another study both PD and other anxious patients at rest had lower pCO_2s than controls, and the anxious groups did not differ from each other (van den Hout et al., 1992). On the other hand, a number of studies have failed to find pCO_2 differences between PD patient and controls (Holt & Andrews, 1998; Woods et al., 1986).

Only few studies have measured pCO_2 in anxious patients outside the laboratory. This was done by using transcutaneous pCO_2 measurement, which is an alternative to capnometry for estimating arterial pCO_2 levels (Garssen et al., 1994). Like capnometry, this method has been validated to reproduce arterial levels accurately. Typically, the sensor is placed on the skin of the forearm. One part of the sensor heats the skin to about 41° Celsius to stimulate evaporation of CO_2 molecules from the blood through the skin. Another part of the sensor is a selective membrane that allows CO_2 molecules to pass through, and the concentration of the gas is then determined within the sensor. Since the diffusion process is slow, changes in arterial pCO_2 are registered with a delay of about 2 min, and sharp changes are blunted or entirely filtered out (Hoffmann et al., 1990). Using this method, pCO_2 was monitored ambulatorily in patients with PD in three studies. Results showed that by far not all naturally occurring panic attacks were accompanied by hyperventilation: 3 out of 5 (Hibbert & Pilsbury, 1988), 7 out of 15 (Hibbert & Pilsbury, 1989), or 1 out of 24 (Garssen et al., 1996). The vastly differing results between studies cast some doubt on the reliability of the measurement. Our own experimentation with this method has shown certain unreliabilities and difficulties in calibration, and we ultimately abandoned this approach. Our preliminary data using ambulatory capnometry indicate large changes during exposure to driving in driving phobics and fluctuations of pCO_2 levels during day and night in panic patients, even when they do not report panic attacks (see Recent Studies section below).

Respiratory Pattern Variability Analysis by Complex Demodulation

Variable respiration has been observed by clinicians in anxious patients for a long time. In early spirograms of psychiatric patients, "psychoneurotic" patients were observed to sigh frequently (Finesinger, 1943). Thus, although tidal volume and respiratory rate (and minute volume, their product) have not been as consistently indicative of respiratory abnormalities in anxiety states as has pCO_2, the variability of tidal volume and respiratory rate have been found to be abnormal in anxious subjects (Abelson et al., in press; Martinez et al., 1996; Papp, 1995; Stein et al., 1995).

For the quantification of breath-to-breath within-subject variability, the most commonly used measures have been the standard deviation or the root mean square successive difference statistic (rMSSD) for breath-by-breath tidal volume and total cycle time series. We use complex demodulation to quantify respiratory variability. This nonlinear time-domain method of time series analysis was developed for quantifying nonstationary oscillations in defined frequency ranges (Bloomfield, 1976). To understand the advantages of complex demodulation, let us consider a variable like tidal volume. The standard deviation or the coefficient of variation (standard deviation divided by the mean) of a sequence of consecutive tidal volumes does not distinguish between the contribution of slow changes over the entire time window and faster changes that might occur, say, between consecutive volumes. A measure like the rMSSD statistic depends only on consecutive volumes and thus indexes only these faster changes. However, "faster" is imprecisely specified since the unit of measurement is a discrete event (a single respiratory cycle) whose time scale depends on the respiration rate in the time window being analyzed. Complex demodulation of tidal volumes that have been expressed as an equidistant time series (using spline interpolation and resampling), on the other hand, is able to quantify stability in defined frequency bands independent of variability in event frequency. Furthermore, complex demodulation in such a time series can be applied in a parallel fashion both to discrete variables such as tidal volume and to continuous variables such as skin conductance level. Finally, unlike spectral analysis, complex demodulation is effective in characterizing nonstationary variability that drifts in frequency and amplitude or occurs in bursts (Hayano et al., 1994; Wilhelm et al., 1997). Another advantage that makes complex demodulation our analysis of choice for ambulatory data is that it provides continuous values for the entire recording with the same time resolution as the variable it is based on. Thus, averages for different period lengths and segments can easily be recomputed.

The methodology for measurement of calibrated respiration (for example, tidal volume, minute ventilation, and inspiratory flow rate) has been described in detail in our previous chapter in this book series (Wilhelm & Roth, 1996). In our current studies, instead of the ambulatory Respitrace™ device we use the inductive plethysmography circuits integrated into the "polysomnography module" of the Vitaport 2 (Becker Meditec, Germany) to measure thoracic and abdominal breathing activity. For the assessment of breath-to-breath within-subject variability, tidal volume and instantaneous respiratory rate values for each breath are converted into equidistant time series using cubic spline interpolation and resampling at 4 Hz. Then, complex demodulation is applied to these time series, with a bandpass of 0.004-0.14 Hz (corresponding to period lengths of 6.6–240 sec) and a transition band width of 0.033 Hz. Our recent studies assessing respiratory variability in anxious patients using complex demodulation indicate abnormally high tidal volume variability in PD patients during quiet sitting (Wilhelm et al., in press-c; Wilhelm et al., in press-d) and during recovery from hyperventilation (Wilhelm et al., in press-a).

Transfer Function Assessment of Respiratory Sinus Arrhythmia

Symptoms of anxiety suggest autonomic dysfunction, and many psychotropic agents used to treat anxiety and affective disorders have strong autonomic effects. Autonomic dysregulation also has been implicated in the increased cardiovascular morbidity in these disorders (Barefoot et al., 1996; Kawachi et al., 1995). One type of autonomic variable often examined in clinical research is cardiac vagal tone, indexed by parameters of heart-rate variability (Friedman & Thayer, 1998). Specifically measures of respiratory sinus arrhythmia (RSA) that quantify oscillations in heart rate or heart period (HP) accompanying respiration have been employed. The basal (tonic) vagal firing rate of the cardiac vagal motor neurons located at the Nucleus Ambiguus (vagal tone) is modulated with a respiratory-related phasic signal by the output of the central respiratory generator. As a result, the tonic HP is periodically shortened during inspiration when phasic vagal firing is attenuated. The magnitude of this phasic modulation of vagal firing is related to tonic vagal firing, and thus allows estimation of vagal tone.

Quantifications of respiratory HP oscillations include peak-to-trough measurement of HP concurrent with respiratory cycle (Grossman et al., 1990a), computation of variance in HP after polynomial filtering (Porges & Byrne, 1992), and computation of spectral power of HP variability in the frequency band associated with respiration (Womack, 1971). These and other "classical" RSA measures are variations of mathematical transformations of HP variability and have been shown to be essentially equivalent (Grossman et al., 1990b). The validity of RSA as a measure of vagal control has been established pharmacologically and by physical manipulations (Porges et al., 1982). Reductions in RSA have been reported in patients with GAD

(Thayer et al., 1996) and a trend for vagal reduction was found in PD (Yeragani et al., 1993). In a sample of undiagnosed volunteers trait anxiety was associated with a reduction in vagal control (Watkins et al., 1998).

In spite of its widespread use, quantification and interpretation of cardiac vagal control remains a complex issue fraught with pitfalls (Grossman, 1992; Jennings & McKnight, 1994). Several researchers (Grossman et al., 1991; Kollai & Mizsei, 1990; Saul et al., 1991) have noted problems in the use of classical RSA measures for estimating vagal control since they neglect respiratory confounds. Since RSA is caused largely by reductions in vagal outflow to the sino-atrial node during inspiration, the amount of RSA is proportional to the depth of inspirations. Thus, deeper breathing induces larger HP oscillations without any underlying change in tonic vagal outflow to the heart (which is indicated by tonic heart rate not changing). In addition, respiratory rate decrease can also increase RSA without underlying changes in tonic vagal outflow to the heart. This is due to the low-pass filter characteristics of the vagal-to-cardiac nerve transmission (Saul et al., 1991).

Theoretically, the best way to avoid respiratory rate and tidal volume confounds when attempting to measure cardiac vagal control under changing stimulus conditions that are known to induce respiratory changes would be to hold respiratory rate and tidal volume constant, which is nearly impossible even by using a ventilator. More practical is the use of paced breathing procedures for controlling respiratory rate (Grossman et al., 1990a; Wilhelm et al., 1998), or, if this is not possible, by calibrating RSA for changes in respiratory rate using a 3-step paced breathing procedure (described below) and adjusting RSA values post-hoc. The confounding influence of tidal volume on cardiac vagal control assessment can be reduced by dividing RSA values by tidal volume (since their relationship is close to linear), or better, by using transfer function analysis relating lung volume changes to HP oscillations.

Our own latest analyses support the usefulness of RSA when corrected for the confounding factors respiratory rate and tidal volume (Wilhelm et al., 2000b; Wilhelm & Roth, 1997; Wilhelm & Roth, 1998a). In the analysis of a recent study, quietly sitting PD patients had lower RSA (adjusted for respiration) than controls; GAD patients were intermediate (Wilhelm et al., 1999b). RSA was also reduced in a previous study of patients with a diagnosis of flight phobia while they reported high anxiety levels during a flight (Wilhelm & Roth, 1998a).

Transfer function RSA is computed by using a computer program written in MATLAB (Wilhelm et al., 1999a) which was customized for ambulatory data. Raw signals of the two respiratory bands are converted to lung volume change using regression weights derived from fixed volume bag calibrations, and resampled to 4 Hz. The beat-by-beat values of HP are edited for outliers due to artifacts or ectopic myocardial activity (any spikes in signals can distort the spectral analyses), linearly interpolated, and converted into instantaneous time series with a resolution of 4 Hz.

RSA values are then calculated for specified epochs of the ambulatory data (typically for consecutive 5-min epochs). Using transfer function analysis, RSA is estimated as the magnitude of the transfer function relating heart period oscillations to lung volume oscillations at the peak respiratory frequency.

The computation procedure for this is as follows: HP and lung volume (LV) time series are first linearly detrended, and the power spectral densities (P_{HP} and P_{LV}) are derived for each period using the Welch algorithm (Welch, 1967), which ensemble averages successive periodograms. Averages are derived from spectra estimated for 60-sec data segments, overlapping by half. For each 60-sec segment, 256 points are analyzed, which includes 240 sampled points with zero padding. The segments are Hanning windowed and subjected to Fast Fourier transform. Estimates of power are adjusted to account for attenuation produced by the Hanning window. The products of the segments of P_{LV} and P_{HP} are averaged to form $P_{LV,HP}$, the cross spectral density of P_{LV} and P_{HP}. The transfer function $T_{LV,\,HP}$ is computed as the quotient of $P_{LV,HP}$ and P_{LV}. Transfer function RSA is the value of $T_{LV,\,HP}$ at the respiratory frequency. The respiratory frequency is identified as the greatest local maximum in the 0.13-0.50 Hz lung volume power spectral density function (corresponding to a range of respiratory rates from 7.8 to 30 breaths/min). Spectral coherence at this frequency is required to be at least 0.5 (this makes sure that measured HP oscillations are truly due to respiratory sources and not due to ectopic beats or other non-RSA variation within the respiratory frequency range, an often neglected criteria). For comparison, the conventional RSA measure, high frequency power of heart period, is computed by summing P_{HP} values over the frequency band associated with respiration (0.13-0.50 Hz), and resulting values are transformed using the natural logarithm. (Note: often the lower limit of the respiratory frequency band is set to 0.15. However, our data indicates that a significant proportion of subjects at certain times have respiratory rates smaller than 9 breaths/min.)

Both estimates of RSA can be adjusted for the confounding effect of within-subject/between-task variation in respiratory rate (Grossman et al., 1991). This is achieved by a paced breathing RSA calibration task: Subjects hear a tape recording of tones with increasing and decreasing pitch modulated sinusoidally at 9, 12, and 15 cycles/min with a duration of 2 min for each pace. They are instructed to breathe in as the pitch rises and out as it falls. For each individual, regression coefficients relating respiratory rate to transfer function RSA values are computed. We have used this procedure successfully for adjusting RSA values during spontaneous breathing for the confounding effect of changes in respiratory rate (Wilhelm et al., 1998). This procedure will remove error variance and enhance the sensitivity of the RSA measure to indicate parasympathetic activation differences within and between individuals. Subjects are to maintain the baseline pCO_2 level (displayed by the capnometer), since reductions in arterial pCO_2 (and central respiratory drive) can lead to reductions in RSA (Al-Ani et al., 1996). Reductions in pCO_2 levels are likely with paced breathing at a rate greater than 15 breaths/min if no feedback about pCO_2 levels is provided.

Controlled Assessment Outside the Laboratory

Most 24-hr monitoring studies attempt to measure representative physiological changes (for example, heart rate, heart rate variability, blood pressure) during normal daily activities of individuals. Unfortunately, wearing a monitoring device provides individuals with anxiety disorder an additional excuse to avoid anxiety producing activities. Thus, patient reports indicate that daily routines are often altered during 24-hr assessment periods as compared to control periods without full assessment (Margraf et al., 1987). Agoraphobics avoid leaving their houses, and social phobics do not want to be seen in public wearing something unusual that would draw attention to them. Another problem in 24-hr assessment is the disturbance of physiological recording by physical activity, such as walking. First, physical activity can cause measurement artifacts. Second, physical activity causes profound changes in physiological systems that can be misinterpreted as indicators of a disease state (for example, hypertension or anxiety).

To help circumvent these problems, we have recently employed a semi-structured assessment strategy in 24-hr monitoring studies. For our current assessment of PD patients we have developed a protocol that includes several controlled baseline assessments ("basal activation test", BA test) and anxiety provocations ("hyperventilation test", HV test) spread out over the 24-hr period. Patients are prompted by a programmable watch with LCD display to perform these structured activities at certain times during the day. The instruction and timing of the tasks is provided by audiotapes. The BA and HV tests serve as standardized assessment periods that minimize the confounding effects of physical activity or social interaction, and allow a straightforward analysis of baseline and reactivity parameters similar to laboratory protocols.

Basal Activation Test

We designed the Basal Activation Test (BA test) as a standardized and reliable baseline assessment of physiological parameters outside the laboratory. Subjects first walk for 3 min at their normal pace and then sit quietly with eyes open for 8 min. Before and after the test, subjects fill out current state and symptom questionnaires. Walking serves as an initial benchmark of moderate physiological activity and induces a modicum of alertness (sleep, or even sleepiness, may lie on a different activational continuum from wakefulness). The period of quiet sitting after walking is long enough to ensure reliable assessment of baseline physiological function.

The BA test is a modification of our previous test procedure (Roth et al., 1998a) which used talking rather than walking as a pre-relaxation benchmark. We had reason to think that a monologue at home alone would be less activating than one in the laboratory with the experimenter listening (Linden, 1987). Our pilot data indicate that walking raises skin conductance levels to about the same degree as talking.

A standardized benchmark activation level allows us to calculate individual change measures (activation minus baseline) helping to reduce inter-individual variance in skin conductance level (SCL), a measure of sympathetic activation. In addition, we found that the slope of SCL decline after walking discriminates best between anxious and control groups when skin conductance vs. the logarithm of time is used to calculate individual regression lines, and when slopes are covaried with the y-intercept. Slopes of SCL decline in anxious patients are consistently less steep than slopes in comparison groups, in spite of test variations (for example, using speaking, loud noise, or walking as a benchmark). Our recent results (Roth et al., 1998a) document that differential slope decline is demonstrable only if groups begin at a level of moderate activation, such as that usually present at the onset of laboratory testing. After a longer time of sitting in the laboratory, slopes in all groups tend towards similar low values. Thus, we think that for repeated testing over 24 hours, it is best to always begin the test at relatively activated benchmark levels like those produced by a short walk.

Hyperventilation Test

We designed the Hyperventilation Test (HV test) as a standardized and reliable assessment of physiological reactivity to a respiratory stressor outside the laboratory. Subjects first breathe deeply at a rate of 1 breath every 3.3 sec for 3 minutes (equivalent to 18 breaths/min) paced by a audio-cassette recording. After that they breathe normally for 8 minutes. Subjects receive feedback during the 3 min of fast breathing from a portable capnometer device that displays end-tidal pCO_2 levels on an LCD display. This feedback signals them to increase or decrease their depth of breathing in order to quickly reach and maintain an end-expiratory pCO_2 level of 20 mm Hg. When the breathing tones stop (after 3 min), subjects are instructed to sit quietly and resume normal breathing for the following 8 min. Before and after the test, subjects fill out current state and symptom questionnaires. Our data indicate that subjects can quite consistently reach the target pCO_2 of 20 mm Hg during 3-min hyperventilation (a steep drop occurs in the first minute, and then the level is stable during minute 2 and 3).

Recent experiments have questioned the importance of hyperventilation to panic: hyperventilation is a relatively weak provocation of panic (Gorman et al., 1988; Gorman et al., 1994; Papp et al., 1997) and spontaneous panic attacks are often unaccompanied by transcutaneously measured pCO_2 reduction (Garssen et al., 1996; Hibbert & Pilsbury, 1989; Hibbert & Pilsbury, 1988). Yet empirically, lower end-tidal pCO_2 has repeatedly, but not invariably, emerged as a difference between anxious patients and comparison groups during recovery from hyperventilation (and in some studies in the baseline periods before hyperventilation as noted in the section "End-tidal PCO_2"). Slowed recovery of pCO_2 levels after voluntary hyperventilation compared to healthy controls has been observed in hyperventilation syndrome patients (a diagnosis showing large overlap with PD) (Brodtkorb et al., 1990; Han et al., 1997; Hardonk & Beumer, 1979; Stoop et al., 1986) and in PD patients panicking during hyperventilation (Gorman et al., 1988; Maddock & Carter, 1991). Negative studies (for example, Rapee et al., 1992) had shorter hyperventilation (< 3 min) or recovery periods (< 5 min) than positive ones. Our own recent study found that slow pCO_2 recovery after hyperventilation was a physiological feature specific to PD patients, compared to social phobia patients or controls (Wilhelm et al., in press-a), and it was accompanied by increased skin conductance levels and heart rates, and by increased reports of shortness of breath and anxiety.

We expect that during 24-hr assessment in PD patients, the BA test measures are likely to change with fluctuations in state anxiety, while the HV test measures will be more trait-like, being more constant upon repeated testing and be more independent of the self-reported psychological state. We base this prediction on reports of an increase in the number of abnormal responses to CO_2 inhalation in relatives of PD patients who at the time of testing never had PD (Bellodi et al., 1998; Cavallini et al., 1999; Perna et al., 1996; Perna et al., 1995). Such findings are compatible with inherited, and possibly enduring, abnormalities of respiratory regulation in PD. Thus, the HV test measures may also fail to normalize as much as the BA test with clinical improvement after treatment or spontaneous recovery.

Recent Studies
Repeated Exposure in Driving Phobia

Study Goal

The fear of driving study (Alpers et al., 2000b) conducted in our laboratory pursued two general goals: assessment of changes in psychophysiological measures with exposure to phobic situations and of changes as people overcame their fear. The study employed state of the art ambulatory recording technology for prolonged monitoring outside the laboratory. In this study, subjects' range of activities was supervised by the experimenter who rode along as a passenger. To our knowledge, it is the first study to continuously assess end-tidal pCO_2 of anxiety disorder patients outside the laboratory. The study provides an example of how psychophysiological monitoring can provide additional information about progress achieved during exposure treatment in a clinical setting.

Study Background:
Much is known about physiological reactions when people experience anxiety, but most observations are based on laboratory induction of emotions. Laboratory paradigms are limited in their ecological validity and ability to elicit strong and distinguishable emotions. For example, film clips or exposure using imagery scripts are of limited potency and it is sometimes difficult to discern which emotions were elicited (Boiten, 1998). Therefore, our study was designed to observe experiential and physiological changes associated with exposure to a real-life phobic situation.

Driving phobia is a clinically relevant fear which can have a serious impact on patients' lives. Exposure to feared situations is the treatment of choice for situational phobias, and profound reductions in the level of anxiety with repeated exposure sessions have been demonstrated many times (Barlow et al., 1998). The treatment's efficacy is well established in a series of well controlled studies (DeRubeis & Crits-Christoph, 1998). Yet, its mechanisms are not completely understood. It is generally assumed that physiological habituation processes play a key role in the improvement within and across exposure sessions (Foa & McNally, 1996).

Exposure to driving phobic situations is especially suitable for ambulatory monitoring since it does not entail much exercise activation, which can hamper interpretation of physiological results in other anxiety producing situation, for example, in a shopping mall. That emotional experience and exercise generally produce indistinguishable physiological activation has long been known (Cannon & Britton, 1927) and several approaches have been developed to quantify emotional activation on the background of physical activity induced activation, for example, by calculating "additional heart rate" (Blix et al., 1974; Myrtek et al., 1994; Wilhelm & Roth, 1998c). The advantage of the driving phobia paradigm is that during exposure to driving situations patients experience considerable levels of anxiety yet the assessment of physiological parameters will be minimally affected by bodily movement and exercise activation. In addition, since driving involves little social interaction and speaking, subjects can continuously breathe through the nose. PCO_2, the most direct measure of hyperventilation, is the gold standard to determine if breathing in excess of metabolic demand occurs when patients with anxiety disorders experience high levels of anxiety.

Methods

Subjects

Driving phobics were recruited by newspaper advertisement. Participants had to be between 18 and 65 years old. All participants were required to have a valid state driver's license, automobile registration, and insurance as required by the law. Some potential participants had to be excluded due to severe medical conditions. Diagnostic assessment was done with a structured clinical interview (First et al., 1995). Symptoms of driving phobia were inquired about in more detail and a driving history was taken.

In order to assess the effects of task performance independent from phobic anxiety, we monitored the physiology of healthy control subjects when driving in the same situations. For each patient a control subject was recruited matched by gender and age. Twenty-nine driving phobics and 25 healthy controls participated in the ambulatory monitoring of at least one driving session. Twenty phobics completed three sessions of freeway driving, and three completed three sessions of driving over a bridge. Eighteen controls completed two sessions of freeway driving, and two completed two sessions of driving over a bridge.

Procedure

Phobic subjects underwent three exposure treatment sessions. In most subjects the feared driving situation that was chosen for exposure treatment was freeway driving. Most of the controls underwent two monitoring sessions, while a few underwent only one session. The second monitoring session was undertaken in order to assess novelty and habituation effects in a non-phobic group. Even in non-phobic participants, being observed when driving and wearing the monitoring device might result in nervousness or excitement during the initial monitoring session, which would complicate the interpretation of observed habituation effects in phobics.

All exposure or monitoring sessions followed the same procedure: (1) laboratory preparation (sensor check, walking activation calibration, Respitrace calibration) and a 5 min quiet sitting baseline, (2) walking from the hospital to the car and driving to the feared situation, (3) driving exposure part one (outbound leg), which lasted 25–30 min in most freeway situations, (4) driving exposure part two (inbound leg), (5) drive back to the hospital, and (6) quiet sitting baseline (5 min), (7) paced breathing RSA calibration (9/13.5/18 cpm for 3 min each), (8) bike ergometer physical activity calibration (Wilhelm & Roth, 1998c), with the sequence: sitting on bike seat, pedalling at 0 Watt, 25 Watt, and 50 Watt, and sitting on bike seat, for 3 min each, (9) second Respitrace calibration. Subjects were prompted for Subjective Units of Distress ratings (SUD ratings) at the end of relevant tasks and every 5 min during the driving. SUD ratings were taken for "anxiety", "excitement", "heart pounding or racing", "breathlessness", and "sweating".

The patients were instructed to follow the same route and drive with approximately the same speed during each of their exposure sessions. The driving routes were individually tailored to the most difficult situation the patient felt able to face. The matched control subject followed the same route as the corresponding patient.

Details of the recording in the car
The Vitaport 2 recording device can be carried on a belt without interfering with driving. Table 1 depicts the channel configuration used for this study.

Electrodes for recording electrodermal activity were small (6 mm diameter) reusable Ag/AgCl well electrodes. They were attached to the middle phalanx of the 4th and 5th digit and covered with adhesive tape. A temperature sensor was attached to the tip of the 5th digit of the left hand. A photoplethysmographic sensor for recording the finger pulse was attached to the 4th finger. The experimenter explained how to best hold on to the steering wheel to ensure safe driving without applying pressure to sensors. Respiratory activity was measured with calibrated elastic bands around chest and abdomen (Respitrace), which were calibrated for each subject using fixed volume bags. Nasal cannuli for the pCO_2 recording and the cables for EOG electrodes (placed vertically above eyebrow and below lower eye-lid) were secured behind the ears so that they would not obstruct the driver's visual field.

Table 1. Channels recorded by the Vitaport 2 during driving. Note: Channel 9-14 are used as control for physical activity and other interfering variables. In addition, salivary cortisol was collected at certain times during the procedure.

No.	Channel	Samplerate (Hz)	Sample Measures
1	Electrocardiogram (chest)	400	Heart rate, RSA, T-wave amplitude
2	Electrodermal activity (left hand)	25	Skin conductance level, non-specific fluctuation
3	Thermometer (left hand)	2	Skin temperature (vasoconstriction)
4	Respiration (thorax)	25	Respiratory rate, tidal volume (and their variability)
5	Respiration (abdomen)	25	Same as above
6	Expired air pCO_2 (nostrils)	25	End-tidal pCO_2
7	Plethysmogram (left hand)	200	Pulse wave amplitude, pulse transit time
8	Electro-oculogram (vertical)	25	Spontaneous eye-blink rate
9	Accelerometer (left wrist)	25	Movement
10	Accelerometer (right foot)	25	Movement
11	Accelerometer (car frame)	25	Movement
12	Thermometer (bag)	2	Environmental temperature
13	Sound (throat)	25	Vocalization
14	Marker (bag)	10	Button presses for indicating phases or special events
		839	Size of data file for 120 min recording about 9 Mbyte

Preliminary Results and Examples of Recorded Data

Our main focus in preliminary analyses was the effect of the repeated exposure sessions on respiration. The results indicate that exposure to feared driving situations causes immediate, marked changes in measures of respiratory physiology (Alpers et al., 2000a). While driving increases respiration rate equally in both groups, tidal volume is increased only in driving phobics, resulting in greater minute ventilation and lower pCO_2 (35 mm Hg at baseline to 28 mm Hg during the first 30 min of exposure). Patient reports of less anxiety during the driving task after repeated exposure sessions are reflected in simultaneous changes in these physiological measures towards healthy control levels. These results demonstrate that hyperventilation does play a role in anxiety and that ambulatory monitoring can document the changes taking place during behavior therapy.

Figure 3 shows a plot of heart rate over time during exposure session 1 and 2 from a 55 year old woman with driving phobia. The plot represents the entire recording period of about 2 hours and 45 min and is typical for patients in this study. In the first session baseline heart rate is somewhat elevated from a normal resting heart rate. Physical exercise produces strong activation in both sessions. In the first session heart rate increases sharply at the beginning of the exposure but subsequently decreases. In the second session, there is less heart rate activation, beginning with baseline and sustained throughout the exposure session. There is usually little change in heart rate from session 2 to 3. Although the course of driving was kept constant for each individual between sessions the naturalistic setting caused some variation in the duration of certain tasks. In this subject, the outbound leg of the first exposure session was longer than usual because of slow traffic. This also demonstrates how important the proper marker settings are for extraction of appropriate segments for the data analysis.

Figure 4 shows the results of an analysis of the raw expired pCO_2 waveform for end-tidal pCO_2 plateaus in the same subject during the first two exposure sessions. The capnometer values before exposure are on the lower end of normal resting values, especially for session 1. In both sessions pCO_2 drops during approach to the freeway and is lowest during driving on the freeway. During the exposure to freeway driving, pCO_2 values do not recover. The steep drop that can be seen at the end of the recording is due to a paced breathing task (9/13.5/18 breaths/minute, for a total of 9 min). Although subjects were instructed to breathe as shallowly as possible, the instruction to follow the tones played back from an audiotape led to increased minute ventilation and synchronous decreases in pCO_2 (pCO_2 values were not displayed to the subject nor experimenter during this task). This demonstrates that the Capnocount can respond quickly to changes in ventilation. The exercise calibration that followed produced small increases in pCO_2; the large increases in heart rate indicate higher metabolic demand and thus more CO_2 production. Overall, pCO_2 reduction is usually greater during session 1 than 2, but there is not much change between sessions 2 and 3.

Minute ventilation, as shown in Figure 5, changes greatly with physical activity. A comparison with heart rate and pCO_2 data for this subject makes it clear that minute ventilation is more responsive to metabolic demand and less reflective of psychological stress than is pCO_2.

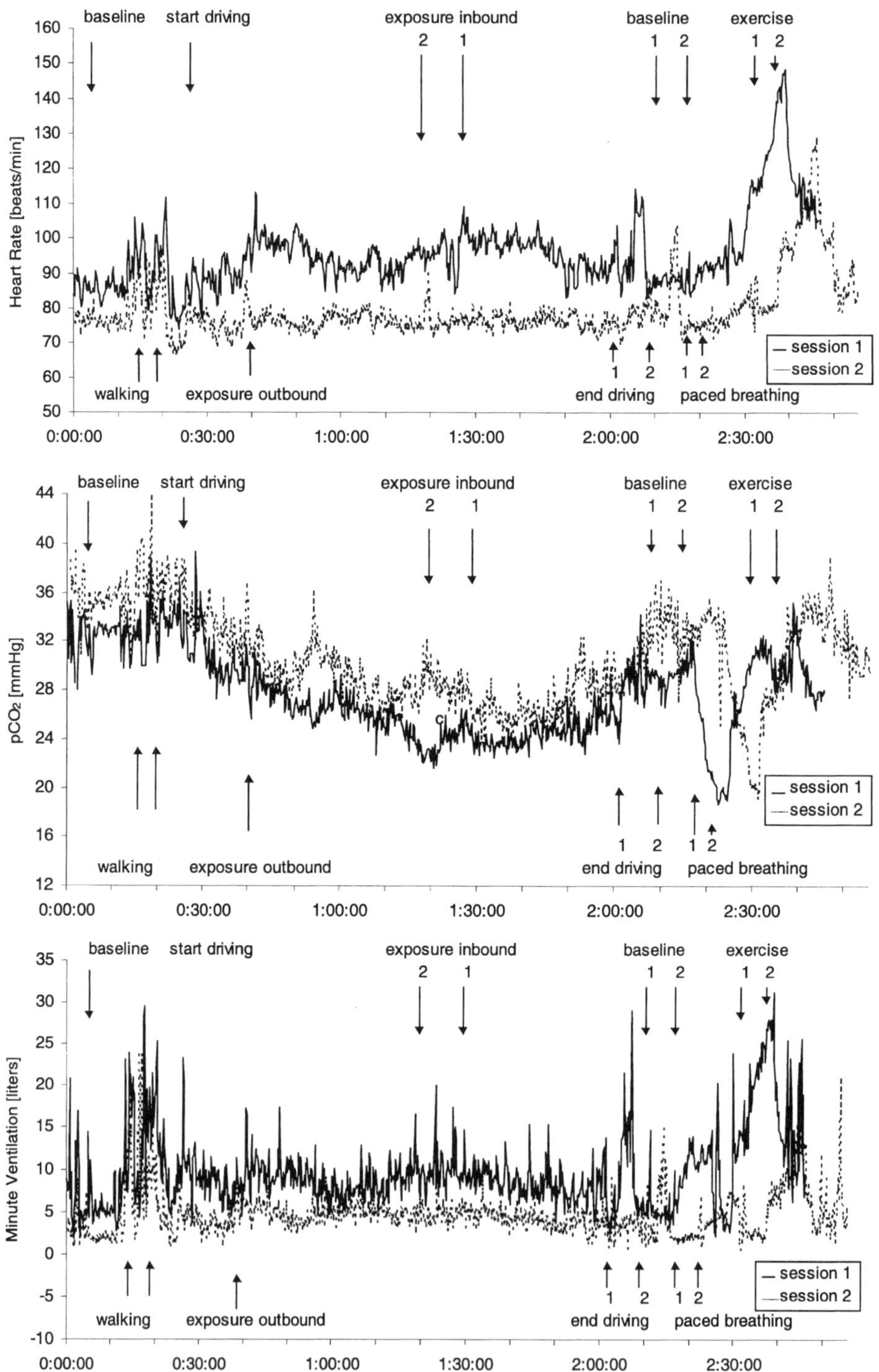

Figures 3-5: Heart rate, end-tidal pCO2, and minute ventilation during the first two driving exposure sessions for a driving phobic patient (subject 28)

4-hr Monitoring in Panic Disorder

Study Goal

The goal of this study is to assess 24-hr respiratory and autonomic patterns in patients with a DSM-IV diagnosis of PD (American Psychiatric Association, 1994) before and after treatment. We are employing the Vitaport 2 technology (Becker Meditec, Germany) and customized software developed in our laboratory (FW). Patients receive respiratory control training with concurrent feedback of end-tidal pCO_2 and respiratory rate over the course of 4 weeks. We assess a wide variety of physiological parameters in addition to self-reports of mood and symptoms immediately before and after the 4-week treatment and at follow-up. It is paradoxical that reported symptoms of increased sympathetic autonomic nervous system activation or respiratory disturbance are a basis of DSM-IV diagnoses of PD, while actual measurements of these physiological changes have not found a place in the clinic, for either assessing individual patients or documenting the efficacy of therapies.

Study Background

PD patients suffer from recurrent, sudden episodes of intense anxiety accompanied by a variety of somatic symptoms. Clinical reports and systematic studies indicate that dyspnea (shortness of breath) is – together with palpitations – the cardinal complaint among panic patients. It was shown that feelings of dyspnea are also elevated during non-panic periods and during laboratory baselines in this patient group. Our recent laboratory experiments (Roth et al., 1998a; Roth et al., 1998b; Wilhelm et al., in press-a; Wilhelm et al., in press-b; Wilhelm & Roth, 1997; Wilhelm & Roth, 1998a; Wilhelm et al., in press-c; Wilhelm et al., in press-d) and studies of other research groups (Abelson et al., in press; Gorman et al., 1994) indicate prominent respiratory abnormalities such as lowered end-tidal pCO_2 and increased breath-by-breath tidal volume variability in PD patients at baseline, in response to panic attack provocations (such as CO_2 inhalations), and during extended recovery from hyperventilation. Not much is known about respiratory patterns of panic patients outside the laboratory (an exception is Martinez et al., 1996), but we expect that the abnormalities found in laboratory studies will be present to some degree during daily activities and during sleep. The respiratory control treatment is designed to normalize the respiratory pathophysiology of panic patients and will serve as a demonstration of how a detailed 24-hr assessment of respiratory and autonomic parameters can be utilized to validate the effectiveness of anxiety therapy.

Respiratory control training using pCO_2 feedback has been successfully applied to a variety of disorders with known respiratory aspects, such as asthma and epilepsy (Fried, 1993). A breathing training without pCO_2 feedback to patients was successfully applied in PD patients, in whom it effectively reduced self-reported anxiety, global ratings of distress, and panic attack frequency (Clark et al., 1985). Data from our laboratory indicate that instructions to breath slowly and shallowly can paradoxically lead to lowering of end-tidal pCO_2. Thus, direct visual feedback of the level of pCO_2 reached during the voluntary breathing maneuvers of respiratory control training should enhance its efficacy. Increasing end-tidal pCO_2 levels should not only normalize respiratory pathophysiology but also the acid-base balance in the blood and increase the delivery of O_2 to the brain and body tissues (Nutt et al., 1999), resulting in a reduction of physical symptoms.

Methods

Subjects

In this ongoing study, patients with a diagnosis of PD with or without agoraphobia between the ages of 18 and 60 are recruited by newspaper advertisement. Potential participants are excluded if they have severe medical conditions. Diagnostic assessment is done with a structured clinical interview (First et al., 1995). In order to assess the effects of daily activity independent from a trait of PD or state of panic anxiety, we also monitor physiological changes in healthy control subjects matched by gender and age. Our goal is to recruit 40 panic patients and 20 controls. Half of the patients will be randomized to immediate treatment, the other half to a delayed (by 4 weeks) treatment control group.

Procedure

The 24-hr recording begins in the laboratory and ends a day later when the subject returns to the laboratory. The laboratory part of the 24-hr assessment is necessary for informing subjects about details of the following recording, the setup of electrodes and recording devices, the calibration of electrodes and physiological response, and for initial testing with the BA and HV tests. The laboratory procedures and durations are described in detail below. In general, subjects report to the laboratory at either 8 or 10 a.m. and return the following day at 9 or 11 a.m. The first laboratory session lasts about 2 hours, and the second about 1.25 hours.

Details of the 24-hr monitoring

The channel configuration used for this study was similar to the driving phobia study (Table 1). However, the photoplethysmogram and EOG were omitted, the car frame accelerometer was placed on the trunk, and a sensor at the neck was used to indicate ambient light changes (indoors vs. outdoors, day vs. night). At a total sample rate of 618 Hz, the file size is approximately 68 Mbytes. Subjects wear the sensors and ambulatory recording devices (Vitaport 2 and Capnocount, contained in a waist pack) an entire day and night, returning the next day to the laboratory for detachment of the sensors. Subjects are asked to follow their normal daily routine.

About every two hours subjects are signaled by a programmable watch to interrupt their activity for about 13 minutes to perform either the BA test or HV test.

Subjects receive a detailed handout for the ambulatory recording with an emphasis on how to maintain the functioning of the devices. For example, subjects are reminded that the devices are sensitive to pressure, jolting, and exposure to water. For the sleep recording, a handout contains another set of instructions and diagrams. For example, subjects are instructed to make sure the capnograph is not covered with any blanket or pillow during the night since this would impede the necessary air exchange for self-calibration of the device. The subject finds a detailed description on how to change the water filter and the nasal cannula of the capnograph after 12 hr of recording. The handout also contains a list of troubleshooting instructions for situations such as beeping of the capnograph alarm (indicating obstruction of the sample line), loosening of electrodes, and other technical problems. Additionally, the subject can page the experimenter at any time during the recording for advice.

Success of this demanding 13-channel configuration for 24-hr monitoring periods depends largely on the adequate preparation of the recording devices, rigorous application of electrodes and sensors, and detailed instructions to subjects. Several months were spent to develop and pilot the specific setup and procedures. Due to space constraints we cannot convey all this information here and have to refer the interested reader to communication with the first author by e-mail.

Preliminary Results and Examples of Recorded Data

The data collection for this study was in an early phase at the time of writing. Results from the first few PD patients that completed therapy indicate that patients find the rationale of the pCO_2 feedback assisted breathing therapy convincing, are highly compliant with the home exercise regimen (which is monitored by the capnometer recordings during each exercise), and show increases in baseline pCO_2 and decreases in anxiety over the course of therapy (Wilhelm et al., 2000c).

Figure 6 shows the results of an analysis of the raw expired pCO_2 waveform for end-tidal pCO_2 plateaus over 24 hours for a 50 years old woman with a diagnosis of PD. Data from individual breaths were averaged minute-by-minute. The data indicates great variability in pCO_2 levels throughout the day in this patient. One can clearly see steep drops in pCO_2 to about 20 mm Hg during the 5 HV tests that were performed during the recording day (at about 10 a.m., 12:30 p.m., 4:30 p.m., 8:30 p.m., and 10 a.m.). Apparently, in this patient pCO_2 decreased during sleep.

Figure 7 depicts the end-tidal pCO_2 levels for a control participant. The 24-hr data shows on average higher pCO_2 values during the day than for the patient depicted in Figure 8. In addition, there is a marked increase in pCO_2 for this control subject during the night. Figure 8 shows the minute ventilation values corresponding to the

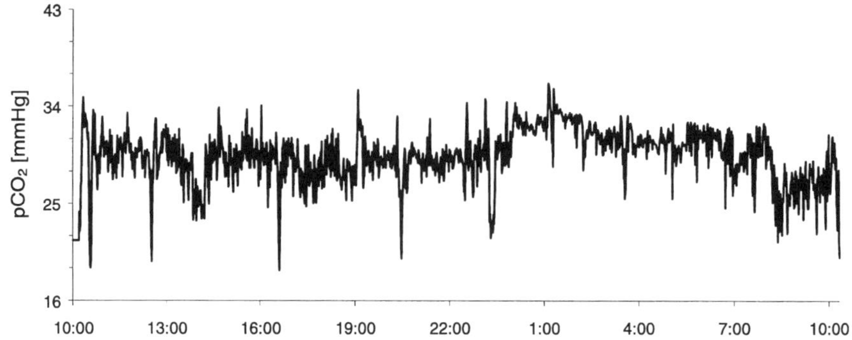

Figure 6. End-tidal pCO2 during the first 24-hr monitoring for a panic disorder patient (subject 10)

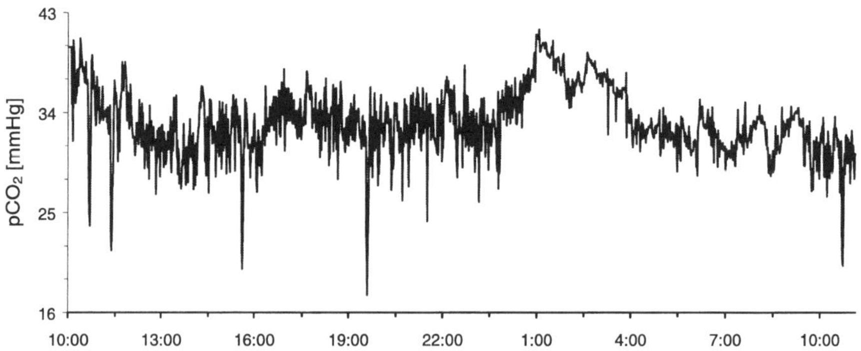

Figure 7. End-tidal pCO2 during the first 24-hr monitoring for a control subject (subject 8)

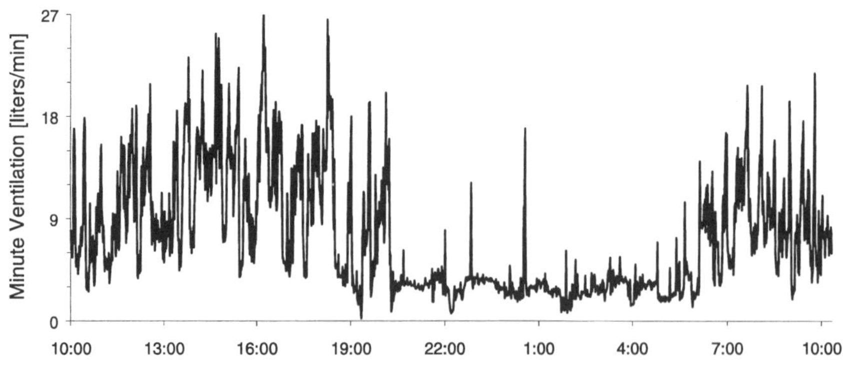

Figure 8. Minute ventilation during the first 24-hr monitoring for the panic disorder patient depicted in Figure 6 (subject 10)

pCO_2 recording depicted in Figure 6. As one can see, minute ventilation is highly variable during the day. Since most increases are likely due to exercise activation, it is not clear without detailed analysis of accelerometry information which segments of the data indicate hyperventilation. Figure 9 shows the skin conductance level of a control participant during the 24-hr recording. Skin conductance level is quite variable during the day, and asymptotically reaches a minimum during the night.

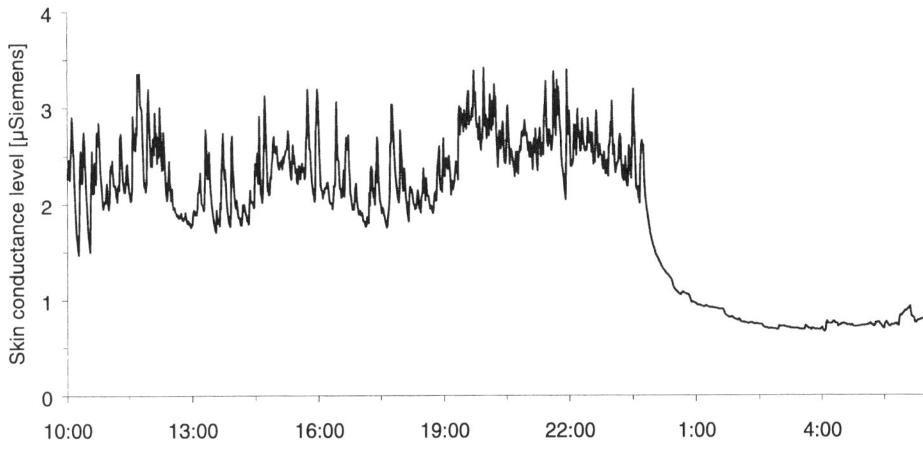

Figure 9. Skin conductance level during the first 24-hr monitoring for a control subject (subject 6)

Outlook

With the rapid advances in microelectronics, devices measuring a wide variety of bodily functions and motoric behaviors in addition to self-report data over periods of hours or days are now available. Existing physiological monitors are so rugged, portable, and automatic that they can record accurately from moving subjects in various settings of daily life. We expect that within the next 10 years they will become more inexpensive, easy to use, and unobtrusive. "Wearable computers" with electrophysiological sensors integrated in clothing to provide real-time feedback about physiological activation are currently being developed (Picard, 1997).

Still, conducting the type of multi-channel ambulatory monitoring studies we described and making the outlined measurements is highly demanding for both patient and experimenter. Because of the number of channels and computed measures, the greatest effort follows the actual recording. In the past years we have developed an integrated system of software programs tailored to analyze a variety of physiological channels with an unprecedented level of detail, so that an array of parameters especially meaningful for anxiety assessment can be extracted from the raw signals (Wilhelm et al., 1999a). Data reduction and computation of breath-by-breath respiratory parameters is especially difficult. Respiration parameters (for example, tidal volume and respiratory rate) have a large range of normal values so that automatic exclusion of outliers is not a viable option (see, for example, our critique of an automated respiratory measurement and analysis system, Wilhelm & Roth, 1998b). Instead, analysis has to be based on full disclosure of the raw waveforms and intelligent judgements about when to exclude artifactual breaths or entire segments of data. We have developed a suite of sophisticated software programs to assist in this task that enables us to acquire physiological data never collected before in patients outside the laboratory. In the future, artificial intelligence methodology may reduce the time required for artifact editing and vastly expand the scope of research projects, or even allow the application of respiratory monitoring to the clinic.

Portable biofeedback systems that target specific physiological systems to assist in anxiety treatment can be developed or are already available. For example, Grossman et al.. (1985) describe a small portable monitor that provides paced breathing tones whenever the patients respiratory rate (measured with a strain gauge) exceeds certain preprogrammed limits. The portable capnometer used in some of our studies can be programmed to beep when end-tidal PCO_2 or respiratory rate change beyond preprogrammed thresholds for longer than a specified period of time. In both devices, physiological measurements are stored in memory for later download and evaluation by the therapist or patient. Thus, ambulatory or portable physiological measuring devices have the potential of extending the therapeutic endeavors of psychologists and psychiatrists far beyond the confines of their consulting rooms (Wilhelm & Roth, submitted).

Given the evidence of respiratory dysregulation at least in a subgroup of anxiety patients, a convincing therapy of anxiety disorders would have to show that these abnormalities are normalized as well. Although even very short cognitive-behavioral treatments for PD have been shown to be quite effective in terms of normalizing self-reported indicators of the disease (for example, Clark et al., 1999), whether physiological measures have been normalized to the same degree has been ignored. The published success rates of cognitive-behavioral treatments are directly or indirectly based on self-reports, which easily may have been biased by the specific demand characteristics of this type of therapy or by nonspecific factors such as exaggerating distress to qualify for therapy, and minimizing distress at the end of therapy to please the therapist. We have shown in this chapter that physiological ambulatory 24-hr monitoring can add another dimension to therapy outcome assessment.

Acknowledgment

Preparation of this chapter was supported by grant NIH/MH56094 and the Department of Veterans Affairs. The authors would like to thank Christiane Melzig for her help in setting up the 24-hr monitoring study.

References

Abelson, J.L., Weg, J.G., Nesse, R.M., Curtis, G.C. (in press). Persistent respiratory irregularity in patients with panic disorder. *Biological Psychiatry.*

Al-Ani, M., Forkins, A., Townend, J., Coote, J. (1996). Respiratory sinus arrhythmia and central respiratory drive in humans. *Clinical Science, 90*, 235–241.

Alpers, G.W., Wilhelm, F.H. (2000). Ambulatory respiratory and autonomic monitoring in anxiety disorders. *Paper presented at the Anxiety Disorders Association of America, 20th National Conference, Washington, USA.*

Alpers, G.W., Wilhelm, F.H., Roth, W.T. (2000a). Do measurements of end-tidal pCO2 during phobic exposure correspond to measurements of minute ventilation? *Paper presented at the 7th Annual Meeting of the International Society for the Advancement of Respiratory Psychophysiology, San Diego, USA*

Alpers, G.W., Wilhelm, F.H., Roth, W.T. (2000b). Psychophysiological measures can index change in behavior therapy. *Psychophysiology, 37*, S8.

American Psychiatric Association (1994). *Diagnostic and Statistical Manual of Mental Disorders, Fourth Edition.* Washington, DC: American Psychiatric Association.

Barefoot, J.C., Helms, M.J., Mark, D.B., Blumenthal, J.A., Califf, R.M., Haney, T.L., O'Connor, C.M., Siegler, I.C., Williams, R.B. (1996). Depression and long-term mortality risk in patients with coronary artery disease. *American Journal of Cardiology, 78*, 613–617.

Barlow, D.H., Esler, J.L., Vitali, A.E. (1998). Psychosocial treatments for panic disorders, phobias, and generalized anxiety disorder. In *A guide to treatments that work.* New York, NY, USA: Oxford University Press, pp 288–318.

Bass, C., Gardner, W.N. (1985). Respiratory and psychiatric abnormalities in chronic symptomatic hyperventilation. *British Medical Journal, 290*, 1387–1390.

Bellodi, L., Perna, G., Caldirola, D., Arancio, C., Bertani, A., Di Bella, D. (1998). CO2-induced panic attacks: a twin study. *American Journal of Psychiatry, 155*, 1184–1188.

Blix, A.S., Strømme, S.B., Ursin, H. (1974). Additional heart rate: An indicator of psychological activation. *Aerospace Medicine, 45*, 1219–1222.

Bloomfield, P. (1976). Complex demodulation. In P. Bloomfield (Ed.), *Fourier analysis of time series: An introduction.* New York: Wiley, pp 118–150.

Boiten, F. (1998). The effects of emotional behavior on components of the respiratory cycle. *Biological Psychology, 49*, 29–51.

Brodtkorb, E., Gimse, R., Antonaci, F., Ellertsen, B., Sand, T., Sulg, I., Sjaastad, O. (1990). Hyperventilation syndrome: clinical, ventilatory, and personality characteristics as observed in neurological practice. *Acta Neurologica Scandinavia, 81*, 307–313.

Cannon, W.B., Britton, S.W. (1927). The influence of motion and emotion on medulliadrenal secretion. *Amercian Journal of Physiology, 79*, 433–465.

Cavallini, M.C., Perna, G., Caldirola, D., Bellodi, L. (1999). A segregation study of panic disorder in families of panic patients responsive to the 35% CO2 challenge. *Biological Psychiatry, 46*, 815–820.

Clark, D.M. (1986). A cognitive approach to panic. *Behavior Research and Therapy, 24*, 461–470.

Clark, D.M., Salkovskis, P.M., Chalkley, A.J. (1985). Respiratory control as a treatment for panic attacks. *Journal of Behavior Therapy and Experimental Psychiatry, 16*, 23–30.

Clark, D.M., Salkovskis, P.M., Hackmann, A., Wells, A., Ludgate, J., Gelder, M. (1999). Brief cognitive therapy for panic disorder: a randomized controlled trial. *Journal of Consulting and Clinical*

Psychology, 67, 583–589.

DeRubeis, R.J., Crits-Christoph, P. (1998). Empirically supported individual and group psychological treatments for adult mental disorders. *Journal of Consulting and Clinical Psychology, 66*, 37–52.

Fahrenberg, J., Foerster, F., Smeja, M., Müller, W. (1997). Assessment of posture and motion by multichannel piezoresistive accelerometer recordings. *Psychophysiology, 34*, 607–612.

Finesinger, J.E. (1943): The spirogram in certain psychiatric disorders. *American Journal of Psychiatry, 100*, 159–169.

First, M.B., Spitzer, R.L., Gibbon, M., Williams, J.B.W. (1995). *Structured Clinical Interview of DSM IV Axis I Disorders.* New York: Biometrics Research Department.

Foa, E.B., McNally, R.J. (1996). Mechanisms of change in exposure therapy. In R.M. Rapee (Ed.), *Current controversies in the anxiety disorders.* New York: Guilford, pp 229–343.

Fried, R. (1987): *The hyperventilation syndrome: research and clinical treatment.* Baltimore: Johns Hopkins University Press.

Fried, R. (1993). *The Psychology and Physiology of Breathing.* New York: Plenum.

Friedman, B., Thayer, J. (1998). Autonomic balance revisited: panic anxiety and heart rate variability. *Journal of Psychosomatic Research, 44*, 133–151.

Gardner, W.N. (1994). Diagnosis and organic causes of symptomatic hyperventilation. In B.H. Timmons & R. Ley (Eds.), *Behavioral and psychological approaches to breathing disorders.* New York: Plenum Press, pp 99–112.

Garssen, B., Buikhuisen, M., Hornsveld, H., Klaver, C., van Doornen, L. (1994). Ambulatory measurement of transcutaneous PCO2. *Journal of Psychophysiology, 8*, 231–240.

Garssen, B., Buikhuisen, M., van Dyck, R. (1996). Hyperventilation and panic attacks. *American Journal of Psychiatry, 153*, 513–518.

Gerlach, A.L., Wilhelm, F.H., Gruber, K., Roth, W.T. (in press). Psychophysiology and subtypes of social phobia: the role of blushing. *Journal of Abnormal Psychology.*

Gilbert, C. (1999). Hyperventilation and the body. *Accident and Emergency Nursing, 7*, 130–140.

Gorman, J.M., Fyer, M.R., Goetz, R., Askanazi, J., Liebowitz, M.R., Fyer, A.J. (1988). Ventilatory physiology of patients with panic disorder. *Archives of General Psychiatry, 45*, 31–39.

Gorman, J.M., Papp, L.A., Coplan, J.D., Martinez, J.M., Lennon, S., Goetz, R.R., Ross, D., Klein, D.F. (1994). Anxiogenic effects of CO2 and hyperventilation in patients with panic disorder. *American Journal of Psychiatry, 151*, 547–553.

Grossman, P. (1992). Respiratory and cardiac rhythms as windows to central and autonomic biobehavioral regulation: selection of window frames, keeping the panes clean and viewing the neural topography. *Biological Psychology, 34*, 131–161.

Grossman, P., de Swart, J.C., Defares, P.B. (1985). A controlled study of a breathing therapy for treatment of hyperventilation syndrome. *Journal of Psychosomatic Research, 29*, 49–58.

Grossman, P., Karemaker, J.K., Wieling, W. (1991). Prediction of tonic parasympathetic cardiac control using respiratory sinus arrhythmia: The need for respiratory control. *Psychophysiology, 28*, 201–216.

Grossman, P., Stemmler, G., Meinhardt, E. (1990a). Paced respiratory sinus arrhythmia as an index of cardiac parasympathetic tone during varying behavioral tasks. *Psychophysiology, 27*, 404–416.

Grossman, P., van Beek, J., Wientjes, C. (1990b). A comparison of three quantification methods for estimation of respiratory sinus arrhythmia. *Psychophysiology, 27*, 702–714.

Han, J.N., Stegen, K., Simkens, K., Cauberghs, M., Schepers, R., Van den Bergh, O., Clement, J., Van de Woestijne, K.P. (1997). Unsteadiness of breathing in patients with hyperventilation syndrome and anxiety disorders. *European Respiratory Journal, 10*, 167–176.

Hardonk, H.J., Beumer, H.M. (1979). Hyperventilation syndrome. In P.J. Vinken &G. W. Bruyn (Eds.), *Handbook of Clinical Neurology.* Amsterdam: North-Holland Publishing Company, pp 309–360.

Hayano, J., Taylor, J.A., Mukai, S., Okada, A., Watanabe, Y., Takata, K., Fujinami, T. (1994). Assessment of frequency shifts in R-R interval variability and respiration with complex demodulation. *Journal of Applied Physiology, 77*, 2879–2888.

Hegel, M.T., Ferguson, R.J. (1997). Psychophysiological assessment of respiratory function in panic disorder: evidence for a hyperventilation subtype. *Psychosomatic Medicine, 59*, 224–230.

Hibbert, G., Pilsbury, D. (1989). Hyperventilation – Is It a Cause of Panic Attacks. *British Journal of Psychiatry, 155*, 805–809.

Hibbert, G.A., Pilsbury, D. (1988). Hyperventilation in panic attacks. Ambulant monitoring of transcutaneous carbon dioxide. *British Journal of Psychiatry, 153*, 76–80.

Hoffmann, U., Essfeld, D., Stegemann, J. (1990). Comparison of arterial, end-tidal and transcutaneous PCO2 during moderate exercise and external CO2 loading in humans. *European Journal of Applied Physiology, 61*, 1–4.

Hofmann, S.G., Newman, M.G., Ehlers, A., Roth, W.T. (1995).: Psychophysiological differences between subgroups of social phobia. *Journal of Abnormal Psychology, 104*, 224–231.

Holt, P.D., Andrews, G. (1998). Hyperventilation and anxiety in panic disorder, social phobia, GAD, and normal controls. *Behavior Research and Therapy, 27*, 453–460.

Jennings, J.R., McKnight, J.D. (1994). Inferring vagal tone from heart rate variability [editorial; comment]. *Psychosomatic Medicine, 56*, 194–196.

Kawachi, I., Sparrow, D., Vokonas, P.S., Weiss, S.T. (1995). Decreased heart rate variability in men with phobic anxiety (data from the Normative Aging Study). *American Journal of Cardiology, 75*, 882–885.

Klein, D.F. (1992). False suffocation alarms, spontaneous panics, and related conditions. An integrative hypothesis. *Archives of General Psychiatry, 50*, 306–317.

Kollai, M., Mizsei, G. (1990). Respiratory sinus arrhythmia is a limited measure of cardiac parasympathetic control in man. *Journal of Physiology (London), 424*, 329–342.

Ley, R. (1985). Blood, breath, and fears: A hyperventilation theory of panic attacks and agoraphobia. *Clinical Psychology Review, 5*, 271–285.

Linden, W. (1987). A microanalysis of autonomic activity during human speech. *Psychosomatic Medicine, 49*, 562–578.

Maddock, R.J., Carter, C.S. (1991). Hyperventilation-induced panic attacks in Panic Disorder with Agoraphobia. *Biological Psychiatry, 29*, 843–854.

Margraf, J., Taylor, C.B., Ehlers, A., Roth, W.T., Agras, W.S. (1987). Panic attacks in the natural environment. *Journal of Nervous and Mental Disease, 175*, 558–565.

Martinez, J.M., Papp, L.A., Coplan, J.D., Anderson, D.E., Mueller, C.M., Klein, D.F., Gorman, J.M. (1996). Ambulatory monitoring of respiration in anxiety. *Anxiety, 2*, 296–302.

Munjack, D.J., Brown, R.A., McDowell, D.E. (1993). Existence of hyperventilation in Panic Disorder with and without Agoraphobia, GAD, and normals: Implications for a cognitive theory of panic. *Journal of Anxiety Disorders, 7*, 37–48.

Myrtek, M., Deutschman-Janicke, E., Strohmaier, H., Zimmerman, W. (1994). Physical, mental, emotional, and subjective workload components in train drivers. *Ergonomics, 37*, 1195–1203.

Nutt, D.J., Ballenger, J.C., Lepine, J.-P. (1999). *Panic disorder: clinical diagnosis, management and mechanisms*. London: Martin Dunitz.

Papp, L.A. (1995). Respiratory neurobiology of panic. In G.M. Asnis & H.M. Van Praag (Eds.), *Panic disorder – clinical, biological and treatment aspects*. New York: John Wiley and Sons, pp 255–275.

Papp, L.A., Martinez, J.M., Klein, D.F., Coplan, J.D., Norman, R.G., Cole, R., de Jesus, M.J., Ross, D., Goetz, R., Gorman, J.M. (1997). Respiratory psychophysiology of panic disorder: three respiratory challenges in 98 subjects. *American Journal of Psychiatry, 154*, 1557–1565.

Perna, G., Bertani, A., Caldirola, D., Bellodi, L. (1996). Family history of panic disorder and hypersensitivity to CO2 in patients with panic disorder. *American Journal of Psychiatry, 153*, 1060–1064.

Perna, G., Cocchi, S., Bertani, A., Arancio, C., Bellodi, L. (1995). Sensitivity to 35% CO2 in healthy first-degree relatives of patients with panic disorder. *American Journal of Psychiatry, 152*, 623–625.

Picard, R.W. (1997). *Affective computing*. Cambridge, MA: MIT press.

Porges, S.W., Byrne, E.A. (1992). Research methods for measurement of heart rate and respiration. *Biological Psychology, 34*, 93–130.

Porges, S.W., McCabe, P.M., Yongue, B.G. (1982). Respiratory-heart rate interactions: Psychophysiological implications for pathophysiology and behavior. In J.T. Cacioppo &R.E.

Petty (Eds.), *Perspectives in Cardiovascular Psychophysiology.* New York, NY: Guilford Press, pp 223–264.

Rafferty, G., Saisch, S., Gardner, W. (1992). Relation of hypocapnic symptoms to rate of fall of end-tidal PCO2 in normal subjects. *Respiratory Medicine, 86*, 335–340.

Rapee, R. (1986). Differential response to hyperventilation in panic disorder and generalized anxiety disorder. *Journal of Abnormal Psychology, 95*, 24–28.

Rapee, R.M., Brown, T.A., Antony, M.M., Barlow, D.H. (1992). Response to hyperventilation and inhalation of 5.5% carbon dioxide-enriched air across the DSM-III-R anxiety disorders. *Journal of Abnormal Psychology, 101*, 538–552.

Roth, W.T., Margraf, J., Ehlers, A., Taylor, C.B., Maddock, R.J., Davies, S., Agras, W.S. (1992). Stress test reactivity in panic disorder. *Archives of General Psychiatry, 49*, 301–310.

Roth, W.T., Trabert, W., Wilhelm, F.H. (1994). Do benzodiazepines impede exposure treatment of specific phobias. *Talk presented at the Anxiety Disorders Association of America, 14th National Conference, San Diego, USA.*

Roth, W.T., Wilhelm, F.H., Trabert, W. (1998a). Autonomic instability during relaxation in panic disorder. *Psychiatry Research, 80*, 155–164.

Roth, W.T., Wilhelm, F.H., Trabert, W. (1998b). Voluntary breath holding in panic and generalized anxiety disorders. *Psychosomatic Medicine, 60*, 671–679.

Saul, J.P., Berger, R.D., Albrecht, P., Stein, S.P., Chen, M.H., Cohen, R.J. (1991). Transfer function analysis of the circulation: unique insights into cardiovascular regulation. *American Journal of Physiology, 261*, H1231–1245.

Stein, M.B., Millar, T.W., Larsen, D.K., Kryger, M.H. (1995). Irregular breathing patterns during sleep in patients with panic disorder. *American Journal of Psychiatry, 152*, 1168–1173.

Stoop, A., de Boo, T., Lemmens, W.H.F. (1986). Hyperventilation syndrome: Measurement of objective symptoms and subjective complaints. *Respiration, 49*, 37–44.

Thayer, J.F., Friedman, B.H., Borkovec, T.D. (1996). Autonomic characteristics of generalized anxiety disorder and worry. *Biological Psychiatry, 39*, 255–266.

van den Hout, M.A., Hoekstra, R., Arntz, A., Christiaanse, M., Ranschaert, W., Schouten, E. (1992). Hyperventilation is not diagnostically specific to panic patients. *Psychosomatic Medicine, 53*, 182–191.

Watkins, L.L., Grossman, P., Krishnan, R., Sherwood, A. (1998). Anxiety and vagal control of heart rate. *Psychosomatic Medicine, 60*, 498–502.

Welch, P.D. (1967). The use of fast Fourier transform for the estimation of power spectra: a method based on time averaging over short modified periodograms. *IEEE Transactions on Audio and Electroacoustics, 15*, 70–73.

Whittal, M.L., Wilhelm, F.H., Taylor, C.B., Roth, W.T. (1996). Agoraphobic avoidance: The relationship with panic expectancy, social anxiety, and physiological activation. *Poster presented at the 30th Annual Convention of the Association for Advancement of Behavior Therapy, New York, USA.*

Wilhelm, F.H., Berkowitz, J., Hansen, M., Grossman, P., Roth, W.T, Gross, J.J. (1998). RSA estimation during spontaneous breathing using a paced breathing calibration. *Psychophysiology, 35*, S88.

Wilhelm, F.H., Gerlach, A.L., Roth, W.T. (in press-a). Slow recovery from voluntary hyperventilation in panic disorder. *Psychosomatic Medicine.*

Wilhelm, F.H., Gevirtz, R., Roth, W.T. (in press-b). Respiratory factors in clinical psychophysiology and biofeedback. *Verhaltenstherapie.*

Wilhelm, F.H., Gross, J.J., Kochar, A.S., Roth, W.T. (2000a). Sympathetic-parasympathetic coactivation during touch. *Psychophysiology, 37*, S105.

Wilhelm, F.H., Grossman, P., Gerlach, A.L., Roth, W.T. (2000b). Improving the clinical sensitivity of noninvasive assessment of cardiac vagal control. *Psychophysiology, 37*, S105.

Wilhelm, F.H., Grossman, P., Roth, W.T. (1997). Assessment of heart rate variability under nonstationary conditions: complex demodulation vs. spectral analysis. *Psychophysiology, 34*, S96.

Wilhelm, F.H., Grossman, P., Roth, W.T. (1999a). Analysis of cardiovascular regulation. *Biomedical Science Instrumentation, 35*, 135–140.

Wilhelm, F.H., Meuret, A.E., Roth, W.T. (2000c). A new treatment for panic disorder: PCO2 and respiratory rate feedback assisted breathing training at home. *Talk presented at the 7th Annual Meeting of the International Society for the Advancement of Respiratory Psychophysiology, San Diego, USA.*

Wilhelm, F.H., Roth, W.T. (1996). Ambulatory assessment of clinical anxiety. In J. Fahrenberg & M. Myrtek (Eds.), *Ambulatory assessment: Computer-assisted psychological and psychophysiological methods in monitoring and field studies.* Hogrefe & Huber Publishers, Göttingen, Germany, pp 317–345.

Wilhelm, F.H., Roth, W.T. (1997). Acute and delayed effects of alprazolam on flight phobics during exposure. *Behavior Research and Therapy, 35*, 831–841.

Wilhelm, F.H., Roth, W.T. (1998a). Taking the laboratory to the skies: ambulatory assessment of self-report, autonomic, and respiratory responses in flying phobia. *Psychophysiology, 35*, 596–606.

Wilhelm, F.H., Roth, W.T. (1998b). Trusting computerized data reduction too much: a critique of Anderson's ambulatory respiratory monitor. *Biological Psychology, 49*, 215–219; discussion 221–222.

Wilhelm, F.H., Roth, W.T. (1998c). Using minute ventilation for ambulatory estimation of additional heart rate. *Biological Psychology, 49*, 137–150.

Wilhelm, F.H., Roth, W.T. (submitted). The somatic symptom paradox in DSM-IV anxiety disorders: suggestions for a clinical focus in psychophysiology. *Biological Psychology.*

Wilhelm, F.H., Trabert, W., Roth, W.T. (1999b). Autonomic, hemodynamic and respiratory instability in panic and generalized anxiety disorders. *Talk presented at the Anxiety Disorders Association of America, 19th National Conference, San Diego, USA.*

Wilhelm, F.H., Trabert, W., Roth, W.T. (in press-c). Characteristics of sighing in panic disorder. *Biological Psychiatry.*

Wilhelm, F.H., Trabert, W., Roth, W.T. (in press-d). Physiological instability in panic disorder and generalized anxiety disorder. *Biological Psychiatry.*

Womack, B. (1971). The analysis of respiratory sinus arrhythmia using spectral analysis and digital filtering. *IEEE Transactions on Biomedical Engineering, 18*, 399–499.

Woods, S.W., Charney, D.S., Loke, J., Goodman, W.K., Redmond, D.E., Heninger, G.R. (1986). Carbon dioxide sensitivity in panic anxiety. Ventilatory and anxiogenic response to carbon dioxide in healthy subjects and patients with panic anxiety before and after alprazolam treatment. *Archives of General Psychiatry, 43*, 900–909.

Yeragani, V.K., Pohl, R., Berger, R., Balon, R., Ramesh, C., Glitz, D., Srinivasan, K., Weinberg, P. (1993). Decreased heart rate variability in panic disorder patients: a study of power-spectral analysis of heart rate. *Psychiatry Research, 46*, 89–103.

Chapter 20
Cardiovascular Reactivity to Work Stress Assessed by Ambulatory Blood Pressure, Heart Rate, and Heart Rate Variability

Tanja G.M. Vrijkotte, Harriëtte Riese, and Eco J.C. de Geus
Department of Biological Psychology, Vrije Universiteit, Amsterdam, The Netherlands

Introduction

Prospective studies have shown that high work stress is associated with increased risk for cardiovascular disease (Bosma, Peter, Siegrist & Marmot, 1998; Lynch, Krause, Kaplan, Salonen & Salonen, 1997; Siegrist, Peter, Junge, Cremer & Seidel, 1990). Despite the epidemiological evidence, the pathophysiological pathways underlying this relationship are still unclear. Exaggerated autonomic nervous system reactivity to work stress has been proposed as a possible etiological mechanism (Everson et al., 1997). Subjects who experience their work as stressful will be repeatedly exposed to protracted periods of emotional upheaval with autonomic activation. If this is accompanied by prolonged increases in heart rate (HR) and blood pressure (BP) this may cause target organ damage (Georgiades, Lemne, De Faire, Lindvall & Fredrikson, 1997) and increase the risk for atherosclerosis (Lynch, Everson, Kaplan, Salonen & Salonen, 1998). Ambulatory monitoring gives us the opportunity to test this hypothesis in a real life work setting. In fact, ambulatory monitoring may be the only alternative to study work stress in an ecologically valid way, because it is difficult or even impossible to envisage a laboratory test battery that could simulate the complex psychological factors involved in the work environment.

This chapter reports on the Amsterdam Work Stress Study where we used 24-hour registrations of continuous HR and intermittent BP on workdays and one non-workday in male white-collar workers and female nurses to investigate the relation between subjective work stress and cardiovascular activation during the workday. Using the data from this study, three main questions will be addressed. First, we tested the validity of the Root Mean Square of Successive Differences (RMSSD) as an index of ambulatory changes in respiratory sinus arrhythmia (RSA), by comparing it to the two "classical" indices of RSA, high frequency band (0.15–0.40 Hz) spectral power and peak-to-through RSA from the combined respiration signal and the Inter Beat Interval (IBI) time series. Next test-retest reliability of three indices of cardiovascular reactivity to a work setting were assessed. Reactivity was defined as either work period versus sleep period on the workday, work period versus leisure period on the workday or workday versus non-workday differences. Finally, in the male white-collar workers the effects of chronic work stress will be examined on reactivity of ambulatory BP, HR, and RMSSD. Increasing evidence shows that work stress effects could be more pronounced during the process of unwinding after work than during the actual work time (Suadicani, Hein & Gyntelberg, 1993; Siegrist, Peter, Junge, Cremer & Seidel (1990). Therefore, special attention will be paid to the processes of recovery during the evening and sleep.

The Amsterdam Work Stress Study

The Amsterdam Work Stress Study examines the relation between work stress and risk factors for cardiovascular disease in two different populations. One population consists of young female nurses (33.7 ± 8.1 y) working at three hospitals in Amsterdam (Riese, van Doornen, Houtman & de Geus, 2000) and the other of middle aged (47.2 ± 5.3 y) male white-collar workers, all working at the same large computer company (Vrijkotte, van Doornen & de Geus, 2000). Non of the subjects received treatment for hypertension, hyperlipidemia or diabetes mellitus, and all subjects were free of overt cardiovascular disease.

Ambulatory registration

Male participants underwent ambulatory monitoring on two workdays, Monday and Thursday, and one non workday (Saturday or Sunday) of the same workweek and always in that order. Female participants were monitored on a workday (third morning shift 7:30 am – 4:15 pm) and one non workday. BP was recorded by a Spacelabs 90207 device at 30-minutes interval only during waking hours. HR and RMSSD were measured continuously for a 24-hour period by the VU-AMS (version 4.6, TD-FPP, Vrije Universiteit, Amsterdam). The VU-AMS has 2 channels for ECG and ICG registration. The memory capacity is 2 MB. The ECG-signal, derived from three electrodes, is led into a differential amplifier, with an input impedance higher than 1 MW, and a CMRR of 70 dB. The amplified ECG is past through a bandpass filter of 17 Hz. The R-top is recognized with a level detector with automatic level adjustment. The output of the level detector is connected to an interrupted request line of the microprocessor. At each R-top, a millisecond counter is read and reset, yielding the raw inter-beat-interval (IBI). From the raw IBI's VU-AMS updates a running average of HR and RMSSD. To get an impression of the physical activity during the registration, the VU-AMS also monitors the amount of body movement (motility) of the subject by an active acceleration sensor. Because the device is always placed on the hip this indexes gross body movements, for instance, transitions in posture and activity. Motility has a range of 0 to 3.2 gsec with a resolution of 0.008 gsec. More information about the VU-AMS can be found on the internet page: www.psy.vu.nl/vu-ams. Reliability and validity aspects and recording methodology of the VU-AMS have been described previously (de Geus & van Doornen, 1996).

Average HR, RMSSD and motility over 30-second periods were stored throughout the 24-hour recording time. Approximately every 30 minutes (10 minutes randomized) the participants were prompted by an audible alarm from the VU-AMS, to fill in a diary. They were instructed to write down time, activities, body postures in chronological order and also consumed cups of coffee, glasses of alcohol and smoked cigarettes. Posture and activity information from the diary were combined with the motility signal using an interactive graphical program and stationary fragments (same posture, same activity) were coded for posture, activity, day and time of the day. Mean values for HR and RMSSD for these coded fragments were calculated by the program and stored simultaneously with start and end time and duration of the period. Each BP value from the Spacelabs device was similarly coded.

Comparison of RMSSD with HF and RSA

Although HR is sometimes measured intermittently, for instance when derived from ambulatory BP monitors, many studies have measured continuous HR. This allows for the additional computation of heart rate variability in the respiratory range (RSA) that is widely regarded to index vagal influences on the myocard (Hayano et al., 1991). The Framingham Heart Study (Sing et al., 1998) has identified decreased vagal tone as a determinant of the progression of hypertension. Apart from its effects on BP, low cardiac vagal tone may predispose to myocard infarction and sudden death by compromising the electrical stability of the heart and by increasing HR, which is a risk factor for cardiac disease independent of BP (Palatini & Julius, 1997). Not surprisingly, low vagal tone has been found to be associated with higher risk for cardiac disease (Liao et al., 1997; Tsuji et al., 1996).

In laboratory settings, RSA is either derived by peak-valley estimation (Katona & Jih, 1975) that uses the time series of IBIs in combination with the respiration signal, or by various quantification techniques that use only the IBI time series, like spectral analysis (Akselrod, Gordon, Madwed, Snidman, Shannon & Cohen, 1985), time domain filtering (Porges & Bohrer, 1980) or Wavelet time-frequency analyses (Houtveen & Molenaar, 2000). Although some disagreement has risen over which method "best" indexes RSA (Byrne & Porges, 1993) these measures have in fact shown excellent correspondence in various resting and task conditions (Grossman, van Beek & Wientjes, 1990; Hayano et al., 1991; Houtveen & Molenaar, 2000).

Ambulatory recording equipment is available that allows computation of all these time-domain and frequency based RSA measures. However, the practical value of these measures in ambulatory research is quite restricted. Valid use of spectral powers, for instance, depends on thorough inspection of each 2 to 3-minute IBI series that are typically used as input. A single missed beat can seriously distort the spectrum (Hilton, Ryan & Beattie, 1997). Reliable peak to through assessment of RSA requires visual inspection of the combined respiration signal with the IBI time series to remove breathing artefacts (de Geus et al., 1995; Grossman et al., 1990).

Therefore, current methods available to extract RSA from continuous ambulatory HR data are very time consuming and almost unfeasible in epidemiology-scaled ambulatory studies in which large amounts of data are collected. A solution would be to use simple time domain measures like the RMSSD as a proxy for vagal tone. Below we test the validity of this approach by comparing ambulatory RMSSD to spectral high frequency power (HF) and peak-to-through RSA from the combined respiration signal and IBI time series.

Twelve women (mean age 37.5 ± 4.5) were selected from the female population. Ambulatory registration of HR for 24 hour was performed by the VU-AMS on a workday and a non-workday. Every 30 (± 10) minutes a beat to beat registration of 5 minutes was registered in which IBIs of consecutive R-peaks were recorded. By means of diary information and a motility signal, the 5 minutes periods were coded for posture (lying, sitting, standing, physical active).

For each of these 5 minutes periods we determined the RMSSD, the peak-to-through RSA and LF, HF and total spectral power. Full description of the methods to derive these measures are described in de Grossman, van Beek & Wientjes (1990) and Mulder (1988). Briefly, peak-to-through RSA combines the respiratory time intervals and the IBIs to obtain the shortest IBI during heart rate acceleration in the inspirational phase (which was made to included 750 milliseconds from the following expiration to account for phase shifts) and the longest IBI during deceleration in the expirational phase (including 750 milliseconds from the following expiratory pause/inspirational phase). The difference between the longest and shortest interval is used as an index of RSA. When no phase-related acceleration or deceleration was found, the breath was assigned a RSA score of zero. Frequency domain analysis of the interbeat intervals was done with the CARSPAN program that is based on sparse Discrete Fourier Transformation and that yields a power-frequency spectrum from 0.01 to 0.50 Hz. The spectrum is based on a series of equidistant samples representing HR. Three frequency bands were deemed of interest: the total power (TF), the power in the frequency band around the intrinsic blood pressure oscillations (0.07–0.14 Hz: MF) and the high frequency band that reflects vagal influence only (0.15–0.40 Hz: HF)

Table 1 shows the Pearson's correlation coefficients between the different indices of vagal tone within each subject with all values, regardless of posture, included. Within-subjects correlation between RMSSD and HF varied between .58 and .92 with median .82. Within subjects correlation between RMSSD and RSA varied between .39 and .89 with median .74. For HF and RMSSD between subject correlations were also calculated, and this was done separately for each posture. High between subject correlation of HF with RMSSD was found throughout: during sitting .91, during physical activity .71., and during sleep .73.

From the male population, a random subset of the 34 participants were selected for detailed RSA analysis. Twenty four hour continuous IBI time series were available on two workdays (Monday and Thursday) and a non-workday. Five minutes epochs from the morning, afternoon, evening and night periods were selected.

Table 1. Within-subject correlations

Subject	RMSSD HF Power	RMSSD MF Power	RMSSD TF Power	RMSSD RSA	RSA HF Power
1	0.71	0.67	0.62	0.74	0.92
2	0.92	0.35	0.60	0.89	0.88
3	0.58	0.51	0.55	0.39	0.62
4	0.75	0.42	0.55	0.79	0.94
5	0.82	0.51	0.78	0.86	0.92
6	0.83	0.38	0.61	0.82	0.86
7	0.83	0.38	0.67	0.74	0.90
8	0.81	0.29	0.50	0.44	0.50
9	0.64	0.19	0.32	0.66	0.72
10	0.70	0.33	0.38	0.67	0.74
11	0.91	0.49	0.72	0.69	0.70
12	0.91	0.16	0.43	0.86	0.87
Median	0.82	0.38	0.58	0.74	0.87

Diary and motility signal were used to assure that the subjects were sitting (lying during sleep). Figure 1 shows the between subject relationship between ambulatory RMSSD and HF as a function of period of the day. Correlations between RMSSD and HF were all highly significant and varied between .54 (Monday morning) and .95 (Non workday sleep) with median value of .89. On all three days, the correlations were lowest during the morning and highest during the night.

From these two studies we conclude that RMSSD is an efficient alternative to RSA or HF to index vagal tone in ambulatory studies.

Reliability of HR, RMSSD and BP reactivity

Ambulatory monitoring studies have concentrated on HR and BP levels, because of the predictive power of these variables for CVD risk (Palatini & Julius, 1997; Kamarck et al., 1998; Mallion, Baguet, Siche, Tremel & De Gaudemaris, 1999). The quantification of BP, HR and their reactivity measures in an ambulatory setting is not as straightforward as in laboratory experiments. There is limited control over known sources of variation in cardiovascular activity during the day other than psychosocial demands like physical activity, posture, food intake, time of day, ambient temperature. Sophisticated statistical analysis have recently been applied to partial out the variance associated with these factors (Fahrenberg & Myrtek, 1996; Kamarck et al., 1998). Fortunately, previous studies have shown that most of the variance due to physical activity in ambulatory signals can be captured largely by looking at posture (Myrtek, Fichtler, Strittmatter & Brugner, 1999; Pieper, Warren & Pickering, 1993; Steptoe, Roy & Evans, 1996). The use of diaries and/or accelerometers are essential in retrieving this information so controlling for influence of physical activity is possible. After controlling for these confounding factors,

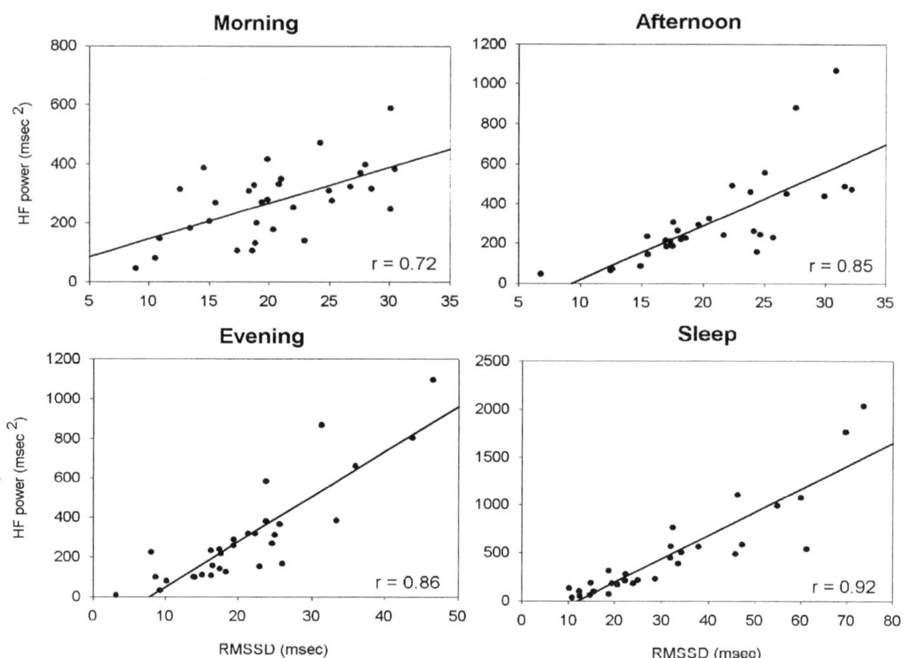

Figure 1. Correlation between two indices of vagal tone, Root Mean Square of Successive Differences (RMSSD) and high frequency (HF) power as a function of period of the day.

indices of real life stress reactivity, like work-sleep or work-leisure or workday-non workday differences will have high ecological validity. However, surprisingly little information is available on the temporal stability of these posture/activity controlled indices of real life stress reactivity.

There is an extensive literature exploring the temporal stability of cardiovascular reactivity in the laboratory (Manuck, Kamarck, Kasprowicz & Waldstein, 1993). Test-retest reliability of cardiovascular reactivity to laboratory stressors is low to moderate, with correlations on average in the .40 to .50 range. As Manuck (1994) stated in his review, reactivity is a more generalized propensity to respond to behavioral stimuli and therefore reactivity should be determined by aggregating subjects' responses over several tasks and several sessions. With this in mind, one would predict high temporal stability of ambulatory reactivity indices like the work period minus leisure period or work period minus sleep period, provided measurements were taken on comparable work-days. In principle, the difference between the average HR level at work and that during sleep can be regarded as the aggregation of the responses to many repeated stressors during the workday.

Ambulatory registrations from the sedentary male populations were used to test this hypothesis. Data from two workdays of the same work week, Monday and Thursday, were compared for the 109 male subjects to assess temporal stability. Mean values of HR, RMSSD and BP for the different periods work, leisure and sleep (the latter only for HR and RMSSD) were determined as well as three reactivity scores: (1) work period minus leisure period (same day), (2) work period minus sleep period (same day), and (3) work period on a workday minus leisure period on a non workday.

The total amount of minutes spent in the activities other than sitting were comparable on Monday and Thursday (see Figure 3). Subjective report of mood, as assessed by the Profile Of Mood States (POMS) (Wald & Mellenbergh, 1990) showed no differences between the workdays in either positive or negative mood. Moreover, test-retest correlations were .58 for positive and .64 for negative mood. Thus, the assumption seems tenable that these workdays yielded comparable levels of work stress both at a group and at an individual level.

Figure 2 shows the relationship between Monday and Thursday for the four ambulatory cardiovascular variables obtained during work period. It is clear from this figure that the correlation between the two workdays is high for all four variables. Table 2 gives the corresponding correlation coefficients, also during leisure period and sleep period, and the reactivity indices. According to Bland and Altman (1986), high correlation coefficients do not always indicate a high repeatability. They recommend coefficient of repeatability (C_{rep}), which describes the range of within

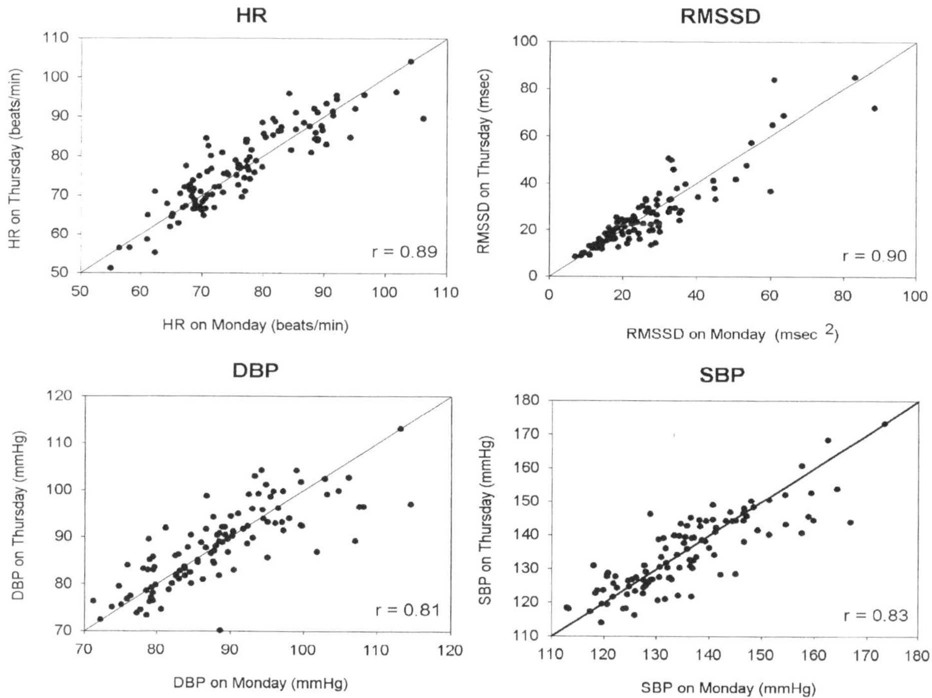

Figure 2. Monday to Thursday test-retest correlation for HR, RMSSD, DBP, and SBP during the work period.

Table 2. Pearson correlation coefficient (r) and coefficient of repeatability (Crep) between Monday and Thursday as a function of period of the day. Mean values are the means of Monday and Thursday.

	All values included			Only sitting values included		
	Mean	r	C_{rep}	Mean	r	C_{rep}
HR (beats/minute)						
work period	79.5 ± 10.1	.88	10.2	77.1 ± 9.9	.89	9.5
leisure period	79.1 ± 9.4	.62	18.5	75.3 ± 9.2	.79	12.6
sleep period	63.8 ± 7.6	.83	9.2	63.8 ± 7.6	.83	9.2
reactivity $_{(work-sleep)}$	15.6 ± 7.9	.75	11.9	13.3 ± 7.7	.76	11.1
reactivity $_{(work-leisure)}$	1.8 ± 5.5	.59	11.2	0.65 ± 6.6	.50	15.5
reactivity $_{(workday- non workday)}$	-0.6 ± 9.0	.85	10.3	1.5 ± 7.6	.83	9.5
RMSSD (msec)						
work period	24.2 ± 9.4	.75	14.6	24.3 ± 9.8	.85	14.4
leisure period	24.8 ± 9.4	.75	14.6	25.0 ± 10.6	.79	11.2
sleep period	31.1 ± 15.1	.81	20.6	32.9 ± 15.1	.81	20.5
reactivity $_{(work-sleep)}$	10.4 ± 15.9	.72	23.8	9.6 ± 16.0	.71	24.4
reactivity $_{(work-leisure)}$	0.3 ± 6.5	.20	21.2	0.5 ± 5.4	.28	16.4
reactivity $_{(workday-non workday)}$	-0.002 ± 8.0	.80	15.7	-.008 ± 9.2	.79	16.5
DBP (mmHg)						
work period	88.3 ± 8.6	.83	10.4	87.9 ± 8.6	.81	11.2
leisure period	85.2 ± 9.0	.84	10.7	84.5 ± 9.1	.83	11.2
reactivity $_{(work-leisure)}$	3.5 ± 6.5	.48	12.9	3.1 ± 4.3	.36	11.9
reactivity $_{(workday-non workday)}$	5.3 ± 5.8	.62	10.4	5.7 ± 6.7	.68	11.3
SBP (mmHg)						
work period	135.7 ± 11.4	.83	14.1	134.6 ± 11.6	.83	14.2
leisure period	133.9 ± 11.7	.82	14.8	132.4 ± 11.5	.82	14.4
reactivity $_{(work-leisure)}$	2.2 ± 6.5	.50	15.1	1.9 ± 5.2	.30	15.2
reactivity $_{(workday-non workday)}$	5.0 ± 6.5	.60	14.1	5.3 ± 7.4	.63	14.2

which 95% of repeated measurements will fall. The coefficient is calculated as 2 x standard deviation of the differences. A wide range relative to the mean indicates low repeatability. The C_{rep} are the lowest for HR and DBP, followed by SBP and RMSSD. Repeatability as a function of posture is described in Table 3. As expected the repeatability was highest during sitting and decreased during physical activity. Based on these findings we expected the repeatability to be higher when only sitting values were included, because it would reduce variance due to differences in physical activity. This was not the case, however, repeatability was the same as when periods with physical activity were included. Probably this reflects the finding that the activity patterns were on average the same on the two workdays (Figure 3). Also we selected a sedentary population: subjects were sitting almost 70% of their time during the work period. Nonetheless, in populations

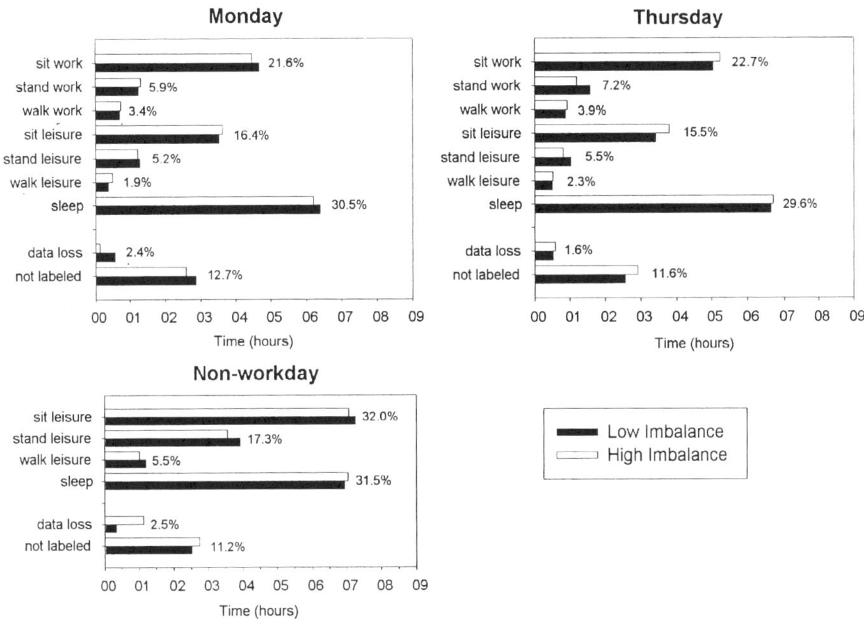

Figure 3. Amount of time spent in different postures during two workdays and one non-workday as a function of effort-reward imbalance.

that are more physically active, like nurses, it could be still be meaningful to select only sitting periods.

The correlation coefficients of the reactivity measures are not as high as the absolute levels but are all highly significant ($p < .001$, except for RMSSD: $p = .05$). The C_{rep} are relatively high compared to the mean reactivity scores, indicating low repeatability. At first glance, the reactivity index obtained by subtracting the non workday from the workday levels seems the best choice in terms of repeatability. However, note that the reactivity values for Monday and Thursday use the same non-workday baseline. For a more fair comparison to the other two reactivity indices we should have repeated the non-workday measurement twice, taking one as baseline for Monday and the other as a baseline for Thursday. In fact, because mean reactivity scores are clustered around zero for $HR_{(work\text{-}leisure)}$, $HR_{(workday\text{-}non\ workday)}$, $RMSSD_{(work\text{-}leisure)}$ and $RMSSD_{(workday\text{-}non\ workday)}$ their repeatability will not be very good.

In conclusion, the repeatability of absolute HR, RMSSD, SBP and DBP in this sedentary white-collar population is high when mean values over relatively long periods, like work or leisure or sleep period, are compared. Repeatability of reactivity scores is low, but test-retest reliability still compares favourable to test-retest reliability of the reactivity of these variables to laboratory stressors. The most optimal reactivity scores are those that contrast day time levels to baseline values at sleep; these yield non-zero reactivity scores for most of the subjects and have the highest repeatability.

Table 3. Pearson correlation coefficient and coefficient of repeatability (Crep) between Monday and Thursday as a function of posture.

	Mean	r	C_{rep}
HR (beats/minute)			
sitting	76.4 ± 9.1	.87	9.7
standing	83.9 ± 9.9	.71	13.7
physical active	90.7 ± 10.1	.66	17.7
RMSSD (msec)			
sitting	25.3 ± 11.8	.83	13.8
standing	26.1 ± 12.6	.84	23.5
physical active	23.3 ± 10.6	.77	17.1
DBP (mmHg)			
sitting	86.4 ± 8.5	.85	9.6
standing	88.2 ± 9.4	.76	12.6
physical active	89.0 ± 9.5	.74	15.2
SBP (mmHg)			
sitting	133.8 ± 11.5	.87	10.8
standing	137.0 ± 12.7	.73	16.9
physical active	139.7 ± 14.0	.73	21.4

Work stress effects on cardiovascular reactivity

Work stress assessment

Although ambulatory monitoring has intrinsic ecological validity, to be useful in stress research it must also have content validity in that it discriminates between subjects who experience their work as high or low stressful. Previous analyses of our male white-collar workers suggest that this is true at least for some aspect of work stress (Vrijkotte, van Doornen & de Geus, 1999; Vrijkotte, van Doornen & de Geus, 2000). The remainder of this chapter will summarize and extend these findings to demonstrate the power of ambulatory recording for psychosocial effects on cardiovascular regulation.

The Effort-Reward Imbalance questionnaire, based on Siegrist's model (Siegrist & Peter, 1994), was used to measure perceived chronic work stress. This model defines chronically stressful experiences at work in terms of a mismatch between high effort spent and low reward received in occupational life. This mismatch is expressed by two summary measures of work stress: imbalance and overcommitment. Of 109 subjects, 23 (21%) experienced a mismatch between extrinsic effort (demanding aspects of the work environment) and reward (esteem reward, monetary gratification and status control) and were classified as high imbalance. Overcommitment states an individual's style of coping with work demands. This component is by itself a mismatch score because those individuals who score high tend to spend an inadequate amount of effort that is not met by the externally defined rewards. Overcommitment was dichotomized so that subjects in the upper tertile were considered high in overcommitment. The groups did not differ in possible confounding factors like: age, body mass index, consumed cups of coffee and glasses of alcohol, smoking, years of services, habitual physical activity. Support for the use of this work stress model comes from the Kuopio Ischaemic Heart Disease Risk Factor Study in which men with high stress induced blood pressure reactivity who also experienced high work demands (Everson et al., 1997) or had low socioeconomic status (Lynch, Krause, Kaplan, Salonen & Salonen, 1997) had the greatest atherosclerotic progression in four years.

Effect of posture

As we mentioned before, posture is the most important confounding factor and our results confirmed this. Ambulatory HR and BP levels increased from lying (only HR) to sitting to standing to walking ($p < .001$) (Table 3). RMSSD also showed a main effect of posture ($p < .001$), but this was completely due to a higher RMSSD during lying (sleep) compared to sitting, standing, and walking (Table 3). This means that any ambulatory cardiovascular differences between the work stress groups could reflect different activity patterns during the ambulatory monitoring days. However, a comparison of the time (number of minutes) spent in different postures showed that the work stress groups did not differ in the total duration of sitting, standing, physical active, and lying (only during sleep) during the various periods of the three days (Figure 3). In fact, statistical analyses on (1) values during sitting-lying only and (2) all values, i.e., regardless of posture, gave essentially the same results. Only the latter values will be presented.

Effect of work stress

On the workdays, DBP and SBP were significantly higher (3.1 and 1.8 mmHg, respectively) during work compared to leisure period (Figure 4). This work-leisure reactivity was, however, independent of work stress. Workday versus non-workday showed that DBP and SBP were lower during the non-workday, even during leisure period on the workdays. On average these DBP/SBP differences were 4.2/3.6 mmHg. And again, this was not different for the high and low imbalance groups.

Within each workday no significant differences between HR and RMSSD during leisure and work periods were found, suggesting that HR and RMSSD reactivity to work was protracted in leisure time. On all days sleep HR was significantly lower and sleep RMSSD significantly higher than the levels during the day. Average reactivity of HR and RMSSD derived by subtracting the non workday from the workday level was very low. Again, for HR and RMSSD, reactivity computed as work minus sleep appears most useful.

The $RMSSD_{(work\text{-}sleep)}$ reactivity was not different between the imbalance groups but the high imbalance group had a higher $HR_{work\text{-}sleep}$ reactivity compared to the

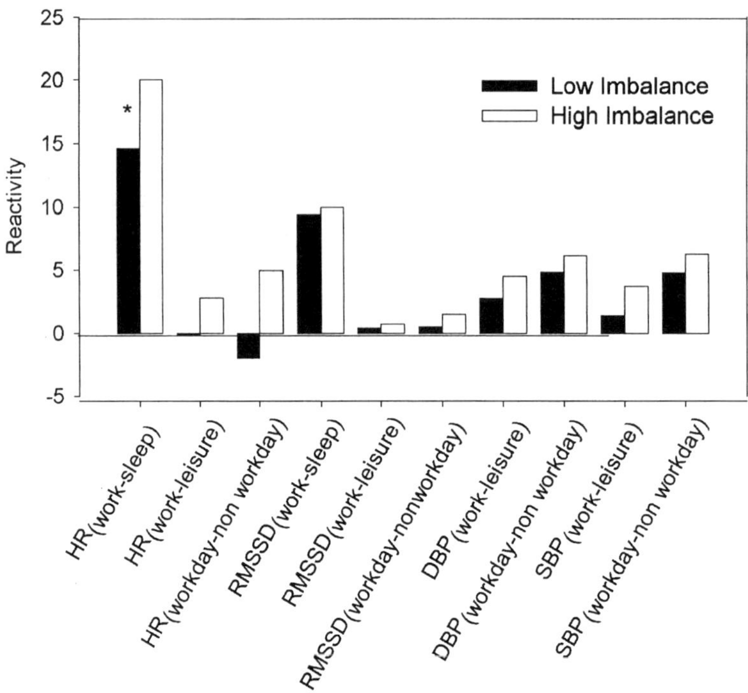

Figure 4. Cardiovascular reactivity to the work period as a function of effort-reward imbalance. Mean reactivity over the two workdays is shown. HR difference in beats/minute, RMSSD difference in msec, BP difference in mmHg. * Sigificant ($p < .05$)

low imbalance group. This difference was on average 6.8 bpm. Higher HR reactivity of this high work stress group remained evident throughout the leisure time period.

Neither overcommitment, the other aspect of work stress in the Siegrist model, nor the interaction of overcommitment with imbalance, had an effect on SBP, DBP, HR and RMSSD reactivity.

Recovery from work stress

A number of recent findings suggests that slow or incomplete recovery from stress may be as important to disease risk as reactivity during stress (Siegrist, Peter, Junge, Cremer & Seidel, 1990; Suadicani, Hein & Gyntelberg, 1993). McEwen used the term 'allostatic load' to refer to the chronic overactivity of stress-related physiological systems, and has argued that chronic allostatic load is frequently manifest as failure to recover following termination of demands (McEwen, 1998). Ambulatory recording provides an excellent setting to test slow recovery processes during sleep after the workday. Our previous analyses showed that HR not only increased more during the workday in the high imbalance group, but also stayed higher during leisure time after work. Overall sleep levels, however, were again comparable. This

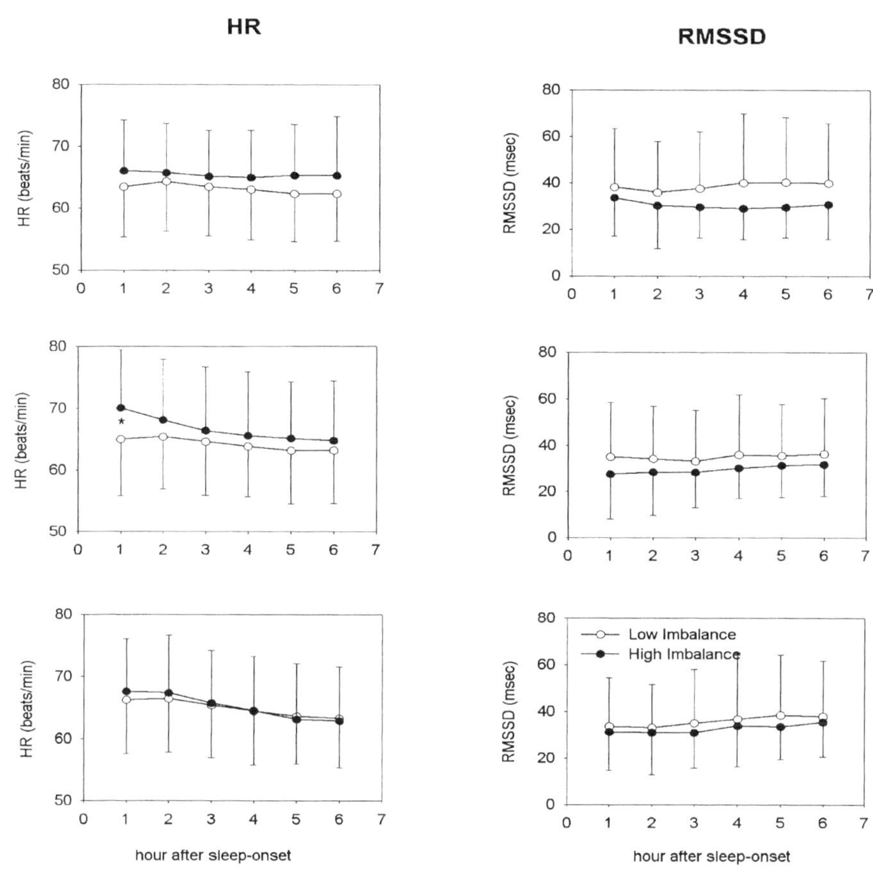

Figure 5: HR and RMSSD (mean and SD) during sleep on Thursday for the high and low imbalance group. * Sigificant (p < .05)

work stress effects disappear gradually in the course of the night. To test this idea, one hour mean values for HR and RMSSD after time to bed were calculated and compared between the work stress groups. Because overcommitment is characterized by worrying and the inability to withdraw from work obligations, we further expected this scale to show the largest sensitivity to individual differences in recovery.

The results, first of all, showed that alcohol and coffee consumption during the day affected HR and RMSSD during the first three hours of sleep. After adjusting for these confounders, HR was higher during the first hour of sleep in the high imbalance group, although significant only on Thursday (Figure 5). RMSSD was not significant different between the imbalance groups. Most surprisingly, overcommitment did not show any effect on HR and RMSSD.

Our results provide only partial support for the importance of compromised recovery to explain the effects of work stress on cardiovascular health. With longer exposure to work stress, however, the high HR found during work, leisure and the first hours of sleep may extend to the whole sleep and possibly non workdays. At some point the overall level of HR may increase to a point where HR dynamics are reduced and work stress is associated with decreased rather than increased HR response to work. This gradual change from HR reactivity to tonic increases in HR with loss of HR dynamics was already proposed by Siegrist (two-stage model of cardiovascular reactivity), with a putative down-regulation of cardiac beta-receptors as an underlying mechanisms (Siegrist & Klein, 1990). Indeed, down-regulation of beta-receptors has been linked previously to chronic stress (Dimsdale, Mills, Patterson, Ziegler & Dillon, 1994) and to diminished HR responses to stress (Eisenhofer, Lambie & Johnson, 1985; Mills, Dimsdale, Ziegler, Berry & Bain, 1990).

Conclusion

In conclusion, 24 hour registration of HR, RMSSD and BP produces reliable and valid information about individual differences in physiological responses to work stress. Also detailed analyses of cardiovascular recovery processes can be made. RMSSD appears to be an efficient index of RSA to index vagal tone in large scale ambulatory studies. Posture and activity are important confounding factors in ambulatory cardiovascular registrations and on-line analysis of posture and motion, described in chapter 13, 14, and 15, would facilitate data analysis and would produce more accurate posture and activity related data. The test-retest reliability of absolute HR, RMSSD and BP during various periods of the day is high. The test-retest reliability of often used ambulatory reactivity measures is lower, but higher than most reliability scores found in the laboratory. The highest and most reliable reactivity scores are obtained by taking mean values during sleep as a baseline. Finally, ambulatory HR reactivity discriminates between high and low chronic work stress. The higher HR found in the high imbalance group during work and leisure period and during the first hours of sleep clearly shows that "real life" work stress has "real life" physiological consequences.

References

Akselrod, S., Gordon, D., Madwed, J.B., Snidman, N.C., Shannon, D.C. & Cohen, R.J. (1995). Hemodynamic regulation: investigation by spectral analysis. *American Journal of Physiology, 249(4),* 867–75.

Bland, J.M. & Altman, D.G.(1986). Statistical methods for assessing agreement between two methods of clinical measurement. *Lancet, 8(1),* 307–10.

Bosma, H., Peter, R., Siegrist, J. & Marmot, M. (1998). Two alternative job stress models and the risk of coronary heart disease. *American Journal of Public Health, 88*, 68–74.

Byrne, E.A. & Porges, S.W. (1993). Data-dependent filter characteristics of peak-valley respiratory sinus arrhythmia estimation: a cautionary note. *Psychophysiology, 30(4),* 397–404.

Everson, S.A., Lynch, J.W., Chesney, M.A., Kaplan, G.A., Goldberg, D.E., Shade, S.B., Cohen, R.D., Salonen, R. & Salonen, J.T. (1997). Interaction of workplace demands and cardiovascular reactivity in progression of carotid atherosclerosis: population based study. *British Medical Journal, 314,* 553–558.

Dimsdale, J.E., Mills, P., Patterson, T., Ziegler, M. & Dillon, E. (1994). Effects of chronic stress on beta-adrenergic receptors in the homeless. *Psychosomatic Medicine, 56,* 290–295.

Eisenhofer, G., Lambie, D.G. and Johnson, R.H. (1985). Beta-adrenoceptor responsiveness and plasma catecholamines as determinants of cardiovascular reactivity to mental stress. *Clinical Science, 69,* 483–492.

Fahrenberg, J. & Myrtek, M. (eds) (1996). *Ambulatory assessment: Computer-assisted psychological and psychophysiological methods in monitoring and field studies.* Seattle, WA: Hogrefe & Huber.

Georgiades, A., Lemne, C., De Faire, U., Lindvall, K. & Fredrikson, M. (1997). Stress-induced blood pressure measurements predict left ventricular mass over three years among borderline hypertensive men. *European Journal of Clinical Investigation, 27,* 733–739.

Geus, E.J.C. de, Willemsen, A.H.M., Klaver, C.H.A.M & van Doornen, L.J.P. (1995). Ambulatory measurement of and respiratory sinus arrhythmia and respiration rate. *Biological Psychology, 41,* 205–227.

Geus, E.J.C. de & Doornen. L.J.P. van (1996). Ambulatory assessment of parasympathetic/ sympathetic balance by impedance cardiography. In: J. Fahrenberg, M. Myrtek (eds). *Computer-assisted Psychological and psychophysiological methods in monitoring and field studies.* Seattle, WA: Hogrefe & Huber Publishers, 141–163.

Grossman, P., Stemmler, G. & Meinhardt, E. (1990). Paced respiratory sinus arrhythmia as an index of cardiac parasympathetic tone during varying behavioral tasks. *Psychophysiology, 27(4),* 404–416.

Grossman, P., van Beek, J. & Wientjes, C. (1990). A comparison of three quantification methods for estimation of respiratory sinus arrhythmia. *Psychophysiology, 27(6),* 702–14.

Hayano, J., Sakakibara, Y., Yamada, A., Yamada, M., Mukai, S., Fujinami, T., Yokoyama, K., Watanabe, Y. & Kazuyuki, T. (1991). Accuracy of assessment of cardiac vagal tone by heart rate variability in normal subjects. *American Journal of Cardiology, 67,* 199–204.

Hilton, M., Ryan, P. & Beattie, J. (1997). Spectral analysis of heart rate variability: the impact of R-wave measurement error. *American Journal of Cardiology, 79(6):*844–845

Houtveen, J., Molenaar, P.C.M. (in press). Comparison between the Fourier and Wavelet methods of spectral analysis applied to stationary and non-stationary heart period data. *Psychophysiology.*

Kamarck, T.W., Shiffman, S.M., Smithline, L., Goodie, J.L., Paty, J.A., Gnys, M. & Yi-Kuan Jong, J. (1998). Effects of task strain, social conflict, and emotional activation on ambulatory cardiovascular activity: Daily life consequences of recurring stress in a multiethnic adult sample. *Health Psychology, 17(1),* 17–29.

Kamarck, T.W., Debski, T.T. & Manuck, S.B. (2000). Enhancing the laboratory-to-life generalizability of cardiovascular reactivity using multiple occasions of measurements. *Psychophysiology, 37,* 533–542.

Katona, P.G. & Jih, F. (1975). Respiratory sinus arrhythmia: noninvasive measure of parasympathetic cardiac control. *Journal of Applied Physiology, 39 (5),* 801–805.

Liao, D., Cai, J., Rosamond, W.D., Barnes, R.W., Hutchinson, R.G., Whitsel, E.A., Rautaharju, P. & Heiss, G. (1997). Cardiac autonomic function and incident coronary heart disease: a population-based case-cohort study. *American Journal of Epidemiology, 145,* 696–706.

Llabre, M.M., Ironson, G.H. & Spitzer, S.B. (1988). How many blood pressure measurements are enough? An application of generalizability theory to the study of blood pressure reliability. *Psychophysiology, 25,* 97–106.

Lynch, J.W., Krause, N., Kaplan, G.A., Salonen, R. & Salonen, J.T. (1997). Workplace demands, economic reward, and progression of carotid atherosclerosis. *Circulation, 96,* 302–307.

Lynch, J.W., Everson, S.A., Kaplan, G.A., Salonen, R. & Salonen, J.T. (1998). Does low socioeconomic status potentiate the effects of heightened cardiovascular responses to stress on the progression of carotid atherosclerosis? *American Journal of Public Health, 88,* 289–394.

Mallion, J.M., Baguet, J.P., Siche, J.P., Tremel, F. & De Gaudemaris, R. (1999). Clinical value of ambulatory blood pressure monitoring. *Journal of Hypertension, 17(5),* 585–95

Manuck, S.B., Kamarck, T.W., Kasprowicz, A.S. & Waldstein, R.R. (1993). Stability and patterning of behaviorally evoked cardiovascular reactivity. In J. Blascovich, E.S. Katlin (eds), *Cardiovascular reactivity to psychological stress & disease.* (pp. 111–134). Washington DC: American Psychological Association.

Manuck, S.B. (1994). Cardiovascular reactivity in cardiovascular disease: "Once more unto the breach". *International Journal of Behavioral Medicine, 1(1),* 4–31.

Markovitz, J.H., Raczynski, J.M., Wallace, D., Chettur, V. & Chesney, M.A. (1998). Cardiovascular reactivity to video game predicts subsequent blood pressure increases in young men: The CARDIA study. *Psychosomatic Medicine, 60,* 186–191.

Mills, P.J., Dimsdale, J.E., Ziegler, M.G., Berry, C.C. & Bain, R.D. (1990). Beta-Adrenergic receptors predict heart rate reactivity to a psychosocial stressor. *Psychosomatic Medicine, 52,* 621–623.

Mulder, L.J.M. (1988). *Assessment of cardiovascular reactivity by means of spectral analysis.* Doctoral Thesis. Groningen: Universiteitsdrukkerij R.U.G

Myrtek, M., Fichtler, A., Strittmatter, M. & Brügner, G. (1999). Stress and strain of blue and white collar workers during work and leisure time: results of psychophysiological and behavioral monitoring. *Applied Ergonomics, 30,* 341–351.

Palatini, P. & Julius, S. (1997). Heart rate and the cardiovascular risk. *Journal of Hypertension, 15,* 3–17.

Pieper, C., Warren, K. & Pickering, T.G. (1993). A comparison of ambulatory blood pressure and heart rate at home and work on work and non-work days. *Journal of Hypertension, 11,* 177–183.

Porges, S.W., Bohrer, R.E., Cheung, M.N., Drasgow, F., McCabe, P.M. & Keren, G. (1980). New time-series statistic for detecting rhythmic co-occurrence in the frequency domain: the weighted coherence and its application to psychophysiological research. *Psychological Bulletin, 88(3)*:580–7

Riese, H., van Doornen, L.J.P. & Houtman, I.L.D. (2000). Job strain and risk indicators for cardiovascular disease in young female nurses. *Health Psychology, 19,* 429–440.

Siegrist, J. & Klein, D. (1990). Occupational stress and cardiovascular reactivity in blue-collar workers. *Work & Stress, 4(4),* 295–304.

Siegrist, J. & Peter, R. (1994). Job stressors and coping characteristics in work-related disease: issues of validity. *Work & Stress, 8,* 130–140.

Siegrist, J., Peter, R., Junge, A., Cremer, P. & Seidel D. (1990). Low status control, high effort at work and ischemic heart disease: Prospective evidence from blue–collar men. *Social and Science in Medicine, 31,* 1127–1134.

Sing, J.P., Larson, M.G., Tsuij, H., Evans, J.C., O'Donnell, C.J. & Levy, D. (1998). Reduced heart rate variability and new-onset hypertension: Insights into pathogenesis of hypertension: The Framingham Heart Study. *Hypertension, 32,* 293–297.

Steptoe, A., Roy, M.P. & Evans, O. (1996). Psychosocial influences on ambulatory blood pressure over working and non-working days. *Journal of Psychophysiology, 10,* 218–227.

Suadicani, P., Hein, H.O. & Gyntelberg, F. (1993). Are social inequalities as associated with the risk of ischaemic heart disease a result of psychosocial working conditions? *Arterosclerosis, 101,* 165–175.

Tsuji, H., Larson, M.G., Venditti, F.J., Manders, E.S., Evans, J.C., Feldman, C.L. & Levy D. (1996). Impact of reduced heart rate variability on risk for cardiac events. *Circulation, 94,* 2850–2855.

Vrijkotte, T.G.M., van Doornen, L.J.P. & de Geus, E.J.C. (1999). Work stress and metabolic and hemostatic risk factors. *Psychosomatic Medicine, 61,* 796–805.

Vrijkotte, T.G.M. & van Doornen, L.J.P. & de Geus, E.J.C. (2000). Effects of work stress on ambulatory blood pressure, heart rate, and heart rate variability. *Hypertension, 2000, 35,* 880–886.

Wald, F.D.M. & Mellenbergh, G.J. (1990). De verkorte versie van de Nederlandse vertaling van de Profile of Mood States (POMS). *Nederlands Tijdschrift voor de Psychologie, 45,* 86–90.

Chapter 21
Objective Characteristics of Jobs Affect Blood Pressure at Work, after Work, and at Night

Renate Rau
Department of Work and Organizational Psychology, University of Technology Dresden, Germany

Introduction

Five years ago, we discussed methods and results of psychophysiological analysis of stress and strain in real life work situations (Rau & Richter, 1996). Based on Hacker's (1985, 1986) action regulation theory we reported results of stress/strain analyses according to all components of sequential completeness which should be included in all work activities (Frese & Zapf, 1994; Hacker, 1985; 1994; 1998; Miller et al., 1960; Volpert, 1987;). These components were goal setting, preparing and organizing the tasks, executing, and feedback. The strain analysis of the reported studies was related exclusively to the working time and thus to short-term effects of work load, such as fatigue, boredom, vigilance, etc. The methodological framework of the analysis and assessment of such short term effects is defined in the ISO 10075 (International Organization for Standardization ISO 10075, 1991; ISO 10075–2, 1994). The study of such short-term effects can only be a first step towards discovering possible effects of work stress on health. The aim for an enlargement of the stress/strain paradigm from short-term effects to long term effects was not achieved with our first studies reported 1996 (Rau & Richter). However, study of the effects of work stress during the time after work including the night is necessary when the workplace is seen as a potential source of stressors that might contribute to the development of heart disease risk factors. Furthermore, the time between work and night has to be considered since within this time further strained or relaxing activities can be carried out by the subjects. Since methods for an ambulatory monitoring of psychophysiological data have been become available, a growing number of studies include cardiovascular changes over 24 hours including ordinary work, leisure and night time. However, up to now the major interest has only been the analysis psychophysiological changes during work. Whereas there is a growing interest in recovery processes during the night, the time between work and night has hardly been examined (see studies regarding the time after work and night, for example, Frankenhaeuser, 1993; Landsbergis et al., 1994; Lundberg et al., 1992; Pickering, 1993; Rau, 1998; Schnall et al., 1998; Theorell, Knox et al., 1985; Theorell,

Ahlberg-Hulten et al., 1993; Theorell, Perski et al., 1988).

The study of work-related determinants of coronary heart disease has been mostly influenced by the job demand/decision latitude model proposed by Karasek and co-workers (Karasek, 1979; Karasek & Theorell, 1990). Data reported by Theorell et al. (1991), Pickering, Schnall et al. (1991), Rau (1996), Schnall et al. (1998) and Belkic, Emdad & Theorell (1998) indicate that sympathetic nervous activity may be increased during occupational stress. In their studies, occupational stress was evaluated as 'high job strain', which is a combination of high demands at work with low decision latitude or control. Considerable evidence exists linking the exposure to "job strain" to hypertension (Peter & Siegrist, 2000; Pickering, 1993; Rau et al., in press; Schnall et al., 1998; Theorell, Ahlberg-Hulten et al., 1993; van Egeren, 1992). In a prospective cohort study (Whitehall II) 6895 male and 3413 female civil servants were tested during three phases between 1985 and 1993 (Bosma, Stansfeld & Marmot, 1998). It was found that low job control (but not job demand or social support) increased the risk of coronary heart disease (angina pectoris, severe pain across the chest, ischemia). Both self-reported and independently (by personnel managers) assessed job control showed roughly similar associations with coronary heart disease.

Data of the reported studies regarding job demand and job control were mainly based on subjective work analyses (such as JCQ, Karasek et al., 1998). Therefore, some researchers have started to employ analytic techniques to overcome self-report bias and to obtain more objective measures of job characteristics (for example, Pieper, LaCroix & Karasek, 1989; Theorell et al., 1991; Landsbergis et al., 1994). The average scores of psychosocial work characteristics for a particular job title are used for individuals with that job title (Johnson et al., 1990; DOT 1979). For example the Swedish classification system (Johnson et al., 1990) consists of the following three psychosocial work characteristics: psychological demands, control, and social support, as well as the two physical work characteristics: physical job demands, and hazardous work. One of the ideas of this system is that it gives the researcher the possibility of avoiding individual bias that could be influenced by personality. However, with the changes in work organization (for example, flexibility of working time, lean production) and the development of new occupations, the use of occupational group-based classification systems is becoming increasingly problematic. The classification system is based upon the idea that an occupation does not change over time and that, for instance, all secretaries who have been working at least twenty years in that occupation and who are older than 45 years have the same level of job control and psychological demands. However, the national occupational averages may have changed substantially over the intervening period. Additionally, Schwartz, Pieper and Karasek (1988) have already reported that a large within variance exists in job characteristics. Therefore, an alternative operationalization of job strain other than the occupational classification system is indicated. Before discussing alternative methods, changes in the world of work are represented, since these changes require the development and use of objective methods of analysis.

Changes in the world of work

During the last two decades we have observed rapid changes in work organization and work content, such as:

- Psychomental work load has risen while bodily activity has decreased.
  Therefore, musculoskeletal diseases constitute one of the modern threats to employees' health (Levi, Sauter & Shimomitsu, 1999). Several studies have shown that physically monotonous and repetitive work, but also psychosocial factors at the work place, are associated with musculoskeletal diseases (for example, Lundberg, Dohns et al., 1999; Moon & Sauter, 1996; Sandsjö et al., 2000; Hägg, 2000). For monotonous and repetitive work, employees typically have hardly any influence and control over their work situation and seem to be exposed to higher levels of chronic stress (Sjøgaard, Lundberg & Kadefors, 2000). Lundberg et al. (1994) found enhanced effects of a mental stressor on trapezius electromyogram when this stressor was combined with physical load.
- Increasing flexibility of work time, characterized on one hand by a shortening of work time to part time jobs and on the other hand by the increased use of overtime in organizations.
  It is not surprising that the effect of overtime on health has been studied regarding cardiovascular risks (Starrin et al., 1990; Uehata, 1991; Harmar and Ilmarinen, 1999), depression (for example, Kawakami & Haratani, 1999), non-insulin dependent diabetes mellitus (for example, Proctor et al., 1996), and fatigue (Schorr, 1991) in a similar way to the work already done in stress research.
  Beside an increase of overtime work, there is also a shift towards contingent work arrangements. The traditional long-term contracts with an implicit understanding of ongoing employment are gradually disappearing (Lewis & Cooper, 1999; Levi, Sauter & Shimomitsu, 1999; McLean Parks, Kidder & Gallgher, 1998). Because of the temporary character of their employment, temporary employees are generally expected to express less favorable job attitudes and less commitment to the organization (Pearce, 1998). Often, they have little control over the termination, the duration and the content of their work (Beard & Edwards, 1995). Low control, unpredictable work situation, roll ambiguity, uncertain personal income due to the temporary work can contribute to job strain, impaired well being and diseases (Martens et al., 1999; Sverke, Gallagher & Hellgren, 2000). When contingent work is voluntarily chosen by employees themselves (for example, for a better balancing of work and family roles), this can also have positive effects. More research is needed for evaluation of the different natures of contingent work.
- The introduction of new systems of work organization like lean production, total quality management, etc., which lead to major changes in work design.
  Landsbergis, Cahill and Schnall (1999) reviewed studies which examined the impact of new systems of work organization like Japanese production management/lean production on work content and job stress. Thirteen studies tested effects of lean production in the car industry. Lean production in the car industry is based on detailed standardization and short work cycles (about 60 seconds) and accompa-

nied by high work intensity and low decision latitude and only a modest and/or temporary increase of decision authority and skill levels. Landsbergis, Cahill and Schnall (1999) concluded that work in lean production systems can be considered to have high job strain. Additionally, lean production is designed to remove activities (for example, walking space at work stations; walking time) and time (waiting time, slack time, etc., up to seconds) or more generally to remove indirect work between subtasks that is not absolutely essential to production. Thus, employees do not have the possibility to carve out some time for buffering activities like rest, bodily activities or social activities.

- Use of information and communication technology (ICT).
  The use of ICT often leads to an increased work intensity during decreased time for a task, greater attentional demands, emotional loading interruptions and higher demands on the cognitive system as a result of increased processing of information (Carayon & Zijlstra, 1999; Roe, Zijlstra & Leonova, 1996). Furthermore, there is a tendency towards a reduction of resting periods by the reduction of subtasks that require low concentration. Resting periods are also reduced when task execution is controlled by the computer, for example, when inputting information into forms. Immediately after one task is finished, the computer is ready to start the next task (Baitsch et al., 1991).
- Qualifications become obsolete during a vocational biography.
  Therefore, life-time learning is required (Bergmann, 1998). The best solution for such life-time learning is qualification by working. But with the introduction of new work organization systems like lean production, increases in skill levels are very modest (Landbergis, Cahill & Schall, 1999). An additional problem in industrial societies is that people's abilities for life-time learning are reduced with the duration and frequency of unemployment (Bergmann, 1996).
- Under the headline of new work organization systems, the introduction of small group activities (for example, total quality control, total quality management) which, in contrast to employers, has fewer or no positive effects for the employees, must also be discussed (Imai, 1986).

The question is here, whether group work is a result of the team concept or of workers collectivity. Workers' collectivity means groups which are constructed by workers themselves to improve their social support at work. In contrast, the team concept is based on socially engineered groups that have been constructed to maximize productivity and to maintain managerially oriented norms and values (Johnson & Hall, 1995). Thus, the team concept might encourage workers to treat each other as competitors rather than as coworkers. This increases the risk of social stress.

When we look at the changes in the world of work, it is not surprisingly that employees today complain less about physical load, but rather about work-related psychical stress (Sauter et al., 1999). Therefore, the analysis of work places that lead to psychical stress and in the longer term to job strain and an increased risk of disturbed well-being or the development of risk factors for diseases is not finished yet.

However, inherent to the introduction of new systems of work organization is the change of work design. The question is, can we influence work design towards healthy work by considering the employer's aim of improved productivity, quality and profitability? This is a very complex question. To find first answers it should be examined whether there are objective methods of analysing and designing work places and whether these are suitable for the job demand/control model of Karasek (1979). Confirmation to the job demand/control model is preferred because most studies done according to job strain are based on this model. Such confirmation would also allow us to examine whether the findings of a relationship between psychosocial work characteristics (as a rule analysed by questionnaires) and job strain can be confirmed by using an objective method of work analysis. Such a method is the Task Diagnostic Survey (Rudolph et al., 1987; Hacker et al., 1995) which is based on action regulation theory (Hacker, 1985, 1998). Job demands and decision latitudes across different work settings can be compared by means of this method, applied to each individual work place. In contrast to the occupational group-based classification system, the Task Diagnostic Survey allows the analysis and evaluation of specific workplaces, and thus the potential source of stressors.

Ambulatory blood pressure monitoring in strain research

The effects of the exposure to job strain can not only be examined during working time. If this exposure plays a role in the development of sustained hypertension, it should be possible to demonstrate that job strain can cause a rise in blood pressure not only during work but also during leisure time and at night. The examination of the relationship between job strain and blood pressure changes should be based on ambulatory blood pressure monitoring. This method has the advantage that there is no observer bias and the number of readings is greatly increased. Additionally, this method is more ecologically valid than casual measure of blood pressure since blood pressure is measured during a person's normal daily activities including work (Schnall, Landsbergis & Baker, 1994). However, the reliability of ambulatory blood pressure can be less than that of casual measures when some conditions such as setting, body position and physical activity, external noise (that affect blood pressure taking), etc., are not controlled for (Fahrenberg, 1996; Fahrenberg & Myrtek, 2001; Käppler, 1994; Pickering, 1991; Schmidt & Jain, 1996). In a study with 178 normotensive and borderline hypertensive men, it was shown that physical job demands affect the blood pressure even at times without any motor activation (Rau et al., in press). Hierarchical regression analyses yielded highly significant effects of physical job demands on blood pressure during work in sitting position and during the night in men (R^2 ranged between .05 and .08 for diastolic blood pressure and between .07 and .10 for systolic blood pressure).

Studies analysing the effect of an exposure to high job strain on leisure-time and night time have come to different and partly contradictory results. Data reported by Theorell et al. (1991), Pickering, Schnall et al. (1991), and Fox, Dwyer and Ganster (1993) indicate that sympathetic nervous system activity may increase at work with high job strain and remain elevated at night, thus hampering nocturnal rewind. In borderline hypertensives, Theorell et al. (1991) did not find an association between exposure to job strain and systolic blood pressure, while diastolic blood pressure was elevated at work and during sleep in those with high job strain occupations. The effect of exposure to job strain on ambulatory blood pressure was investigated in a three-year follow-up study by Schnall et al. (1998). Using 24 hour ambulatory blood pressure monitoring on two occasions 3 years apart, they found that the group having high job strain at both baseline and follow-up had higher systolic (11 mmHg) and diastolic (7 mmHg) blood pressure at work and at home as compared to the group that did not have high job strain at either assessment. On the other hand, in longitudinal studies by Theorell, Knox, Svensson, and Waller (1985), Theorell et al. (1988), and Landsbergis et al. (1994), high demands combined with a low decision-latitude (high 'job strain') were associated with elevated ambulatory systolic blood pressure at work but not during leisure time. An explanation for the different results of the relationship between job strain and cardiovascular activity during the time after work might be the relatively undifferentiated use of the labels "leisure time" and "time at home". The activities after work consist both of stressing activities and of passive relaxation. Therefore, the labels "leisure time" and "time at home" have to be explained in future studies. Additionally, there are only a few studies that consider the effect of the exposure to job strain on the ability to relax or the data about sleep quality beside the effect on cardiovascular changes at night. Since the prospective Rotterdam Civil Servant Study (van Diest & Appels, 1994), it is known that patients who had a myocardial infarction report for the time before their infarct that they felt excess fatigue. These feelings were attributed to prolonged overwork by many patients. This corresponds with the results by Ertel et al. (2000). For so called 'high-tech jobs' they found a significant correlation between working hours per week and a disturbed relaxation ability.

Ambulatory assessment of a working day - an empirical study

The aim of the present study is to explore the effect of objectively measured exposure to job strain on the cardiovascular reactions at work, after work and during sleep following a working day. The following hypotheses were tested:

H 1: The exposure to high job strain as compared with exposure to low job strain is associated with an increased cardiovascular activation at work, after work and a delayed cardiovascular recovery at night.

H 2: Negative health consequences on sleep such as reduced relaxation ability and sleep disturbances are expected for employees who are exposed to high job strain.

Method

Subjects

117 women aged between 20 and 60 years were tested. The women were employed in white-collar jobs and included software engineers as well as employees in public services. In order to recruit them, contact with the leadership of the company and with the "Betriebsrat" (this is a committee of chosen agents who represent the interests of employees facing the leadership of the company) was necessary to get the permission for the study within the companies and during working time. Afterwards women were recruited through oral presentations at the companies and written presentations by using the internal company e-mail systems. As a rule we recruited all women of a division within a department. All women were paid 50 DM for participating in the study.

The sample was reduced because only women regularly working 40 hours per week with complete data from the ambulatory assessment were included in the statistical analyses; 105 women fulfilled both conditions.

There was a further down sizing of the sample because of the classification according to the exposure to job strain. The method of classification is described in the next section. After that, the sample will be described which was finally used in the statistical analyses.

Objective task analysis

The classification of the exposure to high versus low job strain was based on the quadrant model of Karasek (1979). In the present study the operationalization of the job demands and job decision latitude that creates the risk of job strain was not based on dichotomizing self-reports of job demands and decision latitude, but on objectively measured work characteristics using the Task Diagnosis Survey (TDS: Hacker et al., 1995). The TDS scales were rated by experts, one occupational psychologist and one or two colleagues of each subject. The Task Diagnosis Survey is based on Hacker's model of action regulation (Hacker, 1985, 1994). This survey consists of the following five work-related dimensions:

Table 1: Description of the sample

	All subjects	Subjects working full time and having complete data
	n	n
High job strain group	17	17 [a]
Low job strain group	44	41 [a]
No exposure to high or low strain	52	47
Missing	4[b]	12
N	117	105

Note. [a] subjects used in further analyses (N = 58)

[b] missing because subjects did not work regular time on the day of 24-hour assessment.

- technological and organizational work characteristics (12 scales for temporal degrees of freedom, procedural degrees of freedom, quantity/quality-conflicts, work-related decision processes, feedback, partial activity, work cycle time, possibility of prediction, information about organization, information about results, etc.),
- work-related cooperation and communication (three scales for amount of cooperation, kind of cooperation, kind of communication),
- mental regulation requirements (one scale for the level of mental operations),
- learning potential (two scales for qualification application, requirement to learn new things),
- responsibility (two scales for responsibility for results, processes or people, and individual versus group responsibility for results).

The evaluation of analysed work dimensions is supported by thresholds for each of the TDS scales. Thresholds are defined as the lowest scale value that should be met in order to avoid fatigue, stress, monotony, psychosomatic complaints, or losing skills. These lowest scale values are empirically tested values of the TDS. If all of the scale-thresholds are linked, a profile will be visible. In the TDS, this profile is known as the "minimal profile".

In addition to the use of the TDS, women were asked about their regular working hours and about their overtime work (in hours per week).

In this study, *employees were classified as exposed to "high job strain"* when the objective task analyses yielded scores of decision latitude and job demand below their threshold values defined by the TDS. In detail, the *decision latitude* was determined by the TDS scale "procedural degrees of freedom". This scale measures the objective possibilities of determining the working procedures. When the procedure is fixed, for instance, an employee has no freedom to decide what is to do and how something is to be done, or to choose the sequence of working procedures, then the scale 'procedural degrees of freedom' does not meet the threshold value and has to be evaluated as below the minimal profile.

Job demands were determined by the TDS scale "temporal degrees of freedom". This scale asks about employees' possibility of planning the time for executing the subtasks within a day or within a week. Indirectly, this is a question of work intensity. When the time for each step is strongly limited and the technical-related phases of each step are short (ranged between three and a maximum of 30 minutes), the scale "temporal degrees of freedom" does not meet the threshold value and has to be evaluated as below the minimal profile.

The question of overtime work provides additional information for the operationalization of job demand. Employees may tend to work longer, when time pressure occurs because the daily amount of work can not be executed during regular working hours. Therefore, women were additionally classified as exposed to *"high job strain"*, when the scores of the "procedural degrees of freedom" scale were below the "minimal profile" and excessive work was done, defined by doing overtime work.

When the scores of the scales "procedural degrees of freedom" and "temporal degrees of freedom" are higher than the thresholds for the minimal profile and women do not work overtime, *employees are classified as exposed to "low job strain"*.

Women who were exposed to neither high nor to low job strain (n = 47) were not included in the statistical analyses. A total of 17 women were classified as exposed to high job strain and 41 women were classified as exposed to low job strain. The sample which is used in the statistical analysis consists of 58 women (see Table 1).

Chi-squared analyses and t-tests were conducted comparing women exposed to high job strain and women exposed to low job strain on a number of demographic measures. The two job strain groups did not significantly differ on age, bodymass index or number of children (see Table 2). However, the number of smokers tended to be higher in the low strain group [n = 12 (29.3%), non-smokers, n = 29 (70.7%)] compared with the number of smokers in the high strain group [n = 1 (5.9%); non-smokers, n = 16 (94.1%)], χ^2 (1, N=58) = 3.78, $p < .10$.

Ten of the 58 women were on anti-hypertensive medication (five in the low and five in the high strain group). A chi-squared analysis was performed to examine hypertensive and normotensive status as a function of the exposure to low and high job strain. Analysis revealed no significant difference (χ^2 1, N=58) = 2.50, *ns*).

The women who were hypertensives or on anti-hypertensive medication were excluded from all statistical analyses of physiological data.

Procedure

All women were tested during 24 hours on a normal working day. Women performed their regular work for eight hours, with leisure time in the afternoon and the evening, and then they slept. Women arrived at the laboratory which was set up in the companies between 7 and 8 am. The ambulatory equipment was put on and then they were given instructions for blood pressure reading (keep the arm as motionless as possible) and for answering the diary questions on the handheld computer (see next section). After the whole procedure, which took around 15 minutes, women were dismissed.

After the 24 hours of ambulatory assessment, women returned to the laboratory again. The physiological data and the handheld computer data were transferred to the laboratory computer. Based on this

Table 2. Age, Bodymass Index (BMI), number of children based on the exposure to low and high job strain.

	Job Strain	
	Low (n = 17)	High (n = 41)
Age		
M	40.6	39.9
SD	9.12	12.57
t (58)	- 2.35 ns	
BMI		
M	24.2	26.1
SD	3.64	5.85
t (58)	1.52 ns	
Children [a]		
no	1	4
one	27	6
more than one	15	2
χ^2 (2, N=46)	4.53 ns	

Note. [a] 12 women did not answer the question for children

data, women were questioned about their activities, special emotions, and stress they experienced within the last 24 hours. The whole procedure took 30 minutes in the laboratory.

Women were asked to complete questionnaires regarding sociodemographic data, relaxation ability and sleep disturbances. Relaxation ability was assessed using the FABA-Questionnaire (Richter et al., 1996). In this questionaire critical values are defined to identify subjects with a disturbed relaxation ability. The critical values differ depending on gender and age (younger group: < 30 years, middle-aged group: 30 – 50 years, older group: > 50 years).

Sleep disturbances were evaluated using the Sleep Wake Experience List (van Diest, 1990), which asks the women for their sleep experiences during the last three months. This questionnaire also defined critical values for each dimension (for example, falling asleep, waking up during the night etc), and for the general diagnosis of a sleep disturbance. These critical values are independent of gender and age.

Recording of setting and variables of introspection

Before the day of ambulatory assessment, task analysis and an interview about normal daily activities were carried out in order to define specific individual programs for questions of the setting on the handheld computers. Women were asked about their regular activities at work and at home as well as about people they are usually in contact with. Handheld computers (PSION 3a) were used as computer diaries. Women kept these computer diaries to record their location (for example, at work, at home, in the garden, etc.), body position (standing, sitting, lying), and activities (an individual checklist was presented with the activities which had been identified during pre-interview, for example, reading, repairing something, doing the housework, etc.) during the whole day until going to bed. In addition, women repeatedly answered questions concerning perceived control, perceived stress and moods. The control and the stress dimension were rated on seven-point scales from "*not at all*" to "*completely*". Positive and negative affect ratings were used for indicating mood. The items for positive and negative affect were drawn from the "PA/NA-model" by Schallberger and Pfister (in press). This instrument is based on a 2-factor model of affect which is similar to that of Watson and Tellegen (1985). Questions for affects were bipolar and were rated on seven-point scales from "-3" (for example "sad") to "+3" (for example "very happy"). The questions on the handheld computer had to be answered hourly by the women over the whole 24 hour period with the exception of the night. Women were called to answer the questions by the computer's alarm-beep.

Recording of blood pressure

Blood pressure readings were taken by the Korotkoff-method using ambulatory monitoring systems (BOSO TM2420). A microphone was placed over the arteria brachialis of the left arm under the blood pressure cuff. The blood pressure monitor was programmed to take blood pressure every 15 minutes throughout the day and every 60 minutes throughout the night. A shorter interval of blood pressure taking during night would be disturbing for the night sleep. In addition, heart rate and motor activity were continuously recorded using a two-channel ambulatory monitoring system (Minilogger, MedNATIC). Heart rate recordings were taken (in bpm) by a modified Lead 1 derivation from Nehb (cf. Halhuber et al., 1986). Motor activity was recorded by means of an activity sensor attached to the left thigh. The 24 hour data were stored in the memory unit of the equipment system and then transferred to a computer which then constructed an individual data file. Artifacts (defined for systolic blood pressure (SBP) and diastolic blood pressure (DBP) as any of the following: SBP < 50 mmHg, SBP > 250 mmHg, DBP > SBP, DBP < 30 mmHg, DBP > 150 mmHg, HR < 40 bpm) were excluded. Posture (supine, sitting, standing) and levels of physical activity have a strong influence on ambulatory blood pressure and heart rate (Pickering, 1991). To ensure the comparability between work and home data, all analyses are based on data recorded only in the sitting, standing or lying position, and excluding physical activity (in analysing data of the activity sensor).

Statistical Analyses

For data analysis, the 24-h-measurements were divided into 5 periods:

- *work* was defined as all the time spent doing paid work;
- *journey to and from work*;
- *leisure time* was defined as consisting of a number of occupations in which an individual may indulge of his own free will. Leisure time can be spent in recreation, relaxation, self-improvement, or social participation (Dumazedier, 1960);
- *obligatory time* was defined as time spent for household duties, child care, social work (for example, taking care for the elderly or ill, political work, work in a club, etc.) or vocational advanced training, but also for hygiene, eating (Hoff, 1986; Opaschowski, 1997);
- *night* was defined as time spent in bed without any activities (lights out).

Time at work was defined from women's handheld computers and the setting protocols based on post-exploration (just after the 24 h ambulatory monitoring). Nighttime was defined as all sleeping hours judged from participants' handheld computers, the post-exploration and the motor activity data. All readings for systolic and diastolic blood pressure, and for heart rate within each period of time (work, obligatory time, leisure time, night) were averaged to represent that period. Furthermore, a value representing the nocturnal change in the blood pressure in relation to the mean level during the daytime was calculated. The reason is that sleep has the effect of decreasing ("dipping") blood pressure by an average of 10 to 15 percent of the daytime level in most individuals. However, some people's blood pressure does not dip over night or the blood pressure decrease is relatively small. Non-dipping is believed to be pathologic because it exposes the patient to a higher blood pressure load throughout the 24-h day (Käppler, 1994; Dimsdale & Heeren, 1998). Studies using dipping as a parameter differ according to the definition for the time frame of dipping, and for the physical activity during the daytime. Most investigators contrast the daytime blood pressure with the night-time blood pressure, using limited intervals, for example, between 6 am to 10 pm for daytime and 10 pm to 6 am for night-time (for example, Ferrara et al., 1998; Uzu et al., 1999; Weir et al., 1998). However, Nystrom et al. (1996) found that such standardized day and night-time limits may lead to misclassification. Another important effect on blood pressure is the physical activity. Examining the effect of daily activity on nocturnal blood pressure fall, del Arco-Galan & Suarez (1994) and Leary et al. (2000) reported that the classification of non-dippers is dependent on their physical activity during the day. However, most published studies do not report how this activity problem was dealt with. Due to the problems with time limits and activity, the present study used a more precisely defined time frame and took into account the physical activity by excluding the blood pressure of segments with activity (for instance, segments with movement like walking, physical work, and all motor activity recorded by the activity sensor that was > 15 %, were excluded) before averaging the daytime blood pressure. Daytime starts with the beginning of the ambulatory measurement. Night-time starts with the time of going to bed, no activities (for example, sex, reading), and 'lights out', and finishes next morning with time given by subject's alarm clock or by getting up. Due to this restriction on data without activity, the 10% difference was used as a boundary for the classification of dipper and non-dipper (instead of the 15 % difference, which is also frequently used). At first the nocturnal reduction rates (NRR) of SBP and DBP were calculated according to the following formula: *NRR (%) = [(daytime mean - nighttime mean) / daytime mean] x 100*. Then the women were divided into two groups according to the presence (dipper) or absence (non-dipper) of a reduction in both systolic and diastolic blood pressure during the night by an average of more than 10% of the daytime blood pressure.

Between-group differences were performed to assess the relations between job strain (yes versus no) and blood pressure, sleep characteristics as well as the introspective variables (for example, affect, perceived control, etc.). Between-group differences for continuous variables were assessed by using ANOVA and two-sample *t*-tests, and those for discrete variables were assessed by using chi-squared tests. All ANOVAs with blood pressure included the women's age and the bodymass index as covariates.

Results

Objective task analyses depend on strain

The results of the multivariate variance analyses of the five work-related dimensions with the exposure to high or low job strain yielded highly significant differences in all dimensions with the only exception being the dimension "responsibility" (see Table 3). This means that the task design of women who were exposed to low job strain was significantly better than that of those exposed to high job strain. In detail, the scores of all scales of the dimensions "work-related cooperation and communication", "mental regulation requirements" and four of the eleven scales describing the "technical-/organizational work characteristics" dimension were higher for women who were exposed to low job strain than those exposed to high job strain. Women did not differ in the possibility of applying their qualifications depending on the job strain exposure, but in their possibility of learning new things by carrying out the job (see line E in Table 3). Women of the high job strain group as compared with those of the low job strain group had significantly fewer possibilities to learn new things.

Comparing the scores of the low strain group with the minimum task requirements, six of all 21 scores did not obtain the threshold of the minimal profile. These six scales were all scales of only one dimension, the technical and organizational

Table 3: Results of MANOVA for the five work-related dimensions (A-E) and the general job quality (F), as well as of the between group differences for each scale

Work-related dimensions (A - E) and pertinent scales	TDS Scale		Strain		ANOVA			
	Max	Mp	Low M	High M	df1	df2	F	p
A) Technical/organizational work characteristics	Pillai-test:				13	44	15.33	.000***
work cycle time	4	3	5.40	3.38	1	57	57.34	.000***
sequential completeness	4	2	3.56	2.00	1	57	81.59	.000***
number sub-tasks	4	2	2.12	2.29	1	57	2.01	.162
organization tasks	5	3	2.68	1.00	1	57	16.31	.000***
possibility of prediction	4	3	2.78	2.42	1	57	13.99	.000***
information about organization	3	2	2.76	2.82	1	57	0.22	.642
information about results	3	2	1.83	1.00	1	57	21.22	.000***
procedural degrees of freedom	6	3	3.40	2.14	1	57	93.08	.000***
temporal degrees of freedom	5	3	3.63	2.12	1	57	40.45	.000***
work-related decision processes	5	4	3.03	1.07	1	57	48.34	.000***
feedback	5	4	4.03	4.66	1	57	8.30	.006**
quantity/quality-conflicts	3	3	1.60	1.65	1	57	0.06	.813
physical demands	4	4	2.20	2.21	1	57	0.002	.962
B) Work-related cooperation and communication	Pillai-test:				3	54	18.65	.000***
amount of cooperation	5	3	3.47	2.31	1	57	31.32	.000***
kind of cooperation	9	4	4.68	3.59	1	57	5.72	.020*
kind of communication	6	3	3.13	2.00	1	57	28.48	.000***
C) Responsibility	Pillai-test:				2	55	1.07	.351
responsibility for results, processes or people	5	2	2.98	2.71	1	57	1.85	.180
individual vs. group responsibility for results	5	2	2.22	1.94	1	57	0.93	.339
D) Mental regulation requirements								
mental demands	10	5	5.30	2.95	1	57	66.30	.000***
E) Learning potential	Pillai-test:				2	55	12.06	.000***
qualification application	3	2	2.41	2.41	1	57	0.10	.991
requirement to learn new things	4	2	3.39	2.35	1	57	24.43	.000***
F) General job quality (all scales of TDS)	Pillai-test:				21	36	10.55	.000***

Note. n = 41 for the exposure to low job strain; n = 17 for the exposure to high job strain; *p<.05; **p<.01; *** p< .0001; Max = maximum of scale (the minimum of each scale is zero); Mp = threshold value of TDS which define the minimal profile; the minimal profile should be met in order to avoid fatigue, stress, monotony, psychosomatic complaints, or to lose skills; underlined are values which are below the Mp.

work characteristics. In contrast, 13 of all scores of the high strain group in four of the five dimensions did not obtain the minimal profile. This means that the task design of women who were exposed to high job strain lead to a higher risk of negative strain outcomes than that of those exposed to low job strain.

The question about overtime showed that 3 (of 14) women of the high job strain group and 9 (of 41) women of the low job strain group worked long hours. In detail, the three women of the high job strain group did an averaged overtime of 32.3 minutes a week (*min* = 0 hours, *max* = 5 hours a week). The nine women of the low job strain group did an averaged overtime of 52.7 minutes overtime a week (*min* = 0 hours, *max* = 10 hours a week). It is important to note that all women of the low strain group had adequate procedural degrees of freedom (basis for their classification as exposed to low job strain was that the procedural degrees of freedom were above the TDS minimal profile), whereas the procedural degrees of freedom for women who were exposed to high job strain were too low. All in all, neither did the two strain groups differ in the question whether they did overtime work (χ^2 (2, N = 58) = 1.36, *ns*) nor in the question about the amount of overtime (t (58)= - 0.52; *ns*).

Physiological changes depend on the exposure to job strain

The results of examining the question of differences in cardiovascular activation depending on the exposure to job strain are based on a reduced sample because women who were on anti-hypertensive medication had to be excluded from the statistical analyses. Furthermore, the number of women differs slightly in the five tested time intervals because of missing values. Such missing values resulted from the fact that not all women passed all time intervals during the day (for example, some women had no leisure time) or women's body activation was too high during one or more daily interval and thus the data of such intervals had to be excluded from physiological data analyses.

Daily blood pressure was influenced by the exposure to job strain. Results of ANOVA shown in Table 4 yielded significant differences in systolic and diastolic blood pressure during work and obligatory time with higher blood pressure values for the women who were exposed to high job strain compared with those exposed to low job strain. Additionally, systolic and diastolic blood pressure during the night differed significantly between the women of the high job strain group and the low job strain group with higher values for the high job strain group. There was no significant difference in the time (latency) required to attain the lowest systolic and diastolic blood pressure between women exposed to high job strain and those exposed to low job strain [SBP-latency, high job strain: 3 hours and 5 minutes; low job strain: 2 hours and 54 minutes; F (1, 34) = 0.10, ns; DBP-latency, high job strain: 2 hours and 29 minutes; low job strain: 3 hours 12 min; F (1. 34)=0.92, *ns*]. However, the lowest diastolic blood pressure obtained, but not the lowest systolic blood pressure, was significantly higher in women exposed to high job strain than in those exposed to low job strain (see Table 4). The analysis of the lowest systolic blood pressure yielded only a marginally significant difference depending on the exposure to strain.

Table 4. Analyses of variance for blood pressure by exposure to job strain

Daily segments and job strain	SBP		DBP	
	M	SD	M	SD
Work				
high	129.54	13.84	89.15	10.74
low	116.02	10.43	81.52	8.58
F (1, 45) =	10.88 **		6.39 *	
Obligatory time				
high	131.47	23.00	91.57	15.09
low	117.35	12.56	80.71	11.03
F (1, 45) =	5.88 *		6.14 *	
Leisure time				
high	118.77	17.22	81.83	13.88
low	114.50	14.58	77.71	11.49
F (1, 42) =	0.18 ns		0.45 ns	
Recovery period				
high	116.30	17.73	73.63	16.26
low	102.10	9.95	67.50	9.68
F (1, 40) =	6.57 *		3.85 (*)	
Night				
high	110.02	17.14	78.10	12.08
low	100.25	9.99	67.26	8.40
F (1, 43) =	4.42 *		4.37 *	
Lowest value				
high	99.00	20.23	65.7	13.86
low	89.41	11.40	59.4	8.75
F (1, 43) =	3.09 (*)		3.62 (*)	
NRR				
high strain	14.76	8.99	13.49	10.41
low strain	15.05	6.60	16.00	5.25
F (1, 44) =	0.004 ns		0.96 ns	

Note. NRR = Nocturnal Reduction Rate

Neither a significant difference in the nocturnal reduction rate for the systolic blood pressure nor for the diastolic blood pressure were observed depending on strain.

Heart rate recorded during work, leisure time, obligatory time, night and during recovery, as well as the lowest heart rate, the latency to attain this lowest heart rate and the nocturnal reduction rate did not differ between women who were exposed to high and those exposed to low job strain (F ranged between 0.02 and 3.10, p between .086 and .374).

Altogether, 14 of 45 normotensive women were classified as non-dipper (for 3 women dipping-status could not be determined). A significantly higher percentage of women exposed to high strain were non-dippers, n = 6 (54,5%) [dippers, n = 5 (45.5%)] as compared with women exposed to low strain, non-dippers, n = 8 (23.5%), dippers, n = 26 (76.5%), χ^2 (1, N = 45) = 3.73, $p < .05$.

Changes of mood depend on strain

Daily mood was not influenced by strain. For the Positive and the Negative Affectivity, no significant differences were observed between women of the high job strain group and the low job strain group (see Table 5). However, women who were exposed to high job strain perceived significantly more stress and less control during their obligatory time than women exposed to low job strain. In addition, the women of the high job strain group perceived significantly less control during their leisure time than those of the low job strain group.

Evaluation of sleep and relaxation ability

The distribution of subjects with sleep disturbances such as insomnia did not differ depending on strain, χ^2 (1, N = 54) = 0.28, *ns*. However, significantly more women with disturbed relaxation ability were found in the high strain group than in the low strain group. Furthermore, significantly more women exposed to high job strain had problems falling asleep than those exposed to low strain group (see Table 6).

Table 5. Results of MANOVA for rating mood, stress, and control during the three daily segments work, obligatory and leisure time, and one measurement point before going to bed, as well as of the between group differences for each scale

Variable	Exposure to job strain		ANOVA			
	Low	High				
	M	M	df1	df2	F	p
Work		Pillai-test:	4	53	0.71	ns
Positive Affectivity	1.77	1.78	1	57	0.004	ns
Negative Affectivity	1.86	1.83	1	57	0.04	ns
perceived stress	2.63	2.99	1	57	0.81	ns
perceived control	6.28	6.01	1	57	1.72	ns
Obligatory time		Pillai-test:	4	48	2.15	(*)
Positive Affectivity	0.81	1.02	1	53	0.78	ns
Negative Affectivity	1.74	1.92	1	53	0.66	ns
perceived stress	2.42	3.24	1	53	4.12	*
perceived control	6.07	5.58	1	53	2.98	(*)
Leisure time		Pillai-test:	4	45	1.90	ns
Positive Affectivity	0.80	1.14	1	49	1.10	ns
Negative Affectivity	1.93	2.02	1	49	0.13	ns
perceived stress	2.13	1.88	1	49	0.40	ns
perceived control	6.22	5.80	1	49	4.32	*
Before going to bed		Pillai-test:	4	48	0.37	ns
Positive Affectivity	0.08	0.44	1	57	0.85	ns
Negative Affectivity	1.74	1.82	1	57	0.07	ns
perceived stress	2.03	2.29	1	57	0.45	ns
perceived control	5.69	5.88	1	57	0.22	ns

Note. Rating the items for the positive affect and negative affect was based on bipolar seven point scales ranged between -3 to +3.The lower the score the more negative the experience. Rating the items for perceived stress and control was based on unipolar seven point scales ranged between not at all (1) to completely (7). (*) $p < .10$; * $p < .05$

Table 6. Relaxation ability and problems falling asleep as related to job strain exposure

	Exposure to job strain	
	Low	High
Disturbed relaxation ability		
Yes	3	6
No	37	11
χ^2 (1, N = 57)	6.93**	
Problems to fall asleep		
Yes	2	5
No	38	12
χ^2 (1, N = 57)	6.60**	
Reduced sleeping duration		
Yes (< 7 hours)	16	6
No (> 7 hours)	24	11
χ^2 (1, N = 57)	0.11	

Note. One of the 58 women did not complete the questionnaires.
** $p < .001$.

However, the sleep duration rated by the Sleep Wake Experience List (van Diest, 1990) with a limit of seven hours (less than seven hours sleep duration is a short sleep duration; sleep duration is regarded normal if subjects slept 7–8 hours) did not differ depending on the exposure to job strain. The shortest rated sleep duration which was found in the high job strain group was six hours and in the low strain group five hours.

The sleep duration was not only rated by questionnaire for the last three months, but also tested for the night of ambulatory monitoring. There were no differences

Table 7: Duration of daily segments as related to the job strain exposure

Daily segment and level of job strain	Duration (in min)	
	M	SD
Obligatory time		
Low	270	66.7
High	260	66.1
t (57)	-0.52 ns	
Time for household duties		
Low	117	62.0
High	121	57.3
t (57)	- 0.22 ns	
Leisure time		
Low	142	81.9
High	121	64.0
t (57)	- 0.93 ns	

found in the sleep duration during the monitored night between the two job strain groups, t (58) =-1.41, *ns*. Women exposed to high job strain spent seven hours and 11 minutes in bed (lights out, no motor activity), and women exposed to low job strain spent seven hours and 20 minutes in bed.

It has to be examined whether the burden following the working time caused the disturbed recovery. Therefore, the amount of leisure time, obligatory time, and time for household duties were examined between the two job strain groups. The results of variance analyses (Table 7) showed no differences in the amount of the leisure time, obligatory time, and time within the obligatory time for household duties.

Discussion

Objectively assessed job strain

By using an objective method of analysing psychosocial work characteristics and conditions of work places, a configuration of subscales for classifying work places was defined according to the exposure to high versus low job strain. Based on this classification, it was examined whether the other work characteristics tested by objective work analysis (Task Diagnosis Survey, Rudolph et al., 1985; Hacker et al., 1995) differ between the two job strain groups. Work places with a potential to expose employees to high job strain showed deficits in four of the five work related dimensions tested by TDS (a total of 66.7 % of all tested subscales were below the minimal profile). Special emphasis should be given to the low rated subscales of sequential completeness, organization tasks, possibility of prediction, work-related decision processes, feedback and quantity/quality-conflicts as well as all subscales of the dimension work-related cooperation and communication. Each of the work characteristics defined by these subscales needs to be re-designed since the values did not meet the threshold values of the minimal profile. This minimal profile of the Task Diagnosis Survey (Rudolph et al., 1985; Hacker et al., 1995) defines the values that should be attained in order to exclude the probability of negative short-term effects such as fatigue, monotony, stress or psychical saturation.

Work places of both the women exposed to low job strain as well as the women exposed to high job strain were characterized by too low physical demands (TDS-subscale "physical demands" asked for posture and movement-activity). Low physical demands, combined with time pressure and lack of influence over one's work (high job strain), are seen as high risk for muscular problems, for example, lower back, shoulder and neck pain (Lundberg, Dohns et al. 1999; Sandsjö et al., 2000; Wærsted, 2000). Therefore, the low physical demands have to be evaluated as an additional stress factor for women who were exposed to high job strain. However, independently of the exposure to low or high job strain, chronic under-activity has generally been considered to contribute to health problems (see the allostasis model of McEwan, 1998; Sjøgaard, Lundberg & Kadefors, 2000).

It should be noticed that in contrast to the demand for work-related life-time learning (Bergmann, 1998; Joint Employment Report, 2000), the high job strain work places required significantly lower cognitive levels and also a lower learning potential as compared with the low job strain work places. This is in accordance with the hypothesis of Karasek and Theorell (1990, p 100) that "accumulated level of unresolved strain ... appears to restrict a person's ability to learn solutions to new problems". Whereas Karasek and Theorell mean an intraindividual subjective process, the result of the present study show a relationship between learning potential and the exposure to job strain that was assessed independently from subjects' experiences.

Exposure to job strain and psychophysiological changes during the day and the night

As expected (hypothesis H 1), high job strain was of importance to both systolic and diastolic blood pressure levels during daily life. Heart rate was not influenced by job strain. Consistent with the studies by Theorell et al. (1991), Light, Turner and Hinderliter (1992), Landsbergis et al. (1994), Cesana et al. (1996), Schnall et al. (1998) and Laflamme et al. (1998), high as compared to low job strain was associated with elevated blood pressure at work and at night (see also review article by Theorell & Karasek, 1996). Most of these published studies were based on self-report data of job strain. In contrast, the present study classified the exposure to high versus low job strain by using objective measures of job characteristics. Therefore, the problem of self-report bias did not affect the analysis of job characteristics.

In support of hypothesis H 1, job strain was not only important for blood pressure at work, but also for the blood pressure level during the period after work. However, it is not the leisure time which shows a significant relationship to job strain, but the obligatory time, which includes further burden like household duties, child care or care of elderly and ill, etc. This observation is in accordance with the study published by Theorell et al. (1991). They reported job strain effects of diastolic (but not systolic) blood pressure only at night and during work but not during leisure. However, it remains unclear how these authors defined leisure time. It seems that their label "leisure time" was used for both obligatory time and leisure time. In contrast to Theorell et al. (1991) and in support of the observations of the present study, Landsbergis et al. (1994) reported significant associations between job strain and systolic (but not diastolic) blood pressure at work and at home. However, as discussed above for the results by Theorell et al. (1991), the study by Landsbergis et al. (1994) also used a not well-defined label. Time at home consists of a number of occupations. For example, time can be spent in relaxation and self-improvement or on household duties. Returning to the findings of the present study, job strain only affected the blood pressure during the time which consisted of further burden (for example, household duties, children care, etc.) but not during the free available time (leisure). An explanation might be that rewind from job-dependent strain was only possible during leisure time. Or, in other words, women seemed to prefer activities during their leisure time which were able to compensate job strain effects.

The finding of a raised blood pressure during work depending on job strain must not be interpreted negatively. Normally, job strain activates the sympathetic system (for example, blood pressure rise) and the hypothalamic pituary adrenal axis (Pickering, 1991). When job strain has passed, the activation level should return to base-line levels. The cardiovascular system is only potentially harmed if blood pressure or heart rate rewind after work (after stressor) is delayed or incomplete (see review of arousal and physiological toughness by Dienstbier, 1991 or discussion of allostasis and allostatic load by McEwen & Seeman, 1999). In the present study, it was found that the systolic and diastolic blood pressure, but not the heart rate during the night, decreased in women exposed to high job strain significantly less than that of the women exposed to low job strain. In addition, the lowest systolic and diastolic blood pressure differs slightly between the two job strain groups, with higher blood pressure values for women exposed to high job strain. However, the nocturnal reduction rates for systolic and diastolic blood pressure and for heart rate did not differ depending on job strain. Only the classification of women into dippers and non-dippers yielded significant effects. Relatively more women of the high strain group were classified as non-dippers compared with those of the low strain group. One explanation for this contradictory result might be the boundary for the dipper versus non-dipper classification. This boundary was a decrease during the night by an average of more than 10% of the daytime blood pressure. If a stronger decrease is defined, or more than 15 %, the result will probably be lost. On the other hand, the variance in blood pressure during the night might be increased, because the body position during the night was not controlled for (there was no device available for recording body position).

Pickering (1968, 1991) showed that the position lying on the left (blood pressure cuff below heart level) or on the right side (blood pressure cuff above heart level) affects the blood pressure level. This dependence on body position leads to the question whether the above results found for the nocturnal blood pressure can be discussed regarding job strain. However, if one assumes that the nocturnal body position is randomized over all tested subjects, the result has to be interpreted as a relationship between the exposure to job strain and the nocturnal blood pressure change. It is unlikely that women exposed to high job strain prefer the left side for sleeping, while women exposed to low job strain prefer the right side for sleeping. Thus, the inactivation of the blood pressure during the night has to be seen as less efficient in women exposed to high job strain than in those exposed to low job strain. Both repeated elevations of blood pressure over weeks, months, or years and the inability to recover blood pressure after the acute job strain might accelerate hypertension and at least atherosclerosis (McEwen, 1998). The results of this study indicate that sympathetic nervous system activity may increase at work in high strain jobs and remain elevated at night, thus hampering rewind. Thus job strain has to interpreted as a risk factor for cardiovascular health.

Evaluation of sleep and relaxation ability

In accordance with these physiological findings is the observation that more women of the high job strain group reported a disturbed relaxation ability and problems with falling asleep, thus corroborating hypothesis H 2. This suggests that the normal restoration processes that take place during sleep are impaired in women with high job strain. Van Diest & Appels (1991) have already discussed problems initiating and maintaining sleep as potential risk indicators for coronary artery diseases. Especially their research according to the concept of vital exhaustion showed the various relations between sleep and cardiovascular diseases (Appels, Falger & Schouten, 1993; Appels, 1997). For example, problems falling asleep and, in particular, feeling exhausted upon waking up in the morning were predictive for a first, non-fatal myocard infarct (Appels & Schouten, 1991). For men, conflicts at work were conducive to first acute myocardial infarction through their associations with exhaustion (Falger & Schouten, 1992).

Conclusion

The effects of job strain can not be examined during work time alone since during that time we can only assess the response to work stress. The question whether the response to work stress recovers after work stress has finished, required the assessment of job strain over the whole day. If job strain plays a role in the development of sustained hypertension, it should be possible to demonstrate that job strain can cause a rise in the blood pressure not only during work but also during leisure time and night. This could be demonstrated by the results of the present study. The exposure to high job strain was associated with higher blood pressure during work, obligatory time and night as compared to the exposure to low job strain. Furthermore, the ability to relax and to fall asleep were related to job strain. Thus, the results give support to the 'old' statement by Karasek (1979) that the combination of low decision latitude with high job demands (job strain) will lead to negative psychical and physical health outcomes.

As long as the evaluation of job strain was biased by subject's self-report, the question of what is to be done first, modify employees' behavior or re-design work places, remained open. Because in the present study the exposure to job strain has been independently assessed by external observers, the results support the demand for a change in designing work places towards healthy jobs.

References

Appels, A. (1997). Exhausted subjects, exhausted systems. *Acta Physiologica Scandinavica. Supplementum, 640,* 153–154.

Appels A. & Schouten, E. (1991). Waking up exhausted as risk indicator of myocardial infarction. *American Journal of Cardiology, 68*, 395-398.

Appels, A., Falger, P.R. & Schouten, E.G. (1993). Vital exhaustion as risk indicator for myocardial infarction in women. *Journal Psychosomatic Research, 37*, 881-890.

Baitsch, C., Katz, C., Spinas, P. & Ulich, E. (1991). *Computerunterstützte Büroarbeit: Ein Leitfaden für Organisation und Gestaltung.* Zürich: Verlag der Fachvereine.

Beard, K.M. & Edwards, J.R. (1995). Employees at risk: Contingent work and the psychological experience of contingent workers. In C. L. Cooper & D. M. Rousseau (Eds.), *Trends in organizational behavior* (Vol. 2), (pp. 109–126). Chichester: Wiley.

Belkic, K., Emdad, R. & Theorell, T. (1998).Occupational profile and cardiac risk: possible mechanisms and implications for professional drivers. *International Journal of Occupational Medicine and Environmental Health, 11,* 37–57.

Bergmann, B. (1996). Zukunft der Erwerbsarbeit: Arbeit und Arbeitslosigkeit Hinweise aus ostdeutschen Problemsichten. In W. Hacker (Ed.). *Erwerbsarbeit der Zukunft – auch für "Ältere"?*, (pp. 29–41). Zürich: vdf.

Bergmann, B. (1998). Tätigkeitsanforderungen im Verlauf der Berufsbiografie. *Zeitschrift für Arbeits- und Organisationspsychologie, 42*, 2–14.

Bosma, H., Stansfeld, S.A. & Marmot, M.G. (1998). Job control, personal characteristics, and heart disease. *Journal of Occupational Health Psychology, 3*, 402–409.

Carayon, P. & Zijlstra, F. (1999). Relationship between job control, work pressure and strain: Studies in the USA and in the Netherlands. *Work and Stress, 13*, 32–48

Cesana, G., Ferrario, M., Sega, R., Milesi, C., De Vito, G., Mancia, G. & Zanchetti, A. (1996). Job strain and ambulatory blood pressure levels in a population-based employed sample of men from northern Italy. *Scandinavian Journal of Work, Environment and Health, 22*, 294–305.

del Arco-Galan, C. & Suarez, F.C. (1994). Nocturnal fall in arterial blood pressure in normotensive subjects: individual characteristic or the effect of daily activity? [On-line]. *Medicina Clinica (Barcelona), 102,* 616–618. Abstract from: Item UI 942 682 03

Dimsdale, J.E. & Heeren, M.M. (1998). How reliable is nighttime blood pressure dipping? *American Journal of Hypertension, 11*, 606–609.

DOT- Dictionary of Occupational Titles (1979). US Department of Labor (Eds.).

Dumazedier, J. (1960). Current problems of the sociology of leisure. *International Social Science Journal, 12*, 522–531.

Ertel, M., Pech, E. & Ullsperger, P. (2000). Telework in perspective – new challenges to occupational health and safety. In L. Isaksson, C. Hogstedt, Eriksson, C. & T. Theorell (Eds.), *Health effects of the new labour market* (pp. 169–177). New York: Kluwer Academic/Plenum Publishers.

Joint Employment Report (2000). *Commission of the European Communities.* COM (2000), 551 final, Vol I, Brüssel, 6.9.2000 [On-line]. Available: http://europa.eu.int/eur-lex/en/com/pdf /2000/act0551en01/com2000_0551en01_1.pdf.

Fahrenberg, J. (1996). Concurrent assessment of blood pressure, physical activity, and emotional state in natural settings. In J. Fahrenberg & M. Myrtek (Eds.). *Ambulatory Assessment. Computer-assisted psychological and psychophysiological methods in monitoring and field studies* (pp.165–187). Seattle, Toronto, Bern, Göttingen: Hogrefe & Huber.

Fahrenberg, J. & Myrtek (2001). Ambulantes Monitoring and Assessment. In F. Rösler (Ed.), *Enzyklopädie der Psychologie, Biologische Psychologie, Vol. 4* (pp. 657–798), Göttingen: Hogrefe.

Falger, P.R. & Schouten, E.G. (1992). Exhaustion, psychological stressors in the work environment, and acute myocardial infarction in adult men. *Journal Psychosomatic Research, 36*, 777–786.

Ferrara, A.L., Pasanisi, F., Crivaro, M., Guida, L., Palmieri, V., Gaeta, I., Iannuzzi, R. & Celentano, A. (1998). Cardiovascular Abnormalities in Never-Treated Hypertensives According to Nondipper Status. *American Journal of Hypertension, 11*, 1352 – 1357.

Fox, M.L., Dwyer, D.J. & Ganster, D.C. (1993). Effects of stressful job demands and control on physiological and attitudinal outcomes in a hospital setting. *Academy of Management Journal, 36*, 289–318.

Frankenhaeuser, M. (1993). Current issues in psychobiological stress research. In M. Vartiainen (Ed.), *European views in psychology – keynote lectures* (pp. 1–11). Lecture conducted at the Third European Congress of Psychology, Tampere, Finland.

Frese, M. & Zapf, D. (1994). Action as the core of work psychology: a German approach. In Dunnette, M.D., Hough, L.M. & Triandis, H.C. (Eds.), *Handbook of industrial and organizational psychology* (pp. 271–340), Vol. 4, Palo Alto, CA: Consulting Psychologists Press, (second edition).

Hacker, W. (1985). *On some fundamentals of action regulation.* In Ginsburg, G.P., Brenn, J. & von Cranach (eds.), Discovery strategies in the psychology of action. European Monographs in Social Psychology, 35 (pp. 63–84), London: Academic Press.

Hacker, W. (1986). *Arbeitspsychologie.* Bern: Huber.

Hacker, W. (1994). Action regulation theory and occupational psychology. Review of German empirical research since 1987. *The German Journal of Psychology, 2,* 91–120.

Hacker, W. (1998). *Allgemeine Arbeitspsychologie.* Psychische Regulation von Arbeitstätigkeiten. Bern: Huber.

Hacker, W., Fritsche, B., Richter, P. & Iwanowa, A. (1995). *Das Tätigkeitsbewertungsverfahren TBS-L.* Zürich: Verlag der Fachbuchvereine.

Hägg, G.M. (2000). Human muscle fibre abnormalities related to occupational load. *European Journal of Applied Physiology, 83,* 159–165.

Halhuber, M.J., Günther, R. & Ciresa, M. (1986). *EKG-Einführungskurs.* Leipzig: Barth.

Harma, M.I. & Ilmarinen, J.E. (1999). Towards the 24-hour society – new approaches for aging shift workers? *Scandinavian Journal of Work, Environment, and Health, 25,* 610–615.

Hoff, E.-H. (1986). *Arbeit, Freizeit und Persönlichkeit: Wissenschaftliche und alltägliche Vorstellungsmuster.* Bern: Huber.

Imai, M. (1986). *Kaizen (Ky'zen) The Key to Japan's Competitive Success.* New York: Random House Business Division.

ISO 10075 (1991). *Ergonomic principles related to mental work-load – General terms and definitions.* Genf: International Organization for Standardization.

ISO 10075–2 (1994). *Ergonomic principles related to mental work-load – Part 2: Design principles.* Genf: International Organization for Standardization.

Johnson, J.V., Stewart, W., Fredlund, P., Hall, E.M. & Theorell, T. (1990). *Psychosocial job exposure matrix: an occupational aggregated attribution system for work environment exposure characteristics.* Stress research reports; no 221. Stockholm: National Institute for Psychosocial Factors and Health.

Johnson, J.V., Hall, E.M. (1995). Class, work and health. In B.C. Amick, S. Levine, A.R. Tarlov & W.D. Chapman (Eds.), *Society and Health* (pp 247–271). New York: Oxford University Press.

Käppler, C. (1994). *Psychophysiologische Bedingungsanalyse von Blutdruckveränderungen im alltäglichen Lebenskontext.* Frankfurt a. M.: Peter Lang.

Karasek, R. (1979). Job demands, job decision latitude, and mental strain: implications for job redesign. *Administrative Science Quarterly, 24,* 285–307.

Karasek, R.A. & Theorell, T. (1990). *Healthy work.* New York: Basic Books.

Karasek, R., Brisson, C., Kawakami, N., Houtman, I. & Bomgers, P. (1998). The job content questionnaire (JCQ): an instrument for internationally comparative assessments of psychosocial job characteristics. *Journal of Occupational Health Psychology, 3,* 322–355.

Kawakami, N. & Haratani, T. (1999). Epidemiology of job stress and health in Japan: review of current evidence and future direction. *Industrial Health, 37,* 174–186.

Kawakami, N., Araki, S., Takatsuka, N., Shimizu, H. & Ishibashi, H. (1999). Overtime, psychosocial working conditions, and occurrence of non-insulin dependent diabetes mellitus in Japanese men. *Journal Epidemiology, Community and Health, 53,* 359–363.

Laflamme, N., Brisson, C., Moisan, J., Milot, A., Masse, B. & Vezina, M. (1998). Job strain and ambulatory blood pressure among female white-collar workers. *Scandinavian Journal of Work, Environment and Health, 24,* 334–343.

Landsbergis, P., Schnall, P., Warren, K., Pickering, T.G. & Schwartz, J.E. (1994). Association between ambulatory blood pressure and alternative formulations of job strain. *Scandinavian Journal of Work, Environment and Health, 20*, 349–363.

Landsbergis, P., Cahill, J. & Schnall, P. (1999). The impact of lean production and related new systems of work organization on worker health. *Journal of Occupational Health Psychology, 4*, 108–130.

Leary, A.C., Donan, R.T., MacDonald, T.M. & Murphy, M.B. (2000). Physical activity level is an independent predictor of the diurnal variation in blood pressure. *Journal of Hypertension, 18*, 405–410.

Lewis, S. & Cooper, C.L. (1999). The work-family research agenda in changing contexts. *Journal of Occupational Health Psychology, 4*, 382–393.

Levi, L., Sauter, S.L. & Shimomitsu, T. (1999). Work-related stress – it's time to act. *Journal of Occupational Health Psychology, 4*, 394–396.

Lundberg, U., Mardberg, B. & Frankenhaeuser, M. (1992). The total workload of male and female white collar workers as related to occupational level, number of children and age. *Journal of Psychology, 33*, 1–15.

Lundberg, U., Kadefors, R., Melin, B., Palmerud, G., Hassmen, P., Engström, M. & Dohns, I. E. (1994). Psychphysiological stress and EMG activity of the trapezius muscle. *International Journal of Behavioral Medicine, 1*, 354–370.

Lundberg, U., Dohns, I.E., Melin, B., Sandsjo, L., Palmerud, G., Kadefors, R., Ekstrom, M. & Parr, D. (1999). Psychophysiological stress responses, muscle tension, and neck and shoulder pain among supermarket cashiers. *Journal of Occupational Health Psycholology, 4*, 245–255

Martens, M.F.J., Nijhuis, F.J..N.; Van Boxtel, M.P.J. & Knottnerus, J.A. (1999). Flexible work schedules and mental and physical health. A study of a working population with non-traditional working hours. *Journal of Organizational Behavior, 20*, 35–46.

McEwen, B.S. (1998). Protective and damaging effects of stress mediators. *The New England Journal of Medicine, 338*, 171–179.

McEwen, B.S. & Seeman, T. (1999). Protective and damaging effects of mediators of stress. Elaborating and testing the concepts of allostasis and allostatic load. *Annals of the New York Acadamy of Science, 896*, 30–47.

McLean Parks, J., Kidder, D.L. & Gallgher, D.G. (1998). Fitting square pegs into round holes: Mapping the domain of contingent work arrangements onto the psychological contract. *Journal of Organizational Behavior, 19 (Special Issue)*, 697–730.

Miller, G. A., Galanter, E. H. & Pribram, K. (1960). *Plans and the structure of behavior.* New York: Holt.

Moon, S.D. & Sauter, S.L. (Eds.) (1996). *Psychosocial aspects of musculoskeletal disorders in office work.* London: Taylor & Francis.

Nystrom, F., Malmstrom, O., Karlberg, B.E., Ohman, K.P. et al. (1996). Twenty-four hour ambulatory blood pressure in the population. *Journal of Internal Medicine, 240*, 279–284.

Opaschowski, H.W. (1997). *Einführung in die Freizeitwissenschaft.* Leske & Budrich: Opladen.

Pearce, J.L. (1998). Job insecurity is important, but not for the reasons you might think: The example of contingent workers. In C. L. Cooper & D. M. Rousseau (Eds.), *Trends in organizational behavior* (Vol. 5), (pp. 31–46). Chichester: Wiley.

Peter, R. & Siegrist, J. (2000). Psychosocial work environment and the risk of coronary heart disease. *International Archives of Occupational Environment and Health, 73, Suppl:* S 41–45.

Pickering, G.W. (1968). *High blood pressure.* London: Churchill.

Pickering, T.G. (1991). *Ambulatory monitoring and blood pressure reliability.* London: Science Press.

Pickering, T.G. (1993). Applications of ambulatory blood pressure monitoring in behavioral medicine. *Annals of Behavioral Medicine, 15*, 26–32.

Pickering, T.G., Schnall, P.L., Schwartz, J.E. & Pieper, C.F. (1991). Can behavioral factors produce a sustained elevation of blood pressure? Some observations and a hypothesis. *Journal of Hypertension, 9 (suppl 8)*, 566–568.

Pieper, C., LaCroix, A.Z. & Karasek, R.A. (1989). The relation of psychosocial dimensions of work with coronary heart disease risk factors: A meta-analysis of five United States data bases. *American Journal of Epidemiology, 129*, 483–499.

Proctor, S.P., White, R.F., Robins, T.G., Echeverria, D. & Rocskay, A.Z. (1996). Effect of overtime work on cognitive function in automotive workers. *Scandinavian Journal of Work, Environment and Health, 22*, 124–132.

Rau, R. & Richter, P. (1996). Psychophysiological analysis of strain in real life work situations. In J. Fahrenberg & M. Myrtek (Eds.). *Ambulatory Assessment. Computer-assisted psychological and psychophysiological methods in monitoring and field studies* (pp. 271–285). Seattle, Toronto, Bern, Göttingen: Hogrefe & Huber.

Rau, R. (1996). Psychophysiological assessment of human reliability in a simulated complex system. *Biological Psychology, 42*, 287–300.

Rau, R. (1998). Ambulantes psychophysiologisches Monitoring zur Bewertung von Arbeit und Erholung. *Zeitschrift für Arbeits- und Organisationspsychologie, 42*, 185–196.

Rau, R., Georgiade, A., Lemne, C., de Faire, U. & Fredrikson, M. (in press). Psychosocial work characteristics and perceived control in relation to cardiovascular rewind at night. *Journal of Occupational Health Psychology.*

Richter, P., Rudolph, M. & Schmidt, C.F. (1996). *Fragebogen zur Diagnostik belastungs-relevanter Anforderungsbewältigung (FABA).* Frankfurt: SWETS.

Roe, R., Zijlstra, F.R.H. & Leonova, A.B. (1996). *Interruptions in mental information work – effects on work activity and psychological well-being.* WORC Report 96.06.003/4, Tilburg: Work and Organisation Centre.

Rudolph, E., Schönfelder, E. & Hacker, W. (1987). *Tätigkeitsbewertungssystem für geistige Arbeit mit/ohne Rechnerunterstützung (TBS-GA).* Berlin: Psychodiagnostisches Zentrum an der Humboldt Universität (im Vertrieb Göttingen: Hogrefe).

Sandsjö, L., Melin, B., R.D., Dohns, I. & Lundberg, U. (2000). Trapezius muscle activity, neck and shoulder pain, and subjective experiences during monotonous work in women. *European Journal of Applied Physiology, 83*, 235–238.

Sauter, S.L., Hurrel, Jr., J.J., Fox, H.R., Tetrick, L.E. & Barling, J. (1999). Occupational health psychology: an emerging discipline. *Industrial Health, 37*, 199–211.

Schallberger, U. & Pfister, R. (in press). Flow-Erleben in Arbeit und Freizeit: Eine Untersuchung zum "Paradox der Arbeit" mit der Experience Sampling Method (ESM). *Zeitschrift für Arbeits- und Organisationspsychologie.*

Schmidt, T. & Jain, A. (1996). Continuous assessment of finger blood pressure and other haemodynamic and behavioral variables in everyday life. In J. Fahrenberg & M. Myrtek (Eds.). *Ambulatory Assessment. Computer-assisted psychological and psychophysiological methods in monitoring and field studies* (pp. 189–213). Seattle, Toronto, Bern, Göttingen: Hogrefe & Huber.

Schnall, P.L., Landsbergis, P.A., Baker, D. (1994). Job Strain and Cardiovascular Disease. *Annual Review of Public Health, 15,* 381–411.

Schnall, P.L., Pieper, C., Schwartz, J.E., Karasek, R.A., Schlussel, Y., Devereux, R.B., Ganau, A., Alderman, M., Warren, K. & Pickering, T. G. (1990). The relationship between "job strain", work place diastolic blood pressure, and left ventricular mass index. *JAMA, 263*, 1929–1935.

Schnall, P.L., Schwartz, J.E., Landsbergis, P.A., Warren, K. & Pickering, T.G. (1998). A longitudinal study of job strain and ambulatory blood pressure: results from a three-year follow-up. *Psychosomatic Medicine, 60*, 697–706.

Schorr, J. (1991). *The overworked American – the unexpected decline of leisure.* New York: Basic Books.

Schwartz, J. E., Pieper, C. F., Karasek, R. A. (1988). A procedure for linking psychosocial job characteristics data to health surveys. *American Journal of Public Health, 78*, 904–909.

Sjøgaard, G., Lundberg, U. & Kadefors, R. (2000). The role of muscle activity and mental load in the development of pain and degenerative processes at the muscle cell level during computer work. *European Journal of Applied Physiology, 83*, 99–105.

Starrin, B., Larsson, G., Brenner, S.O., Levi, L. & Petterson, I.L. (1990). Structural changes, ill health, and mortality in Sweden, 1963–1983: a macroaggregated study. *International Journal of Health Services, 20*, 27–42.

Sverke, M, Gallagher, D. C. & Hellgren, J. (2000). Alternative work arrangements. In L. Isaksson, C. Hogstedt, Eriksson, C. & T. Theorell (Eds.), *Health effects of the new labour market.* New York: Kluwer Academic/Plenum Publishers.

Theorell, T., Knox, S., Svensson, J. & Waller, D. (1985). Blood pressure variations during a working day at age 28: Effects of different types of work and blood pressure level at age 18. *Journal of Human Stress, 11*, 36–41.

Theorell T., Perski, A., Akerstedt, T., Sigala, F., Ahlberg-Hulten, G., Svensson, J. & Eneroth, P. (1988). Changes in job strain in relation to changes in physiological state: A longitudinal study. *Scandinavian Journal of Work, Environment & Health, 14*, 189–196.

Theorell, T., de Faire, U., Johnson, J., Hall, E., Perski, A. & Stewart, W. (1991). Job strain and ambulatory blood pressure profiles. *Scandinavian Journal of Work, Environment and Health, 17*, 380–385.

Theorell, T., Ahlberg-Hulten, G., Jodko, M., Sigala, F. & Torre, B. (1993). Influence of job strain and emotion on blood pressure in female hospital personnel during workhours. *Scandinavian Journal Work Environ Health, 19*, 313–318.

Theorell, T. & Karasek, R.A. (1996). Current issues relating to psychosocial job strain and cardiovascular disease research. *Journal of Occupational Health Psychology, 1*, 9–26.

Uehata, T. (1991). Long working hours and occupational stress-related cardiovascular attacks among middle-aged workers in Japan. *Journal of Human Ergology, 20*, 147–153.

Uzu, T., Fujii, T., Nishimura, M., Kuroda, S., Nakamura, S., Inenaga,T. & Kimura, G. (1999). Determinants of Circadian Blood Pressure Rhythm in Essential Hypertension. *American Journal of Hypertension, 12*, 35–39.

van Diest, R. (1990). Subjective sleep characteristics as coronary risk factors, their association with Type A behavior and vital exhaustion. *Journal of Psychosomatic Research, 34*, 415–426.

van Diest, R. & Appels, W.P. (1994). Sleep physiological characteristics of exhausted men. *Psychosomatic Medicine, 56*, 28–35.

van Egeren (1992). The relationship between job strain and blood pressure at work, at home, and during sleep. *Psychosomatic Medicine, 54*, 337–343.

Volpert, W. (1987). Psychische Regulation von Arbeitstätigkeiten. In Kleinbeck, U. & Rutenfranz, J. (Eds.), *Enzyklopädie der Psychologie, Arbeitspsychologie, Vol. 1* (pp. 1–42), Göttingen: Hogrefe.

Watson, D. & Tellegen, A. (1985). Toward a consensual structure of mood. *Psychological Bulletin, 98*, 219–235.

Wærsted, M. (2000). Human muscle activity related to non-biomechanical factors in the workplace. *European Journal of Applied Physiology, 83,* 151–158.

Weir, M.R., Reisin, E., Falkner, B., Hutchinson, H.G., Sha, L. & Tuck, M.L. (1998). Nocturnal Reduction of Blood Pressure and the Antihypertensive Response to a Diuretic or Angiotensin Converting Enzyme Inhibitor in Obese Hypertensive Patients. *American Journal of Hypertension, 11*, 914–920.

Chapter 22
Heart Rate Monitoring in an Academic Test Situation

Hans Zeier, Alexandra Haeseli, and Joachim Fischer
Swiss Federal Institute of Technology, Department of Behavioral Sciences, ETH Zürich, Switzerland

Introduction

Ambulatory monitoring is a powerful method for measuring physiological correlates of stress responses in real life situations (Zeier, 1992). For such studies, heart rate monitoring is a reliable and frequently used parameter. This is mostly due to the fact that the electrocardiogram (ECG), which is used for the measurement of heart rate, is the strongest bioelectrical signal produced by the body and, therefore, can be detected easily. In addition, heart rate is very sensitive to physiological and psychological stress factors, thus being a general indicator of physical, emotional and mental load. Finally, highly miniaturised devices are now commercially available. They allow continuous recordings for 24 h or more with almost no disturbance of the subject.

To assess the potential health impact of chronic or acute stress, it is highly desirable to perform long-term ambulatory monitoring of physiological variables. Ambulatory recording of the ECG is well established in Internal Medicine to detect cardiac arrhythmia. The method is also used to assess cardiac responses to physical exercise. Less data are available from everyday situations for example, working in a stressful environment such as an intensive care unit. In these situations the interest is more focussed on changes in heart-rate or heart-rate variability rather than the detection of arrhythmia. To allow segregation of the effects of physical activity from the effects of psychological arousal or stress, it is mandatory to obtain a reliable estimate of the physical activity. Ideally the recording device should be small to minimise disturbance of the subject.

The present paper demonstrates an application of long-term heart rate monitoring to an academic test situation. Emphasis is made to procedures for detecting artifacts and to elucidate methods for discriminating between heart rate responses caused by physical and mental activation, respectively.

Academic test situations are an everyday situation, which may be perceived as stressful by the individual. Often, the test results have far-reaching consequences for the professional career of the tested individuals. The chosen written academic exams in this study represents a typical real-life situation with a good validity and reliability. This is the reason why investigators interested in psychophysiological responses to stressful life situations frequently use exams as an independent variable. The dependent variables such as heart rate or levels of stress hormones are usually measured immediately before, during and after such a test situation. However, as for example, Scheuch et al. (1985) have shown, anticipatory stress responses can lead to elevated heart rates several hours before an exam takes place. Therefore, it appears advisable to perform such monitoring over a longer time period before and after the investigated test situation. Furthermore, prolonged monitoring also allows to monitor the recovery processes. This may be an important research objective since recovery responses were found to be impaired following an academic test situation (Spangler, 1997). Adequate recovery from acute stress is an important determinant of the long term consequences and health burden of stress (McEwen, 1998).

Methods

Subjects

The subjects were 14 male students, recruited among 148 participants of a post-graduate course leading to a Masters Degree in Science Education at the Swiss Federal Institute of Technology Zurich. Selection criteria were good health and no or only very little consumption of cigarettes and alcohol. The subjects were between 23 and 36 years old (M = 26.1; SD =3.5) and gave written informed consent to participating in the study. There were no financial incentives offered.

Study design

The study was performed during a one-week training seminar at a secluded boarding school in Zuoz, situated in the Swiss alps at an altitude of 1600 m. The setting of the seminar subjected all participants to the same circadian activity pattern with approximately equal awakening times, scheduled meals, and daily activities.

Continuous heart rate measurements were taken on a previous control day, and on the second, third and fifth day of the seminar. Recording started at 14.30 and lasted until 10.30 on the following morning. On the control day, individually arranged about three months before the training seminar, heart rate measurements were taken over the same time period in order to familiarize the subjects with the recording device and to let them experience wearing the device overnight. At this time baseline information and psychological traits were assessed with standardized questionnaires. During the seminar, participants assembled in a lecture hall together with the other students (total n=158) from 17.00 to 18.00 to complete an academic task on all three recording days. This task was a written examination on recording day 1, a lecture on recording day 2, and the Raven intelligence test (Raven, 1979) on recording day 3. The written examination was announced beforehand and required about one week of studies for preparation. Test performance on this examination was evaluated in a criterion-oriented way (criterion-reference test) by com-

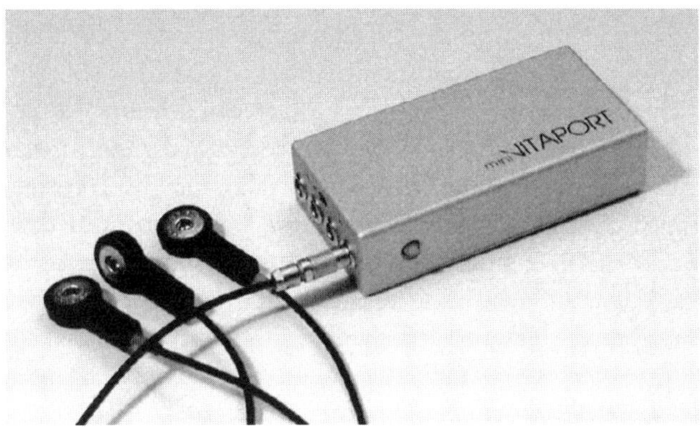

Figure 1. Mini-Vitaport of the ambulatory recording system Vitaport with attached electrode cable for picking up the electrocardiogram (ECG) signal.

paring the actual answers of each examinee with model solutions previously defined (Jäger, 1988, Jäger et al., 1989, Klauer, 1987). The criterion-oriented design of the examination aimed to provide maximal transparency. Its result counted 20% towards the final post-graduate grade. In contrast to the examination, participants were not informed about the Raven intelligence test. They expected a normal lecture as on recording day 2. In this way, we minimized the anticipatory reaction.

Immediately before the academic tasks at 17.00, subjects completed a set of questionnaires assessing different state aspects (Haldemann, 1999). Furthermore, subjects had also to note their principal activities and other events in a structured daily log-sheet.

Recording equipment

As recording device the Mini-Vitaport (Jain et al., 1996) was used (Figure 1). This battery-powered device has a size of 2 x 4,5 x 8,5 cm and a weight of 125 g. It is some kind of actometer with extended features, having a microprocessor, a solid state memory of one megabyte and four analogue input channels for recording heart rate, physical activity, electrodermal activity (EDA), and respiration. A further analogue input channel monitors the voltage of the battery. This information is useful for identifying recording problems. A digital input channel serves as event marker, allowing to register the occurrence time of important incidents by pressing a button. The device can compute and store values averaged across predefined time intervals (for example, 1 s, 1 min) and the standard deviations of all recorded parameters. Due to its small size and weight, it can easily be worn underneath clothing during almost all daily activities.

After amplification the signals are A/D converted and then further computed by the microprocessor for on-line data reduction. Different types of filters and processing procedures (moving average, high pass, integral, R-R-interval, etc.) can be set according to specific needs. The time base is one millisecond and stored as real time. Sampling and storage rates, as well as the type and settings of data processing are specified by a special software (Vitagraph) of the Vitaport system (Stephan et al., 1989, Jain et al., 1996) on a host computer for each channel separately and are downloaded to the recorder prior to measurement. After pre-processing, data are stored digitally with 8 or 16 bit resolution on the inbuilt solid-state memory. The critical limitation for recording duration is the capacity of the standard 1,5 volt battery (type micro/AAA), allowing a recording time of up to about 24 hours. If battery power falls below 1.2 volts, the microprocessor is switched off and no further recording is made. This procedure saves enough energy for keeping the recorded data stored in the memory for at least an additional 24 hours. A further but usually not critical limitation is the one-megabyte storage capacity. This limitation has to be accounted for by choosing appropriate recording and data reduction parameters. For downloading the recording parameters and for checking the quality of the signals before starting a recording session, the device is connected by an optically insulated interface to a standard serial input port of the host computer.

On the heart rate channel, a hardware trigger detects the QRS-complex of the ECG. The intervals between succeeding heart beats can either be stored directly as R-R-interval recording or indirectly as calculated heart rate per minute, averaged over a preselected interval. If rather short intervals are selected (for example, 500 ms), it is possible that there are intervals where no heartbeat occurs. In such intervals, the heart rate value of the preceding interval will be stored. Physical activity is assessed with a uniaxial motion detector (sensitive in one dimension of space). It is built into the recording device in a way that it detects accelerations applied in the direction of its smallest size. Since the output of this sensor is dependent on the angle between its sensitivity axis and the gravitational force, it is advisable to use the standard deviations and not the raw values of this signal as an indicator of physical activity. Skin conductance is measured with a DC current of a constant voltage of 0.5 volt and respiratory movements with a strain gauge belt fixed around the subject's chest or upper abdomen.

In the present study, heart rate and physical activity were recorded. The recording device Mini-Vitaport was worn beneath the clothes with a cushioned belt in front of the subject's chest. The subjects were allowed to remove the device briefly for taking showers and to change the positioning during the night if this increased the comfort of sleeping. The ECG signal was picked up by a modified Lead 1 derivation. Disposable electrodes were attached below the clavicle on the subject's left and over the lowest rib on the subject's right side. A third electrode, attached over the lowest rib of the subject's left side, served as ground. Heart rate was computed and stored at 500 millisecond intervals. The signal of the acceleration sensor was sampled with 16 Hz and averaged over successive 250 millisecond intervals. The standard deviations of these mean values were stored and used as a gross indicator of physical activity. The recording device was fixed on the subjects in such a way that the stored values represent the horizontal component of their body movements.

Data analysis

The individual recording sessions were first plotted with the Vitagraph software (Figure 2) for visual inspection. The signals were checked for recording failures and artifacts. Recording failures occur if one ore more electrodes lose their contact with

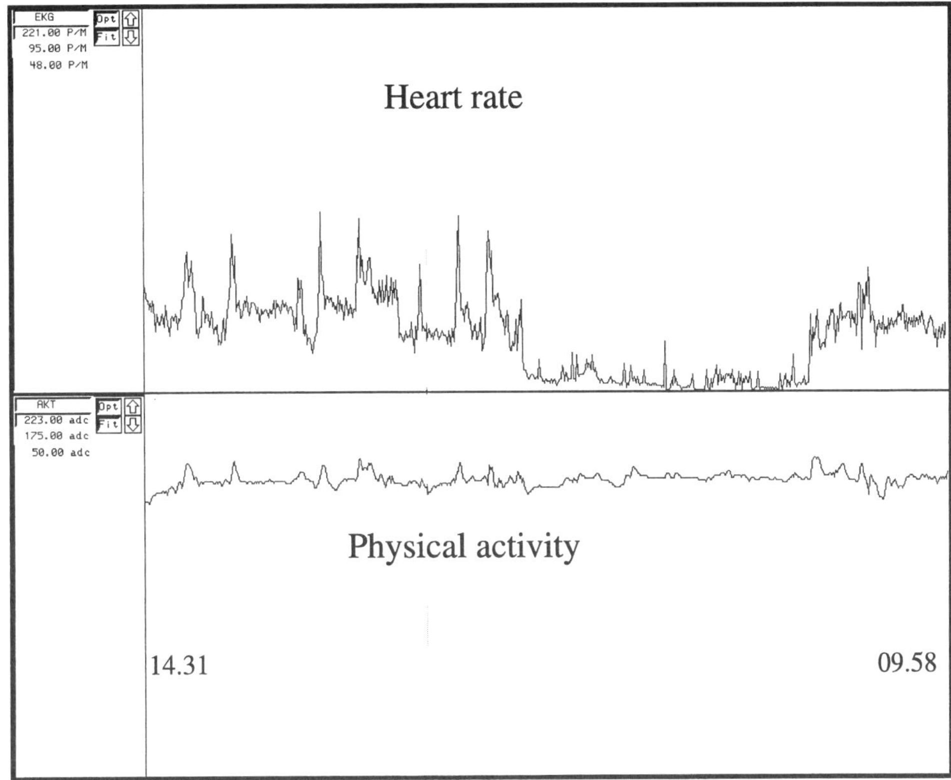

Figure 2. Example of an individual session, plotted with the Vitagraph software of the ambulatory recording system Vitaport. The session started at 14.31 and ended at 9.58 on the following morning.

the skin, battery power falls below the critical level of 1.2 volts, subjects disconnect the recording device, or the device suffers from other technical problems. Recording failures were treated as missing data in all subsequent analyses. Artifacts in heart rate recordings are usually due to mechanical impacts on the ECG electrodes, leading to small movements between electrodes and underlying skin. Artifacts in physical activity recordings are very rare and may only occur if the recording device is too loosely fixed on the body.

Using the standard Vitagraph software, a single value was defined as artifact and replaced by the average of the previous 32 seconds (64 values) if it showed an instantaneous jump of more than 25 percent above or below this moving average. Such a jump corresponds to a sudden increase in heart rate from 100 to 125, or a sudden decrease from 100 to 75 – a condition most likely resulting from movement artifacts or arrhythmias but not from normal physiological or psychological processes. As a next step, mean values of successive one-minute intervals were computed for each recording session and converted into an ASCII-file. This file was then imported into the SPSS program (Statistical Package for Social Sciences, version 9).

In order to identify data periods with significant physical activity as walking, running, or doing sports, an activity threshold was defined for every individual recording session. This threshold was determined by visual inspection of the activity data. The threshold was set at a rather low level in order to achieve that practically all one-minute intervals were marked as period with physical activity where the subject was not sitting or lying but being in upright position and doing some physical activity. In this way even minor physical activity such as walking around in a room was detected.

The large amount of data was further reduced into reasonable units by computing mean values of successive one-hour blocks. In order to have data with equal recording time for all subjects, only the data recorded between 15.00 and 09.00 of the following day were used. This procedure summarized the data into 18 blocks of one hour.

From the heart rate data an individual day-time-baseline and night-time-baseline were determined for each recording day. For this purpose, 5-minute moving average values were computed. Day-time-baseline was defined as lowest 5-minute average occurring between 15.00 and 22.00. During this period all subjects were awake. Night-time-baseline was defined as lowest 5-minute average occurring between 01.00 and 05.00. The time course of the individual changes in heart rate during the recording days is represented by the differences against this day-time-baseline. This procedure compensates individual differences in the level of the resting heart rate.

Statistical significance of differences between the corresponding one-hour blocks across the recording days was tested with one-way ANOVAs (analysis of variance). Multiple post hoc comparisons were performed with Scheffé tests. This conservative approach was chosen to ensure that differences between the three recording sessions were not overestimated. The time course within the recording sessions was not analysed (for example, by means of multiple ANOVAs with repeated measures) because differences in heart rate and physical activity between different time periods such as day and night are obvious.

Results

Detection of recording failures and artifacts

The 14 subjects cooperated very well. Most reported that the measurement interfered little with their activities and that they were unaware of the system after a short adaptation period. Therefore, not many recording failures were found. Most of them occurred for a short time when a subject disconnected the recording device for taking a shower or when battery power was falling below the critical limit.

An example of the corrections made by the applied procedure for detecting artifacts is shown in Figure 3. Using the criterion mentioned above, five percent of the heart rate data was identified as artifact and, therefore, replaced by the average of the previous 32 seconds. On the data indicating body movements, the correction procedure detected practically no artifacts. This is to be expected, since it is a mechanical measurement being hardly susceptible to artifacts.

Heart rate baselines

The heart rate baselines are shown in Table 1. In accordance with the marked difference in physical load between day and night, night-time-baselines were significantly lower than day-time baselines. However, neither day-time-baselines nor night-time-baselines showed any statistical differences across the three recording days. On the control day, day-time-baseline was significantly lower as on the three recording days. Night-time-baselines showed the same trend, although the difference did not reach statistical significance. The lower heart rate on the control day is primarily due to the difference in altitude. Zurich is situated on 400 m above see level, Zuoz on 1600 m. A possible effect of adjustment to the seminar environment could only be minimal and would be masked by the stronger impact of the difference in altitude. On the three recording days, day-time-baselines and night-time-baselines were highly correlated with each other, with r = .65 to .77 remarkably higher than on the preceding control day (r = .43).

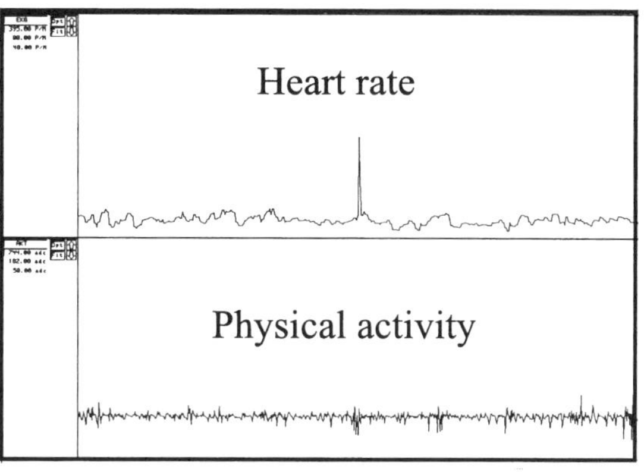

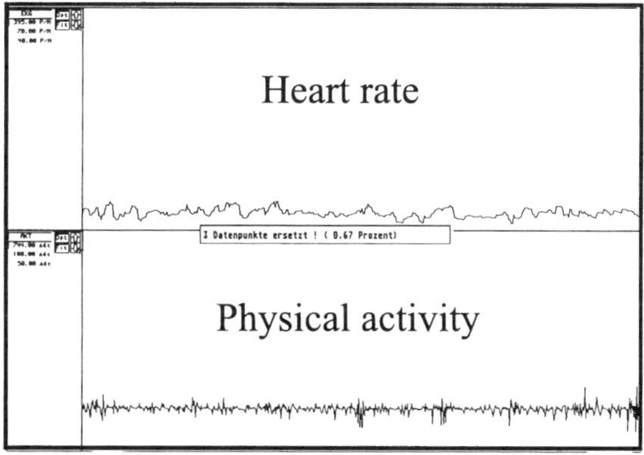

Figure 3. Example of the corrections made by the applied artifact detection procedure on heart rate data (above: raw data; below: data corrected for artifacts).

Table 1. Means of the heart rate baselines in beats per minute with standard deviations on the control day (C) and the three recording days (1, 2, 3).

	N	Control day (Zurich)	Day 1 (Zuoz)	Day 2 (Zuoz)	Day 3 (Zuoz)	Statistical significance
Day-time-baseline	14	53.6 ± 4.9	64.5 ± 8.0	67.0 ± 8.0	63.1 ± 9.8	C to 1,2,3 *
Night-time-baseline	14	43.6 ± 5.8	52.5 ± 10.3	48.4 ±4.6	52.9 ± 11.1	n.s.
Statistical significance	14	***	***	***	***	
Paired samples correlations	14	.43	.65*	.72**	.77**	

* p < .05; ** p < .01; *** p < .001; n.s.: not significant

Effect of academic tasks

The increase in heart rate above day-time-baseline occurring during the academic tasks performed on the three recording days is shown in Table 2, as well as the measurements indicating physical activity. Heart rate was significantly higher when the subjects completed the written examination or the intelligence test than when they were just listening to a lecture. However, there was no significant difference between examination and intelligence test. The higher heart rates found during examination and intelligence test must be due to mental load and performance stress, since the subjects were sitting in a lecture hall and did not have any physical load. This is reflected by the activity measurements, being low during all three academic tasks, and therefore, do not show any statistical differences. During examination, activity measurements are slightly but not significantly higher than during the two other academic tasks. This may indicate that during examination subjects showed some motor restlessness and were sitting less quietly. However, this physical activity is far below a level which would have to be considered as a relevant physical load.

Table 2. Increase in heart rate above daytime-baseline and physical activity on the three recording days (mean ± standard deviation).

	N	Day 1 (Examination)	Day 2 (Lecture)	Day 3 (Intelligence test)	Statistical significance
Heart rate increase (beats per m.)	14	21.4 ± 10.0	10.6 ± 6.5	18.7 ± 6.7	2 to 1,3 *
Physical activity (arbitrary units)	14	7.6 ± 6.3	4.9 ± 3.0	5.2 ± 3.3	n.s.

* $p < .05$; n.s.: not significant

Time course of heart rate and physical activity

The time course of the changes in heart rate against day-time-baseline, as well as the time course of physical activity, are shown in Figure 4 plotted as mean values per hour. As to be expected, physical activity shows a clear-cut difference between day and night. On the other hand, there were no statistical differences between any one-hour means of the three recording days. However, there is a trend towards higher physical activity between 19.00 and 20.00 on recording day one. During this recreational period immediately after dinner most participants were practising some sports, apparently with a little more vigour on day one than on day two or three.

In heart rate, there were some statistically significant differences between the three recording days. First, the above-mentioned effects of the academic tasks (tests versus lecture), performed between 17.00 and 18.00, can also be seen in these curves. Second, in the time between 20.00 and 21.00, there was a significant increase in heart rate on recording day one, while physical activity was as low as during the two other recording days. Between 20.00 and 21.00 on the first recording day, participants were rehearsing in front of each other for oral presentations they had to

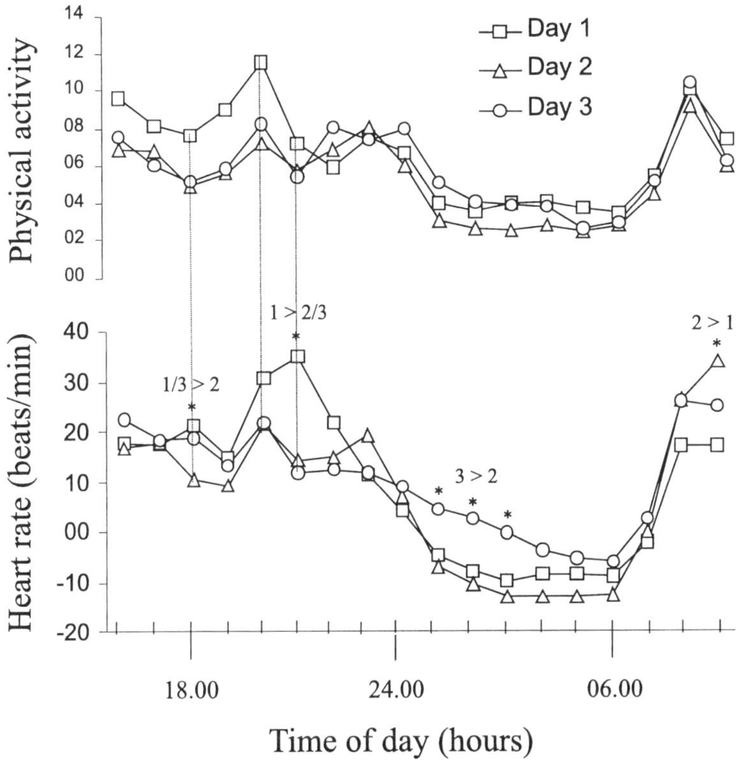

Figure 4. Time course of the changes in heart rate against day-time-baseline, and time course of physical activity, plotted as mean values per hour (* p < .05).

present during the following day. It is remarkable, that this kind of peer viewed public speaking situation led to a much higher increase in heart rate than either the academic test or the intelligence test. Third, on recording day three, between 24.00 and 03.00, heart rate was significantly higher than on the two other recording days. Recording day three included the last evening of the seminar where participants were going out for celebrating a party and most of them went to bed later than during the previous days. Fourth, between 08.00 and 09.00, heart rate was significantly higher on recording day two than on recording day one. behavioral data revealed no reason for this difference.

Time course of activity corrected heart rate

The time course of changes in activity corrected heart rate against day-time-baseline is shown in Figure 5 plotted as mean values per hour. Overall, 17 percent of the one-minute intervals were identified as data periods with physical activity above the individually defined threshold. As correction procedure, these intervals were excluded from the analysis comparing heart rates of the three recording days. The remaining data depicted in Figure 5 demonstrate that the correction did not relevantly

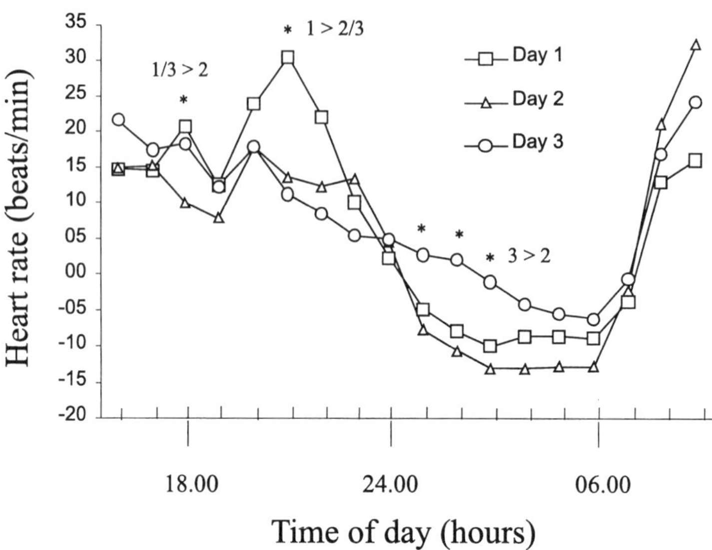

Figure 5. Time course of changes in activity corrected heart rate against day-time-baseline, plotted as mean values per hour (* $p < .05$).

change the effects shown in Figure 4, thus indicating that emotional and mental load but not physical load were the major sources of the increase in heart rate occurring during the time periods with the stressors academic test, intelligence test and public speaking.

Discussion

The ambulatory monitoring method applied in this study provided reliable heart rate recordings over prolonged periods of time. Artifacts occurred only in minor proportion of the data (about five percent) and could be eliminated by interpolation. Due to the small size and weight of the recording device, subjects reported almost no disturbance by the recording procedure and most of them stopped thinking about the recording after a short adaptation period. Even the overnight recordings could be performed without major problems. Sleeping comfort was achieved by the cushioned fixation of the recording device and the possibility to eliminate occurring pressure by moving the device to either side of the chest. Sufficient adaptation to the recording situation is achievable after one recording session. Day-time-baselines and night-time-baselines showed a high correlation for all three recording days. The lower correlation between day-time-baselines and night-time baselines on the control day can be considered as a first night effect.

Despite a limited correspondence between the output of the uniaxial acceleration sensor and the amount of physical activity, overall variation was sufficient as the recordings clearly showed the expected results: There was a marked difference between day and night, and periods with physical exerce could be identified. Furthermore, during the three recording days the time course of the activity curves was very similar, following to the circadian schedule of daily activities. As to activity, there were no statistically significant differences across the three observation days in any of the 18 computed one-hour data blocks. Nevertheless, a trend towards higher physical activity during the academic examination probably indicates that during the examination subjects showed more motor restlessness (for example, sitting less quietly) than during the two other academic tasks. However, this physical activity was far below a level which would have to be considered as a relevant physical load. A further trend suggested that subjects were exercising more actively during the recreational period of recording day one (following the examination) than on the following recording days.

Segmentation of records to separate data periods with or without physical activity could be achieved with a simple procedure by visually determining individual activity thresholds on plotted activity graphs. This procedure allowed to judge, whether a sudden rise in heart rate was caused by physical load, that is, increased metabolic requirements, or whether this change was possibly attributable to regulative arousal accompanying an emotional response or a mental effort.

Heart rate recordings showed the expected increase during an academic test situation. However, although statistically significant, this increase was rather small and only about half as much as the observed increase caused by a simple public speaking situation, where subjects were rehearsing oral presentations with peers. The small effect is probably due to the special type of examination applied. For study preparation, students had a catalogue of questions, and, for the examination, a selection of them was presented. Apparently, this procedure has the intended effect of being less stressful than usual examinations. The major reason for lower stress could be that this examination procedure gives to the students clear expectations about the questions they will get, thereby reducing uncertainty and test anxiety.

Activity correction of heart rate was not necessary for the academic tasks investigated in the present study since subjects were sitting in a lecture hall. However, recording physical activity ascertained that the observed increase of the heart rate during the recreational period of the first recording day was due to public speaking stress rather than physical activity.

Heart rate monitoring combined with some physical activity assessment is a simple but reliable method to identify emotional and mental stress episodes in real-life situations. Disturbance of subjects can be avoided or minimized by using highly miniaturised recording devices. Future developments may lead to devices not bigger than an electrode clip. At present, reducing energy consumption is the major problem, and, it is likely that the battery will always remain the largest component in highly miniaturised recording devices.

Acknowledgements

The following student co-workers whose contribution is greatly appreciated collected the data presented here: A. Abd-el-Razik, M. Haldemann and P. Kunz. Our special thanks go to Prof. K. Frey who organized the seminar in Zuoz and made it possible to perform the recordings.

References

Haldemann, M. (1999). *Salivary cortisol concentrations after awakening, stress-induced psychophysiological reactions to an academic examination, and test performance.* Diss. rer nat. ETH Zürich.

Jäger, R.S. (1988). *Psychologische Diagnostik.* München: Psychologie Verlags Union.

Jäger, R.S., Horn, H. & Ingenkamp, K. (Eds.). (1989). *Test und Trends 7.* Weinheim: Beltz.

Jain, A., Martens, W.L.J., Mutz, G., Weib, R.K. & Stephan, E. (1996). Towards a comprehensive technology for recording and analysis of multiple physiological parameters within their behavioral and environmental context. In J. Fahrenberg & M. Myrtek (Eds.), *Ambulatory assessment: computer-assisted psychological and psychophysiological methods in monitoring and field studies* (pp. 215–235), Göttingen: Hogrefe & Huber Publishers.

Klauer, K.J. (1987). *Kriteriumsorientierte Tests.* Göttingen: Hogrefe.

McEwen, B.S. (1998). Protective and damaging effects of stress mediators. *New England Journal of Medicine, 338*, 171–179.

Raven, J.C. (1979). *Standard progressive matrices / Raven Matrizen Test (SPM). Leistungs- und Fähigkeitstest: Intelligenztest für Kinder bis Erwachsene.* Bern: Verlag Hans Huber.

Scheuch, K.H., Schröder, H. & Gruber, G. (1985). Factors of influence on the adaptation dynamic illustrated on the course of vegetative parameters within examination investigations. In F. Klix, R. Näätänen & K. Zimmer (Eds.), *Psychophysiological approaches to human information processing* (pp. 393–400), Amsterdam: North-Holland.

Spangler, G. (1997). Psychological and physiological responses during an exam and their relation to personality characteristics. *Psychoneuroendocrinology, 22*, 423–441.

Stephan, E., Mutz, G., Langer, S., Schmitz, D. & Wemschulte, B. (1989). A portable microprocessor-controlled psychophysiological data-acquisition-system. *Journal of Psychophysiology, 3,* 338.

Zeier, H. (1992). *Psychophysiologische Stressforschung. Methodik und Ergebnisse einer Untersuchung bei Flugverkehrsleitern.* Bern: Verlag Paul Haupt.

Chapter 23
On-line Measurement of Additional Heart Rate. Methodology and Applications

Michael Myrtek and Friedrich Foerster
Forschungsgruppe Psychophysiologie, Department of Psychology, University of Freiburg, Germany

Introduction

In the foregoing book of this series, we described a special ambulatory monitoring device for the on line measurement of additional heart rate (non-metabolic heart rate) or emotional arousal (Myrtek, Brügner & Müller, 1996a, 1996b). Heart rate was measured by means of an electrocardiogram (ECG) and served as an overall strain indicator, reflecting physical, emotional, and mental strain components simultaneously. Motion detectors measured physical activity. Both parameters were analyzed on line on a one minute basis. The values of heart rate and physical activity of each minute were compared with the values of the previous minutes. If the heart rate of a given minute exceeded the rate of the previous minutes without an accompanying increase of activity, an increase in heart rate elicited by emotional factors was assumed (Myrtek et al., 1988). The occurence of this event triggered a feedback signal (beeper) with the purpose of prompting the subject to respond to several predefined questions. The questions, concerning his or her subjective state and current behavior, were displayed on the screen of the monitoring device.

This method is theoretically based on studies dealing with the synergism of multiple stressors. Several authors have demonstrated that heart rate reactivity in a stressor combination, for example, work on a bicycle ergometer and mental arithmetic, was higher than heart rate reactivity either in the ergometer or in the arithmetic condition (Bartenwerfer, 1963; Blix, Stromme & Ursin, 1974; Roth, Bachtler & Fillingim, 1990; Turner, Carroll, Hanson & Sims, 1988). In an own laboratory study, we used the stressors mental arithmetic, cold pressor, and low grade ergometric exercise (Myrtek & Spital, 1986). Heart rate reactivity was significantly higher for all stressor combinations as compared to heart rate reactivity of the single stressors. The combination of all three stressors yielded the highest heart rate reactivity which was significantly higher than each double stressor combination. Generally, heart rate reactivity elicited by a stressor combination was nearly an additive combination of the respective reactivity elicited by the single stressors.

In our studies cited in this chapter, we used a small computer called MULTI-TALENT (MT, Zak Company, Simbach, Germany). Unfortunately, this device has no longer been produced for several years. Therefore, it was not possible for other users to administer our method. In the meantime, we have however adapted the algorithms to the recorders VITAPORT-II (TEMEC Instruments B.V., Kerkrade, NL.; Becker Meditec, Karlsruhe, Germany) and VARIOPORT (Becker Meditec, Karlsruhe, Germany). A description of these recorders is given by Stephan, Mutz, Feist, and Weiss in the present book. Subjective state and current behavior of the subjects are recorded with the hand-held computer Psion 3a, which is connected to the recorder. An additional development is that posture and motion are assessed by calibrated accelerometry now. This method will be described by Foerster in the present book. A detailed description containing all information about hardware, algorithms, application of electrodes, examples for the recording of behavior and subjective state, primary and secondary data analyses, norm values, and so on is provided in the forthcoming book "Freiburger Monitoring System (FMS)" (Myrtek, Foerster & Brügner, in press). In the following paragraphs, we will present an overview of the methods used and some applications.

Method

The aim of our method is to gather information about physiological reactivity, subjective state, and behavior in everyday life. Mostly, the recording of these parameters lasted for 23 hours in our studies. Especially relevant is the assessment of the differing work-load components (physical, emotional, and mental) because several of our studies dealt with stress and strain at the work place. Moreover, in studies dealing with heart disease patients, information about the ST segment amplitude as an indicator of blood supply to the heart muscle is valuable.

Assessment of the different work-load components

Total work load

Heart rate is the parameter most often used to assess total work load. Our laboratory study cited above showed that heart rate reflected both psychological and physical work load (Myrtek & Spital, 1986). The ECG, which is used for the measurement of heart rate, is a very strong biological signal and, therefore, can be detected with ease. To analyze the aforementioned work-load components, however, still other parameters must be assessed.

Physical work load

During ascending ergometric exercise, physical work load (watt) and oxygen uptake are linearly correlated. When emotional and mental work load are absent during ergometric exercise, physical work load and heart rate are linearly correlated, too. Under conditions of everyday life, measurements of oxygen uptake are difficult to obtain because subjects are forced to wear a mask. Several authors tried, therefore, to assess physical work load on the basis of the subjects' physical activity. Most important for this approach is a strong correlation between physical activity and oxygen uptake. By means of accelerative sensors, very high correlations between oxygen uptake and physical activity during treadmill ergometric exercise were observed under laboratory conditions (Tryon, 1991).

Mental work load

According to many authors, a decrease in heart rate variability is an indicator of mental work load (Hecker, 1988; Meshkati, 1988; Wilson, 1988). We have shown in the above cited laboratory study that the decrease of heart rate variability (operationalized by the mean squared successive differences, MSSD) during mental arithmetic was higher than during a cold pressor test (Myrtek & Spital, 1985). Attenuation of the T wave amplitude of the ECG is also claimed to be an indicator of mental work load. However, our extensive studies with many different samples have shown that T wave amplitude is not a valid indicator (Myrtek et al., 1996b).

Emotional work load

As already mentioned, our method is based on the simultaneous on line comparison of heart rate and physical activity in order to assess heart rate increases which are not caused by physical activity (additional heart rate, emotional arousal). The algorithms used are described below.

Base line

Physiological changes at work have to be related to a suitable base line because individual differences in physiological parameters, for example, heart rate, are highly dependent on the actual physical condition of the subjects. In our studies, the mean values of the physiological parameters assessed during deep sleep are used for base line measurements because heart rate at night generally reveals high stability coefficients (Fahrenberg, Foerster, Schneider, Müller & Myrtek, 1985; Myrtek, Brügner, Fichtler & Müller, 1994a). In our studies, the hour of the night in which the heart rate mean reaches a minimum was assessed for each subject. The mean values of all physiological parameters for this hour, with exception of additional heart rate, were the base lines for the respective parameters assessed during work.

Measurement of the physiological variables

ECG leads

ECG was recorded bipolarly with monitoring electrodes (Red Dot) attached on the chest of the subject. The first ECG lead was placed in a way to allow for a high R wave amplitude (mostly V_4) in order to facilitate the recognition of heart rate during on line analysis. The second lead was placed analogue to V_5. This lead served the analysis of the ST segment amplitude. The negative electrodes for this lead are placed on the sternum beneath the fossa jugularis one below the other. Five electrodes, including a ground electrode (on the processus xiphoideus), were needed for each record. It is important to test the quality of ECG lead attachment with an oscilloscope or when using VITAPORT-II or VARIOPORT with the VITAGRAF software. Furthermore, the ECG leads were tested in different body positions (supine, sitting, standing) to guarantee an optimal data quality for the analyses.

Physical activity

In our studies using the MT-device, physical activity was measured by two motion detectors (accelerative sensors, Zak Company, Simbach, F.R.G.). The detectors were placed on the chest below the clavicle and on the thigh above the knee. Both detectors were coupled to give a common signal and were connected by wires to the analogue device of the MT. Each detector was sensitive to all three dimensions of space (three axes with piezo ceramic elements). The signal of the detectors was amplified and rectified in the analogue device. With the new devices (VITAPORT-II or VARIOPORT), the placement of the detectors was changed to the sternum and the thigh in order to assess posture and motion (see Foerster, this Volume). For overall physical activity, the sensor output is combined on-line by vectorial addition.

On line analysis of additional heart rate

To understand the algorithm for additional heart rate (AHR) and the algorithm for feedbacks, three requirements should be considered:

1. Additional heart rate is an increase of the heart rate relative to the constitutional as well as the situational heart rate level. Therefore, the heart rate changes caused by physical activity due to metabolic demands have to be eliminated from the current heart rate.
2. The feedback signals prompting the subjects to rate their behavior should be continuously distributed throughout the day. Regular and nearly equidistant intervals between the feedback minutes would help to assess the behavior without gaps.
3. Besides feedback minutes initiated by AHRs (so-called "true feedbacks"), feedbacks without AHRs should be prompted (so-called "random feedbacks").

On line analysis of heart rate and physical activity was performed continuously by the MT-device with a sampling rate of 256 Hz. The R waves of the first ECG lead were detected with the help of amplitude, slope, and curvature parameters which were continuously adapted to the changing shape of the QRS-complex (moving average of 10 QRS-complexes). Mean heart rate for each minute was computed from the number of R waves and stored. The impulses of the motion detectors were integrated for each minute and stored simultaneously.

For additional heart rate, the following parameters are relevant:

- Current heart rate of minute i:
- Heart rate level for minute i, defined as the moving average of the 3 minutes before the current minute:

$$HRL_i = (HR_{i-1} + HR_{i-2} + HR_{i-3}) / 3 \quad (1)$$

- Heart rate change of minute i:

$$HRC_i = HR_i - HRL_i$$
$$= HR_i - (HR_{i-1} + HR_{i-2} + HR_{i-3}) / 3 \quad (2)$$

- Physical activity of minute i: ACT_i
- Metabolic heart rate change caused by physical activity during minute i.: HRM_i

$$HRM_i = ACT_i / CDIV_i \quad (3)$$

- Parameter $CDIV_i$ is variable during on line analysis according to rule 2 (see above; distribution of all feedbacks in the time domain) and rule 3 (see above; distribution of the number of "true feedbacks" in relation to the number of "random feedbacks"). This individual adaptation was reversed in the statistical analyses by setting CDIV to a fixed value of 30 in order to compare different subjects.
- Minimal heart rate change in minute i to classify this minute for a true feedback minute $HRPLUS_i$:

$$HRPLUS_i = (90 + ACT_i) / CDIV_i$$
$$= HRM_i + 90/CDIV_i \quad (4)$$

  with parameter $CDIV_i$ as mentioned above. Accordingly, in case of no physical activity, the minimal heart rate change is $90/CDIV_i$. Because $CDIV_i$ is limited to ≤ 30, the amount of HRPLUS is minimally 3 bpm.
- For additional heart rate of minute i (AHR_i), a score is formed defined as the factor, by which the current heart rate change (HRC_i) exceeds the minimal required heart rate change ($HRPLUS_i$):
-

$$AHR_i = HRC_i / HRPLUS_i$$
$$= \{HR_i - (HR_{i-1} + HR_{i-2} + HR_{i-3}) / 3\}$$
$$/ \{(90+ACT_i) / CDIV_i\} \quad (5)$$

  Note: In order to get integer numbers, AHR_i was multiplied by 10.
- For a minute with true feedback, current heart rate change (HRC_i) has to be higher than or equal to the minimal required heart rate change ($HRPLUS_i$):

$$HRC_i \geq HRPLUS_i \quad (6)$$

- Or, in other words, current heart rate (HR_i) has to be greater than the minimal required heart rate change ($HRPLUS_i$) above the heart rate level for minute i

(HRL_i):

$$HR_i \geq HRL_i + HRPLUS_i \quad (6a)$$

- Or, with additional heart rate:

$$AHR_i \geq 1 \quad (6b)$$

- Not regarded as true feedbacks are minutes with a strong increase in physical activity. It is required that current physical activity of minute i (ACT_i) is not higher than 10 units above the activity level (mean activity of the preceding 3 minutes):

$$ACT_i \leq (ACT_{i-1} + ACT_{i-2} + ACT_{i-3}) / 3 + 10 \quad (7)$$

- Moreover, minutes fulfilling the requirements for a true feedback minute but following a minute with high physical activity and high heart rate are excluded. This means that the heart rate of a true feedback minute has to be higher than the heart rate of the preceding minute:

$$HR_i > HR_{i-1} \quad (8)$$

- The continuous distribution of feedback signals throughout the day (rule 2) is controlled by parameter $CDIV_i$. Basically, after 10 - 20 minutes after the last feedback a new feedback is required. If too few minutes do fulfill the criteria (6) – (8), the minimal requirement according to (6) is lowered. This means that the minimal required heart rate change will be reduced by augmenting parameter $CDIV_i$. For adaptation of parameter $CDIV_i$, the relation between the minutes already recorded and those minutes fulfilling criterion (6), that is, AHR ? 1, is considered:

$$\begin{aligned} &\text{If } N_{total} / N_{AHR\geq 1} < 5 \\ &\text{then } CDIV_i = CDIV_i - 1 \\ &\text{If } N_{total} / N_{AHR\geq 1} > 10 \\ &\text{then } CDIV_i = CDIV_i + 1 \end{aligned} \quad (9)$$

  whereby $CDIV_i$ is limited to the interval [1, 30]. The starting point at the beginning of the recording is $CDIV_0 = 23$. If there is no minute fulfilling the criteria (6) – (8), that is, no „true feedback“ possible in the prescribed interval of 10 – 20 minutes after the last feedback, then nevertheless a feedback is given in minute 20. These feedbacks are treated as „random feedbacks“.
- For reasons of comparison but also to avoid possible conditioning, “random feedbacks” are given with no indication of an emotional event after three “true feedbacks”. These “random feedbacks” are given randomly in the interval of 10 – 20 minutes after the last feedback. If in this minute for “random feedback” the criteria (6) – (8) are fulfilled (“true feedback”), then the next following minute is used for “random feedback”.
- If the relation between “true” and “random feedbacks” is smaller than 5 : 2, then no further “random feedbacks” are given with the exception that within the interval of 20 minutes no “true feedback” is possible. In this case a “random feedback” is given in minute 20.

The numerical values of additional heart rate for single minutes vary according to the algorithm between "0" and "HRPLUS" (formula 5) and are not, therefore, normally distributed. However, averaging the values over many minutes as done for such segments as daytime, night time, etc., yields a normal distribution. These algorithms used in our studies were developed empirically in several small studies, whereby considerations of the amount of heart rate increases during emotional states played a significant role.

Heart rate variability (MSSD)

Mental work load is operationalized in our studies by the mean squared successive differences (MSSD). The difference between the instantaneous heart rates (bpm) over two successive RR intervals is computed and squared. These squares are summed up and divided by the number of the differences. Finally, the square root is formed:

$$MSSD = \sqrt{\{\Sigma_{i=2,\ldots,n} (HR_i - HR_{i-1})^2 / (n - 1)\}} \qquad (10)$$

The dimension of the MSSD is beats per minute (bpm). We have not used the instantaneous heart rates in all of our studies, choosing instead to use the RR intervals directly (8.3 ms/min, caused by the off-line sampling rate of 120 Hz).

$$MSSD_{RR} = \sqrt{\{\Sigma_{i=2,\ldots,n} (RR_i - RR_{i-1})^2 / (n - 1)\}} \qquad (10a)$$

P wave amplitude

In several of our studies, the P wave amplitude was shown to be a valid indicator of sympathetic activation (Myrtek et al., 1996b); this parameter might be valuable for field studies and stress-strain research. Naturally, P wave amplitude is correlated with additional heart rate and physical activity because both parameters are associated with sympathetic activation. Therefore, an increase of the P wave amplitude is an indicator of both emotional/mental and physical strain. A detailed description of the measurement is given by Myrtek et al. (in press).

ST segment amplitude and ischaemic episodes

In cardiology, depression of the ST segment amplitude is an indicator of an insufficient blood supply to the heart (Deanfield et al., 1984; Gabbay et al., 1996). However, this interpretation deserves some caution. In our studies, we observed a significant depression of the ST segment amplitude in some of our healthy 11-year old schoolboys. This depression, however, was also dependent on the body position. Similar results were reported by Csapo (1980) and Eggeling et al. (1988). It is interesting to note that women showed more ST segment depression than men in our studies.

Only constant or descending ST segment depressions are relevant in cardiology. Therefore, the normal slope of the ST segment of a subject is used for the interpretation of ST segment depression. During on line analysis of the ECG, ST segment amplitudes of each heart cycle are measured 80, 100, 120, and 140 ms after the tip of the R wave. Reference points for the ST segment are measured 76 and 60 ms prior to the tip of the R wave. During off-line analysis the measurements of the ST segment are related to the so-called PQ knot, formed as the mean of the two points lying prior to the R wave. To serve as a reference, the two points forming the PQ knot should not show a difference greater than 0.035 mV. Otherwise, this heart cycle is omitted. For each minute of the record, the four ST segment amplitudes of all heart cycles are averaged.

The difference is subsequently computed between the 140 ms point and the 80 ms point for each minute, whereby the amplitude of the 120 ms point should be > -0.5 mV and < +0.7 mV. These minutes are averaged and represent the normal ST segment slope of the subject. The point of reference for ischaemic ST segment depressions is the ST segment amplitude 100 ms after the R wave. Ischaemic depression is postulated when the 100 ms point is ≤ -0.1 mV and the slope of the ST segment of this minute is not greater than the normal slope plus one SD of the slope. These minutes are marked in the record.

For clinical purposes, the determination of ischaemic episodes is recommended. The first minute with an ischaemic depression marks the beginning of an episode. The end of an ischaemic episode is characterized by the minute which is followed by two minutes without ischaemic depression. Single minutes in which there is no ischaemic depression but which do occur within an episode do not interrupt the episode. Important parameters for ischaemic episodes are the number of episodes, the minimal, mean, and maximal duration of the episodes as well as the minimal, mean, and maximal amplitude of the ST segment.

Assessment of behavior and subjective state

A feedback signal was emitted by the device every 10 to 20 minutes, resulting in an average of four feedback signals per hour requiring subjects´ response. Subjects did not know that the feedback signals were triggered by their heart rate; they were only told that the signals served to monitor their daily activities. They had the possibility of canceling the feedback algorithm, for example, during the night. The average record had a length of 23 hours, whereby one additional hour is needed for attaching and detaching the device. On average there was eight hours of sleeping time, leaving 15 hours for feedbacks. With an average of four feedbacks per hour, maximally 60 feedbacks were obtained, resulting mostly in about 40 true and 20 random feedbacks.

The subject was requested by the acoustic feedback to describe his or her actual situation and subjective state. Questions were presented on the LCD-display of the device and were answered by moving a cursor and then pressing a key. Because there were four feedbacks per hour, questions had to be limited to a minimum and always had to be tailored to the respective subject samples. It took about 15 to 20 seconds to answer the questions, which were posed from the start of the monitoring till going to bed. Subjects were requested to start the feedback signals again upon awakening. By branching out the questions it was also possible to ask about more complicated issues.

Subjects were well instructed in the use of the device, and all questions together with the possible answers were demonstrated prior to ambulatory monitoring. In addition, a sheet of paper with the questions and the different answers was available. In the studies with patients, subjects were requested to activate the system by themselves if they perceived chest pain. These self-activations of the system were handled in the same way as were the true or random feedback signals, whereby the next feedback was given 10 to 20 minutes after the self-activation.

To give an impression of the questions posed, we provided an example of a study with schoolboys. (Myrtek, Scharff, Brügner & Müller, 1996). In this study, we were especially interested in the TV consumption of the boys. At each signal, they were asked to provide the following information for the minute immediately prior to the beep: Feelings of excitement/arousal, enjoyment of the situation, physical activity, their whereabouts with subsequent questions tailored to the respective situation, and social circumstances. In the case of TV viewing, the boys were asked to disclose the TV station and type of program being broadcasted. All TV stations available in the town were listed on the screen of the device as were the different types of programs.

Data analysis

Artifact control of the physiological data is done with an interactive graphic program which shows all parameters of the 1387 minute record. Data which are thought to be artifacts are eliminated.

For behavioral categorization of the record, all variables of each feedback minute together with the variables of the previous and the following minute are assigned to a category according to the different behavioral information, for example, "daytime", "nighttime", "at work", "at home", etc. If the variables of two or more subsequent feedback minutes are classified in the same category, the variables of all minutes between the two feedback minutes are also assigned to that category. The variables assigned to each category are then averaged for each subject. Statistical analysis is done on these means, and is carried out mostly using MANOVAs (general linear model analysis) in a two- or higher-factorial design (SAS Institute, 1993). Wilks' Lambda is used to determine the F-values.

Evaluation of the method

The main advantage of our method is the rather simple recording technique because only heart rate and physical activity have to be recorded. Compared to other biosignals, both parameters can be recorded nearly without any artifact. Moreover, the subjects are not hampered by the equipment and not aware of the measurement itself. Both parameters, heart rate and physical activity, are able to differentiate over a wide range of physiological activation.

In laboratory experiments as well as in field studies it was shown that additional heart rate is a valid indicator of emotional strain or the emotional work-load component (Myrtek et al., 1996b). It was also demonstrated that physical activity assessed by the device is an indicator of the physical work-load component. Finally, it was demonstrated that heart rate variability is an indicator of mental work load.

However, minor disadvantages in the assessment of the emotional work-load component should be mentioned. Increases in heart rate due to emotional factors accompanied by increasing physical activity cannot be assessed with this method. Moreover, additional heart rate is not only a consequence of emotional factors but also mental factors, at least at the beginning of a task (Myrtek, Dieterle & Brügner, 1990). On the other hand, it is assumed that mental work load does not increase additional heart rate much because the correlation between MSSD and additional heart rate is low, as shown by within-subject correlations. Finally, various emotions are accompanied by various heart rate increases, resulting in the fact that emotions with stronger increases of heart rate are assessed more easily (Cantor, Zillmann & Day, 1978; Caprara et al., 1987; Eisenberg et al., 1988).

Applications

The starting point for the development of this method was a clinical research question on the effects of emotional arousal on myocardial functions. The method, however, is also fruitful for studies on emotions as well as for research in ergonomics. Several samples were used for the assessment of the different work-load components.

Contingencies between ECG changes and cardiac perception in patients

In the foregoing book of this series (Myrtek et al., 1996a), we commented on a study with 30 patients suffering from cardiac neurosis and 20 control patients with no heart-related physical complaints. In this study, the physiological, psychological, and behavioral contingencies of emotional arousal and heart pain were analyzed (Myrtek et al., 1995). It was shown that cardiac perception in these patients was determined by psychological factors and had no physiological origin. In a second study with 35 asymptomatic and 35 symptomatic myocardial infarction patients, the hypothesis was tested that the phenomenon of asymptomatic myocardial infarction might be only the result of an insufficient duration or severity of the myocardial ischaemia (Myrtek, Fichtler, König, Brügner & Müller, 1994b). This hypothesis was not substantiated. However, symptomatic patients were characterized by psychological factors such as complaints of poor health and emotional lability.

In another study with 223 coronary heart disease (CHD) patients, the associations between ischaemia, ventricular premature contractions (VPC), objective emotional/mental arousal, and anginal pain were investigated (Myrtek, Frölich, Fichtler & Brügner, 2000). The hypothesis of this study was that during ischaemic episodes or VPCs „objective emotional/mental arousal“ is more pronounced than during comparable episodes without these events. Objective emotional/mental arousal was indicated by additional heart rate. Forty-nine patients revealed ischaemic episodes and 115 patients VPCs. Emotional/mental arousal was higher during ischaemic episodes as compared to control minutes whereas minutes with VPCs showed no diff-ference. No differences between ischaemic episodes or VPCs and the respective control minutes were observed for anginal pain. Objective emotional/mental arousal was associated in this study with ischaemia but not with arrhythmia, thus partly confirming the hypothesis stated. Because anginal pain is, as shown, not related to objective cardiac events, detection of CHD has to rely on medical examinations.

Interoception of emotional arousal

We already reported five studies with nearly 500 subjects which investigated the perception of emotional events in everyday life (Myrtek & Brügner, 1996). Comparisons of true feedbacks with random feedbacks did not show significant differences for excitement and enjoyment ratings in any of the normal samples and in one patient sample.

In a new study presented in this Volume (Myrtek, Zanda & Aschenbrenner), we studied 50 female and 50 male students with our monitoring device. Following the feedback, the subjects were asked to report their emotions directly (happiness, anger, anxiety/fear, sadness, surprise, disgust, no emotion). Results show that the frequency of the emotions was not different between true and random feedbacks, indicating that the subjects were not able to discriminate well between events with and without emotional arousal. The results further show that cognitive schemata and personality dimensions are more important in emotion perception of everyday life than emotionally caused physiological activation.

Ergonomic studies

We also reported on a study with 23 train drivers (Myrtek et al., 1994c). Speed of the train, mode of driving, and stress of the situation were rated by two observers who accompanied the drivers in the cabin. Starting the train and coming to a halt showed greater emotional work load as compared to cruising. Several discrepancies were seen between work load as indicated by the physiological parameters and corresponding stress ratings by the observers or by the drivers.

In the study with 50 female and 50 male students, we investigated the influence of sex, level of chronic study stress (stressed vs. non-stressed), and study subject ("soft science" vs. "hard science") on physiological reactivity, behavior, and psychological parameters during everyday life (Myrtek, Hilgenberg, Brügner & Müller, 1997). The physiological and psychological parameters were assessed with our device both while at the university and at home. The following hypotheses were tested: (1) time spent at the university as compared to staying at home will show generally higher physiological reactivity, (2) men more than women will show higher physiological reactivity while at the university, (3) chronically stressed as compared to non-stressed students will reveal higher physiological reactivity while at the university, and (4) students studying "hard science" as compared to students studying "soft science" are presumed to be more chronically stressed by their studies and, therefore, will show higher physiological reactivity while at the university.

Comparisons between study-related and leisure activities revealed no differences in physical activity, but heart rate (indicating total work load) and P wave amplitude responses (indicating sympathetic activation) were higher while studying, especially for men, thus confirming the first two hypotheses. Study-related activities also showed a tendency for higher responses in heart rate variability, indicative of increased mental load. Students studying "soft science" revealed higher additional heart rate (indicating emotional work load) than students studying "hard science". We expected higher physiological reactivity in chronically stressed as compared to non-stressed students and higher reactivity in students studying "hard science" as compared to students studying "soft science". However, these hypotheses were not confirmed.

In the study by Myrtek, Fichtler, Strittmatter, and Brügner (1999) with 29 blue and 57 white collar workers, behavior, level of subjective stress, and objective strain during work and leisure time was investigated. Analysis of the physiological parameters for the working hours from 8 h to 16 h revealed differences between the hours for physical activity, heart rate, and additional heart rate but not for heart rate variability. Between 12 h and 13 h, physical activity was somewhat lower and additional heart rate higher, presumably caused by the lunch break. Physical activity and heart rate were higher for blue than white collar workers due to the different tasks of the workers. Self-reports of excitement and enjoyment during the working hours showed no main effects in the MANOVA. Comparison between total working time and leisure time revealed lower physical activity and heart rate but higher additional heart rate for leisure time. In the self-reports, however, leisure time was rated less exciting and more pleasant than working time. There was no indication of higher emotional strain for one or the other group, but mental strain at work was somewhat higher for the blue collar workers. In a questionnaire, white collar workers reported having significantly more stress at work and outside work than blue collar workers. Analysis of the behavior during leisure time (physical activity, activity, social contacts) showed only minor differences between the groups.

Effects of television viewing

In a study with preschool children (six years), 18 boys and 18 girls were recorded with our device in their home environment while viewing different television films (Wilhelm, Myrtek & Brügner, 1997). Two cartoons designed for children of this age and a sequence of commercials were presented in a balanced order. One cartoon consisted of many action scenes ("Ghostbusters") the other reported the story of "Unlucky Jack". Heart rate and additional heart rate were significantly higher for Ghostbusters than for Unlucky Jack, the commercials appearing between both cartoons. Generally, girls displayed a higher heart rate than boys, but during Ghostbusters heart rate was higher in boys. For the commercials, a significant interaction sex x type of commercial was found. Girls´ heart rate was higher for commmercials designed for girls (e.g., Barbie) than for sex neutral commercials (e.g., Smarties). Children with light TV consumption (rated by their parents) showed significantly more additional heart rate than children with heavy TV consumption. This result means that heavy TV viewing is associated with an attenuation of emotional reactivity.

In an extensive study with 100 eleven-year old and 100 fifteen-year old schoolboys, the effects of TV viewing in the home environment on a normal schoolday were investigated (Myrtek & Scharff, 2000). Boys were assigned to either a heavy TV consumption group or light TV consumption group by a median split of the viewing time on the day of recording. Heavy viewers spent about three hours, light viewers one hour for TV viewing. The finding of an attenuation of emotional reactivity (additional heart rate) during TV viewing for heavy viewers as compared to light viewers was substantiated in this study, too. A comparison of school and leisure time showed that additional heart rate was significantly higher during leisure time. The subjective ratings of excitement and enjoyment elicited by the feedback signals of the device, however, revealed higher excitement and less enjoyment during schooltime. Physical activity was significantly reduced in the heavy viewing group. Light viewers had more social contacts with friends than heavy viewers who were alone more frequently. At school heavy viewers had poorer marks especially in the German language.

Summary

As shown by several studies, heart rate is both an indicator of emotional arousal and an indicator of physical activity. It is possible to separate the emotional and physical component if physical activity reflecting the metabolic demand can be measured accurately. With a special ambulatory monitoring device, heart rate and physical activity (recorded with motion detectors) are compared on line. If heart rate of a specific minute exceeds the rate of the previous minutes without an accompanying increase of physical activity, an emotional event (additional heart rate) may be assumed. In such a case, the subject is requested by a beep signal to answer relevant questions of how he or she feels, about what he or she is doing, etc. Until now the device used in our studies was not available for other research groups because the device was no longer produced by the company. Now we have adapted the algorithms to the widespread VITAPORT II and VARIOPORT devices. In this chapter we describe the most important algorithms and the rationale for our ambulatory monitoring.

The method was used in our studies with preschool children, schoolboys of diffferent age, students of both sexes, train drivers, industrial blue and white collar workers, patients with coronary heart disease, and patients suffering from cardiac neurosis. As yet, we have gathered ambulatory monitoring data from more than 1,300 persons. The diversified use shows that the method is useful for many research questions such as cardiac perception in patients, emotions in everyday life, ergonomic studies, effects of television viewing, etc.

Acknowledgements

This research was supported by a grant from the Deutsche Forschungsgemeinschaft (DFG). We thank Marcus Cheetham for improving the English version of this Chapter.

References

Bartenwerfer, H. (1963). Über Art und Bedeutung der Beziehung zwischen Pulsfrequenz und skalierter psychischer Anspannung. *Zeitschrift für experimentelle und angewandte Psychologie*, *10*, 455-470.

Blix, A.S., Stromme, S.B. & Ursin, H. (1974). Additional heart rate - An indicator of psychological activation. *Aerospace Medicine*, *45*, 1219-1222.

Cantor, J.R., Zillmann, D., & Day, K.D. (1978). Relationship between cardiorespiratory fitness and physiological responses to films. *Perceptual and Motor Skills*, *46*, 1123-1130.

Caprara, G.V., D'Imperio, G., Gentilomo, A., Mammucari, A., Renzi, P., & Travaglia, G. (1987). The intrusive commercial: Influence of aggressive TV commercials on aggression. *European Journal of Social Psychology*, *17*, 23-31.

Csapo, G. (1980). *Konventionelle und intrakardiale Elektrokardiographie*. Wehr: Ciba-Geigy.

Deanfield, J.E., Shea, M., Ribiero, P., De Landsheere, C.M., Wilson, R.A., Horlock, P. & Selwyn, A.P. (1984). Transient ST segment depression as a marker of myocardial ischemia during daily life. *American Journal of Cardiology*, *54*, 1195-1200.

Eggeling, T., Günther, H., Treis-Mueller, I., Osterspey, A., Höher, M. & Hombach, V. (1988). ST segment changes in healthy volunteers during Holter monitoring and exercise stress test. *European Heart Journal*, *9* (Suppl. N), 61-64.

Eisenberg, N., Fabes, R.A., Bustamante, D., Mathy, R.M., Miller, P.A., & Lindholm, E. (1988). Differentiation of vicariously induced emotional reactions in children. *Developmental Psychology, 24*, 237-246.

Fahrenberg, J., Foerster, F., Schneider, H.J., Müller, W. & Myrtek, M. (1985). Adequate scaling of heart rate reactions - A comparative study based on resting levels, measures of basal (sleeping) state, vita maxima, and individual range. In: J.F. Orlebeke, G. Mulder & L.J.P. van Doornen (Eds.), *Psychophysiology of cardiovascular control. Methods, models, and data* (pp. 479-490). New York: Plenum.

Gabbay, F.H., Krantz, D.S., Kop, W.J., Hedges, S.M., Klein, J., Gottdiener, J.S. & Rozanski, A. (1996). Triggers of myocardial ischemia during daily life in patients with coronary artery disease: physical and mental activities, anger and smoking. *Journal of the American College of Cardiology, 27*, 585-592.

Hecker, C. (1988). *Feld- und Laboruntersuchungen zu simultan und sukzessiv unterbrochenen Belastungssuperpositionen bei Fahrzeugführung und Kransteuerung.* Fortschritt-Berichte VDI, Reihe 17, Nr.46. Düsseldorf: VDI-Verlag.

Meshkati, N. (1988). Heart rate variability and mental workload assessment. In: P.A. Hancock & N. Meshkati (Eds.), *Human mental workload.* (pp. 101-115). Amsterdam: Elsevier.

Myrtek, M. & Brügner, G. (1996). Perception of emotions in everyday life: studies with patients and normals. *Biological Psychology, 42*, 147-164.

Myrtek, M., Brügner, G., Fichtler, A., König, K., Müller, W., Foerster, F. & Höppner, V. (1988). Detection of emotionally induced ECG changes and their behavioral correlates: A new method for ambulatory monitoring. *European Heart Journal, 9* (Supplement N), 55-60.

Myrtek, M., Brügner, G., Fichtler, A. & Müller, W. (1994a). Test-retest stability of ECG parameters during ambulatory monitoring of patients with ischemic heart disease. *Journal of Ambulatory Monitoring, 7*, 265-279.

Myrtek, M., Brügner, G. & Müller, W. (1996a). Interactive monitoring and contingency analysis of emotionally induced ECG changes: Methodology and applications. In: J. Fahrenberg & M. Myrtek (Eds.), *Ambulatory assessment. Computer-assisted psychological and psychophysiological methods in monitoring and field studies* (pp. 115-127). Göttingen: Hogrefe.

Myrtek, M., Brügner, G. & Müller, W. (1996b). Validation studies of emotional, mental, and physical workload components in the field. In: J. Fahrenberg & M. Myrtek (Eds.), *Ambulatory assessment. Computer-assisted psychological and psychophysiological methods in monitoring and field studies* (pp. 287-304). Göttingen: Hogrefe.

Myrtek, M., Deutschmann-Janicke, E., Strohmaier, H., Zimmermann, W., Lawerenz, S., Brügner, G. & Müller, W. (1994c). Physical, mental, emotional, and subjective workload components in engine drivers. *Ergonomics, 37*, 1195-1203.

Myrtek, M., Dieterle, W., & Brügner, G. (1990). Psychophysiological response patterns to variations of the experimental load of a reaction time task. *Journal of Psychophysiology, 4*, 209-220.

Myrtek, M., Fichtler, A., König, K., Brügner, G. & Müller, W. (1994b). Differences between patients with asymptomatic and symptomatic myocardial infarction: The relevance of psychological factors. *European Heart Journal, 15*, 311-317.

Myrtek, M., Fichtler, A., Strittmatter, M. & Brügner, G. (1999). Stress and strain of blue and white collar workers during work and leisure time: Results of psychophysiological and behavioral monitoring. *Applied Ergonomics, 30*, 341-351.

Myrtek, M., Foerster, F. & Brügner, G. (in press). *Freiburger Monitoring System (FMS). Ein Daten-Aufnahme- und Auswertungs-System für Untersuchungen im Alltag: Emotionale Beanspruchung, Körperlage, Bewegung, EKG, subjektives Befinden, Verhalten.* Frankfurt/M.: Peter Lang.

Myrtek, M., Frölich, E., Fichtler, A. & Brügner, G. (2000). ECG changes, emotional arousal, and subjective state. An ambulatory monitoring study with CHD patients. *Journal of Psychophysiology, 14*, 106-114.

Myrtek, M., Hilgenberg, B., Brügner, G. & Müller W. (1997). Influence of sex, college major, and chronic study stress on psychophysiological reactivity and behavior: Results of ambulatory monitoring in students. *Journal of Psychophysiology, 11*, 124-137.

Myrtek, M. & Scharff, C. (2000). *Fernsehen, Schule und Verhalten. Untersuchungen zur emotionalen Beanspruchung von Schülern.* Bern: Huber.

Myrtek, M., Scharff, C., Brügner, G. & Müller, W. (1996). Physiological, behavioral, and psychological effects associated with television viewing in schoolboys: An exploratory study. *Journal of Early Adolescence, 16*, 301-323.

Myrtek, M. & Spital, S. (1986). Psychophysiological response patterns to single, double, and triple stressors. *Psychophysiology, 23*, 663-671.

Myrtek, M., Stiels, W., Herrmann, J.M., Brügner, G., Müller, W., Höppner, V. & Fichtler, A. (1995). Emotional arousal, pain, and ECG changes during ambulatory monitoring in patients with cardiac neurosis and controls: Methodological considerations and first results. In: D. Vaitl & R. Schandry (Eds.), *From the heart to the brain. The psychophysiology of circulation - brain interaction* (pp. 319-334). Frankfurt/M.: Peter Lang.

Roth, D.L., Bachtler, S.D. & Fillingim, R.B. (1990). Acute emotional and cardiovascular effects of stressful mental work during aerobic exercise. *Psychophysiology, 27*, 694-701.

SAS Institute (1993). *SAS Procedures Guide, Version 6.* Cary, NC: SAS Institute.

Tryon, W.W. (1991). *Activity measurement in psychology and medicine.* New York: Plenum.

Turner, J.R., Carroll, D., Hanson, J. & Sims, J. (1988). A comparison of additional heart rates during active psychological challenge calculated from upper body and lower body dynamic exercise. *Psychophysiology, 25*, 209-216.

Wilhelm, P., Myrtek, M. & Brügner, G. (1997). *Vorschulkinder vor dem Fernseher. Ein psychophysiologisches Feldexperiment.* Bern: Huber.

Wilson, G.F. (1988). Measurement of operator workload with the neuropsychological workload test battery. In: P.A. Hancock & N. Meshkati (Eds.), *Human mental workload.* (pp. 63-100). Amsterdam: Elsevier.

Chapter 24
Interactive Psychophysiological Monitoring of Emotions in Students' Everyday Life. A Replication Study

Michael Myrtek, Denis Zanda, and Eveline Aschenbrenner
Forschungsgruppe Psychopysiologie, Department of Psychology, University of Freiburg , Germany

Introduction

Emotion research has to deal with several problems. The most prominent are the method of emotion induction, the interaction of the different response systems (verbal-cognitive, physiological, behavioral), and the specificity of physiological responses for differing emotions. The validity of emotion induction is equivocal for both laboratory and field studies. In laboratory experiments, different emotional states are elicited by the experimenter with often questionable success. As opposed to field studies, subjects in laboratory experiments know that they will be exposed to special situations which may enhance the correlations between physiological activation and self-reported emotional states. On the other hand, field studies also have limitations because they have to rely on the perception of emotions. In a first paper on the perception of emotions in everyday life (Myrtek & Brügner, 1996), we reported on five ambulatory monitoring studies in which physiological and psychological parameters were assessed simultaneously throughout the day. Emotional events were identified by an increase of heart rate without an accompanying increase in physical activity (emotional or additional heart rate), and, under certain conditions, a feedback signal was given which requested subjects to answer predefined questions. In addition, "random" feedbacks were interspersed between these "true" feedbacks but with no indication of emotional arousal. Subjects in these studies were unaware that the feedback signal was triggered by their own heart rate. Despite great mean differences in emotional heart rate (about 7 bpm) with no differences or even a decline in physical activity, comparisons of the excitement and enjoyment ratings following the true feedbacks (emotional events) with those of following the random feedbacks (neutral situations) did not show significant differences in any of the normal samples and in one of the patient samples. We concluded that the perception of physiological changes as an indicator of emotional arousal in everyday life is quite different from the results suggested by laboratory experiments. Obviously, the identification of emotional arousal in everyday life is much more difficult because we have to account for subjective hypotheses and schemata as proposed by several authors (Myrtek, 1998; Pennebaker, 1982; Rimé, Philippot & Cisamolo, 1990).

The second problem pertains to the interaction of the different response systems. According to the three systems approach (Lang, 1993), verbal reports, behavioral responses, and physiological activity are coupled imperfectly. Alternatively, the view is also held that physiological changes actually cause the emotion (Schachter & Singer, 1962). This emotion perception model assumes that there is activity in different physiological processes which are detected by some higher-order system to generate an emotion report. However, the perception model has been heavily criticized (Reisenzein, 1983).

A third problem deals with the different physiological responses for different emotions. The notion of systematic response profiles associated with various emotions is still a matter of debate. Levenson (1994) states that the emotions anger, fear, and sadness produce larger increases in heart rate than disgust. This author demonstrated that these differences show consistency across subject populations different in profession, age, culture, and gender. As to happiness, Levenson reports that anger and fear produce larger heart rate accelerations than happiness. The issue of physiological response profiles surely is a matter of the chosen time base, too. In a study conducted by Johnsen, Thayer, and Hugdahl (1995), a heart rate acceleration occurred with happy facial expressions, and a heart rate deceleration with angry expressions, contradicting the findings reported by Levenson and those of our first study presented in this paper (Myrtek, Aschenbrenner & Brügner, submitted). Differences in the methods might explain the contrasting results because Johnsen et al. used phasic heart rate changes, based on the 6 s of stimulus presentation which was compared to the 2 s preceding stimulus onset, whereas in our study, the mean heart rate of a whole minute was used.

Our above cited ambulatory studies (Myrtek & Brügner, 1996) did not ask the subjects about their emotional state directly. Therefore, we decided to conduct the present studies in which subjects were asked to indicate whether or not an emotion was present during both feedbacks (true and random). In these studies, too, subjects did not know the nature of the feedbacks. They were only told that the feedbacks served to monitor their daily activities. In the case of a perceived emotion, subjects were asked to disclose the emotion. The following emotions were listed on the display of the device: happiness, anger, anxiety/fear, sadness, surprise, and disgust. Moreover, subjects were encouraged to activate the system by themselves in order to record their psychological state when they perceived an emotion.

A crucial questions is, whether our method can detect emotional arousal validly. The method is based on the decomposition of heart rate, which reflects both the physical (energetical) activity as well as the emotional and mental activation. Several studies using multiple stressors (for example, physical activity and mental stress) have shown that heart rate increase to the stressor combination is a nearly additive combination of the heart rate increases induced by the single stressors (Myrtek & Spital, 1986; Roth, Bachtler & Fillingim, 1990; Turner, Carroll, Hanson & Sims, 1988). Emotional events were operationalized in the present studies by the simultaneous comparison of heart rate and physical activity, yielding the non-metabolic heart rate component. This operationalization is analogous to "additional heart rate", which is defined as heart rate acceleration without a corresponding increase of physical activity indicated by oxygen consumption (Blix, Stromme & Ursin, 1974; Turner et al., 1988). Because of technical reasons, it was not possible to determine oxygen consumption in the field. Instead of oxygen consumption, we therefore used two very sensitive motion detectors in order to differentiate between metabolic and non-metabolic heart rate. This method of detecting emotional events depends on the extent to which physical activity recorded by motion detectors really reflects metabolic demand. Because heart rate is dominated by the metabolic demand (physical activity), we may expect strong correlations between physical activity measured by motion detectors and heart rate, regardless of whether emotional events are present or not. Therefore, the magnitude of this correlation coefficient would reflect the extent to which motion detectors can be used for the detection of rough metabolic demand. Pooled within-subject correlations between heart rate and physical activity, measured by motion detectors based on ambulatory monitoring records with 1387 minutes, revealed coefficients between 0.70 and 0.81 for samples of boys, female and male students as well as white- and blue-collar employees (Myrtek, Brügner & Müller, 1996a). Taking into account that emotionally induced increases in heart rate lower the coefficients, it can be concluded that physical activity measured by motion detectors is a good reflection of metabolic demand.

The strong correlation between physical activity and heart rate is only a prerequisite for the detection of emotional events. Other demonstrations of proof are necessary to endorse the assumption that "emotional heart rate" taps variance caused by emotional arousal. In two laboratory experiments with male students, we were able to show that emotional heart rate was significantly higher when watching an erotic film as compared to a comedy. This finding holds for the student sample watching the films under resting conditions as well as for the second sample watching the films during light but varied ergometric exercise (Myrtek & Brügner, 1996). An ambulatory monitoring study with train drivers showed that emotional heart rate was higher for the driving modes "start" and "braking to stop" as compared to differing train speeds up to 200 km/h (Myrtek et al., 1994). The heightened risk of accidents while driving into and leaving the station may be the reason for the increase in emotional arousal. Further evidence stems from a study with schoolboys (Myrtek, Scharff, Brügner & Müller, 1996c). In this study, boys with light TV consumption were compared to boys with heavy TV consumption. Boys with heavy TV consumption displayed significantly lower emotional heart rate increase while watching TV than boys with light consumption. We argued that the high TV consumption of the former group could be related to emotional bluntness, with no or only small reactions to the often emotional information presented on TV. This finding of a reduced emotional heart rate reaction in heavy TV consumers was replicated in a sample of preschool children (Wilhelm, Myrtek & Brügner, 1997) and in a sample of male students (Myrtek et al., 1996a). Further arguments supporting the view that emotional heart rate is an indicator of emotional arousal derive from special social situations. With student samples, we could show that social contacts with peers revealed lower emotional heart rate reactions than social contacts with strangers (Myrtek et al., 1996a). Other ambulatory monitoring studies with samples of cardiac or rheumatic patients showed that emotional heart rate was higher during contacts with doctors or nurses as compared to contacts with other patients or whilst being alone.

The term "emotional event" or "emotional heart rate" used in the present paper does have some limitations. Increases in heart rate due to psychological reasons not only occur during emotional states but also with increased mental workload, at least at the beginning of a task (Myrtek, Dieterle & Brügner, 1990). However, we do not assume that this latter component is an important factor for emotional heart rate in our ambulatory monitoring studies because heart rate variability, a widely used indicator of mental workload (Meshkati, 1988; Wilson, 1988), does not correlate to a substantial degree with emotional heart rate. The pooled within-subject correlations between emotional heart rate and heart rate variability for the different samples mentioned above only revealed coefficients between -0.03 and -0.10 (Myrtek et al., 1996a). A limitation of the present study is given by the fact that our method cannot be used to detect all emotional events. Emotional arousal with increased heart rate and an accompanying increase in physical activity, caused for instance by behavioral responses, would be overlooked by this method. Taken all together, however, we are convinced that the method used is able to detect a good deal of the variance caused by emotional arousal.

The following ambulatory monitoring studies offer the opportunity to assess the frequency of emotional experience in everyday life in students as well as to subjectively appraise different emotions according to excitement (arousal) and affective valence, the most important emotional dimensions (Bradley, Greenwald & Hamm, 1993; Wundt, 1905). Schwartz, Warren, and Pickering (1994) observed in their 24-

hour blood pressure monitoring study that 65% of all blood pressure readings were neutral. In this study, happiness was the most frequent emotion (12%), followed by anxiety (7%) and anger (1%). In a similar study, Shapiro, Jamner, and Goldstein (1997) also observed that a happy mood was the most prominent mood in subjects' reports. In the experiment by Johnsen et al. (1995) with 96 female students using the Ekman faces, the authors reported the following equation for excitement: fear = angry > surprise > disgust = sad = happy > neutral. For pleasantness the following equation was reported: happiness > neutral > surprise > sad = fear = angry = disgust.

Several personality dispositions are related to emotions. There might be, for example, a "propensity" for high trait anxious persons to view uncertain events as possible threats (Frijda, 1994). Therefore, our subjects filled in several personality questionnaires in which the various personality dimensions might be related to different emotions: Happiness might be related to extraversion, neuroticism (negatively), and trait-anxiety (negatively); anxiety/fear to trait-anxiety, neuroticism, health worries, and physical complaints; anger to anger disposition, anger expression, and anger temperament; and sadness to introversion, neuroticism, and trait-anxiety. No clear expectations can be formulated for the emotions surprise and disgust.

In summarizing, the studies presented address the following questions:

- Frequency of emotions;
- Quality of emotions;
- Physiological profiles of different emotions;
- Accuracy of the perception of emotional arousal; and
- Influence of personality dimensions on the emotions reported.

Method

Subjects and procedure

In the first study (Myrtek et al., submitted), fifty female students (mean age 22.3 years, range 20 to 27) were recruited from all disciplines except psychology by leaflets at the university. They were paid for taking part. In a first session, subjects were informed about the procedure and were asked to complete the following questionnaires: German version of the State-Trait-Anger-Expression Inventory (STAXI; Schwenkmezger, Hodapp & Spielberger, 1992), German version of the State-Trait-Anxiety Inventory (STAI; Laux, Glanzmann, Schaffner & Spielberger, 1981), Freiburg Personality Inventory (FPI; Fahrenberg, Hampel & Selg, 1984), and Life Satisfaction Questionnaire (FLZ; subscale "health satisfaction"; Fahrenberg, Myrtek, Schumacher & Brähler, 2000).

The second session took place in the morning a few days later. Five electrodes for two channel electrocardiogram (ECG), two motion detectors, and a small microphone for speech activity were attached, and the quality of ECG lead attachment was tested with an oscilloscope. Subjects were instructed in the proper use of the device, especially in answering the questions which were posed on the display of the device and announced by acoustic signals. They were asked to return to the laboratory after 23 hours.

In the replication study, fifty male students were recruited and examined in exactly the same way. This student sample had a mean age of 23.3 years (range 20 to 28). The somewhat higher age of the male sample is due to military service prior to their studies.

Apparatus

A description of the method was already given in our previous paper (Myrtek & Brügner, 1996), and methodological questions were discussed in some other publications (Myrtek, 1990; Myrtek et al., 1988; 1996a; 1996b). Therefore, only a brief outline of the method is given in this paper. The device, carried by the subjects in a leather bag, consisted of a small computer equipped with a LCD display and an analogue device which performed the on-line analysis of physical activity, heart rate, and speech activity. Because the connections between the electrodes, motion detectors, or microphone and the device were about 4 m in length, the bag could be placed next to the bed at night, allowing for unrestricted body movement during sleep. Physical activity was measured by two motion detectors (accelerative sensors, sensitive to all three dimensions of space) placed on the chest below the clavicle and on the thigh above the knee. ECG was recorded by two chest leads, whereby the first lead was used to detect the R-wave in the ECG, and the second to analyze the ST-segment amplitude. The microphone was placed on the side of the larynx and mechanically protected by a metal cap. Subjects wore a scarf to conceal the microphone. On-line analysis of physical activity, heart rate, and speech activity was performed continuously with a sampling rate of 256 Hz, and mean values were stored for each minute.

Heart rate (HR) and physical activity (PA) of each minute were compared to the moving average of the previous 3 minutes in order to detect surmised emotional events. An emotional event was postulated if the heart rate of a given minute was at least 3 beats/min greater than the average of the previous minutes with no or only a small increase in physical activity (= 10 units). If physical activity increased, the minimal additional heart rate used to indicate an emotional event increased as well. The algorithm for this procedure was: HR = moving average of HR + HRPLUS, with HRPLUS = (PA + 90)/PAR and PAR = 30 (starting points for HR = 120, PA = 0, and PAR = 23). For example, with PAR = 30 and PA = 0, a minimal heart rate increase (HRPLUS) of 3 beats/min was required to indicate an emotional event; with PAR = 30 and PA = 60 a minimal heart rate increase of 5 beats/min was required. The parameter PAR was adapted individually to optimize the detection of emotional events. Q was the number of elapsed minutes of the recording time divided by the number of possible emotional events as defined above during this time. If Q < 5 then PAR = (PAR – 1); if Q > 10 then PAR = (PAR + 1), only if PAR < 30 (starting point for Q was 8). This means that for subjects with rare emotional events (Q > 10) HRPLUS was lowered (minimally to 3 beats/min) and for subjects with frequent emotional events HRPLUS was raised. This individual optimization was reversed in the statistical analyses by setting PAR to a fixed value of 30 to compare different subjects. The emotional heart rate of the different segments (happiness, anger, anxiety, etc.) represents the mean value of the emotional heart rate for the respective events. These mean values were divided by 3 (to yield the factor by which the minimal heart rate was exceeded) and multiplied by 10 (units of emotional heart rate/min; see also Myrtek & Foerster, this Volume).

A feedback signal was emitted by the computer every 10 to 20 minutes, resulting in an average of four feedback signals per hour requiring subject response. Feedback signals were either triggered by an emotional event as defined above (true feedback) or were given randomly after about two emotionally-triggered signals (random feedback). The number of true and random feedbacks is not fixed totally because of the individual differences in emotional response. Predefined questions were presented on the LCD display of the device and were answered by moving a cursor and then depressing a key. At each signal, the subjects were asked to provide the following information for the minute immediately prior to the beep: feelings of excitement (4-step rating scale: 1 = not to 4 = very excited), enjoyment of the situation (5-step rating scale: 1 = very enjoyable to 5 = very unpleasant), physical activity (lying, sitting, standing, etc.), present location of the subject (at the university, at home, elsewhere), activity (resting, washing, eating, housework, etc.), and social contact (alone, students present, friends present, etc.). The last question pertained to the emotions with 1 = no emotion, 2 = happiness, 3 = anger, 4 = anxiety/fear, 5 = sadness, 6 = surprise, and 7 = disgust. At the end of monitoring, the record of each subject comprising 1387 minutes was transferred to a PC hard disk.

Data analysis

The following physiological parameters were included: physical activity (units/min), heart rate (bpm), emotional heart rate (units/min), heart rate variability (mean squared successive differences, MSSD, bpm), P-wave amplitude (microV), ST-segment amplitude (microV), and speech activity (% activity/min). For categorization of the record (segmentation), all variables of each feedback minute, including those minutes in which subjects activated the system by themselves, were assigned to a category according to the different emotions. The variables assigned to each category were then averaged for each subject. Statistical analysis was applied to these means.

Multivariate comparisons between the different categories were done with the generalized T^2 statistic (Hotelling's T^2; Anderson, 1984), followed by univariate t-tests for dependent samples. Wilks's Lambda was used to determine the F-values. In the correlation analyses, Pearson coefficients were determined. All analyses were done with SAS (SAS Institute, 1993). If not otherwise stated, a level of significance of $p < .05$ is used throughout the text.

Results

Frequency of emotions

In the first study with female students, a mean of 34.9 true feedbacks and a mean of 18.6 random feedbacks was observed. Moreover, the system was activated by 39 women with a mean of 2.6 activations. The replication study with male students revealed a mean of 29.8 true feedbacks and a mean of 15.8 random feedbacks. Self-activation of the system occurred in 31 students with a mean of 1.9 activations. During true feedbacks 61.0% of the female students reported no emotion as compared to 72.7% of the male students. For random feedbacks the figures are 59.1% and 72.4%, respectively. This sex difference is significant ($p = .004$). As shown in Figures 1 to 3, female students reported higher frequencies of anger, anxiety/fear, and sadness than male students. Happiness was the most frequent emotion in all students followed by anger and anxiety/fear. Sadness, surprise, and disgust occurred very infrequently.

A significant difference between true and random feedbacks was observed only for anxiety/fear whereby the frequency for this emotion was higher for true feedbacks. Of the 50 female students, $N = 46$ had social contacts with other students and personal friends. As may be expected, perceived emotions were more frequent in the interaction with friends (63.7% of all feedback minutes plus the minutes with self activation) than in the interaction with other students (30.8%) or being alone (31.5%). MANOVA for the social contacts (friends, students, alone) was significant with $F(2,44) = 34.81$, $p = .0001$. Forty-three of the male students had social contacts with other students and personal friends. Perceived emotions occurred in the interaction with friends with a frequency of 58.2%. During interactions with other students emotions were reported with a frequency of 29.7%, and being alone showed a frequency of 22.7%. MANOVA was significant with $F(2,41) = 30.45$, $p = .0001$.

Subjective quality of emotions

The most frequent emotions were happiness, anger, and anxiety/fear. Figures 4 to 6 show the comparisons for the subjective quality during these emotions. As we might expect, excitement is low for happiness and high for both anger and anxiety/fear, with no significant difference between the latter emotions. Male students

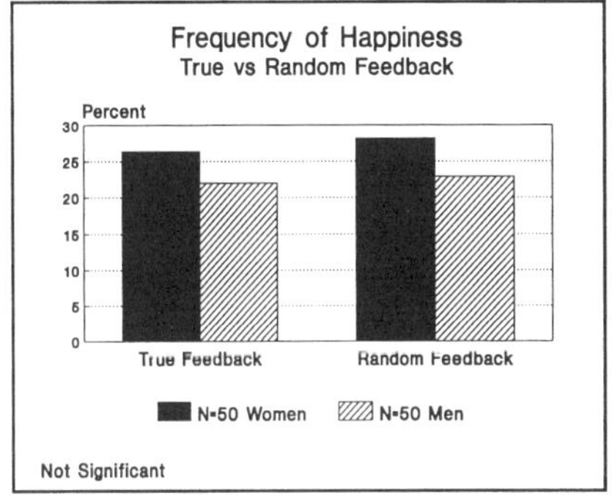

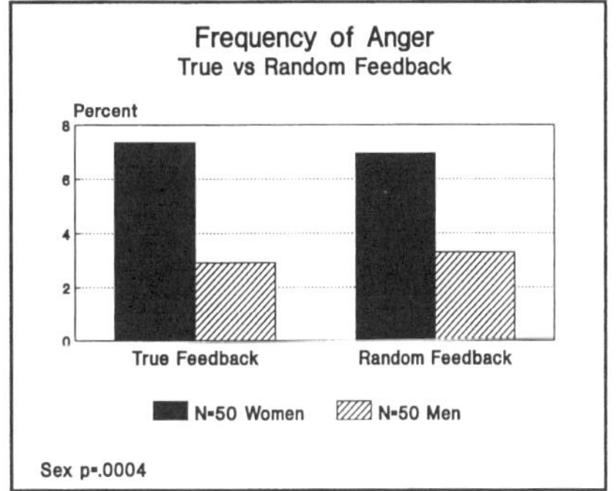

Figure 1. Frequency (% of feedbacks) of happiness and anger during true and random feedback in female and male students.

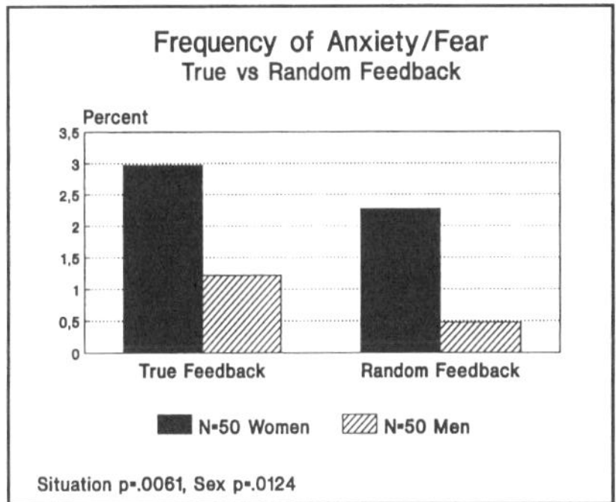

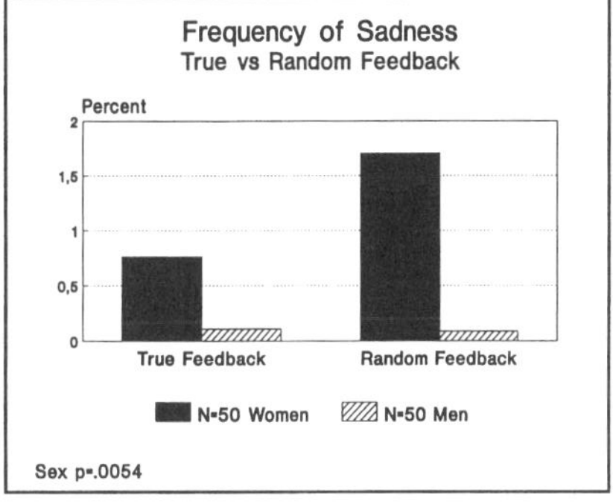

Figure 2. Frequency (% of feedbacks) of anxiety/fear and sadness during true and random feedback in female and male students.

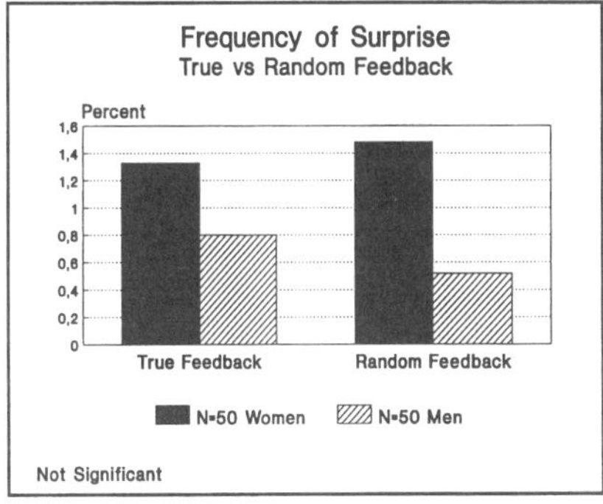

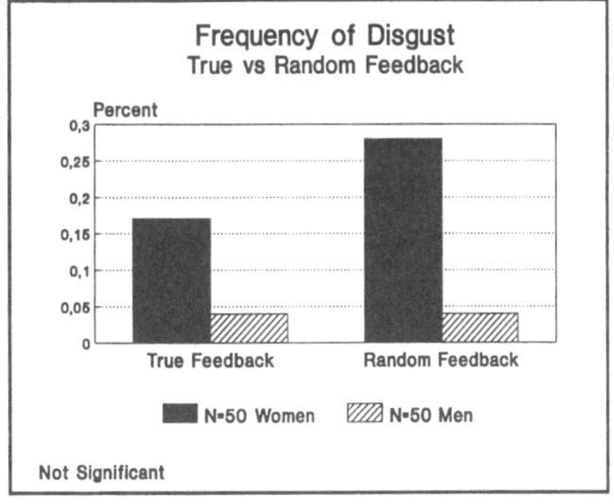

Figure 3. Frequency (% of feedbacks) of surprise and disgust during true and random feedback in female and male students.

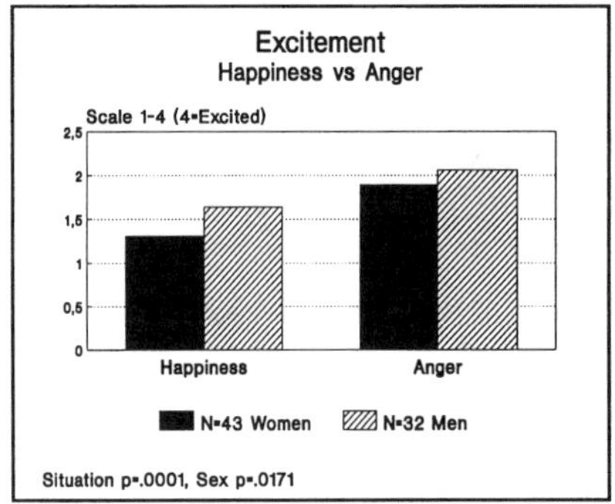

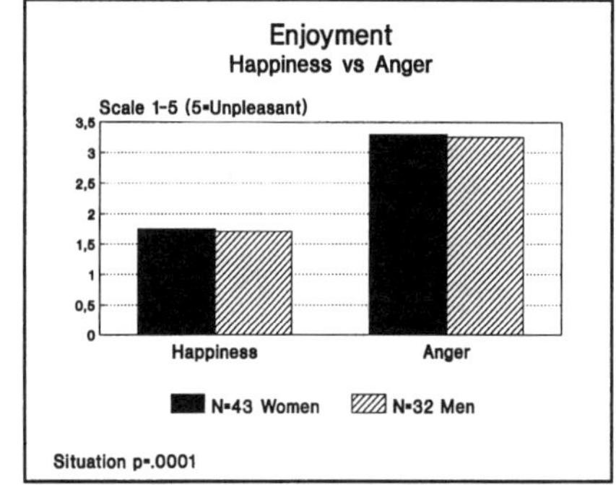

Figure 4. Excitement and enjoyment during happiness compared to anger in female and male students.

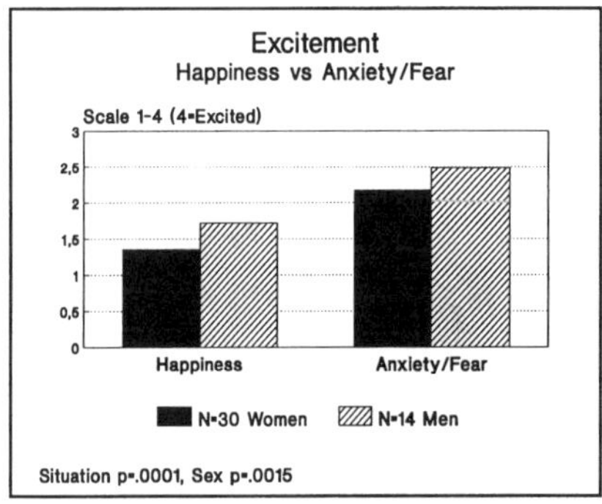

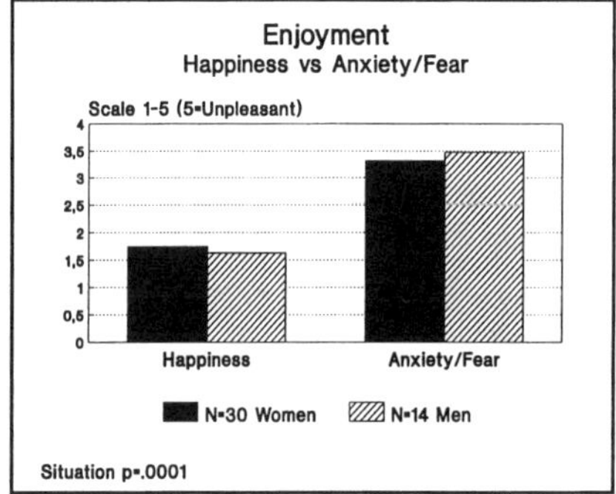

Figure 5. Excitement and enjoyment during happiness compared to anxiety/fear in female and male students.

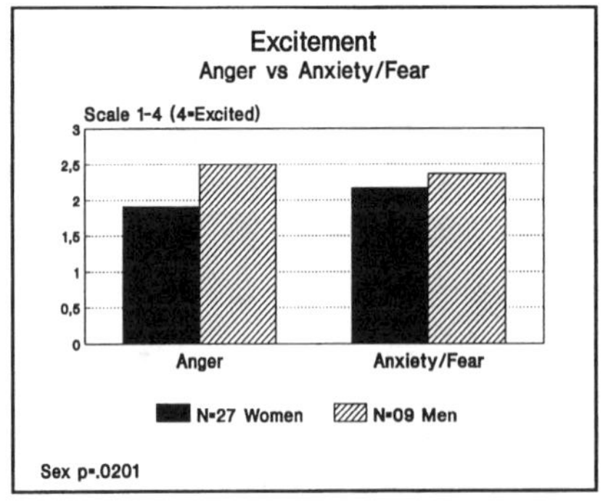

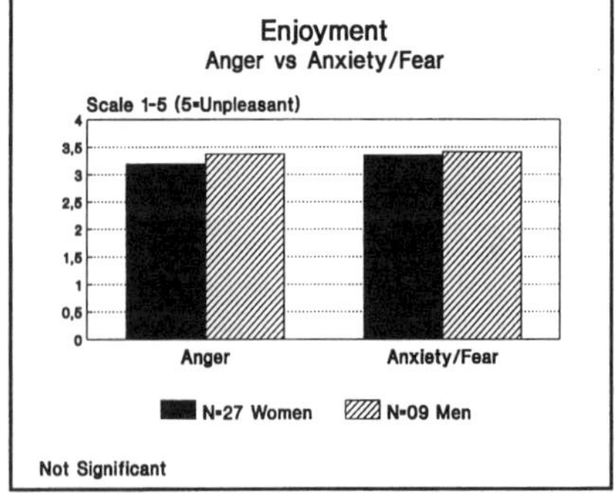

Figure 6. Excitement and enjoyment during anger compared to anxiety/fear in female and male students

are more excited during all emotions than female students. The valence ratings for the three emotions are very similar for both female and male students. Happiness is rated as being enjoyable whereas anger and anxiety/fear as unpleasant. No significant difference between anger and anxiety/fear was observed. We may conclude that the subjective quality of these emotions is rated very similar by both sexes.

Physiological profiles of different emotions

Mean comparisons between feedback minutes without emotions versus feedback

Table 1: Mean comparisons between feedback minutes without perceived emotions versus feedback minutes with emotions.

Happiness	None	Happy	p
Physical activity (units/min)	20.29	25.32	**.021**
Heart rate (bpm)	80.92	86.01	**.009**
Emotional heart rate (units/min)	10.39	9.89	.462
Heart rate MSSD (bpm)	3.97	3.73	.528
P-wave amplitude (microV)	181.02	196.99	**.012**
ST-segment amplitude (microV)	44.72	28.47	**.001**
Speech activity (%/min)	20.01	39.92	**.001**

N = 45; Generalized T^2 statistic: F(7,38) = 13.37, p = .001.

Anger	None	Anger	p
Physical activity (units/min)	19.50	18.99.	.846
Heart rate (bpm)	81.78	84.73	.274
Emotional heart rate (units/min)	10.09	7.86	.128
Heart rate MSSD (bpm)	4.20	3.77	.258
P-wave amplitude (microV)	191.30	189.48	.832
ST-segment amplitude (microV)	53.46	42.53	.077
Speech activity (%/min)	20.65	27.57	.137

N = 31; Generalized T^2 statistic: F(7,24) = 1.47, p = .225.

Anxiety/Fear	None	Anxiety	p
Physical activity (units/min)	19.81	16.73	.654
Heart rate (bpm)	81.32	80.67	.859
Emotional heart rate (units/min)	10.91	16.92	**.046**
Heart rate MSSD (bpm)	3.79	4.46	.337
P-wave amplitude (microV)	202.33	200.09	.868
ST-segment amplitude (microV)	71.38	83.38	.310
Speech activity (%/min)	23.06	25.20	.762

N = 12; Generalized T^2 statistic: F(7,5) = 1.60, p = .312.

Sadness	None	Sadness	p
Physical activity (units/min)	18.14	24.67	.770
Heart rate (bpm)	79.74	79.67	.937
Emotional heart rate (units/min)	10.08	10.00	.939
Heart rate MSSD (bpm)	3.79	3.82	.894
P-wave amplitude (microV)	175.65	172.55	.845
ST-segment amplitude (microV)	34.11	23.53	.614
Speech activity (%/min)	17.17	53.12	.130

N = 03; Generalized T^2 statistic not possible due to sample size.

Surprise	None	Surprise	p
Physical activity (units/min)	20.76	25.04	.552
Heart rate (bpm)	83.25	83.80	.826
Emotional heart rate (units/min)	10.03	8.57	.497
Heart rate MSSD (bpm)	4.77	5.84	.127
P-wave amplitude (microV)	187.76	200.35	.193
ST-segment amplitude (microV)	76.99	69.12	.663
Speech activity (%/min)	21.42	28.18	.191

N = 14; Generalized T^2 statistic: F(7,7) = 0.60, p = .745.

Disgust	None	Disgust	p
Physical activity (units/min)	16.08	21.42	.604
Heart rate (bpm)	81.51	77.25	.387
Emotional heart rate (units/min)	11.01	8.33	.543
Heart rate MSSD (bpm)	4.57	4.18	.550
P-wave amplitude (microV)	197.18	219.61	.222
ST-segment amplitude (microV)	75.27	79.41	.796
Speech activity (%/min)	19.21	27.90	.564

N = 06; Generalized T^2 statistic not possible due to sample size.

minutes with emotions (including minutes with self-activation of the system) were drawn for the physiological parameters. Of the 50 female subjects, 49 reported at least a total of one minute of happiness, 43 anger, 30 anxiety/fear, 14 sadness, 17 surprise, and 6 disgust. Although the differences between minutes with and without emotions were significant for happiness and sadness (generalized T^2 statistic), the results in the univariate analyses were disappointing. Physical activity, heart rate variability (MSSD), and P-wave amplitude were not different between minutes with and without emotions for all of the six emotions in the univariate analyses. Heart rate was lower during surprise. Emotional heart rate was even lower during happiness and sadness. Anger showed a lower ST-segment amplitude as compared to no emo-

Table 2: Mean comparisons between feedback minutes with happiness versus anger versus anxiety/fear.

Happiness versus anger	Happiness	Anger	p
Physical activity (units/min)	23.74	18.99	.230
Heart rate (bpm)	86.74	84.73	.600
Emotional heart rate (units/min)	9.98	7.86	.118
Heart rate MSSD (bpm)	3.81	3.77	.991
P-wave amplitude (microV)	206.89	189.48	.177
ST-segment amplitude (microV)	39.55	42.53	.663
Speech activity (%/min)	41.53	27.57	.009

N = 31; Generalized T^2 statistic: F(7,24) = 1.99, p = .098.

Happiness versus anxiety/fear	Happiness	Anxiety	p
Physical activity (units/min)	25.43	16.73	.247
Heart rate (bpm)	86.12	80.67	.281
Emotional heart rate (units/min)	10.54	16.92	.054
Heart rate MSSD (bpm)	4.12	4.46	.644
P-wave amplitude (microV)	214.14	200.09	.462
ST-segment amplitude (microV)	52.17	83.38.	**.018**
Speech activity (%/min)	32.76	25.20	.311

N = 12; Generalized T^2 statistic: F(7,5) = 074, p = .652.

Anger versus anxiety/fear	Anger	Anxiety	p
Physical activity (units/min)	22.72	18.20	.751
Heart rate (bpm)	90.59	82.88	.393
Emotional heart rate (units/min)	11.87	17.72	.345
Heart rate MSSD (bpm)	3.39	4.78	.197
P-wave amplitude (microV)	189.49	196.88	.741
ST-segment amplitude (microV)	60.38	93.75	.074
Speech activity (%/min)	26.25	21.74	.666

N = 08; Generalized T^2 statistic for physiological parameters: F(7,1) = 0.99, p = .653.

tion. Happiness was accompanied by higher speech activity. With the exception of the ST-segment amplitude and the speech activity, all other significant differences were in an unexpected direction. Table 1 shows the mean comparisons for the male students. Of the 50 students, 45 reported happiness, 31 anger, 12 anxiety/fear, 3 sadness, 14 surprise, and 6 disgust. Generalized T^2 statistic is significant for happiness only. In the univariate analyses only speech activity could be replicated.

Because happiness, anger, and anxiety/fear were the most frequent emotions, we carried out respective mean comparisons between these three emotions. In the female sample, generalized T^2 statistic was significant for happiness versus anger. Minutes with anger revealed greater physical activity, higher heart rate, greater P-wave amplitude, lower ST-segment amplitude, and less speech activity than minutes with happiness. All differences are in the expected direction. In the male sample, generalized T^2 statistic was marginally significant for happiness versus anger (Table 2). The univariate analyses showed that only speech activity was significant, with higher speech activity during happiness. We may conclude that the physiological profiles for the different emotions are rather uncharacteristic and could not be replicated.

Accuracy of the emotional perception

With the exception of anxiety/fear, the frequency of all other emotions showed no differences between true and random feedback. It is conceivable that differences might exist between subjects´ accuracy of the emotional perception, thus obscuring differences between true and random feedback. Accuracy was defined as either the percentage of correctly classified true feedbacks (identification of an emotion) or random feedbacks (reporting that no emotion was present). It was supposed that subjects with good emotional perception would have a high percentage of correct classifications for both true *and* random feedbacks. Therefore, a positive correlation was expected. Moreover, personality dimensions might be relevant for accuracy, for example, higher introversion or neuroticism in subjects with good perception. As can be seen from Table 3, the high correlation of -0.89 for the female and -0.82 for the male students between true and random feedback is quite contrary to our expectation. Obviously, two types of emotional perception exist, "emotional subjects" who always perceive emotions regardless of the physiological arousal and "cool subjects" who seldom perceive emotions. The former are characterized by a greater dis-

Table 3: Correlations between the percentage of correctly classified true feedbacks (emotional arousal present) or the percentage of correctly classified random feedbacks (no emotional arousal present) and personality

	True	Random
Correctly classified random, %	-0.89	----
	-0.82	----
STAXI anger disposition, high = frequent	0.30	-0.28
	0.31	-0.17
STAXI anger temperament, high = hot	0.27	-0.26
	0.33	-0.26
STAXI anger expression, high = expression	0.24	-0.32
	0.27	-0.21
FPI extraversion, high = extraverted	0.20	-0.24
	0.33	-0.37

Note: First line N = 50 women, second line N = 50 men; 0.24 p= .100, 0.28 p = .050, 0.36 p = .010, 0.45 p = .001).

position to experience anger and reveal tendencies toward a "hot" temperament, greater anger expression as well as more extraversion. The latter, however, show the opposite profile: tendencies of a lower disposition toward anger experience, "cool" temperament in regard to anger, lower anger expression, and more introversion.

Correlations between perceived emotions and personality dimensions

Table 4 shows the correlations between the frequency of the perceived emotions (percent of all feedbacks) and the personality dimensions examined. Female and male subjects who frequently stated that they were happy revealed more extraversion and tended toward a "hotter" temperament and higher anger expression. Angry subjects tended toward a "hotter" anger temperament and higher anger expression, too. The most correlations were observed in subjects who frequently stated that they were anxious. These subjects are characterized by a tendency toward greater anxiety, higher disposition to experience anger, and higher anger sensitivity. Moreover, they demonstrate a tendency toward more strain, neuroticism, more physical complaints, and a lower satisfaction with their health. Because the other emotions were rare in both samples, no other correlations between the frequency of these emotions and personality dimensions could be replicated.

Discussion

Most of the feedbacks were not accompanied by an emotion. This is in accordance with the study by Schwartz et al. (1994) cited in the Introduction. In both samples, happiness was the most frequent emotion, followed by anger and anxiety. Schwartz et al. (1994) and Shapiro et al. (1997) also observed that a happy mood was the most prominent mood in subjects' reports. The clear differences in excitement and enjoyment associated with the differing emotions was replicated in the male student sample and both studies are in good accordance with the study by Johnsen et al. (1995; see Introduction).

As mentioned already in the Introduction, there is a controversial debate as to the interaction of the different response systems during an emotion. For Lang (1993) emotional cognitions are not necessarily accompanied by an autonomic arousal. Other authors assume an autonomic arousal for most emotions (Gray, 1994; Levenson, 1994), and still other researchers regard autonomic changes as an important part of emotion perception or even as a cause of emotion (Schachter & Singer, 1962). In our former paper on this topic (Myrtek & Brügner, 1996), we assumed that this latter view is primarily due to the experimental method used because research on emotion has to date mostly been done in the laboratory. We also stated that emotion perception is not necessarily linked to physiological changes but seems essentially to be a function of cognitive schemata, hypotheses, and so on. It was

Table 4: Correlations between perceived emotions (percent of all feedbacks), personality dimensions, and habits.

	Happiness
STAXI anger temperament, high = hot	0.16
	0.27
STAXI anger expression, high = expression	0.25
	0.21
FPI extraversion, high = extraverted	0.28
	0.32

	Anger
STAXI anger temperament, high = hot	0.36
	0.15
STAXI anger expression, high = expression	0.16
	0.31

	Anxiety/Fear
STAI anxiety, high = anxious	0.24
	0.31
STAXI anger disposition, high = frequent	0.28
	0.16
STAXI anger reaction, high = sensitive	0.29
	0.22
FPI strain, high = strenuous	0.22
	0.25
FPI physical complaints, high = frequent	0.22
	0.27
FPI emotional lability, high = labile	0.30
	0.15
FLZ health satisfaction, high = unsatisfied	0.25
	0.15

Note: First line N = 50 women, second line N = 50 men; 0.24 p = .100, 0.28 p = .050, 0.36 p = .010, 0.45 p = .001).

suggested that there is a clear difference between emotional arousal, indicated by physiological changes, and emotion perception. We supposed that most of the emotional events (as indicated by emotional heart rate) obviously do not reach the level of consciousness and, hence, the level of perception, with the exception of those events generating extreme emotional arousal.

The present studies confirm and specify this view. The frequency of the perceived emotions during true feedback (with physiological arousal) and random feedback (without physiological arousal) was not different with the exception of anxiety/fear. This finding indicates that the subjects were not able to differentiate well between these situations with different physiological arousal. In accordance with this result, the physiological profile of feedback minutes without perceived emotions as compared to the profiles of the differing emotions showed no clear differences in both studies and, therefore, could not be replicated. In the female student sample, the mean comparisons between minutes with happiness, anger, and anxiety showed physiological profiles which were in line with expectations but these differences could not be replicated in the male student sample. This finding for the physiological parameters sharply contrasted with the psychological parameters in both studies which were in accordance with the perceived emotions.

The replicated results on the accuracy of emotion perception deserves attention. The correlation between the percentage of correctly classified true feedbacks and the percentage of correctly classified random feedbacks was highly negative, resulting in two types of emotional perception ("emotional" and "cool" subjects). This finding was so unexpected that we searched for other explanations. We thoroughly examined the statistical distribution of both parameters, the possible statistical dependency of both parameters due to the limited number of feedbacks, and the possibility that subjects refused to answer the questions that were posed on the display correctly. All alternative explications could to be ruled out. Therefore, the correlation between the percentages of the correctly classified true and random feedbacks is not due to an artifact. This means that emotion perception is really determined to a great extent by cognitive schemata such as being emotionally "cool" or "hot".

This view is also confirmed by the correlations between the perception of emotions and certain personality dimensions such as anger disposition and anger expression. Subjects who describe themselves as not expressing anger or being seldom angry tend to perceive no emotions. The correlations between specific emotions and personality dimensions agree with this. This is especially true for anxiety. As in the present study, Shapiro et al. (1997) reported a positive correlation between the percentage of anxious mood and trait anxiety. These authors also observed a negative correlation between happy mood and anxiety whereas anger and sadness were positively correlated with hostility.

Research on emotion in everyday life is difficult because inferences have to be made from subjective reports on emotional events. This implies that the subjects can report only those emotional events that they are aware of. Given this fact, the question as to what extent emotions depend on physiological changes cannot be answered with certainty because emotion perception is not necessarily linked to physiological changes. In the present study, this inherent difficulty with self-reports was avoided since our method allowed for the assessment of emotionally-induced physiological activation. Our results show that personality dispositions together with cognitive schemata are especially involved in emotion perception. This does not mean that there are no physiologically discernible affective states. Everybody has perceived such states in his life and the reproducible subjective appraisal of the different emotions show that the subjects share the same emotional experiences.

However, such strong affective states are rare events and not common in everyday life. We suppose that only few subjects if any have experienced such strong affective states during monitoring. Presumably, subjects infer their emotional state by external or internal cues. This assumption would explain both the missing physiological differentiation between the different emotions on the one hand and the reproducible subjective appraisal of the emotions on the other.

The results of the present studies are in accordance with a review on emotion research done by Reisenzein (1983). The author concluded that peripheral arousal is no necessary condition for an emotional state as claimed by the perception model. Our results are also in line with studies on social schemata. Rimé et al. (1990) have shown that people have social schemata about peripheral changes in emotion, and that these schemata are similar across cultures. It might well be "that distinctive patterns of actual peripheral changes occur only during especially intense emotions. These extreme states could constitute exemplars or generate prototypes that would be generalized to less intense states" (p. 46).

Summary

In the present study, emotional arousal was monitored throughout the day with a special ambulatory device. Fifty female and 50 male students received acoustic feedback every 10 to 20 minutes. The feedback was based either on true emotional events (emotional or additional heart rate) or was random without emotional arousal. Following the feedback the subjects were asked to report their emotions. Moreover, subjects were encouraged to activate the monitoring system by themselves whenever they perceived an emotion. The following emotions were listed on the display of the monitoring device: no emotion, happiness, anger, anxiety/fear, sadness, surprise, and disgust.

With the exception of anxiety/fear, the frequency of the emotions was not different between true and random feedbacks, indicating that the subjects were not able to discriminate well between events with and without emotional arousal. Accordingly, the physiological profiles of the differing emotions (physical activity, heart rate, emotional heart rate, heart rate variability, P-wave and ST-segment amplitude, speech activity) compared to conditions with "no emotion" were unclear in both samples. The psychological ratings of excitement and enjoyment for the differing emotions, however, were similar in both the female and male students. Subjects who identified true feedbacks correctly (emotion present) also reported after random feedbacks that they perceived an emotion and subjects who identified random feedbacks correctly (no emotion present) also reported after true feedbaks that they perceived no emotion. This means that some subjects described themselves as "emotional" irrespective of their actual physiological activation, whereas other subjects described themselves as being "cool". Several correlations between personality dimensions and the frequency of the differing emotions were observed. The results show that cognitive schemata and personality dimensions are more important in emotion perception of everyday life than emotionally caused physiological activation.

Acknowledgment
This research was supported by a grant from the Deutsche Forschungsgemeinschaft (DFG).

References

Anderson, T.W. (1984). *Introduction to multivariate statistical analysis* (pp. 164–167). New York: John Wiley Sons.

Blix, A.S., Stromme, S.B. & Ursin, H. (1974). Additional heart rate – an indicator of psychological activation. *Aerospace Medicine, 45*, 1219–1222.

Bradley, M.M., Greenwald, M.K. & Hamm, A.O. (1993). Affective picture processing. In N. Birbaumer & A. Öhman (Eds.), *The structure of emotion* (pp. 48–65). Seattle: Hogrefe & Huber Publishers.

Fahrenberg, J., Hampel, R. & Selg, H. (1984). *Das Freiburger Persönlichkeitsinventar FPI.* Göttingen: Hogrefe.

Fahrenberg, J., Myrtek, M., Schumacher, J. & Brähler, E. (2000). *Fragebogen zur Lebenszufriedenheit (FLZ). Handanweisung.* Göttingen: Hogrefe.

Frijda, N.H. (1994). Varieties of affect: Emotions and episodes, moods, and sentiments. In P. Ekman & R.J. Davidson (Eds.), *The nature of emotion. Fundamental questions* (pp. 59–67). New York: Oxford University Press.

Gray, J.A. (1994). Three fundamental emotion systems. In P. Ekman & R.J. Davidson (Eds.), *The nature of emotion. Fundamental questions* (pp. 243–247). New York: Oxford University Press.

Johnsen, B.H., Thayer, J.F. & Hugdahl, K. (1995). Affective judgement of the Ekman faces: A dimensional approach. *Journal of Psychophysiology, 9*, 193–202.

Lang, P.J. (1993). The three-system approach to emotion. In N. Birbaumer & A. Öhman (Eds.), *The structure of emotion* (pp. 18–30). Seattle: Hogrefe & Huber Publishers.

Laux, L., Glanzmann, P., Schaffner, P. & Spielberger, C.D. (1981). *Das State-Trait-Angstinventar. Theoretische Grundlagen und Handanweisung.* Weinheim: Beltz.

Levenson, R.W. (1994). The search for autonomic specificity. In P. Ekman & R.J. Davidson (Eds.), *The nature of emotion. Fundamental questions* (pp. 252–257). New York: Oxford University Press.

Meshkati, N. (1988). Heart rate variability and mental workload assessment. In P.A. Hancock & N. Meshkati (Eds.), *Human mental workload* (pp. 101–115). Amsterdam: Elsevier.

Myrtek, M. (1990). Covariation and reliability of ECG parameters during 24-hour monitoring. *International Journal of Psychophysiology, 10*, 117–123.

Myrtek, M. (1998). *Gesunde Kranke - kranke Gesunde. Psychophysiologie des Krankheitsverhaltens.* Bern: Huber.

Myrtek, M., Aschenbrenner, E. & Brügner, G. (submitted). Emotions in everyday life. An ambulatory monitoring study with female students. *Biological Psychology.*

Myrtek, M. & Brügner, G. (1996). Perception of emotions in everyday life: studies with patients and normals. *Biological Psychology, 42*, 147–164.

Myrtek, M., Brügner, G., Fichtler, A., König, K., Müller. W., Foerster, F. & Höppner V. (1988). Detection of emotionally induced ECG changes and their behavioral correlates: A new method for ambulatory monitoring. *European Heart Journal, 9* (Supplement N), 55–60.

Myrtek, M., Brügner, G. & Müller, W. (1996a). Validation studies of emotional, mental, and physical workload components in the field. In J. Fahrenberg & M. Myrtek (Eds.), *Ambulatory assessment. Computer-assisted psychological and psychophysiological methods in monitoring and field studies* (pp. 287–304). Seattle: Hogrefe & Huber Publishers.

Myrtek, M., Brügner, G. & Müller, W. (1996b). Interactive monitoring and contingency analysis of emotionally induced ECG changes: Methodology and applications. In J. Fahrenberg & M. Myrtek (Eds.), *Ambulatory assessment. Computer-assisted psychological and psychophysiological methods in monitoring and field studies* (pp. 115–127). Seattle: Hogrefe & Huber Publishers.

Myrtek, M., Deutschmann-Janicke, E., Strohmaier, H., Zimmermann, W., Lawerenz, S., Brügner, G. & Müller, W. (1994). Physical, mental, emotional, and subjective workload components in engine drivers. *Ergonomics, 37*, 1195–1203.

Myrtek, M., Dieterle, W. & Brügner, G. (1990). Psychophysiological response patterns to variations of the experimental load of a reaction time task. *Journal of Psychophysiology, 4*, 209–220.

Myrtek, M., Scharff, C., Brügner, G. & Müller, W. (1996c). Physiological, behavioral, and psychological effects associated with television viewing in schoolboys: An exploratory study. *Journal of Early Adolescence, 16*, 301–323.

Myrtek, M. & Spital, S. (1986). Psychophysiological response patterns to single, double, and triple stressors. *Psychophysiology, 23*, 663–671.

Pennebaker, J.W. (1982). *The psychology of physical symptoms.* New York: Springer.

Reisenzein (1983). The Schachter theory of emotion: Two decades later. *Psychological Bulletin, 94*, 239–261.

Rimé, B., Philippot, P. & Cisamolo, D. (1990). Social schemata of peripheral changes in emotion. *Journal of Personality and Social Psychology, 59*, 38–49.

Roth, D.L., Bachtler, S.D. & Fillingim, R.B. (1990). Acute emotional and cardiovascular effects of stressful mental work during aerobic exercise. *Psychophysiology, 27*, 694–701.

SAS Institute (1990). *SAS procedures guide.* Cary, NC: SAS Institute Inc.

Schachter, S. & Singer, J. (1962). Cognitive, social, and physiological determinants of emotional state. *Psychological Review, 69*, 379–399.

Schwartz, J.E., Warren, K. & Pickering, T.G. (1994). Mood, location, and physical position as predictors of ambulatory blood pressure and heart rate: Application of a multi-level random effects model. *Annals of Behavioral Medicine, 16*, 210–220.

Schwenkmezger, P., Hodapp, V. & Spielberger, C.D. (1992). *Das State-Trait-Ärgerausdrucks-Inventar STAXI.* Bern: Huber.

Shapiro, D., Jamner, L.D. & Goldstein, I.B. (1997). Daily mood states and ambulatory blood pressure. *Pychophysiology, 34*, 399–405.

Turner, J.R., Carroll, D., Hanson, J. & Sims, J. (1988). A comparison of additional heart rates during active psychological challenge calculated from upper body and lower body dynamic exercise. *Psychophysiology, 25*, 209–216.

Wilhelm, P., Myrtek, M. & Brügner, G. (1997). *Vorschulkinder vor dem Fernseher. Ein psychophysiologisches Feldexperiment.* Bern: Huber.

Wilson, G.F. (1988). Measurement of operator workload with the neuropsychological workload test battery. In P.A. Hancock & N. Meshkati (Eds.), *Human mental workload* (pp. 63-100). Amsterdam: Elsevier.

Wundt, W. (1905). *Grundzüge der physiologischen Psychologie.* Leipzig: Engelmann.

Chapter 25
In-Flight Psychophysiological Monitoring

Glenn F. Wilson
Air Force Research Laboratory, Human Effectiveness Directorate, Flight Psychophysiology Laboratory, Wright-Patterson AFB, OH, USA

Introduction

Flying modern aircraft is a complex task which can place extremely high cognitive demands upon crew members. Crew members are required to monitor and process large amounts of information, manage complex sub-systems and often are under time pressure. Most of the required work in the cockpits of modern aircraft is cognitive in nature. Very little physical effort is required so cognitive demands are of concern when evaluating the costs of flying. As with any situation requiring measurement, precise and reliable measures are required. Aviation research presents unique problems to investigators. Ambulatory recording methods are required to monitor crew members performing their jobs during flight. They must be free to move about the aircraft and be able to rapidly egress the aircraft in case of an emergency. There are further limitations in that some aircraft only have space for the pilot as is the case with single seat aircraft. Typical flights may take from one to ten or more hours of constant duty. Few aircraft are instrumented to record performance data which makes data collection difficult. Subjective reports are used to evaluate the crew member's experience with a given aircraft or flight. However, the subjective reports are prone to memory loss and bias and their recording during flight may interfere with the crew member's job performance. Psychophysiological measures have been shown to have utility in flight studies. They are excellent candidates since they can be continuously obtained without interfering with the crew members job. This is very important in aviation where interference with a crew member's task performance could have fatal consequences. Because significant unplanned events often occur during flight, the availability of the continuously recorded physiological data can be advantageous.

The earliest report of physiological recording during flight occurred in 1917 when an Italian physician recorded the pulse rate of a pilot during flight (reported in Roscoe, 1992). During the intervening eighty years numerous investigations of the cognitive aspects of flight on crew members' physiology have been undertaken. Of the psychophysiological measures, heart rate has been the most widely used during flight. Respiration, electroencephalograph (EEG), electrodermal activity (EDA), electrooculograph (EOG) and electromyograph (EMG) have also been used to varying extent (Caldwell et al., 1994; Wilson & Eggemeier, 1991; Wilson, in press). A review of the heart rate literature through the 1980s was written by Roscoe (1992) who was responsible for numerous studies. Landing approach, novel take off situations, flying into unfamiliar airports, in-air refueling, and flying experimental aircraft all were found to effect heart rate. A number of simulated flight studies have been performed as well. Sirevaag, Kramer, Wickens, Reisweber, Strayer and Grenell, (1993) reported that blink closure duration and event related potential amplitude discriminated between two modes of communication in simulated helicopter flights. Veltman and Gaillard (1996) reported significant changes in heart rate and blood pressure related to mental workload demands. Veltman and Gaillard (1998) further found heart rate increases as the difficulty of a 'tunnel in the sky' tracking task increased. Blink rate decreased with increased demands on the visual system to obtain information.

Our flight research has been directed towards understanding operator functional state. The emphasis has been in the area of mental workload during flight. Because piloting and other flight tasks require a variety of cognitive activities, multiple psychophysiological measures are used. By using multiple psychophysiological measures we are better able to understand the cognitive demands of flight on crew members. For example, eye blink rate is sensitive to the visual demands of a task and therefore changes in blink rate are diagnostic. Heart rate is sensitive to the mental workload experienced by an operator but it is not especially diagnostic since several conditions will result in changes in heart rate. For example, both take off and landing increase a pilot's heart rate. We have tried several measures with differing levels of success. They include ECG, EEG, EOG, DC EEG, respiration, EDA, EMG, and actigraphy. Overall, ECG and EOG have produced the most consistent positive results.

Human factors research during flight poses unique problems. Aircraft are typically not equipped to record the performance variables that are required. Flight scenarios are often complicated which impose limits upon subjective recall of events. Performance data may be difficult to interpret and its collection could interfere with the crew member's job. Subjective data collection could also intrude into the primary flight duties and is also liable to bias based upon crew expectations. Ambulatory recording equipment affords continuous psychophysiological recordings. By keeping an accurate time record of flight events, it is possible to correlate the psychophysiological data with mission events. Recording altitude as well as latitude and longitude provides a highly accurate history of each flight. Using these procedures one is able to develop a moment-to-moment view of crew member's responses to the demands of flight. This information can be very valuable with regard to understanding the demands of various flight maneuvers, testing new and modified aircraft, and addressing training issues.

Ambulatory recording of psychophysiological data during flight shares many of the common problems of all ambulatory recording. The major problems found with flight recordings are physiologically related. Movement, muscle, and eye related artifacts are of primary concern. As with most other situations where ambulatory recordings are made the operators must move. This is a necessary part of their jobs. These movements, including those associated with speech, generate artifacts for the other recording modalities. For example, pilots must visually scan for other air traffic. The movements associated with scanning the airspace generates EMG and movement related activity that can interfere with obtaining clean EEG and ECG recordings. Fortunately, there are a number of techniques available for detecting and removing these artifacts. Interference from aircraft electronic systems, such as radio and radar, is often thought to be a major problem with these recordings. However, they are of little concern. These potentially interfering signals are relatively small and their frequency bands are much higher than the low frequency responses of the physiological signals. The availability of small, powerful ambulatory recorders enhances the ability to perform physiological recordings during flight. These devices provide amplification and recording. They may contain microprocessors that allow sophisticated on-line signal processing such as digital filtering.

Flight Studies with Operational Aircraft

In our first study (Wilson, Purvis, Skelly, Fullenkamp & Davis, 1987; Skelly, Purvis & Wilson, 1988), the goal was to use psychophysiological measures to examine the cognitive demands of single seat military aircraft (A-7) air-to-ground training missions. Flight segments having unique cognitive demands during the approximately one hour mission were studied. These included maneuvers such as takeoff, cruise, weapons delivery, and landing. The various segments placed different cognitive demands on the pilots. Since a single seat aircraft was flown, all aspects of the flights were the responsibility of the pilot. This study was further designed to determine the effects of aircraft position in a four aircraft formation. Each of the eight pilots flew twice, once in the lead and once in the wing position. They also flew the same mission in a fixed base simulator. Flying three times in positions having different responsibilities is a unique aspect of this study. It provided the opportunity to examine the effects of different segments of flight but also provided insight into the effects of flying the same segments with different overall responsibilities to the flight of four aircraft. Heart rate, eye blinks and brain activity were recorded on small wearable recorders worn in a pocket of the flight suit of the eight pilots. Del Mar Avionics Model 509 Neurocorders were used in this study to amplify the physiological signals and record them on analog tape for post-flight processing. A voice recorder was used to allow correlation of the physiological signals with mission events.

Heart rate proved to be sensitive to both the varying demands of the different segments of flight and to the different requirements of flying lead, wing, or in the simulator. Heart rates were higher for the more demanding segments such as take off, weapon delivery, and landing. The rates were lower during the less demanding cruise segments. This was true for the two actual flights but not the simulated flight where the rates were stable over the entire mission. The mean heart rates were significantly higher when each pilot was leading the four aircraft formation than when in the wing position or in the simulator. The additional responsibility for the entire formation was associated with higher heart rates even though the missions were the same regardless of the pilot's position in the formation. This is shown in Figure 1 which represents the mean heart rates for the three types of flights. Blink rate tended to be reduced during segments having high visual demand such as landing. Overall, blink durations were significantly shorter for the missions when the pilots flew in the wing position. It was suggested that this was due to the demands of the wing position to keep the lead aircraft in sight at all times in order to maintain proper distance and position.

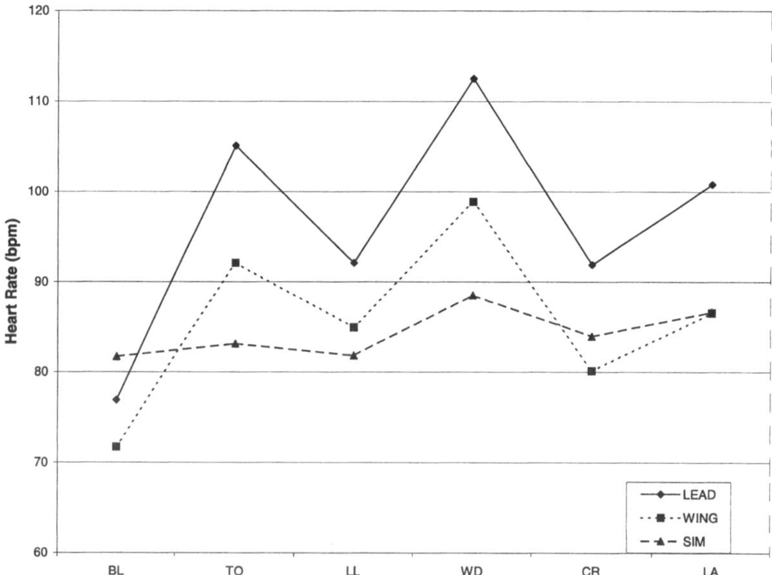

Figure 1. Mean heart rates for A7 pilots flying three different missions. Each pilot flew three times, once in the lead position, once in a wing position, and once in a simulator. The segment labels are BL - Baseline, TO - Take Off, LL - Low Level, WD - Weapons Delivery, CR - Cruise, LA - Landing.

This study serendipitously provided other interesting data. Two in-flight and two simulator emergencies occurred (Wilson, Skelly & Purvis, 1988). One of the in-flight emergencies was a bird strike and the other required an evasive maneuver to avoid a possible collision with another aircraft. The in-flight emergencies were associated with at least a 50% increase in heart rate within 30 seconds of the events. In both cases the pilot's heart rates returned to their pre-event levels within 60 – 80 seconds. This is remarkable when considering that these events occurred during actual flight and could have had very serious consequences. The rapid return to pre-event heart rate levels speaks well for the training and skill of the two pilots. They were able to assess the situation, make corrections and proceed. During the simulator portion of the study there were 'crashes' during two of the missions. Neither of these events was associated with increased heart rates from either pilot. These data point out the sensitivity of heart rate to unusual events. Further, these data were available because of the continuous nature of the physiological recordings with the associated time line.

Our second flight study was designed with several goals in mind (Wilson, 1993). F4 Phantom aircraft were used which have a two person crew, a pilot and a weapons systems officer (WSO). This means that two people are at the same place at the same time but with different jobs. This permits the evaluation of the relative levels of mental workload of the two people during the various aspects of the mission. It should be possible to use psychophysiological measures to differentiate the workload demands of these two positions. Further, the WSO controlled the aircraft for a period of time. They are not trained pilots but are given enough experience in order to return the aircraft to base if the pilot is incapacitated. To compare the similarities between laboratory and flight tasks, the pilots and WSOs were asked to perform a laboratory tracking task prior to each flight. Many experiments have been performed in the laboratory with the goal of extrapolating the results to real-world job performance situations. It was felt that the inclusion of the tracking task would permit a direct comparison between a typical laboratory task having at least one component of the pilot's and WSO's jobs. In addition to the comparison of the two jobs, and laboratory versus flight, these data would also permit replication of the results from earlier flight studies. Several psychophysiological measures were used for comparison with regard to their utility to assess the effects of the various demands placed upon the pilots and WSOs during the mission.

Ten experienced Phantom crews participated in the study which was an air-to-ground training mission. Each crew member was instrumented to collect heart, eye, and respiration data. Subjective estimates of mental workload were also collected after each flight using a ten point scale. The Del Mar Neurocorders were also used in this study. A specially built voice/time code recorder that was connected to the aircraft communication system permitted correlation of the psychophysiological data with the relevant mission events. Two minute epochs, surrounding twelve events of interest, were used to analyze the data. These included both ground and flight segments such as resting baseline, tracking task, take off, bombing range, cruise, and landing.

The heart rate data showed an approximately 43 percent increase from lowest to highest segment (Figure 2). Flight produced higher heart rates than the ground based segments for both pilots and WSOs. The highest heart rates for both crew members was at the bombing range. Take off and landing were the next highest for the pilots while the segment when the WSO was flying the aircraft was the next highest for the WSOs. These results are consistent with the mental demands of the two jobs. Both crew members face high demand levels at the bombing range. The pilots are challenged during take off and landing while the WSOs are primarily performing visual scanning functions. The demands placed on the WSOs during the time when they are actually in command of the aircraft were quite high. On the other hand, heart rate variability analysis performed on the same data in two bands, middle and high, showed few statistically significant effects.

The blink rate analysis revealed periods of increased visual demand for both crew positions. The pilots' data showed significantly reduced blink rates during the tracking task, at the bombing range and while landing. For the WSOs' data, lower blink rates were found during tracking task performance and during the segment when

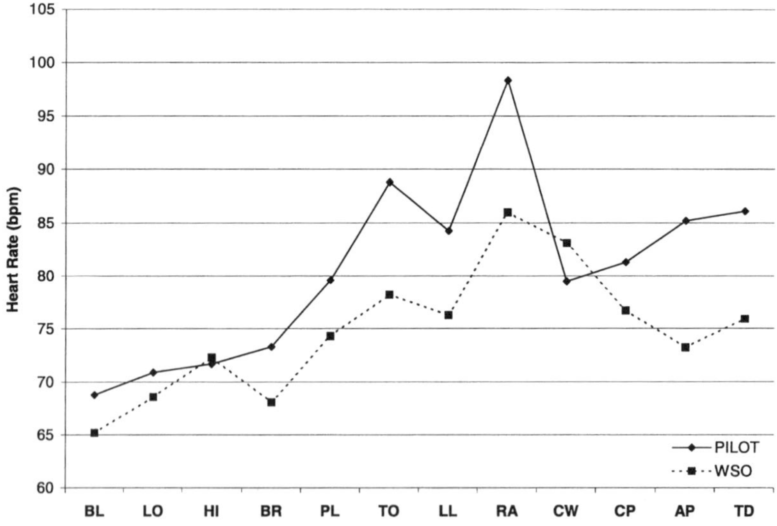

Figure 2. Pilot and WSO mean heart rates for ground and flight segments. Note the higher WSO heart rates during the CW condition. The segment labels are BL - Baseline, LO - Tracking at low difficulty level, HI - Tracking, high difficulty level, BR - Preflight briefing, PL - Preflight checklists, TO - Take Off, LL - Low Level, RA - Bombing Range, CW - Cruise with WSO flying, CP - Cruise with Pilot flying, AP - Approach to landing, TD - Touch Down at landing.

the WSOs were actually flying the aircraft. Respiration rates were significantly higher during the tracking task for both the pilots and WSOs when compared to the other ground segments. During the flights, the pilots' respiration rates were higher at the bombing range while the WSOs' were higher when they were in command of the aircraft. The pilots' subjective mental workload ratings were highest for the segments at the bombing range. In contrast to the heart rate data, the pilots' subjective workload ratings for take off and landing were among the lowest. The WSOs rated the segment when they were flying the aircraft as the most difficult with the bombing range ratings being next highest.

These results demonstrate that the psychophysiological measures are sensitive to the various mental demands experienced by the pilots and WSOs as shown by the differences among the segments. The data indicated that the mental workload of the pilots was greater than that of the WSOs. The measures also differentiated between the demands placed on the pilots and WSOs when performing their different jobs. The comparison of tracking task with flight results showed significant differences. For example, heart rate was higher during the more demanding flight tasks but blink rate was lower during the tracking tasks. The lower blink rates may be due to the nature of the single task tracking situation. Only the tracking task has to be attended while the flight environment is a multi-task situation which demands concurrent attention to several tasks.

The first known airborne evoked potentials (EP) were also recorded during this study (Wilson, Fullenkamp & Davis, 1994). The pilots were presented with tones in an odd ball paradigm. The tones were presented during the baseline, tracking task, cruise with pilot flying, and cruise with the WSO flying. The measures listed above were used to validate the EP results. The goal of this study was two fold. The first was to determine if EPs could be recorded during flight while the pilot was in command of the aircraft. The second goal was to reveal if the information in the EPs was useful in the analysis of mental workload. The baseline segment established the parameters of the EP with no interference from other tasks. The tracking task permitted comparisons with previous laboratory studies. The WSO in command cruise segment was to establish whether or not flight EPs could be recorded. The pilot in command cruise segment was used to determine if the EPs would be sensitive to task demands. The cruise conditions were selected for the EP analysis because they were low workload segments and would not interfere with the safety of flight during the EP collection when the pilot was counting the rare tones. Four EP components were identified: N1, P2, N2, and P3. The amplitude of the P3 component is typically used as the measure of task involvement (Kramer, 1991). However, to reduce artifacts during the flight data collection, a bipolar lead was used which linked Cz and Pz. This reduced the magnitude of the P3 amplitude since its distribution is wide spread over these scalp regions. The N1 amplitudes were significantly smaller during both flight segments compared to all of the ground segments. The P2 component amplitude of the pilot in command cruise segment was significantly smaller than both the ground based and WSO in command cruise segment. The P3 component amplitudes were the same for all conditions. Only the P2 component amplitude discriminated among flying the aircraft, being a passenger in the aircraft, and the ground based segments. However, as noted above, the other psychophysiological measures were also able to discriminate among the various segments and did not require the extensive data processing that was required for the EP signals.

Flight Studies with General Aviation Aircraft

The use of operational pilots and aircraft provides realism to research studies. However, there are often constraints included with their use. For example, the type of mission is typically dictated by the training sequence of the operational unit. There are also constraints on the types of maneuvers that can be used in order to meet the current training needs of the operational unit. This led us to undertake two studies using general aviation aircraft. Aircraft from the local aeroclub were used to provide inexpensive flight time and an adequate supply of trained and certified pilots. Within the limits of safe flight we could design scenarios that permitted us to investigate different aspects of flying that would expand our investigations into the psychophysiology of flight. In the first study (Hankins & Wilson, 1998) we were able to measure the effects of visual flight rules (VFR) versus the more difficult instrument flight rules (IFR) flying. Standard flight maneuvers were used such as take off, landing, touch and go, holding patterns, and instrument flying. The scenario was developed to vary the mental demands on the pilots by using navigation problems. By including IFR conditions we were able to determine the effects of the higher visual demands of instrument flying. In effect we were able to create a 'flying laboratory.' In order to gain the most comprehensive understanding of the relationship between flight dynamics and the pilot's physiology we recorded a number of measures. These measures were heart rate, heart rate variability, eye blinks, horizontal eye movements, EEG from four electrode sites (Fz, Cz, P3, P4) and the pilot's subjective rating of mental workload. Two minute epochs were employed from 19 different segments during ground and flight periods.

The results showed notable heart rate increases during the take offs and landings. The next highest heart rates were found during the IFR flight segments. Interestingly, the high speed IFR segments were associated with the lowest heart rates. This was interpreted as being due to having just performed the same maneuvers at a lower speed. This effect is similar to those reported by Roscoe (1975) and Roman, Older, and Jones (1967) who reported decreased heart rates when repeating maneuvers during flight. The VFR cruise segment was also associated with the lowest heart rates. HRV in the medium and high bands were highly correlated but exhibited few statistically significant effects over the 19 segments. This relative insensitivity of HRV to differentiate among flight tasks is consistent with our earlier flight study and the results of others (Jorna, 1992; Veltman & Gaillard, 1996). Eye blink rate showed a dramatic decline during all of the IFR segments (Figure 3). The pilots wore special goggles that restricted their vision to the inside of the cokkpit to simulate night or bad weather flying. This greatly increased their dependence on information from the instruments since they were not able to look at the ground to confirm their altitude and location. The EEG theta band activity (P3 electrode) increased over the duration of the flights with peaks associated with segments involving increased cognitive activity such as flying arcs and tracking instrument pathways prior to landing. The theta activity showed troughs during landing segments which emphasize eye-hand coordination. The subjective mental workload rating scale (NASA TLX, Hart & Staveland, 1988) was remarkably insensitive to the varying demands of the flight task. The six scales were highly correlated (r = 0.66 to 0.97) suggesting that the TLX may not tap different aspects of the cognitive demands of flying. In order to examine which variables provided convergent data and which were redundant, a correlational analysis was undertaken. This analysis showed the cardiac measures to be highly intercorrelated. A second cluster of highly intercorrelated measures was comprised of the eye measures and the EEG theta band activity. EEG alpha band activity and the subjective ratings were not significantly correlated with any of the other measures. These results can be used to investigate the cognitive aspects of flying and also to reduce the number of psychophysiological measures that are required to fully understand the underlying dynamics.

These results demonstrate the utility of multiple psychophysiological measures to provide insight into the complex cognitive activities required in piloting. By taking advantage of the unique information provided by the different psychophysiological measures, a better composite picture of the demands of piloting can be derived. The patterns of correlated activity across the various measures may contain further information that can be used in the analysis of the demands of piloting. Because of the continuous nature of the psychophysiological data it is possible to continually monitor the effects of flying on the cognitive resources of the pilot.

In a second 'flying laboratory' study, we replicated the conditions of the first study (Wilson, 1999). Few, if any, flight studies have provided direct replication of either earlier studies or replication of individual flights by the same pilots. The same scenario that was used in the Hankins and Wilson (1998) investigation was replicated. Further, the ten new pilots flew the same scenario twice. Additional measures were recorded during these flights. EDA, 29 channels of EEG, actigraphy, aircraft position via GPS, and altitude were new features added to the ECG, EOG, respira-

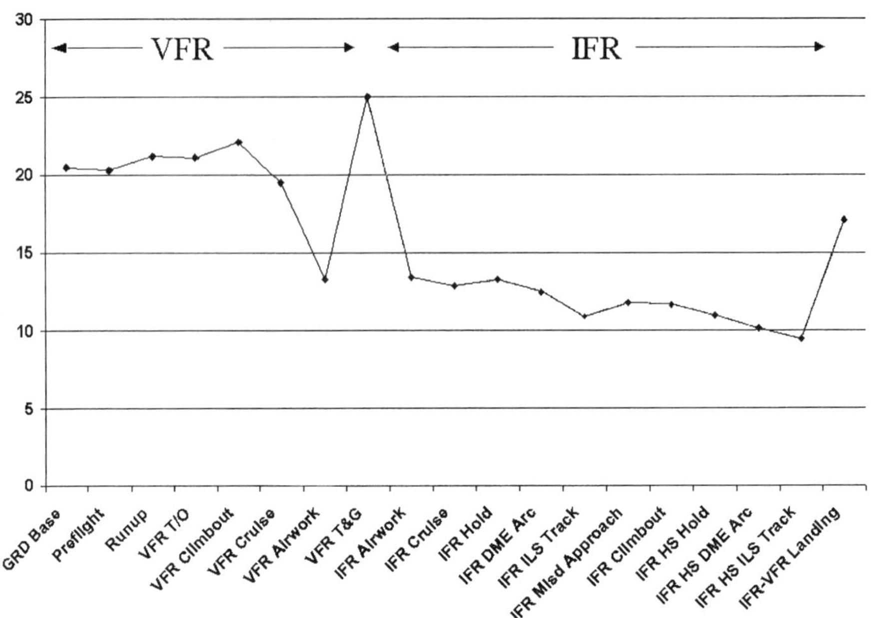

Figure 3. Mean blink rates for IFR and VFR potions of the approximately 90 minute flights. The increased blink rates during the VFR touch and go are due to transition blinks as the pilots looked from inside the cockpit to the runway and back. This is seen to a lesser extent during the final landing but not during the IFR missed approach which did not permit looking outside the cockpit. The decline in blinks during VFR air work is due to the higher visual demands of this segment.

tion, and subjective ratings of mental workload measures of the first study. By colllecting 29 EEG channels we were able to visualize the topographic changes in brain activity during the flight segments. Vitaport II and Smart Helmet recorders were used in this study to collect the psychophysiological data. The approximately 90 minute scenario was divided into 22 two-minute segments for analysis. Artifacts in the physiological data were detected and corrected. The heart rate and eye blink results replicated those from the first study. The EEG results were found to be slightly different from those in the first study. Examination of the data from the two flights of this study showed them to be statistically identical. This reinforces the belief that the day to day psychophysiological dynamics remain constant during a flight task.

The heart rate and EDA results were highly correlated ($r = 0.83$). These data are shown in Figure 4. This is due to the common influence of the autonomic system on both of these systems. The take offs and landings produced the largest responses for both heart rate and EDA. HRV in the middle and high frequency bands again showed significant decreases during only the take off, and touch and go segments.

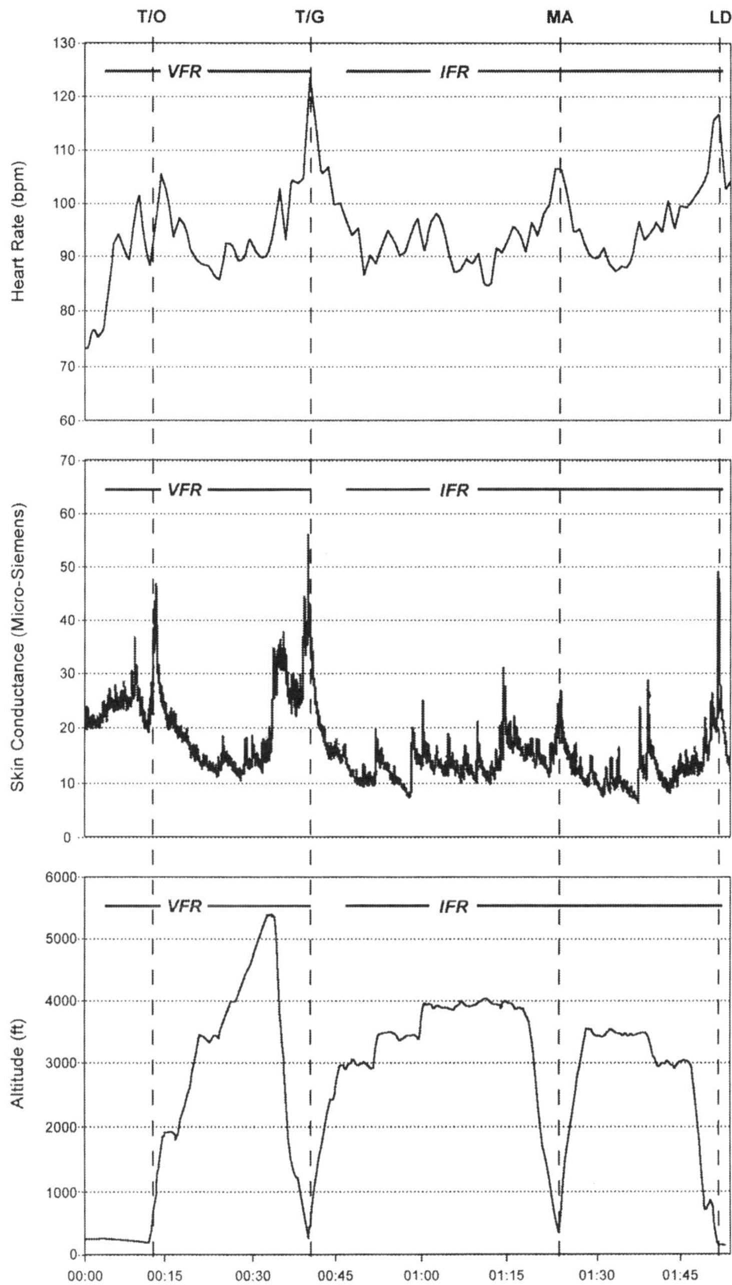

Figure 4. Heart rate, EDA and altitude from one pilot during a general aviation flight scenario. Take off (T/O), touch and go (T/G), missed approach (M/A) and final landing (LD) are noted on the figure. VFR and IFR periods are indicated. The scenario time line is shown on the ordinate.

As reported in the first study, the blink rate dramatically decreased during the IFR flight conditions. This replication further supports the effect of high visual demand upon eye blink activity. The results from this study showed the EEG alpha band activity to decrease over right posterior sites during the IFR segments during landings, missed approaches, and climb outs. The delta band EEG activity at central and parietal scalp sites showed increased activity during touch and go, landings, take offs, and the IFR segments. The topographic analysis of the EEG provided a better picture of the dynamics of the brain activity during the flights than was possible in the first study in which data were recorded from only four scalp sites. The latitude and longitude aircraft position is currently being used to implement a finer grained analysis of the physiological data. The effects of specific events is being examined. This includes the changes in the psychophysiological data associated when the pilots initiated, executed, and terminated climbs, descents, and turns.

The results of this second 'flying laboratory' study again demonstrated the value of multiple physiological measures. Further, the high reliability of the data between the two studies as well as between the two flights of the second study was demonstrated. While more difficult to implement, the 29 channel topographic EEG data provided important information concerning the distribution of the brain's electrical activity over the 90 minute scenario. The high correlation between the heart rate and EDA activity questions the value added by the EDA data. It is more difficult to record than the cardiac data, and if it does not provide further information then its collection may not be justified. However, further analysis examining changes to specific flight maneuvers may show the EDA does provide unique information. The collection of aircraft position via the readily available GPS system and altitude permits close examination of specific responses to particular flight events compared to averaging over a two minute segment.

Model Development

On the basis of the results of previous flight studies using psychophysiological data, a study was undertaken with the Swedish National Defence Research Establishment to develop models of pilot performance (Svensson, Angelborg-Thanderez & Wilson, 1999). Subjective reports from air-to-air training flights were used to develop a model of pilot performance including the effects of mental workload and situation awareness. Performance and subjective data were collected from actual flights. Then heart rate and eye blink measures were recorded in a simulation of the same air-to-air missions. The physiological data were collected using a Vitaport II recorder in Sweden and were sent via the internet to the United States for analysis. As expected, heart rate was a sensitive measure of the cognitive loads experienced by the pilots in the simulated mission. Heart rate was highly correlated with measures of mental capacity. Heart rate increased when the pilot's mental capacity was reduced. Blink rate reliably indexed visual search behavior of the pilots during the simulated missions. During periods of visual search by the pilots, such as when intercepting another aircraft, blink rate decreased, heart rate and blink fixation increased. Blink rate was seen to decrease so that visual information would not be lost during the blink. The increased heart rate was related to the increased mental demands of the task. Because of the similarities of the simulator and flight models, it was concluded that the same model was appropriate in both situations and that the psychophysiological data provided valuable information.

Aircraft Test and Evaluation Using Psychophysiological Measures

Heart rate and eye blink measures were used to evaluate the relative demands of two aircraft mounted sensor systems (Wilson, Badeau & Gawron, 1993). Infrared and radar sensors were used during training of test pilots to demonstrate the relative merits of the two systems. The test aircraft flew a race track path with one type of sensor used to detect a target on each leg. It was concluded that the infrared system was the most demanding because blink rates were lower and heart rates were higher during the infrared portions of the mission. Periods of blink inhibition were seen just before target location in both tasks. These were the times of highest visual demand as the operators were trying to locate the targets and identify the elements of the targets.

Psychophysiological measures have been used in the test and evaluation of new and upgraded aircraft. These include the B-1, C-17, C-130J, and the PACER CRAG upgrade to the KC-135. An interesting application of heart rate data was to use it as a debriefing aid (Rokicki, 1987). During post-flight debriefings, periods of high heart rate were matched with the flight profiles. Periods of the test missions having unexpectedly high values were highlighted and used in the debriefings to pin point unusual events. This was found to be a useful technique to jog the crew members memories concerning unexpected events during the missions.

During the operational test and evaluation of a new transport aircraft, heart rate was recorded from the pilots, copilots, and loadmasters. In the new aircraft, computers were used to perform navigation tasks and resulted in the elimination of the navigator position. This left the pilot and copilot with the total navigation responsibilities for each mission. Because this may have increased the pilot's and copilot's workload to unacceptable levels there were human factors concerns. Heart rate data were used, along with performance and subjective data, to determine if the mental workload was acceptable with only two crew members in the cockpit. The crew members were instrumented with Del Mar ambulatory Holter recorders that they wore in a pocket of their flight suits. The digitized data were sent via the internet to

Wright-Patterson Air Force Base for analysis. During one portion of the evaluation the crews performed a number of touch and go landings. Touch and go maneuvers are practice landings and take offs. The aircraft lands but then accelerates and performs a take off. This provides testing of both landing and take off characteristics. The two pilots traded responsibilities during the several touch and go segments with dramatic changes in their heart rates. Figure 5 shows mean heart rates for one mission. The pilot in command of each landing exhibited increased heart rates while the heart rates of the non-pilot in command did not increase. These data support other reports showing heart rate increases from the pilot in command during high workload maneuvers (Roscoe, 1992; Hart & Hauser, 1987). Compared to laboratory data, the peak heart rates seen during touch and gos are very large, up to 30 beat per minute increases from the pre-landing heart rates. The general decline in the heart rates for both pilots over the approximately more than four hour duration of the mission is often seen. During one flight a crew attempted to land the aircraft on an ice covered runway. This was a very high workload situation and was accompanied by extremely high heart rates in the pilot in command of the aircraft. Peak heart rates of about 175 beats per minute were observed with one minute mean heart rates in the 150 bpm range. The non-pilot in command exhibited much lower heart rates even though he faced the same danger as the pilot in command. This led to the conclusion that it was the mental demands that were the primary drivers of the increased heart rates in the command pilot and not the fear of a crash. During the same series of evaluation tests the aircraft was landed on a short, assault run-

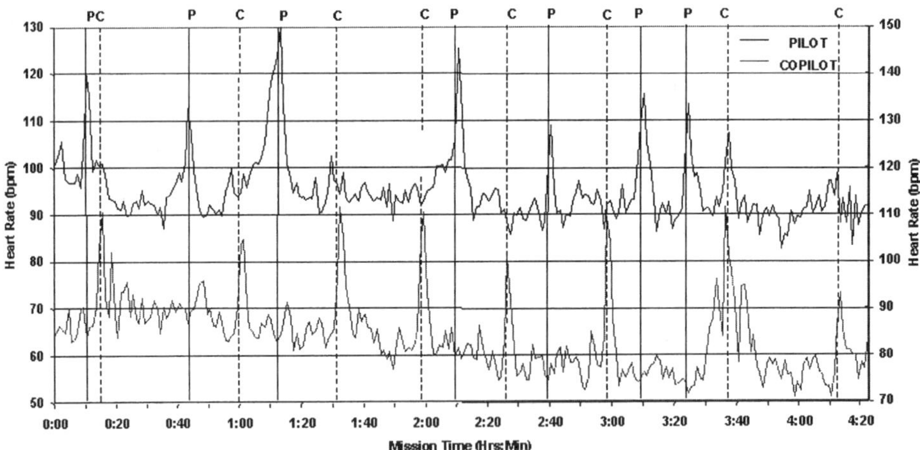

Figure 5. Pilot and copilot one minute mean heart rates for a test and evaluation mission of a new cargo aircraft. The pilot's data are on the top and take off and touch and go events are marked with the vertical lines. The solid lines indicate when the pilot was in command and the dashed lines indicate when the copilot was in command of the aircraft.

way. In the first part of the tests the runway length was painted on a normal runway. The pilot's job was to land the aircraft and come to a complete stop within the boundaries. This is a more difficult task than normal and was associated with higher heart rates. Landing on actual packed earth assault runways was associated with even higher heart rates. One copilot flew with several pilots during the packed earth assault landings. His heart rates were slightly elevated but not to the extend shown by the pilots in command. These results are in contrast to simulated emergency situations during actual flight. These simulated emergencies were typically associated with small increases in heart rate. During one actual in-flight emergency both the pilot's and copilot's heart rates showed notable increases. The use of psychophysiological measures in test and evaluation has value to both the testing and to increasing our knowledge about the human's responses to real world situations.

Operator Functional State Classification

Our current efforts are focused on extending our results to explore the possibility of real time operator functional state classification and its use in adaptive aiding. Because psychophysiological measures provide reliable information concerning the functional state of crew members, it may be possible to use this information to modify the task to meet the momentary needs of the operator. Our first exploration of this concept involved using EEG data to train a classifier to recognize pilot and WSO workload levels using data from the study described above (Wilson & Fisher, 1991). Heart and eye data from ten pilots and eight WSOs were used to train a stepwise discriminant (SWD) classifier to discriminate between pilots and WSOs and to recognize eight different flight segments. The data were randomly divided into training and test sets. The classifier was trained with the training set and then its ability to correctly discern the eight segments was tested by having it classify the test data set. Pilots and WSOs were correctly discriminated with an accuracy of 84 percent. For the pilot's the correct segment of the eight was correctly identified 92 percent of the time with and accuracy of 89 percent for the WSOs. These very high classification rates using the combined heart and eye data suggest that on-line classification is possible with accuracy rates that would be acceptable to the operational community.

Laboratory generated data were used to classify seven different tasks each having two levels of difficulty (Wilson & Fisher, 1995). EEG from nineteen scalp sites was used to train a SWD classifier using the training and testing strategy described above. Principle components analysis was used to derive the EEG bands that were input to the classifier. Overall, 86 percent mean correct classification was achieved with a range of 61 to 95 percent correct. High frequency bands, above 30 Hz, from electrodes located around the sides of the head were the most salient features used by the SWD. These results show that EEG data also contains information that can be used to correctly classifier subject functional state with a very high level of accuracy.

Data from simulated aircraft landings were used by Russell, Wilson and Monet (1996) to test the ability of artificial neural networks (ANN) to use psychophysiological data to correctly classify pilot workload. Five pilots flew a simulated landing approach in cloudy conditions. When the clouds cleared, the pilots found themselves lined up with the center of the runway, 1,064 or 2,128 feet to the left or right of the runway centerline. The larger deviations from the runway centerline were associated with higher pilot workload. Using EEG data from seven electrode sites, heart, eye, and respiration data, the ANN was trained using half of the available data. The remaining data were used to test the accuracy of the trained ANN. Overall, the ANN classifier was able to correctly identify the type of landing offset with a mean accuracy of 83 percent across the five pilots. The range across subjects was 79 to 90 percent correct. These results suggest that ANN classifiers are capable of high levels of accuracy while pilots are engaged in a complex landing task. The use of multiple physiological measures was useful in achieving these levels of accuracy.

Using data from a study of the effects of varying levels of workload on air traffic controllers Russell and Wilson (1998) implemented ANN techniques to determine how well the various levels could be discriminated. Data from seven controllers were used and consisted of EEG from 17 channels distributed over the head following the 10/20 system. The data were divided into five frequency bands. The data were then divided into three sets, training, validation, and test. The validation set was used to avoid overtraining the ANN so that it would not just recognize the training set data. There were two manipulations of the task to control difficulty. The ANN was able to discriminate among the three levels for the two manipulations with accuracies of 86 and 83 percent correct. In a separate condition an effort was made to mentally overload the controllers. The ANN performed very well when identifying the overload condition from the non-overload conditions with an overall mean accuracy of 92 percent correct across the seven controllers. Further refinement of the ANN procedures using feature saliency techniques to reduce the feature set resulted in 98 percent to 100 percent correct classification of this two class problem. These results suggest that very high levels of operator functional state can be achieved during complex task performance if high levels of mental demand are to be identified. This would be the case in most real world situations where the goal is to detect operator functional states that would lead to mental overload conditions and produce errors.

The results of these investigations established that very high levels of operator functional state classification accuracy could be achieved using psychophysiological data. The next step was to use this information to dynamically modify the task to meet the needs of the operator. Many current systems have the capability of modifying themselves. If these changes could be at least partially determined based upon the needs of the operator then errors could be avoided and the overall system performance would be enhanced. In an effort designed to demonstrate the beneficial effects of adaptive aiding based on psychophysiologically determined operator functional state assessment, Wilson, Lambert and Russell (1999) used a multiple task laboratory battery, the Multi-Attribute Task Battery (MATB, Comstock & Arnegard, 1992) to implement adaptive aiding. Seven subjects were trained to stable performance on the MATB. Six EEG channels, ECG, EOG, and respiration were monitored and used as inputs to an ANN. The ANN was trained on data from the three difficulty levels of the task for each subject. The ANN was then used to classify the functional state of the subjects and then to provide adaptive aiding when it determined that the subject was in a high workload condition. Two of the four MATB tasks were turned off to decrease the subject's workload with the aim of improving performance on the remaining tasks. The ANN correctly classified the three difficulty conditions with a mean accuracy of 84 percent. The application of the adaptive aiding resulted in significant improvement in performance on the remaining two tasks. There was a 44 percent reduction in RMS error for the manual tracking task and a mean 33 percent reduction in the error score for the resource management task of the MATB. These results are very encouraging and for the first time show that physiologically determined adaptive aiding improves performance when used to reduce mental workload. Further research is being undertaken to replicate and extend these results. Improvements are being made to the classifier and more complex real world tasks will be used. With the availability of miniature amplifiers having sophisticated signal processing capabilities it is possible to construct wearable operator functional state assessment devices to interface with systems. The operator functional state information can be used to modify system characteristics to meet the immediate needs of the operator. For example, display clutter could be reduced leaving only the critical information necessary to solve a problem. The effect of this adaptive aiding would be to reduce the operator's workload and thereby reduce the probability of error and improve overall system performance.

Summary

The results of our in-flight studies have enhanced our knowledge of the cognitive effects of flight upon crew members physiology. This information can be used to evaluate the cognitive demands of new and modified aircraft and flight procedures on crew members. Our data have shown that the added responsibilities of being in the lead or wing aircraft has direct effects on the pilots' heart and blink rates. We have further demonstrated that flying is associated with significant differences in crew members' physiology when compared to performing a standard laboratory task. The different responsibilities of two crew members in the same aircraft were associated with different response patterns depending on the demands placed on each crew member. We have also demonstrated that EPs can be recorded during flight and that these responses are associated with the demands of flying. Using the 'flying laboratory' concept permitted us to gain more control over the mental demands of our flight scenarios. This resulted in being able to determine the patterns of responses from several psychophysiological systems during flight. Notable among these effects were the dramatic reduction in blink rate during the more visually demanding IFR portions of the flights. Our ability to replicate not only day to day effects but across studies lends support to the use of psychophysiological methods in flight research. The topographical EEG analysis illustrated the benefits of this approach to localize scalp areas showing changes in brain activity which were related to specific aspects of flying. y using a number of physiological measures were are able to determine patterns among these variables and possibly extract more information. We have used psychophysiological measures in the operational test and evaluation of aircraft. This application was found to be beneficial in the testing environment. The real emergency situations encountered during flight have provided unique insights into the dynamics of how pilots mobilize resources to meet sudden demands. The selection of two minute epochs for the analysis of much of the flight data has also been useful. Shorter or longer epochs may not have yielded the same results. Most of the psychophysiological measures that we have tried have proved to provide useful data. There may be redundancy among measures as may be the case with EDA when heart rate data are available. Heart rate variability does not seem to provide useful information in the flight environment.This may be because the multiple task nature of flight overwhelms the dynamic range of heart rate variability. We also have demonstrated that psychophysiological data can be successfully used to classify operators' functional state. This opens the possibility of closing the loop between operators' momentary needs and the demands placed by the system. With new systems gaining more capability with regard to automation it will be possible to tailor the task to the momentary needs of the operator to achieve optimal overall system performance

References

Caldwell, J.A., Wilson, G.F., Centiguc, M., Gaillard, A.W.K., Gundel, A., Lagarde, D., Makeig, S., Myhre, G. & Wright, N.A. (1994). Psychophysiological Assessment Methods. *AGARD Advisor Report, AGARD-AR-324, AGARD, Paris, France.*

Comstock, J.R. & Arnegard, R.J. (1992). The multi-attribute task battery for human operator workload and strategic behavior research. *NASA Technical Memorandum No. 104174.*

Hankins, T.C. & Wilson, G.F. (1998). A comparison of heart rate, eye activity, EEG and subjective measures of pilot mental workload during flight. *Aviation, Space and Environmental Medicine, 69*, 630–367.

Hart, S.G. & Hauser, J.R. (1987). Inflight application of three pilot workload measurement techniques. *Aviation, Space, and Environmental Medicine, 58*, 402–410.

Hart, S.G. & Staveland, L.E. (1988). Development of NASA-TLX (Task Load Index): Results of empirical and theoretical research. In P.A. Hancock & N. Meshkati (Eds.) *Human Mental Workload.* Amsterdam: North Holland Press.

Jorna, P.G.A.M. (1992). Spectral analysis of heart rate and psychological state: a review of its validity as a workload index. *Biological Psychology, 34*, 237–259.

Kramer, A.F. (1991). Physiological metrics of mental workload: A review of recent progress. In Damos, (Ed.) *Multiple-task Performance* (pp. 279–328). London: Taylor and Francis.

Rokicki, S.M. (1987). Heart rate averages as workload/fatigue indicators during OT&E. *Proceedings of the 31 st Annual Meeting of the Human Factors Society, 2*, 784–785.

Roscoe, A.H. (1992). Assessing pilot workload. Why measure heart rate, HRV and respiration? *Biological Psychology, 34*, 259–288.

Russell, C.A., Wilson, G.F. & Monett, C.T. (1996). Mental workload classification using a back propagation neural network. In C.H. Dagli, M. Akay, C.L.P. Chen, B.R. Fernandez & J. Ghosh. *Proceedings of the Artificial Neural Networks in Engineering (ANNIE'96) Conference, 6*, 685–690.

Russell, C.A. & Wilson, G.F. (1998). Air traffic controller functional state classification using neural networks. *Proceedings of the Artificial Neural Networks in Engineering (ANNIE'98) Conference, 8*, 649–654.

Sirevaag, E.J., Kramer, A.F., Wickens, C.D., Reisweber, M., Strayer, D.L. & Grenell, J.F. (1993). Assessment of pilot performance and mental workload in rotary wing aircraft. *Ergonomics, 36*, 1121–1140.

Skelly, J.J., Purvis, B. & Wilson, G. (1988). Fighter pilot performance during airborne and simulator missions: Physiological comparisons. In *Electric and Magnetic Activity of the Central Nervous System: Research and Clinical Applications in Aerospace Medicine,* AGARD Symposium, Trondheim, Norway, 1987, 23–1 to 23–15.

Svensson, E., Angelborg-Thanderz, M. & Wilson, G.F. (1999). *Models of pilot performance for systems and mission evaluation – Psychological and psychophysiological aspects. AFRL/HE-WP-TR-199-0215.* Wright-Patterson AFB, OH: Air Force Research Laboratory.

Veltman, J.A. & Gaillard, A.W.K. (1996). Physiological indices of workload in a simulated flight task. *Biological Psychology, 42*, 323–342.

Veltman, J.A. & Gaillard, A.W.K. (1998). Physiological workload reactions to increasing levels of task difficulty. *Ergonomics, 41*, 656–669.

Wilson, G.F. (1993). Air-to-ground training missions: A psychophysiological workload analysis. *Ergonomics, 36*, 1071–1087.

Wilson, G.F. (1999). Flight Psychophysiology. *Proceedings of the Human Factors and Ergonomics Society 44th Annual Meeting,* 3–33 to 3–36.

Wilson, G.F., Badeau, A. & Gawron, V. (1993). Evaluation of two inflight sensors using heart rate and eye blink measures. *Proceedings of the Seventh International Symposium on Aviation Psychology, 2*, 886–890.

Wilson, G.F. (in press). Psychophysiological Test Methods and Procedures. In S. Charlton & T.O'Brien (Eds.), *Handbook of Human Factors Testing & Evaluation, Second Edition.* Mahwah, New Jersey: Lawrence Erlbaum Associates, Inc.

Wilson, G.F. & Eggemeier, F.T. (1991). Physiological measures of workload in multi-task environments (pp. 329–360). In D. Damos (Ed.) *Multiple-task performance.* London: Taylor and Francis.

Wilson, G.F. & Fisher, F. (1991). The use of cardiac and eye blink measures to determine flight segment in F4 crews. *Aviation, Space and Environmental Medicine, 62*, 959–961.

Wilson, G.F. & Fisher, F. (1995). Cognitive task classification based upon topographic EEG data. *Biological Psychology, 40*, 239–250.

Wilson, G.F., Purvis, B., Skelly, J., Fullenkamp, P. & Davis, I. (1987). Physiological data used to measure pilot workload in actual flight and simulator conditions. *Proceedings of the Human Factors Society*, 779–783.

Wilson, G.F., Skelly, J. & Purvis, B. (1988). Reactions to emergency situations in actual and simulated flight. AGARD Conference Proceedings, *Human Behavior in High Stress Situations in Aerospace Operations, (pp. 9–13). NATO: AGARD.*

Wilson, G.F., Fullenkamp, P. & Davis, I. (1994). Evoked potential, cardiac, blink, and respiration measures of pilot workload in air-to-ground missions. *Aviation, Space and Environmental Medicine, 65*, 100–1005.

Chapter 26
Psychophysiological Monitoring of Air Traffic Controllers: Exploration, Simulation, Validation

Joachim Vogt and Michael Kastner
Department of Organizational Psychology, University of Dortmund, Germany

Introduction

Air traffic controllers (ATCOs) are well studied subjects in psychophysiological research. Their task is to ensure safe separation of aircraft in time and/or space. The combination of high workload, high responsibility for safety and shift-work makes air traffic control (ATC) a stressful job. Martindale wrote in 1977:

"The job of juggling airliners and making snap decisions on which lives depend exacts a steep toll in stress-related diseases, nightmares, and acute anxiety."

Although ATCOs are well-selected with respect to physical and psychological fitness, Baader and Graf found in 1958 among 295 German ATCOs 24 % with gastrointestinal, 20 % with vegetative, 14 % with cardiovascular, and 17 % with multiple complaints. The dramatic air traffic increase during the last decades added to the problem, because it can only partly be compensated by new technologies (SRATM, 2000). Therefore, stress in ATC is an issue of utmost importance.

Many studies have tried to identify the main stressors in ATC aiming at compensatory measures, for example in the break and shift system. Most of these studies have used psychophysiological measures to characterize the effects of the stressors. Table 1 reviews the most important studies and the measures they used.

It is widely agreed upon that the most important factor determining stress levels is the number of aircraft under control (Arad, 1963, 1964; Brookings et al., 1996; Cabon, Mollard, Cointot, Martel & Beslot, 1997; Cobb & Rose, 1973; Costa, 1993; Hurst & Rose, 1978; Laurig, Becker-Biskaborn & Reiche, 1971; Kimbelton, 1970; Melton, Smith, McKenzie, Wicks & Saldivar, 1977; Repetti, 1989, 1993; Rohmert & Rutenfranz, 1972; Rose & Fogg 1993; Smith, Melton & McKenzie, 1971; Smith, 1980; Zeier & Grubenmann, 1990; Zeier et al., 1996; using the number of flight data strips: Reiche, Kirchner & Laurig, 1971). The topography of the airspace sector controlled by radar ATCOs and the visibility for tower controllers has also been considered a stress factor by some authors (Arad, 1963, 1964; Hurst & Rose, 1978;

Table 1. Physiological stress measures in air traffic controllers.
⇧ significant increase, ⇩ significant decrease, ⇳ complex pattern, ⇔ no change during work

Authors	Biosignal		Change during work
Laurig et al., 1971 Rohmert & Rutenfranz, 1972 Henderson et al., 1990 Costa, 1993	Heart rate		⇧
Smith, 1980	Heart rate Blood pressure		⇧ ⇔
Cobb & Rose, 1973	Blood pressure		⇧
Melton et al., 1977	Heart rate (low traffic) Catecholamines Corticosteroids		⇔ ⇧ ⇧
Rose & Fogg, 1993	Heart rate Blood pressure Cortisol	"Responder" classes: Upper sextile Grand mean Lower sextile	 ⇧ ⇧,⇔ ⇔,⇩
Theorell, Perski, Akerstedt, Sigala, Ahlberg-Hulten et al., 1988	Blood pressure Prolactin (in morning blood sample) Cortisol (in morning blood sample)		⇧ ⇧ ⇩
Klimmer, Aulmann & Rutenfranz, 1972	Catecholamines in urine		⇧
Zeier, 1994; Zeier et al., 1996	secretory immunoglobulin A Cortisol		⇧ ⇧
Kan, Malinovskaia, Kuprianov & Denisov, 1984	Catecholamines in urine Potassium in saliva Sodium in saliva		⇳ ⇧ ⇩
Lille & Cheliout, 1982	Heart rate (night vs. day shift) Low frequency EEG		⇧ ⇧
Cabon et al., 1997	EEG, P300 EEG Theta Beta Cortisol		⇩ ⇧ ⇧ ⇧,⇔
McGregor & Stern, 1996	Duration of saccades Amplitude of saccades		⇧ ⇳
Brookings et al., 1996	Heart rate Eye blink frequency Saccades Respiration frequency EEG Theta Beta Delta/Alpha		⇔ ⇩ ⇧ ⇧ ⇧ ⇧ ⇳

Repetti, 1989, 1993). The speed of the aircraft under control (Hurst & Rose, 1978) and the number of conflicting aircraft (Kimbelton, 1970) were only rarely studied. And finally, the information content of radio transmissions (e. g., instruction, information, question, report, inquiry, Reiche et al., 1971; Rohmert & Rutenfranz, 1972), their frequency and duration (Kimbelton, 1970; Hurst & Rose, 1978; Henderson, Bakal & Dunn, 1990; Zeier et al., 1996) were investigated.

However, the number of aircraft under control is the only well-established indicator of ATCO taskload. In a multiple regression analysis performed by Hurst and Rose (1978) 53 % of stress responses were explained by the number of aircraft. Rohmert and Rutenfranz (1972) predicted heart rate changes from traffic volume and duration. The correlation between predicted and measured heart rate changes was 0.5, and the authors concluded, first, that heart rate alone is a satisfactory predictor of response, and that the number of aircraft is the main stressor. Other traffic and airspace features were only sporadically used, and were less predictive or difficult to define, such as quality of radio transmissions.

Finkelman et al. (1979) criticized that there is no theory-led approach to evaluating stressors and stress responses in ATC. In an attempt to close this gap, the following studies were based on the dynaxity model (Kastner, 1986; Kastner, Ademmer, Budde, Hagemann, Udovic & Vogt, 1998), considering two meta-stressors in ATC: Complexity and dynamics. Complexity is a stable feature of a task and is determined by the number of elements (Simon, 1964), their diversity (Schroeder, Driver & Streuffert, 1967), and their interdependence (Dörner, 1976). The dynamics describe the changes of these features over time.

The only study trying to give operational definition to complexity is that of Brookings, Wilson and Swain (1996). They investigated eight ATCOs in a simulation study and varied "traffic complexity". This was defined as the ratio of arriving and departing aircraft, pilot skills, and aircraft types. Following this approach, three studies were conducted to add some empirical evidence to the existing "considerable disagreement about number and relative importance of elements that comprise airspace complexity" (Mogford, Murphy & Guttman, 1994; Brookings et al., 1996).

Exploration study

The aim of the exploration study was to identify the most important stressors in ATC as an input for the simulation study. The exploration study was conducted in April and May of 1996. On the basis of suggestions from experts of the German Air Traffic Control Services (Deutsche Flugsicherung, DFS), Bremen and Frankfurt airports were selected for the study. In Bremen, traffic volume is relatively small but diversity is very high (regular, charter, training, military, private flights; high percentage of visual flight routines). In contrast, traffic volume in Frankfurt is among the highest in Europe but diversity is rather low, since most aircraft are professionally operated.

In addition to the airport, three different ATC areas were studied: Tower (TWR), approach (APP) and area center control (ACC). The tower controllers are responsible for the runway traffic, and arriving or departing aircraft. Their control zone usually has a radius of about 25 nautical miles and extends up to about 2500 ft above ground. They hand over departing aircraft and take over landing aircraft to/from the approach controller. Depending on airspace and flight routes, APP extends up to about 9000 ft. The area center usually covers flight levels up to 24500 ft.

Method

The two factors – airport and ATC area – were fully combined in a 3x2 design with repeated measurements. 36 male, non-smoking ATCOs were recruited for the study, six in each ATC area at Bremen and Frankfurt airports respectively. The age of the ATCOs ranged from 26 to 52 years (M=34), and they had between 2 and 26 years (M=11) of work experience. Age and work experience of the volunteers did not differ significantly between airports or ATC areas.

Preparations for the monitoring were made in a lounge close to the work places. Subjects refrained from drinking coffee or mineral water (to prevent sodium and potassium contamination of saliva, since the electrolytes were used as a salivary indicator of stress) for the duration of the experiment and drank only fruit juice. After arrival and in case of food intake, subjects rinsed their mouths with ion-free water to remove particles. The monitoring procedure was explained to the ATCOs and informed consent was obtained. Figure 1 shows all biosignals monitored throughout the three studies using the Physiologger HD 64180 (MedNATIC Ltd., Munich, Germany). In a pre-interview, a number of control questions were answered regarding pre-existing diseases, medication, sports, caffeine consumption, sleep, etc.

After a relaxation period of at least 30 minutes, five minutes of resting values were recorded. Subsequently, subjects collected the saliva they actually had in the mouth and gave it into a polysterol tube for a baseline sample. This procedure was preferred over the Salivette with respect to the electrolytes, which should be determined in unstimulated saliva (Hinton, Burton, Farmer, Rotheiler, Shewan et al., 1992). The Riva-Rocci blood pressure measurement as the most unpleasant procedure was last in the sequence, which was repeated also during work.

Five minutes after completion of the blood pressure measurement, the ATCO moved to his workplace and took over from his predecessor. This was the first sampling point during work. Six further sampling points followed in 15-minute-intervals. Traffic quantity and quality was obtained from DFS records and the flight data strips. For this reason, all monitoring equipment was synchronized to Greenwich Mean Time. After 90 minutes of work, the ATCO returned to the lounge and the monitoring equipment was removed. A post-interview asked for the representativity of the 90-minute work period and special events. In a stimulus recall interview, radar pictures and radio transmissions of the six sampling points were replayed, and subjective ratings were obtained to gauge levels of experienced stress, concentration, motivation, upset (Hinton & Burton, 1997; Vogt, Hinton & Burton, 1992), complexity and

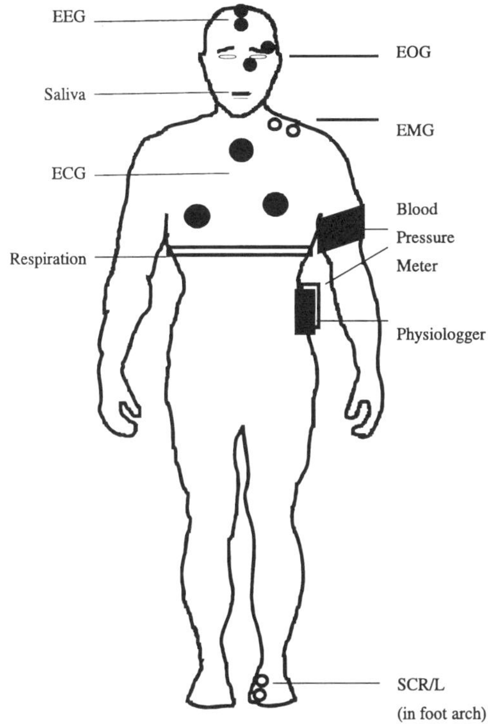

Figure 1. Monitoring equipment used in all three studies: Physiologger HD 64180, MedNATIC Ltd., Munich; automated blood pressure device TM2420, boso Ltd., Jungingen, Germany.

ECG: Electrocardiogramm, 50 Hz, default 0,75 mV
EEG: Electroencephalogramm over Fz Cz, 50 Hz, default 100 μV, only simulation
EMG: Electromyogramm, 5 Hz, default 140 μV, only exploration study
EOG: Electrooculogramm, 10 Hz, default ±0,4 mV
Resp.: Respiration, 5 Hz, default high sensitivity
SCR/L: Skin conductance response and level, 10 Hz, 0,5 μS
BP: Systolic, diastolic blood pressure and pulse, 15-minute intervals in exploration study, 10-minute intervals in simulation and validation study
Saliva: Sodium, potassium, and immunoglobulin A, 15-minute intervals in exploration study, 10-minute intervals in simulation and validation study

dynamics of traffic, and the NASA task load index (Hart & Staveland, 1988).

The five minutes before the resting blood pressure measurement and the two minutes before each blood pressure measurement during work were analyzed with respect to beats per minute, cycles per minute, eye blinks per minute (Stern, 1994), mean muscle tension (corrected according to Strasser, Ernst & Müller, 1992), skin conductance responses above 0.2 μS per minute, and mean skin conductance level. These analyses were performed with the Physiologger Software. The only exception was eye blink detection, which was performed with an in-house Windows program. The saliva samples were stored at –20°C. After they were defrosted, saliva mass was determined, primarily as a control for the immunoglobulin (IgA) measurement but also as a stress indicator on its own (Somer, Ben Aryeh & Laufer, 1993). IgA was determined using low level radial immune diffusion endoplates (Sanofi Diagnostics Pasteur Ltd., Freiburg; since 1997 Beckman Instruments Inc., Chaska, Minnesota; method by Mancini, Carbonara & Heremans, 1965, adopted for saliva according to Kugler, 1990). Before the following flame emission photometry was conducted for sodium and potassium determination, samples were centrifuged at 2000 cycles per minute for three minutes.

Those biosignals, for which some consensus about lower and upper limits exists in the literature were controlled for outliers (Table 2).

Table 2: Upper and lower limits for outlier control in the exploration study.

Biosignal	Upper limit	Lower limit	Controlled	Reference
Heart rate, beats per minute	190	40	Yes	Klinge (1992)
Systolic blood pressure, mmHg	220	70	Yes	
Diastolic blood pressure, mmHg	140	50	Yes	
Respiration, cycles per minute	45	9	Yes	Stern, Ray & Davis (1980)
Saliva mass			No	
Immunoglobulin A, mg/dl			No	Kugler (1994)
Potassium, mmol/l Sodium, mmol/l	25.58 8.70	15.35 0	No	Jenkins (1978)
Potassium, mmol/l Sodium, mmol/l	40.00 25.00	15.00 10.00	No	Löffler (1990)
Skin conductance responses	30	0	Yes	Boucsein (1988)
Muscle tension			No	
Eye blink frequency			No	

Two to five of the 36 subjects (depending on the particular biosignal) had missing values among the seven work samples. However, missing values were spread widely over airports and ATC areas, so that the minimum number of subjects in each cell of the design was five. Only the salivary measures had more missing values since some samples were too small for IgA or electrolyte determination or both due to unstimulated sampling.

Results

Figure 2 shows the mean heart rate of the six TWR-, APP-, and ACC controllers at Frankfurt and Bremen airport during rest, take-over and six work situations. Heart rate was increased in all groups by 10 to 20 bpm at the time of work take-over. Because physical activity (e. g. climbing the pulpit of the tower, moving to the workplace) and mental stress of "taking the picture" were confounded, the take-over sampling point was removed from the subsequent analyses. At the six regular work situations, mean heart rate ranged between 80 and 85 bpm. Only the APP controllers at Bremen reached baseline values by 15 minutes after take-over.

Mean systolic blood pressure and most of the other phasic measures showed a similar pattern. Mean systolic pressure was elevated over baseline in all groups at the time of take-over (Figure 3). In Bremen it continuously decreased and was close to baselines at the end of the 90-minute monitoring session. In Frankfurt it stayed 10-

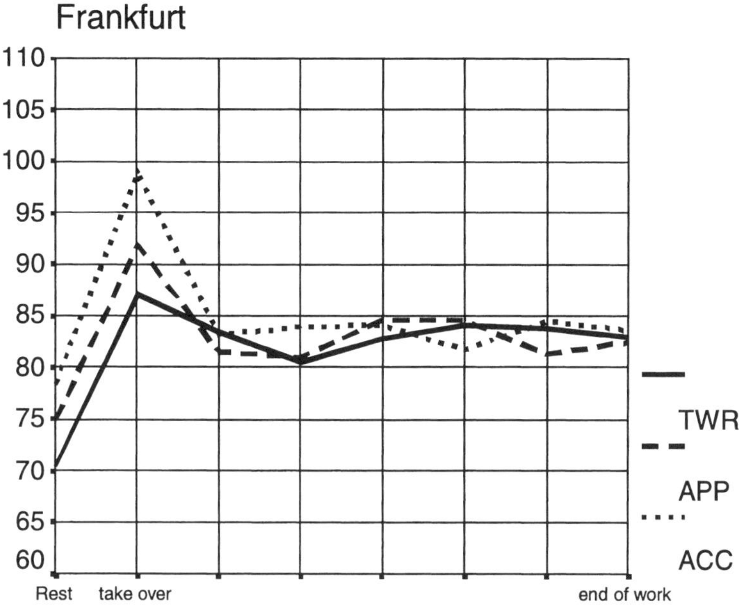

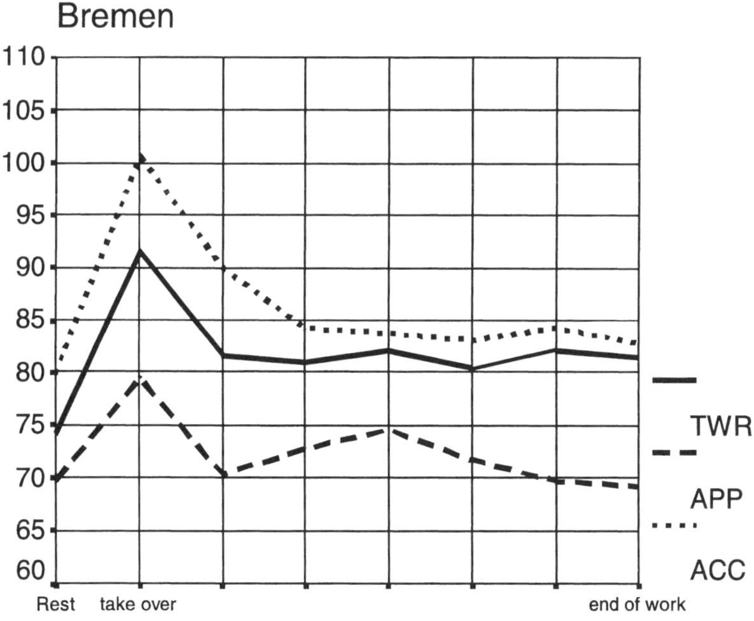

Figure 2. Mean heart rate of six tower, approach and center controllers at Frankfurt and Bremen airport during rest, take-over of work and six work samples.

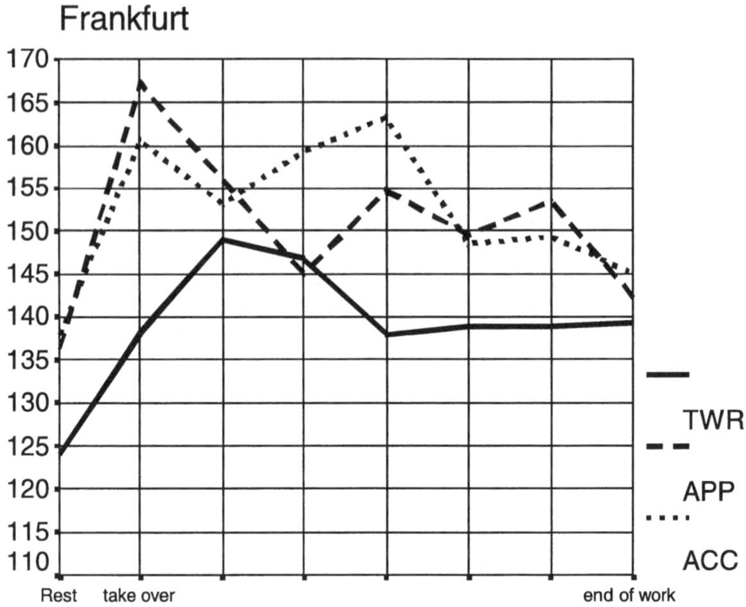

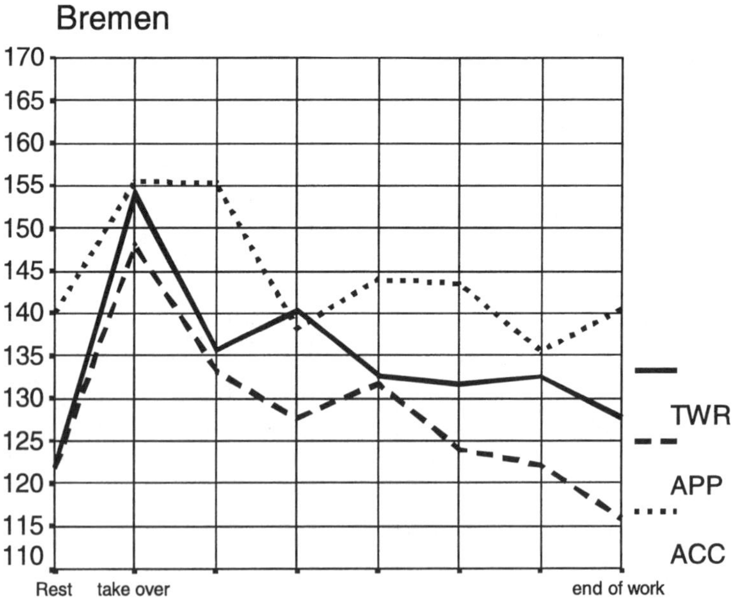

Figure 3. Mean systolic blood pressure of six tower, approach and center controllers at Frankfurt and Bremen airport during rest, take-over of work and six work samples.

Table 3. Significance of MANOVA main and interaction effects in the exploration study.

	Main effect Airport	Main effect ATC area	Main effect Time	Interaction AirP x ATC	Interaction AirP x Time	Interaction ATC x Time
Herat rate	.527	.292	**.000**[4]	.350	.070	**.031**[9]
Pulse	.516	.398	**.000**[4]	.330	**.018**[8]	.179
Systolic	**.025**[1]	.273	**.000**[4]	.415	**.046**[8]	**.002**[9]
Diastolic	**.030**[1]	.633	**.000**[4]	.558	.167	.061
Respiration	.493	**.001**[2]	**.000**[4]	**.005**[6]	.078	.202
Saliva mass	.655	.410	.845	.168	.883	.436
Saliva IgA	.799	.706	**.004**[4]	.629	.200	.857
Potassium	.213	.946	.560	1.00	.369	.803
Sodium	.264	.171	**.027**[4]	.771	.940	**.011**[10]
SCRs	.755	.875	**.000**[4]	.543	.613	.341
EMG	.158	.777	**.001**[4]	.606	.186	.679
Eye blinks	.058	.176	**.001**[4]	.203	**.016**[8]	.217
Concentration	**.008**[1]	.111	5	**.030**[7]	5	5
Upset	.223	**.043**[3]	5	.493	5	5
Motivation	**.005**[1]	.127	5	.063	5	5

[1]Frankfurt ATCOs responded more than their colleagues in Bremen; [2]APP > TWR > ACC; [3]ACC > TWR > APP; [4]Work > Rest, only exceptions: Sodium (stress induced decrease expected) and respiration (probably due to [6]); [5]For the self-report items, no baseline was obtained; [6]Baseline respiration frequency of TWR and APP ATCOs higher in Frankfurt than in Bremen; [7]Frankfurt TWR and APP ATCOs more concentrated than corresponding Bremen groups; [8]Work > Rest in Frankfurt for all groups, in Bremen only for pulse and systolic pressure of TWR ATCOs; [9]Work > Rest significant for all groups in Frankfurt and Bremen TWR ATCOs; [10]Expected sodium decrease during work only for TWR ATCOs.

15 mmHg over baseline. However, the groups exhibited different baseline values. Therefore, multivariate analyses of variances (MANOVA) were conducted to determine whether there were significant differences between groups.

Missing values and outlier control (Table 2) left at least four out of six regular working values of each subject to be averaged and compared to the respective baselines using the MANOVA. Subjects with more missing values were excluded from the analysis. Table 3 shows that nearly all biosignals indicated the expected change over time. The Frankfurt and the tower controllers exhibited stronger responses for some measures than their respective colleagues.

Mean physiological response was next correlated with traffic data (Table 4). Apart from overall traffic volume, the number of light (up to 7 t) and heavy, slow (propeller and turbopropeller up to 640 km/h) and fast as well as level flying and climbing/descending aircraft (vertical traffic) were counted. The difficulty of controlling fast and climbing/descending aircraft is substantial, because it requires fast and three-dimensional information processing (ATCOs either report that they have a three-dimensional representation of the traffic or that they stack up flight levels on a two-dimensional map). Heavy aircraft cause wake turbulence which can affect smaller aircraft behind them. Since the seven traffic variables are not independent, the t-tests for the correlation coefficients were alpha-adjusted according to Holms

Table 4. Coefficients and one-tailed error probabilities for the correlation of mean biosignal responses and self-report with traffic in the exploration study.

	Overall	Light	Heavy	Level	Vertical	Slow	Fast
Heart rate	.39 .014	-.25 .089	.44* .006	-.01 .476	.41* .011	-.57* .004	.58* .004
Pulse	.22 .116	-.11 .269	.25 .087	.20 .134	.43* .007	-.14 .280	.36 .055
Systolic	.30 .048	-.14 .215	.34 .030	.03 .442	.27 .066	-.36 .054	.37 .052
Diastolic	.31 .040	.05 .399	.32 .037	-.23 .100	.09 .308	-.25 .140	.17 .229
Respiration	-.31 .037	-.30 .041	-.27 .060	-.01 .480	-.30 .043	-.47 .014	-.18 .206
Saliva mass	-.10 .286	.03 .429	-.10 .275	.08 .331	.08 .320	.28 .094	.01 .487
Saliva IgA	.33 .055	.21 .161	.29 .078	-.17 .208	.10 .310	.15 .271	.16 .259
Potassium	.23 .462	.28 .115	.03 .452	-.05 .412	.03 .454	.21 .228	.23 .462
Sodium	-.04 .440	.06 .409	-.38 .048	.30 .102	.06 .400	.16 .280	-.04 .440
SCRs	.10 .300	-.18 .162	.13 .241	-.07 .345	.07 .347	-.30 .097	.23 .157
EMG	.17 .167	-.07 .342	.19 .145	-.16 .182	.10 .280	-.32 .079	.19 .199
Eye blinks	.44* .005	.11 .280	.44* .005	-.15 .206	.25 .083	-.15 .257	.45 .020
Concentra-tion	.36 .015	-.04 .420	.38 .011	.10 .278	.50* .001	-.18 .199	.41 .024
Upset	.26 .063	.34 .022	.21 .110	-.06 .359	.02 .450	.21 .158	-.03 439
Motivation	.29 .042	-.29 .042	.35 .019	-.19 .140	.55* .000	-.39 .030	.52* .004

*Coefficients significant with alpha correction.

(Krauth, 1988, i. e. the smallest p-value had to remain under 0.0071, the second smallest under 0.0083, etc).

Mean eye blink frequency increased significantly with traffic volume. No other correlation with traffic volume was statistically significant (Table 4). However, heart rate, blood pressure, as well as self-reported concentration and motivation, tended to increase with traffic volume. The elevation of respiration rate over baseline was unexpectedly smaller under high compared to low traffic conditions. This was likely to be due to either the high baseline values in Frankfurt (Table 3, comment 6) or to the increase in radio transmissions under high traffic, requiring more frequent communication of the controllers. The respiration belt may have failed to detect communication related exchange of air (for recording problems due to speaking and moving see Wientjes, 1992).

Heart rate and eye blink rate increases correlated especially with the number of heavy aircraft. Also the expected blood pressure increase and the sodium decrease occurred under this difficult traffic condition, but it remained below alpha-corrected significance. Moreover, higher concentration and motivation were reported. On the other hand, responses tended to be smaller with greater numbers of light aircraft (Table 4).

Heart rate and pulse responses as well as self-reported concentration and motivation were higher when more vertical traffic (climbing and descending aircraft) had to be controlled. There was no correlation between the number of level flying aircraft and physiological response.

Finally, heart rate responses and reported motivation were significantly correlated with the number of jets. The more propeller aircraft under control, the smaller the heart rate response. Pulse, blood pressure, and eye blink responses, as well as reported concentration also tended to increase with the number of jets.

Discussion of the exploration study

The exploration study produced new evidence that tower controllers are more stressed than their colleagues in the control centers. This finding disproved the common prejudice that radar work is more sophisticated and therefore more stressful than work in control centers (Vogt & Budde, 1997). Moreover, the high and homogeneous levels of traffic in the Frankfurt airspace caused a greater response than its antipole in Bremen. Finally, stress responses tended to correlate with traffic volume, but even more significant correlation coefficients were found considering the number of heavy, fast, climbing and descending aircraft.

However, airport and traffic were confounded in the exploration study. Therefore, a simulation experiment was designed in order to systematically vary traffic features and to draw causal conclusions.

Selection of biosignals for the simulation study

With the exception of saliva mass and potassium concentration, the twelve biosignals indicated the expected stress response during work (Table 3). But only the four cardiovascular measures, respiration rate, and occasionally sodium concentration and eye blink frequency were able to differentiate airports and ATC areas. Moreover, a significant correlation with air traffic was found for heart rate, pulse and eye blink frequency only (Table 4).

The continuously recorded biosignals heart rate, respiration rate, skin conductance responses, eye blink frequency, and mean muscle tension were subjected to a reliability analysis. For this purpose, the five resting minutes were inter-correlated. Again, heart rate proved to be the best indicator with a mean retest-reliability of .95. It was followed by respiration rate (.74), SCRs (.68), and eye blink frequency (.65). Mean muscle tension had the worst reliability (.56).

According to these statistical results, the multi-channel-approach was changed in favor of more efficiency. The monitoring procedure itself was only slightly modified in order to treat all subjects in the same way. However, only the cardiovascular and respiratory measures as well as eye blink frequency were analyzed in the simulation study (Vogt, 1998). From these, only pulse and systolic response are reported in this chapter.

Simulation experiment

An ACC scenario was selected for the simulation since the necessary hardware was available at the ATC academy in Langen and the number of controllers was greater compared to the other areas. The simulated airspace was unknown to all subjects, namely the mirrored Frankfurt West Sector with the control center "UniDO radar" and two airfields. Like in real centers, controllers and pseudo pilots received special instructions, the "UniDO procedures". In order to ensure the planned course of the scenario, a few special instructions had to be included, for example to take over control not before sector entry. The experiment was conducted from February to May 1997.

Discussing the results of the exploration study with ATC experts revealed quickly the number of aircraft and the portion of climbing/descending machines as the first two simulation variables. However, heavy and fast aircraft are not difficult per se. Only in combination with the traffic context, they can become stressors, for example the wake turbulence of a heavy aircraft endangering a light one or a fast aircraft catching up a slower one at the same flight level. Therefore, as the third simulation variable, a meta-stressor was composed called simulated potential conflicts containing cases like these. Finally, pilot errors were included as a fourth simulation variable.

It was expected from previous research that the number of aircraft most probably has the greatest effect. Potential conflicts between aircraft were a very important matter in the discussion with ATCOs and therefore supposed to be nearly as stressful. Considering the results of the exploration study, climbing and descending aircraft were expected to take the third rank of importance. There was no clear hypothesis about the effect size of pilot errors.

Design

There were two levels (high and low) of each of the four variables (Table 5) that were fully combined to a 2x2x2x2 within-subject design. The resulting 16 ATC scenarios were run in sessions lasting 20 minutes each. Each scenario or "run" began with the subject taking over from an assistant, who was always the same person. At this time, the scenario contained already the defined number of level flying, climbing and descending aircraft, which were maintained throughout the run by the simulation software. Conflicts between aircraft were simulated 9 and 19 minutes after system start, as the experimenter handed in flight strips of aircraft unexpectedly entering the airspace. In runs with errors, these were made by the pseudo pilots also 9 and 19 minutes after system start (for example turning right instead of left as the controller said).

The monitoring system was slightly changed compared to the exploration study: Electroencephalography (EEG), rather than EMG, was recorded over Cz and Fz (Figure 1). The change was due to the above mentioned publication by Brookings et al. (1996), who reported that spectral EEG responses differentiated traffic complexity.

Minutes 9 and 19 (at the beginning of which the conflicts and pilot errors occurred in the runs they were due) of each simulation run were analyzed with respect to

Table 5. Four important traffic variables were varied high (+) and low (-) and fully combined. The resulting 16 difficulty levels of air traffic control were used in the simulation study. Example ACVE: 12 aircraft continuously under control, 6 potential conflicts, 2/3 of aircraft in vertical movement (i. e. climbing or descending), 2 pilot errors.

Run acronym	AC VE	AC Ve	AC vE	AC ve	Ac VE	Ac Ve	Ac vE	Ac ve	aC VE	aC Ve	aC vE	aC ve	ac VE	ac Ve	ac vE	ac ve
Number of aircraft permanently under control	+ 12	+ 12	+ 12	+ 12	+ 12	+ 12	+ 12	+ 12	– 6	– 6	– 6	– 6	– 6	– 6	– 6	– 6
Number of potential conflicts	+ 6	+ 6	+ 6	+ 6	– 2	– 2	– 2	– 2	+ 6	+ 6	+ 6	+ 6	– 2	– 2	– 2	– 2
Portion of climbing/ descending aircraft	+ 2/3	+ 2/3	– 1/3	– 1/3	+ 2/3	+ 2/3	– 1/3	– 1/3	+ 2/3	+ 2/3	– 1/3	– 1/3	+ 2/3	+ 2/3	– 1/3	– 1/3
Pilot error (e. g., read back incorrect, direction change without clearance)	+ 2	– 0	+ 2	– 0	+ 2	– 0	+ 2	– 0	+ 2	– 0	+ 2	– 0	+ 2	– 0	+ 2	– 0

physiological responses. At the end of the two minutes, saliva samples were taken and blood pressure was measured. The two values of each run were averaged.

After the simulation run the ATCOs went to the adjacent lounge and relaxed for ten minutes. At the end of the relaxation period, another sampling point was set to make sure that all biosignals had returned to baseline level. A short version of the stimulus recall interview was conducted in the following 10 minutes and after this, subjects returned to the simulator for the next run.

24 ATCOs volunteered for the experiment. Their age ranged from 25 to 41 years with a mean of 32. On average, they had ten years of work experience. At the day of arrival, the ATCO was introduced to the simulating environment and had several training runs to become familiar with the UniDO procedures. The experiment started the following day with informed consent, pre-interview and baseline measurement as described in the exploration study. Eight runs were performed for the rest of the day, interrupted by a lunch break. The whole procedure was repeated the following day. The runs were presented in a random sequence. The baselines of the two days were averaged.

Subjects were eliminated from analysis when 25 % of their data were missing. Probably due to the long monitoring time, this number was especially high for ECG (12 subjects), although sweat-resistant electrodes (H94 by ARBO) were used. Therefore, only the Riva-Rocci results are reported here. EEG measures were also heavily affected. In the case of single missing values, these were estimated either within subject (one missing sampling point in a run replaced by the other) or between subjects (two missing sampling points of a run replaced by the mean of the other subjects for this run). Repeated measurement MANOVA was conducted for the response values (simulation – baseline) and effect sizes for number of aircraft, potential conflicts, vertical (climbing/descending) traffic and pilot errors were determined.

Results

Figure 4 shows mean pulse and systolic responses as a function of run difficulty. The highest difficulty is coded by the capital letters A for 12 aircraft continuously under control, C for six potential conflicts, V for 66 % vertical traffic (i. e. climbing or descending aircraft), E for two pilot errors (Table 5). Low difficulty is indicated by the respective small letters. Column 1 to column 8 represent runs with high number of aircraft, 1 to 4 and 9 to 13 those with six potential conflicts, 5 to 8 and 13 to 16 with only two. The percentage of climbing and descending traffic varied from column pair to column pair and pilot errors occurred in the runs represented by every odd column.

Systolic response to the most difficult run was on average 10 mmHg. The corresponding pulse increase was about 5 and unexpectedly outranked by the response to run ACvE (7 bpm).

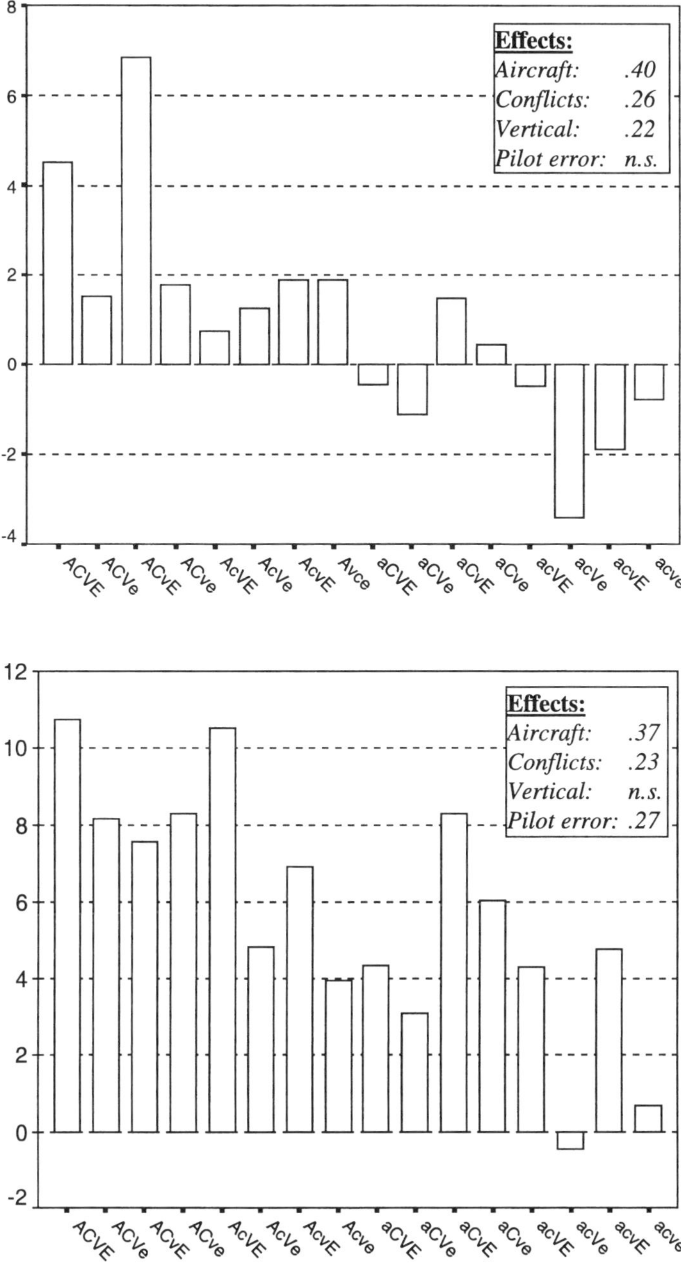

Figure 4. Mean pulse (top) and systolic response (bottom, n=22) as a function of run difficulty. The boxes display significant main effects as well as their effect sizes.
A, a: 12 vs. 6 aircraft continuously under control.
C, c: 6 vs. 2 potential conflicts at the two sampling points.
V, v: Always 66 % vs. 33 % vertical traffic, i. e. climbing or descending aircraft.
E, e: 2 vs. 0 pilot errors at the two sampling points.

Analyses of variances revealed significant main effects of the number of aircraft for both variables. Moreover, pulse and systolic response were significantly affected by the number of potential conflicts. Finally, climbing and descending aircraft had an effect on pulse, and pilot errors on systolic response. Pulse response was unexpectedly lower in runs with a higher portion of vertical traffic (column 1 and 2 compared to 3 and 4, 5 and 6 compared to 7 and 8 , etc.).

Discussion of the simulation study

The number of aircraft under control significantly affected nearly all stress responses and therefore was confirmed as the most important stressor in ATC. However, apart from traffic volume, the probability of potential conflicts had significant effects.

Pilot errors on the other hand affected only single stress responses. This confirms the result of the exploration study that semi-professional and training flights in Bremen were less stressful than the high number of aircraft in Frankfurt. The relevance of climbing and descending aircraft found in the exploration study was not confirmed in the simulation. However, a post-hoc control of real and target traffic showed that the simulation software could not maintain the portion of vertical trafffic, since the subjects extensively used flight level changes to coordinate the traffic. The other simulation variables were successfully maintained by the system (number of aircraft), the experimenter (conflicts) or the pilots (pilot error), and deviations of real and target traffic were below 10 %.

Validation study

The objective of this study was to prove whether the simulation results are valid under real traffic conditions. For this purpose, as many as 1344 different ATC situations were monitored at Munich airport.

The study took place from July to August 1997. 56 male, non-smoking ATCOs in four control areas participated: 13 in the tower, 15 in the approach, 14 in the area center control, and – for the first time – 14 in the upper air control. Age ranged between 25 and 50 years (M=33). Three APP, one ACC and one UAC controller had to be excluded from the analysis due to missing values.

The monitoring protocol was similar to that of the exploration study, apart from an extended duration (240 instead of 90 minutes) and shorter sampling intervals (10 instead of 15 minutes). Moreover, subjective evaluation of each sampling point was not obtained in a stimulus recall interview but rather through the more efficient use of a checklist with nine items, which was filled out after saliva was collected. Physiological responses were obtained as shown in Figure 1.

An observing controller noted the number of aircraft under control, the number of potential conflicts, the portion of climbing and descending aircraft, pilot errors

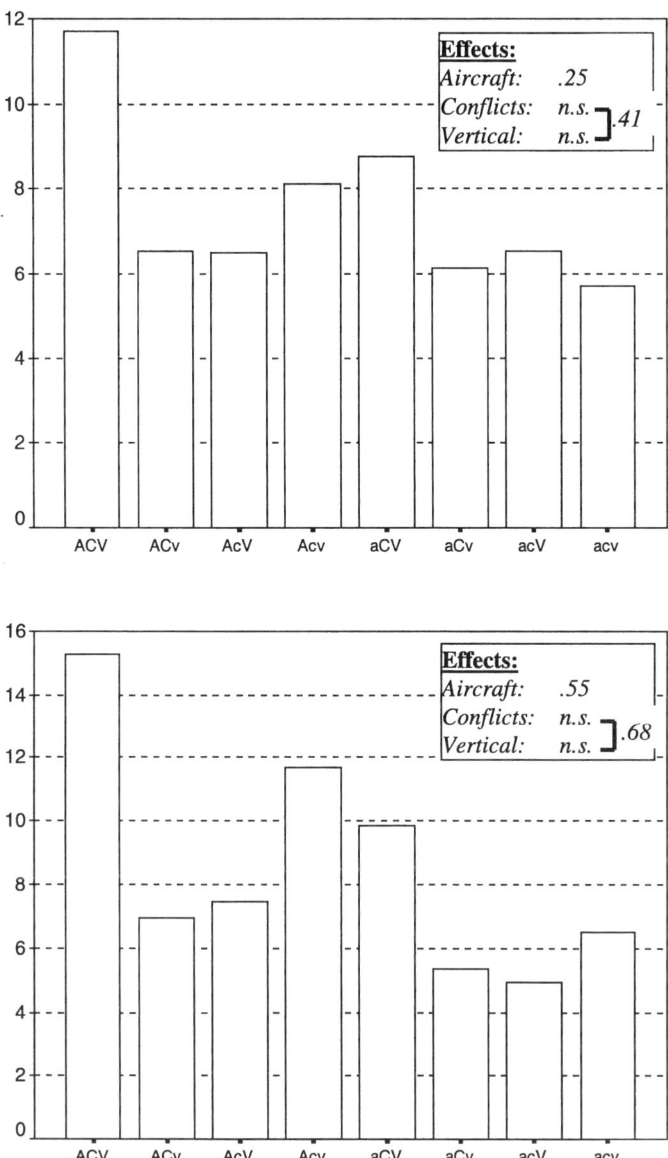

Figure 5. Mean pulse (top) and systolic response (bottom, n=12 ACC ATCOs Munich) as a function of ATC situation difficulty. The boxes display significant effect sizes of main and interaction effects.

A, a: Number of aircraft under control high vs. low after median split.

C, c: Number of potential conflicts high vs. low after median split.

V, v: Vertical traffic (climbing/descending aircraft) high vs. low after median split.

and other features of the traffic situation in 10-minute-intervals. This procedure was preferred over the objective traffic records used in the exploration study, since potential conflicts and pilot errors are not included in these statistics. For the tower control, slightly different definitions had to be used: Since the portion of climbing and descending aircraft would be always 100 %, observers noted the percentage of traffic mixture, which is decisive for climbing behavior (jets performing better than propeller aircraft). The category pilot error was broadened to include unpredictable events, for example misbehavior on the part of airport and apron personnel (e. g., the presence of a non-approved car on the runway). This expert protocol was used to post-hoc classify the 1344 situations: Within each control area, each traffic variable was classified as high or low using a median split. In none of the 1344 situations, the experts found other relevant traffic variables than those from the simulation study. Moreover, pilot errors were very rare, such that the classification was limited to number, conflicts and climbing/descending aircraft. Compared to the simulation study, the following bar graphs are missing every odd column (two pilot errors).

Results

The most difficult type of situation (ACV i. e. aircraft number high, conflicts high and vertical traffic high, equivalent to simulation run ACVe) led to an average pulse response of 12 bpm in the center (Figure 5). As expected, the smallest response occurred in situations of type ACV. Only the number of aircraft had a significant main effect. In contrast to the simulation, there was a significant interaction between the number of conflicts and the portion of climbing and descending aircraft. Pulse response decreased with the portion of vertical traffic only when the number of conflicts was high (column 1 vs. 2 and 5 vs. 6). With only a few potential conflicts, climbing and descending aircraft did not enhance pulse response (column 4 vs. 3 and 8 vs. 7).

A similar but clearer picture was obtained for systolic response.

For the other ATC areas, the predictive power of the (ACC) simulation variables was smaller. Nonetheless, also in APP and UAC the number of aircraft under control was the dominating variable, sometimes with a main effect but mostly in interactions with the other two. Stress responses to TWR work were only affected by the number of aircraft, the (predictable) conflicts, and their interaction.

Discussion of the validation study

The traffic variables were not independent in real traffic situations. They had to be identified post-hoc and were probably inter-correlated (e. g., more conflicts under high traffic conditions). This might explain the importance of interactions in the real traffic situations as compared to the simulation experiment. However, also under real traffic conditions, stress responses were nearly exclusively affected by the number of aircraft under control and potential conflicts.

The role of climbing and descending traffic could not definitely be clarified. They could enhance as well as reduce stress responses in interaction with potential conflicts and number of aircraft. The latter can be explained from an ATC point of view for the upper air control: Flight levels are (apart from speed) extensively used for separating aircraft; making a pilot climb or descend can unwind a difficult situation at a certain flight level.

Pilot errors and other traffic problems did not play a role in the Munich ATC situations.

In contrast to the exploration study, tower work in Munich was not more stressful compared to APP or ACC. This can be explained with the extremely low portion of visual flight routines at Munich airport.

Discussion and practical implications

In all three studies, number was confirmed as the most important stressor in ATC. As a new result, potential conflicts of, for example, fast behind slow or heavy in front of light aircraft were found the second important stressor. Tower work – although maybe less sophisticated – is not less stressful than center work.

On the basis of these results, the DFS developed a new sector categorization scheme: The former wage groups were differentiated into eight categories considering the main stressors identified in our studies. ATCOs at Frankfurt center for example are in the highest rank. Since stress cannot be compensated financially and wages of German ATCOs are rather high (due to privatization in 1993), it was recommended that work times be defined according to the new scheme. Frankfurt controllers are now only 26 hours a week at radar, their colleagues with less traffic load work up to 38 hours. Furthermore, health promotion programs were developed, for example a relaxation instruction booklet with CD, which is readily available to all controllers. This 10-minute exercise significantly enhanced physiological recovery compared to a conventional break (Vogt, Becher & Kastner, 1999).

The use of objective stress measures established acceptance among subjects and management. Moreover, the data were reliable and valid. The mean correlation of heart rate and pulse during the rest and the six working samples in the exploration study can be seen as parallel test reliability and it ranged between 0.80 and 0.90. As a measure of concurrent validity, Cronbach´s alpha was 0.64 for pulse, systolic pressure, experienced concentration and upset. In the reported studies, all physiological measures were able to indicate work stress, some of them could also differentiate ATC areas and situations.

The tripartite methodology (exploration, simulation, validation) proved very useful. In the exploration study, important results could be obtained quickly and subjected to preliminary practical implementation and further scientific investigation. The simulation study revealed causal conclusions and effect sizes, the validation study confirmed their validity also under real traffic situations. The practical consequences will hopefully contribute to manage the future challenges of ATC.

Acknowledgements
The reported studies were conducted on behalf of the German Air Traffic Control Services DFS. Setting an example for theory-to-practice, they requested scientific support for management decisions. Thanks are also due to Caro Zimmermann, Gerd Budde, Tim Hagemann and Andreas Udovic, our co-workers in this research project.

References

Arad, B.A. (1963). *The control load, the control capacity, and optimal sector design.* Washington D.C.: Federal Aviation Administration.

Arad, B.A. (1964). The control load and sector design. *The journal of air traffic control, 5*, 12–31.

Baader, E.W. & Graf, K.O. (1958). *Gesundheitserhebungen bei den Bundesanstalten "Deutscher Wetterdienst" und "Flugsicherung".* Gutachten im Auftrag des Bundesverkehrsministeriums.

Boucsein, W. (1988). *Elektrodermale Aktivität: Grundlagen, Methoden und Anwendungen.* Berlin: Springer.

Brookings, J.B., Wilson, G.F. & Swain, C.R. (1996). Psychophysiological responses to changes in workload during simulated air traffic control. *Biological Psychology, 42*(3), 361–377.

Cabon, P., Mollard, R., Cointot, B., Martel, A. & Besiot, P. (1997). *Elaboration of a method for the assessment of psychophysiological states of ATCOs in simulation.* EEC Report No. 323.

Cobb, S., Rose, R.M. (1973). Hypertension, peptid ulcer and diabetes in air traffic controllers. *Journal of the American Medical Association, 224*, 489–492.

Costa, G. (1993). Evaluation of workload in air traffic controllers. *Ergonomics, 36*(7), 1111–1120.

Dörner, D. (1976). *Problemlösen als Informationsverarbeitung.* Stuttgart: Kohlhammer.

Finkelman, J.M., Zeitlein, L.R., Romoff, R.A., Friend, M.A. & Brown, L.S. (1979). Conjoint effect of physical stress and noise stress on information processing performance and cardiac response. *Human Factors, 21*, 1–6.

Hart, S.G. & Staveland, L.E. (1988). Development of NASA-TLX (Task Load Index): Results of empirical and theoretical research. In P.A. Hancock & N. Meshkati (Eds.), *Human mental workload* (pp. 139–183). Amsterdam. North-Holland.

Henderson, P.R., Bakal, D.A. & Dunn, B.E. (1990). Cardiovascular response pattern and speech: A study of air traffic controllers. *Psychosomatic Medicine, 52*, 17–26.

Hinton, J.W. & Burton, R.F. (1997). A psychophysiological model of psystress causation and response applied to the workplace. *Journal of Psychophysiology, 11*, 200–217.

Hinton, J.W., Burton, R.F., Farmer, J.G., Rotheiler, E., Shewan, D., Gemmell, M., Berry, J. & Gibson, R. (1992). Relative changes in salivary [Na^+] and [K^+] relating to stress induction. *Biological Psychology, 33*, 63–71.

Hurst, M.W. & Rose, R.M. (1978). Objective job difficulty, behavioral response, and sector characteristics in air traffic control centers. *Ergonomics, 21*, 697–708.

Jenkins, G.N. (1978). *The physiology and biochemistry of the mouth.* Oxford: Blackwell.

Kan, L., Malinovskaia, O.O., Kuprianov, V.A. & Denisov, A.F. (1984). Biochemical and psychological indicators in air controllers in the "pre-start" state before beginning work activities. *Kosm-Biol-Aviakosm-Med, 18*, 62–68.

Kastner, M. (1986). Zur Koppelung von Beanspruchungen im Rahmen der Arbeits- und Organisationspsychologie. In H. Methner (Ed.), *Psychologie in Betrieb und Verwaltung* (pp. 43–66). Bonn: Deutscher Psychologen Verlag.

Kastner, M., Ademmer, C., Budde, G., Hagemann, T., Udovic, A. & Vogt, J. (1998). *Belastung und Beanspruchung in den Flugsicherungsdiensten. Arbeitswissenschaftliches Gutachten an die DFS.* Offenbach: Deutsche Flugsicherung.

Kimbelton, S.R. (1970). *An approach to the re-sectorization of the Cleveland area.* Washington D.C.: Federal Aviation Administration.

Klimmer, F., Aulmann, H.M. & Rutenfranz, J. (1972). Catecholamine excretion in urine during mental workload in the air traffic control service. *Internationales Archiv für Arbeitsmedizin, 30*(1), 65–80.

Klinge, R. (1992). *Das Elektrokardiogramm.* Thieme: Stuttgart.

Krauth, J. (1988). Distribution-free statistics: An application-oriented approach. In J.P. Huston (Ed.), *Techniques in the behavioral and neural sciences*, Vol. 2 (p. 37). Amsterdam: Elsevier.

Kugler, J. (1990). *Filminduzierte Änderung der emotionalen Befindlichkeit und Immunglobulin A im Speichel. Ein Beitrag zur Psychoneuroimmunologie.* Dissertation Heinrich-Heine-Universität Düsseldorf.

Kugler, J. (1994). Stress, salivary immunoglobulin A and susceptibility to upper respiratory tract infection. Evidence for adaptive immunomodulation. *Psychologische Beiträge, 36*, 175-182.

Laurig, W., Becker-Biskaborn, G.U. & Reiche, D. (1971). Software problems in analyzing physiological and work study data. *Ergonomics, 14*, 625–631.

Lille, F. & Cheliout, F. (1982). Variations in diurnal and nocturnal waking state in air traffic controllers. *European Journal of Applied Physiology, 49*(3), 319–328.

Löffler, G. (1990). *Physiologische Chemie.* Berlin: Springer.

Mancini, G., Carbonara, A.O. & Heremans, J.F. (1965). Immunochemical quantitation of antigens by single radial immunodiffusion. *Immunochemistry, 2*, 235–254.

Martindale, D. (1977). Sweaty palms in the control tower. *Psychology Today, 10*, 71–75.

McGregor, D.K. & Stern, J.A. (1996). Time on task and blink effects on saccade duration. *Ergonomics, 39*(4), 649–660.

Melton, C.E., Smith, R.C., McKenzie, J.M., Wicks, S.M. & Saldivar, J.T. (1977): *Stress in air traffic personnel. Low-density towers and flight service stations.* Oklahoma City: Federal Aviation Administration.

Mogford, R.H., Murphy, E.D. & Guttman, J.A. (1994). Using knowledge exploration tools to study airspace complexity in air traffic control. *The International Journal of Aviation Psychology, 4*, 29–45.

Reiche, D., Kirchner, J.H. & Laurig, W. (1971). Evaluation of stress factors by analysis of radiotelecommunication in ATC. *Ergonomics, 14*, 603–609.

Repetti, R.L. (1989). Effects of daily workload on subsequent behavior during marital interaction: the roles of social withdrawal and spouse support. *Journal of Personality and Social Psychology, 57*(4), 651–659.

Repetti, R.L. (1993). Short term effects of occupational stressors on daily mood and health complaints. *Health Psychology, 12*(2), 125–131.

Rohmert, W. & Rutenfranz, J. (1972). Benutzerhandbuch zu den Untersuchungen zur psycho-physischen Belastung und Beanspruchung von Fluglotsen. Institut für Arbeitswissenschaft, Technische Hochschule Darmstadt.

Rose, R.M. & Fogg, L.F. (1993). Definition of a responder. Analysis of behavioral, cardiovascular, and endocrine response to varied workload in air traffic controller. *Psychosomatic Medicine, 55*, 325–338.

Schroeder, H.M., Driver, M.J. & Streufert, S. (1967). *Human Information Processing.* New York: Holt, Rinehart & Winston.

Simon, H.A. (1964). The architecture of complexity. *General System Yearbook, 10*, 63–76.

Smith, R.C. (1980). *Stress, anxiety and the air traffic control specialist. Some conclusions from a decade of research.* Oklahoma City: Federal Aviation Administration.

Smith, R.C., Melton, C.E. & McKenzie, J.M. (1971). Affect adjective checklist assessment of mood variations in air traffic controllers. *Aerospace Medicine, 42*(10), 1060–4.

Somer, E., Ben Aryeh, H. & Laufer, D. (1993). Salivary composition, gender and psychosocial stress. *International Journal of Psychosomatics, 40,* 17–21.

Stern, J.A. (1994). Blink rate: A possible measure of fatigue. *Human Factors, 36*, 285–297.

Stern, R.M., Ray, W.J. & Davis, C.M. (1980). *Psychophysiological Recording.* New York: Oxford University Press.

Strasser, J.E., Ernst, J. & Müller, K.W. (1992). *Günstige Bewegungen für die ergonomische Arbeitsgestaltung.* Heidelberg: Dr. Curt Hafner Verlag.

SRATM (2000). *Stress reduction, safety, and efficiency in future air traffic management through flight progress information.* Final report to the EC.

Theorell, T., Perski, A., Akerstedt, T., Sigala, F., Ahlberg-Hulten, G., Svensson, J. & Eneroth, P. (1988). Changes in job strain in relation to changes in physiological state. A longitudinal study. *Scandinavian Journal of Work and Environmental Health, 14*(3), 189–196.

Vogt, J. (1998). *Psychophysiologische Beanspruchung von Fluglotsen.* Universität Dortmund: Dissertation.

Vogt, J., Becher, L. & Kastner, M. (1999). *Kurzentspannung für den Arbeitsplatz.* Dortmund: FUGS e.V.

Vogt, J. & Budde, G. (1998). Psychophysiological Stress of Air Traffic Controllers: Exploration, Simulation, Prediction, Intervention. Proceedings of the *37th Annual Conference of the International Federation of Air Traffic Controllers Associations*, Toulouse.

Vogt, J., Hinton, J.W. & Stewart, R. (1992). Development and testing of an ambulatory stress monitoring system in field settings using electrodermal activity, salivary ionic concentrations ($c[K^+]/c[Na^+]$) and self-report measures. *Proceedings of the Second International Congress of Behavioral Medicine*, Hamburg, July 15th – 18th, 145.

Wientjes, C.J.E. (1992). Respiration in psychophysiology: methods and applications. *Biological Psychology, 34*, 179–203.

Zeier, H. (1994). Workload and psychophysiological stress reactions in air traffic. *Ergonomics, 37*, 525–539.

Zeier, H., Brauchli, P. & Joller-Jemelka, H.I. (1996). Effects of work demands on immunoglobulin A and cortisol in air traffic controllers. *Biological Psychology, 42*, 413–423.

Zeier, H. & Grubenmann, E. (1990). Stressuntersuchung bei Flugverkehrsleitern der Swisscontrol. Interner Bericht, Institut für Verhaltenswissenschaft, Eidgenössische Technische Hochschule Zürich.

Chapter 27
Ecological Momentary Assessments in Aviation The Development of a Pilot Experience Evaluating Device (PEED) for the In-Flight Registration of Flight Phases, Mental Effort, and ReactionTime

Eamonn K.S. Hanson and Jan Bazański
National Aerospace Laboratory, Amsterdam, The Netherlands

Introduction

Research in Aviation Psychology mainly focuses on determining the intentions, actions, errors and capabilities of pilots. This information is used for many different purposes, such as accident and incident analysis, the selection and training of pilots, usability testing of new cockpit interfaces, determining situation awareness or crew decision-making processes (Amalberti & Wioland, 1997; Backs & Boucsein, 2000; Stokes & Kite, 1994). To enable such measurements in the work environment of the pilots (the cockpit), frequent, intensive and precise ambulatory measurements are required (Hart & Wickens, 1990; Jorna, 1997; Hankins & Wilson, 1998). The present chapter describes the development of an ambulatory device that enables estimations of a pilot's mental effort and reaction times during flight.

According to Csikszentmihalyi et al. (1987), and Delespaul (1995), self-reports immediately after events are hardly biased by incorrect recall, and are therefore more valid than questionnaire assessments that may occur hours or even days later. Because the self-reports are performed in an everyday real-life situation, they are considered "*Ecologically Valid*". Schwartz et al. (1998) refer to such measurements as Ecological Momentary Assessments (EMA). In the present study, EMA is used to measure pilot mental effort and reaction times during aircraft operations. For this purpose a device was developed to register pilot inputs during flight. The device is called *Pilot Experience Evaluating Device* (PEED), and was designed by the Polish Air Force Institute of Aviation Medicine (Hanson et al., 1999; Piórko et al., 1998; van der Pal et al., 1999). The device was first tested by aircraft pilots in a fixed base simulator (on the ground), and later in actual flight.

What is going on in the air?

The design of PEED was initiated by the desire to know what is going on during flight. Many aircraft operations (for example, some solo training flight or fighter missions) are performed by a single pilot. This means that there is no observer present to determine if the flight is performed as described in the flight plan. More importantly, the timing of the flight segments (for example, take-off, cruise, approach , etc.) is unknown. Any deviations from operational procedures also may remain unreported, simply because the pilot does not exactly remember the course of events.

An airborne Flight Data Recorder (FDR, or "black box") is probably the first important source of information. The emphasis of the crash and fire protected device is on collecting actual flight conditions of the aircraft, for instance, heading, altitude, airspeed, vertical accelerations, and time (and more recently Cockpit Voice Recordings, information about the engines, flight controls, flaps, etc.). However, this system has drawbacks for Human Factors engineers because pilot perceptions and behavior is not recorded (for example, stick forces or perceived system status). One cannot determine what behavior was actually performed by the pilot, or why. For example, at what moments of the flight did the pilot push or pull the controls of the aircraft? The crash protected flight data recorder (FDR) is only mandatory in civil aircraft, which means the smaller aircraft (not meant for public transportation) usually do not have the device. Many in-flight experiments are performed in such smaller aircraft, and thus its absence is a problem. Airborne Data Measurement and Recording Systems (like the FDR) and airborne recorders that record pilot behavior (such as PEED) both provide information of great importance to the aviation psychologist.

The validity of airborne behavior recordings

In order to determine the external validity of the PEED mental effort ratings, the relation was calculated between the PEED mental effort scores and valid indices of mental effort (Meijman et al., 1986; Mulder et al., 1987). In two experiments described below, it was determined whether the PEED mental effort ratings could be associated with Reaction Times (RTs), the Rating Scale Mental Effort (RSME) and the Middle Frequency band of heart rate (Heart Rate Variability, MF_HRV).

To determine the validity of the PEED flight phase indications, pilot inputs were compared to data recordings from the computer of the fixed base simulator (experiment 1) or airborne data measurement and recording system (experiment 2). As was discussed in the previous paragraph, the PEED self-reports are collected during the flights. PEED inputs were required at specific moments throughout the flight. The moments were indicated by a flash of the LED and by an auditory signal (experiment 1) or were chosen by the pilots after each phase (experiment 2). At these moments the pilots were instructed to indicate the flight phase or the operation they had just performed by pressing a button. The pilots indicated their mental effort by sliding a key of a potentiometer. To decrease the intrusiveness of the measurements, pilots were instructed to ignore the flashes if they felt it necessary.

Since the present version of PEED is only a prototype in an early stage of design, the opinions of pilots about the usability of the device was also collected. The results of the usability testing will be used to improve the design of the device.

Addressing the hierarchical structure of the data

The characteristics of data collection in ambulatory studies may affect the relations between variables, and the hierarchy of the data. Typically, if a variable (for example, mental effort) is measured several times, the measurements within each individual (pilots) may be dependent. The same goes for mental effort measurements within flights, and within flight-phases. If not accounted for adequately, dependency between variables may lead to biased interpretations of the data (Berry, 1997; Jaccard & Wan, 1993). A statistical method that can be used to account for dependency is multilevel analysis, or random coefficient model (Bryk et al., 1992; Goldstein, 1995). Applying this method reduces the risk of Type I error (for instance, bias toward rejecting the null hypothesis) (Schwartz & Stone, 1998).

A second advantage of multilevel analysis, is that it provides a good description of the structure of the data. In some studies it may be worthwhile knowing if a specific effect is mainly caused by differences between pilots, flights, and flight-phases, respectively. For example, it is worthwhile knowing whether changes in a dependent variable (for example, mental effort) is due to differences between pilots, and not to differences between flight-phases. In this example the measure of mental effort is sensitive to between pilot differences (and thus more "trait dependent") and not to differences between flight phases (and thus less "situation dependent"). Such an analysis is of additional value when comparing two measures of mental effort (for example, the RSME versus the PEED measurements).

Variables associated with pilots such as sleep quality (which can be measured once in the morning using a questionnaire) are referred to as units at a higher level or „pilot-level". The variables measured several times per flight (e.g., mental effort) are referred to as lower level units or „flight-phase-level" measurements. If there is not enough variance in the dependent variable at a specific level, it makes no sense distinguishing it as a separate level. For example, little or no variance at the flight level means that there are (very little or) no differences between flights.

In sum, performing a multilevel analysis of the data has two advantages. First, the effects of independent variables on the dependent variables can be determined with a reduced risk of type I error. Second, it can be determined at which level of analysis (for example, pilot, flight or flight-phase levels) effects are found. With this information, it can be determined to what extent the dependent variable may be considered "trait dependent" or "situation dependent". In the results section of the first experiment described in this chapter, a multilevel analysis was performed on indices of mental effort. To enable comparison with more traditional descriptive analyses, Pearson correlations of the variables used in the multilevel analysis have been calculated.

Experiments performed to determine the external validity of PEED, and the structure of the data

The present chapter touches on two important issues: (1) determining the external validity of the PEED mental effort ratings, (2) accounting for hierarchies in the data. The relation between mental effort as rated with PEED, and well-known measurements of mental effort (RSME and MF_HRV) was calculated to determine external validity. The first experiments was performed in a F-16 fixed base simulator, and the second one was performed in a Slingsby T67M200 trainer aircraft (Hanson, 1998). Experiment 1 summarizes the findings of the fixed base simulator experiment, and experiment 2 summarizes the finding of the Slingsby experiment.

Experiments

Experiment 1: Fixed Base Simulator

In the fixed base simulator the following flights were performed: (1) a rate-one turn, (2) a vertical-S delta, (3) a pop-up maneuver,(4) a High Value Asset Combat Air Patrol Air-to-Air (HVA CAP A/A) engagement, and (5) a Surface-to-Air (S/A) treat engagement. Each flight was performed four times (4 runs).

Subjects

Nine male former F-16 pilots (mean age: 35,3) were asked to participate in the study. The last time the pilots had flown a F-16 was (on average) 5 years ago. Nearly all subjects had previous Mid Life Update F-16 (MLU F-16) fixed base simulator experience. Prior to the experiment all subjects were briefed about the MLU F16 fixed base simulator. The subjects did not receive any training (no trial runs) before the tasks were started.

Procedure

The pilots were asked to perform 5 different flights that were repeated four times (run1 – run4), leading to a total of 20 runs for each pilot (5 tasks x 4 runs = 20 runs). Within each flight, a number of flight segments were distinguished. The task order was randomized separately within each pilot. Before each flight, a resting period of 5 minutes was held as a reference period. For the first two flights (rate-one and vertical S-delta) the following 7 segments or pilot operational procedures were distinguished: approach, first half, second half, exit, rest, loading weapons and not specific. In the third flight (pop-up maneuver) 6 flight segments could be distinguished: approach, maneuver, escape, rest, loading weapons, and not specific. In the fourth and fifth flights 9 flight segments or pilot operational procedures were distinguished: observing the horizontal situation display (HSD), observing available weapons, using the head-up display (HUD), combat air patrol (CAP), fire control radar (FCR), intercepting, rest, loading weapons, and not specified. Thus a total of 38 (7+7+6+9+9) flight segments or operational procedures could be distinguished. In total 1368 (38 segments x 4 runs x 9 pilots) relevant segments were used for analysis. During the resting period and after the flight, pilots had to fill in the Rating Scale Mental Effort (RSME), and also respond to the PEED interrogations. To guarantee anonymity, all subjects were given code numbers, which were changed and rehustled after completing the experiment.

Mental effort

Mental effort was indicated by the inter-beat-interval heart rate variability (Mulder et al., 1987) and a subjective index of effort, the Rating Scale Mental Effort (RSME) (Meijman et al., 1985) which were recorded in a VITAPORT-II device.

Sleep quality and mental fatigue

Sleep impairment was measured using the "Groningen Sleep Quality Scale" (Meijjman et al., 1985) and mental fatigue was measured using the Multi-Dimensional Fatigue index (Smets et al., 1995).

PEED mental effort ratings and reaction times

PEED (Pilot Experience Evaluating Device) is an instrument that can be used to register self-reports of mental effort, occurrence of flight phases, and reaction times (see Figure 1). The device can be installed in a cockpit, or strapped to a pilot's leg. The front panel is equipped with a red LED, which flashes when an input of the pilot is required. The pilot's attention is also attracted by a beep (via earphones), which is synchronized with the red diode. The inter-beep interval was set at 60 seconds, after which the pilots had 60 seconds to react by pressing one of the black keys on the panel and sliding the potentiometer to indicate their level of mental effort. Each of the black keys refers to a different flight phase. The green key on the panel is used to initialize the device, and determine the inter-beat-interval.

PEED has 2 operating modes: (1) a *time-sampling* mode, prompting pilot inputs at fixed time intervals (for example, 30, 60, 90, 120 or 300 seconds), and (2) an *event-sampling* mode, which requires pilot inputs as pre-defined events occur (for example, after take-off, landing, etc.).

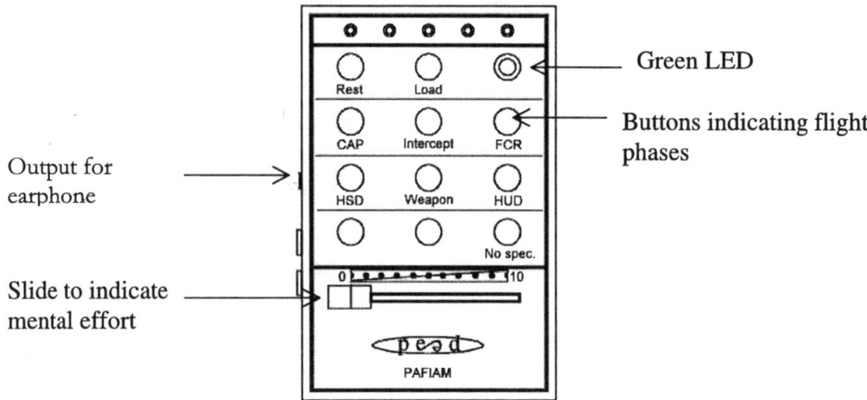

Figure 1. Pilot Experience Evaluation Device (PEED).

Multilevel analysis or random coefficient model

The multilevel analysis was performed as follows. First, a model was tested without independent variables (this is the so-called null-model, see Table 2). From this model the amount of variance (percentages) at each level was determined for both PEED mental effort and the RSME. Second, independent variables at the flight and pilot levels were introduced (model 1, Table 3). Non-significant variables were dropped from the models. All estimates of the regression coefficients were obtained using the program MLn (Woodhouse et al., 1996). The significance of the fixed effects was determined by dividing the estimate by its standard error (Bryk & Raudenbusch, 1996).

Results of Fixed Base Simulator experiment

Of the 1368 flight segments that were distinguished for analysis, 1067 PEED responses were given by pilots. This means that there was 22% missing data. The percentage of flight segments or operational procedures reported correctly by pilots in PEED varied strongly. The percentage correctly reported segments are: 65% (rate-one turn), 63% (vertical S-delta), 58% (pop-up maneuver), 45% (HVA-CAP) and 28% (S/A). The objective data from the fixed base simulator computer was used to determine the flight segments and operational procedures for the remainder of calculations in this chapter.

External validity

The results in Table 1 show a positive relation between PEED mental effort scores and RSME scores (.22), confirming external validity. RSME scores, but not PEED mental effort are negatively associated with mental fatigue (-.37).

Table 1. Pearsons correlations between PEED mental effort scores in the fixed base simulator and reaction time, Inter-Beat-Interval (IBI), heart rate variability (MF_HRV), Rating Scale Mental Effort (RSME) and sleep quality.

	PEED Mental effort	IBI	MF_HRV	RSME	Mental fatigue	Poor sleep
Reaction time	.08 .09	-.05 .32	.03 .48	-.08 .08	-.01 .75	.03 .53
PEED Mental effort		.05 .26	-.05 .28	.22** <.01	-.08 .06	-.02 .66
IBI			-.66** <.01	.02 .67	-.05 .24	.40** <.01
MF_HRV				.03 .44	.12** <.01	-.07 .10
RSME					-.37** <.01	-.07 .08
Mental fatigue						.10* .03

n cases = 524, 9 subjects.
* Correlation is significant at the 0.05 level (2-tailed).
** Correlation is significant at the 0.01 level (2-tailed).

Distribution of variance

To determine whether the hypothesized levels are indeed present in the data, the variance at each level was determined using all available data (see Table 2). Significant variance at a specific level justifies distinguishing that level as a separate level. The calculation shows that there is enough variance to distinguish 3 levels in the PEED mental effort data, and only 2 in the RSME data. There is insufficient RSME variance at the pilot level, which means that differences between pilot mental effort cannot be derived from the RSME data.

For PEED mental effort 21% of the variance is found at the pilot level, 16% at the flight level and 63% at the flight phase level. For RSME most of the variance is also at the flight phase level. This means that changes in RSME scores as well as PEED mental effort scores are strongly determined by differences between flight phases (see Table 2).

Table 2. Distribution of variance over pilot, flight and phase levels determined using a multilevel analysis.

Null model	PEED mental effort var (percentage)	RSME
Pilot level	99.9 (21%)	-
Flight level	173.9 (16%)	78 (13%)
Flight phase level	293.5 (63%)	534 (87%)

n cases = 1067, 9 subjects. Var = Unexplained variance. Values within parenthesis indicate percentages (%) relative to total variance for each dependent variable.

Effects of the experimental manipulation of mental effort

Using a multilevel analysis, it was determined whether RSME and PEED mental effort were higher during the flight task in comparison to a rest period before the task. The size and direction of this experimental manipulation of mental effort is given in Table 3, and is illustrated in Figures 2 and 3. The results show that PEED mental effort was 16.15 units higher during flight in comparison to the resting period before the flight. The RSME scores were 37.58 units higher during the flight in comparison to the resting period.

The multilevel analysis also shows that RSME is positively associated with PEED mental effort (Table 3). RSME and the experimental manipulation explain changes in PEED mental effort. All other variables (for example, IBI, HRV, poor sleep and mental fatigue) are not related to PEED mental effort. Furthermore, using PEED 15% percent of the variance at the pilot level is explained, and 22% and 51% of the variance is explained at the flight and flight phase levels, respectively. Again associations with fatigue (this time poor sleep) are found for RSME and also low physiological arousal. The multilevel analysis shows that RSME is associated with poor sleep (-1.58), HRV (0.30) and the interaction between MF_HRV and run number (MF_HRV*run = -0.08). These associations explain 14% of the variance at the flight level, and 85% at the flight phase level.

Table 3. Estimates of the effects of independent variables on RSME and PEED mental effort, derived from a multilevel analysis.

Model 1	PEED mental effort Var (s.e.)	RSME Var (s.e.)
Intercept	2.18 (3.18)	10.92 (2.08)*
Experimental manipulation	16.15 (1.8)*	37.58 (0.80)*
RSME	0.19 (0.04)*	-
Run		0.67 (0.66)
PEED mental effort	-	0.14 (0.02)*
HRV	-	0.30 (0.05)*
Run HRV	-	-0.08 (0.02)*
Poor sleep	-	-1.58 (0.26)*
Explained variance	**Var (Percentage)**	**Var (Percentage)**
Pilot level	84.9 (15%)	
Flight level	53.6 (22%)	67.2 (14%)
Flight phase level	144.2 (51%)	81.8 (85%)

The top half of the table shows the estimates (magnitude and direction) of the independent variables on PEED mental effort and RSME. The bottom half shows variance at each level. Percentage = decrease in variance as a percentage of variances in null-model. For all *: $p<0.05$ (n cases = 1067, 9 subjects). Non-significant effects were removed from the models (-).

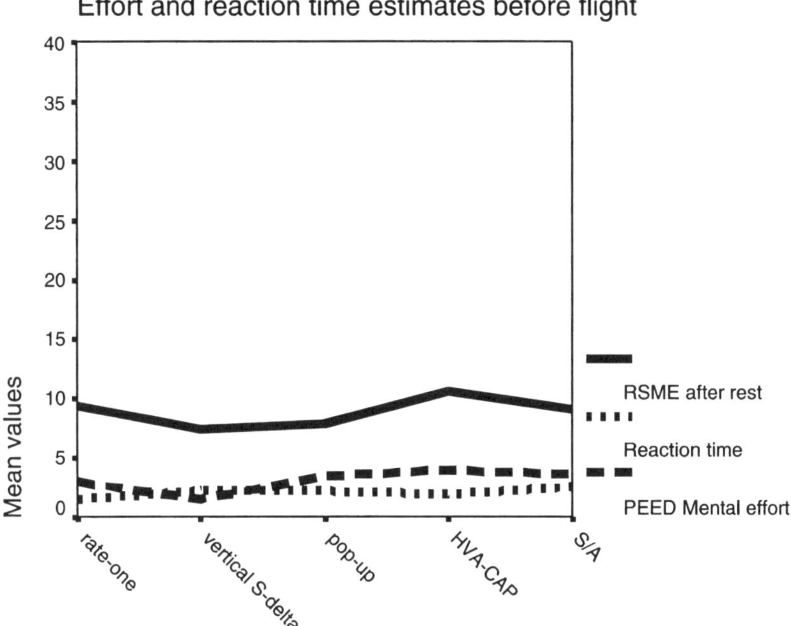

Figure 2. Effort and reaction time estimates before flight (fixed base simulator).

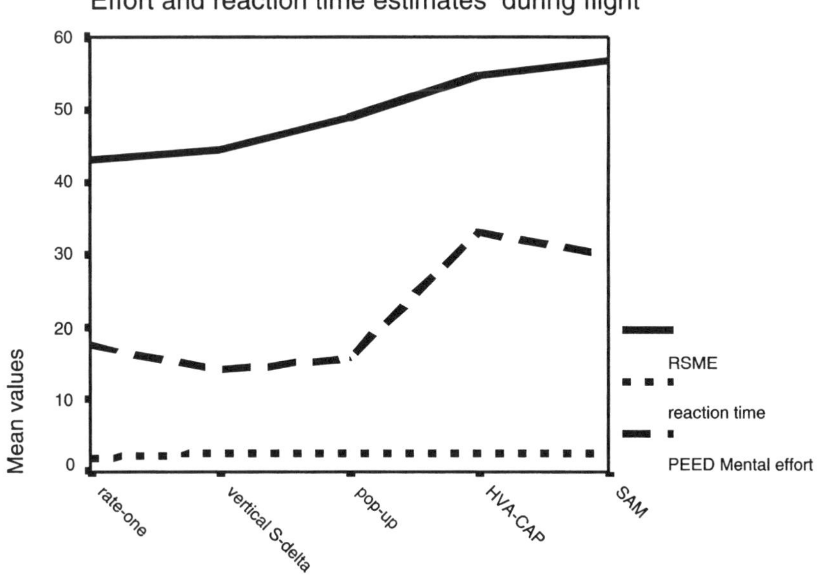

Figure 3. Effort and reaction time estimates during flight (fixed base simulator)

Experiment 2: Slingsby aircraft

In this experiment, performance and mental effort during tasks performed in a Slingsby aircraft were assessed. This was achieved by asking the candidate pilots to perform a number of tasks in two separate flights.

Subjects

Six third and final year Royal Netherlands Military Academy recruits (5 male, 1 female; mean age: 23.3) participated in the study. The candidates received 6 hours of flight training each year the past 3–4 years. The candidates had not yet started the military pilot training. Prior to the experiment, the purpose of the experiment was explained to all pilots. The subjects were capable of performing each maneuver without prior training. The maneuvers are referred to as flight phases (see Figure 4).

Procedure

During the experiment, each candidate-pilot performed 2 flights on the same day, during which the performance of nine maneuvers was assessed (see Figure 4). Subjects were asked to fill in questionnaires about fatigue and sleep quality (Meijman et al., 1985; Smets ct al., 1995), and after each flight they had to fill in a RSME ques-

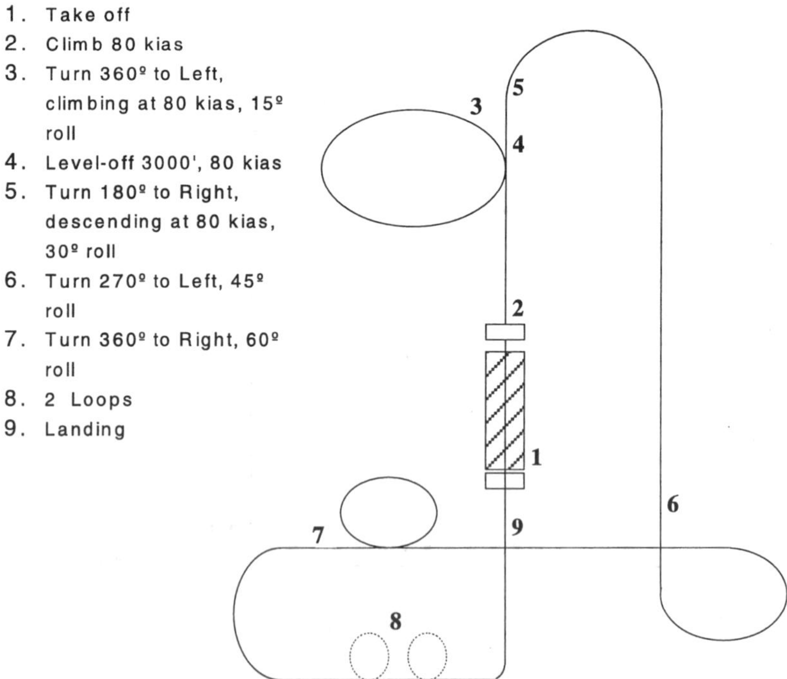

Figure 4. The circuit flown by the candidate-pilots.

tionnaire for all flight-phases. Heart rate was collected using a VITAPORT-II device, and PEED was used to collect on-line self-reports of mental effort. To guarantee anonymity, all subjects were given code numbers, which were changed and rehustled after completing the experiment.

A Slingsby T67M200 aircraft was used in the experiment. The entire flight was a pre-defined circuit, see Figure 4. From this circuit, 9 phases (or maneuvers) were chosen during which aircraft parameters, psychological data (self reports) and physiological data (heart rate and blink rate) were collected. These data were used to derive estimates of mental effort and performance. The candidates were asked to do their best, and they knew that their performance would be rated and debriefed as if they had just taken part in an examination. The candidates did not review the flight profile until 30 minutes before the flight. Thus, all pilots had the same preparation giving them all equal chances. All flights started and ended at Seppe airfield. The experiment was only performed if the lower cloud level was above 500 ft, and a horizon could be found above the clouds. A horizon was needed to optimally accomplish the tasks. The candidates flew in the left seat as pilot in command, and controlled the aircraft at all times (except during take-off and landing). The instructor sat in the right seat, and served as safety pilot and data observer. The instructor initiated the airborne instruments as soon as the relevant maneuvers started, and stopped the airborne registrations at the end of each relevant maneuver.

The following Visual Flight Rules (VFR) fight phases were selected for analysis: (1) take-off, (2) climb of 1000 ft at 80 KIAS (Kts Indicated Air Speed), (3) 360 degrees climbing turn of 1000 ft over left at 80 KIAS and 15 degrees roll, (4) level-off: 80 KIAS, (5) 180 degrees descending turn over right (1000 ft) at 80 KIAS, and 30 degrees roll, 6) 270° turn over left – 45° roll, 7) 360° turn over right, 60 degrees roll, 8) loop, 9) landing. Phases 4 and 5 were combined, thus a total of 8 phases could be distinguished per flight. In total 96 observations or flight phases were evaluated (96 = 8 phases x 2 flights x 6 pilots). These flight phases were chosen because correct execution of them involves a wide range of skills from the pilot. Each of the phases were to be performed at the specified criteria, a verbal warning was given by the instructor if altitude deviated more than 60 ft (250 ft during climb or descent), speed deviated more that 10 kts or heading deviated more than 10 degrees. No other information was given to the pilots during the flight.

Results of Slingsby experiment

From the airborne equipment 96 flight phases were distinguished (96 = 8 phases x 2 flights x 6 pilots). The pilots were only capable of providing PEED inputs in 34 flight phases, indicating 65% missing data. Of the 34 inputs provided by the pilots only 3 (9%) were incorrect.

External validity

In this in-flight experiment PEED mental effort and RSME are not correlated, as can be seen in Figure 5. However PEED mental effort is negatively correlated with inter-beat-interval (-.43). Thus when subjects reported higher PEED mental effort they also had a higher physiological arousal. Subjects that slept poorly invested less mental effort according to PEED, as is indicated by the negative correlation between the two variables (-.39). The results also show that subjects with a higher mental effort as indicated by a IBI, MF_HRV, and RSME have slower PEED reaction times (correlations of -.29, -.29 and -.28, respectively). Reaction times were also slower in subjects with a high mental fatigue and poor sleep quality.

A positive correlation is found between RSME scores and IBI, which means that pilots that reported a higher effort (by filling in the RSME after the flight) had a lower physiological arousal during the flight.

Discussion

In the present chapter a pilot study was performed to establish the validity of PEED, an instrument that can be used to determine pilot mental effort, flight phases and reaction times during flight. It was argued that on-line measurement of mental effort and reaction times might be considered ecologically valid because the

Table 4. Pearsons correlations between PEED mental effort scores in-flight and reaction time, Inter-Beat-Interval (IBI), heart rate variability (MF_HRV), Rating Scale Mental Effort (RSME) and sleep quality.

	PEED Mental effort	IBI	MF_HRV	RSME	Mental fatigue	Poor sleep
Reaction time	.14 .45	-.29* .02	-.29* .02	-.28* .02	-.28* .02	-.36** <.01
PEED Mental effort		-.43** .01	.24 .18	.16 .36	.13 .47	-.39* .02
IBI			.08 .42	.21* .04	.11 .29	.30** <.01
MF_HRV				.24* .02	.35** <.01	.35** <.01
RSME					.10 .34	.30** <.01
Mental fatigue						.83** <.01

n cases = 34, 6 subjects.

* Correlation is significant at the 0.05 level (2-tailed).

** Correlation is significant at the 0.01 level (2-tailed).

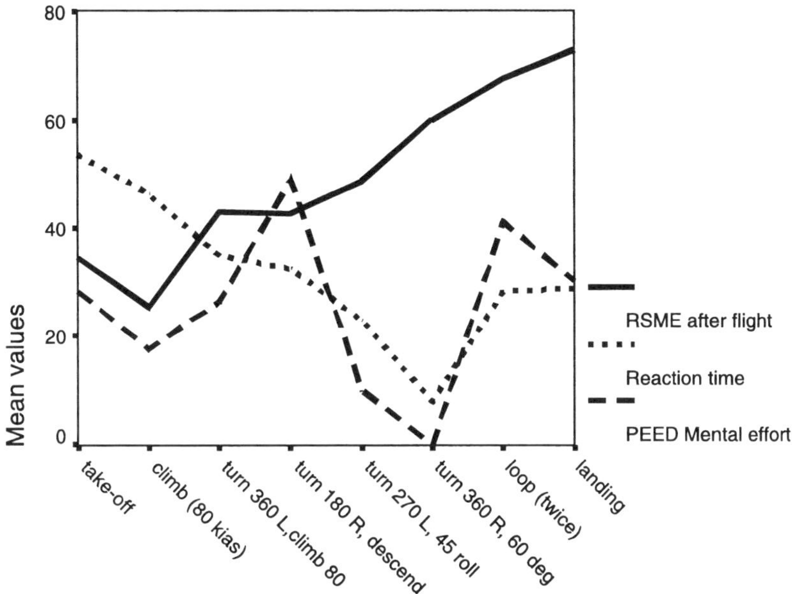

Figure 5. Mental effort and reaction times in Slingsby aircraft.

probability of bias due to impaired recall is reduced. Unfortunately, requiring inputs from pilots during flight may be distracting and form a potential threat to the safety of pilots. To determine the usability of the device, and to test external validity two experiments were performed. The first experiment was performed in a fixed base simulator. The fixed base simulator enabled safe testing of the capabilities of the device. The second experiment was performed during an actual aircraft operation. Because of the small number of participants, it should be emphasized that some correlation coefficients may not have reached significance. In order to increase the confidence in the results, future tests should be performed with a larger group of pilots.

In both experiments Ecological Momentary Assessments (EMA) were performed (using PEED) to register self-reports of flight phases and mental effort. The EMA assessments used in the two experiments differed slightly. In the first experiment EMA was performed according to the principles of *time sampling* (Delespaul, 1995). Every 60 seconds subjects were expected to provide PEED inputs. In the second experiment EMA was performed according to the principles of *event sampling*. Each time a new pre-defined flight phase was entered, subjects were expected to provide PEED inputs. The results show salient differences between the two approaches. Time sampling led to only 22% missing data, whilst event sampling led to 65% missing data. In contrast, identification of flight phases was less precise using the time sampling EMA (28% – 65% correct responses in tasks 1 – 5) in comparison to event sampling (91% correct responses). Thus although event sampling may be associated with more missing data, it is more precise. It should however be noted that the different results could also be caused by the PEED design. As can be seen in Figure 1 the buttons of the device are quite close to each other and errors may occur because buttons are misinterpreted. This may especially apply to the more effortful flights such as the HVA-CAP and S/A engagement. Future innovations of the design should improve this.

The unclear definition of flight segments and operational procedures may also have caused the higher percentage of incorrect responses in the first experiment. For example, in the fixed base simulator experiment, subjects were required to distinguish between "combat air patrol" (see CAP Figure 1) and "intercept". The distinction between the two is subject to personal interpretation. Some operational procedures on PEED (like using FCR, HSD, weapons or HUD) can be interpreted as being part of one of the first two flight segments.

The results also show other important differences between the two approaches (time-sampling versus event sampling). As a result of time-sampling (in the fixed base simulator) experiment PEED reaction times were much quicker (5.8 seconds) than as a result of event sampling (47.3 seconds). It seems that time-sampling forces subjects to react quickly, whilst event sampling provides more freedom, resulting in the longer reaction times. Because event sampling is less compulsory, it interferes less with aircraft operations, and may be considered safer.

After each flight, pilots were asked to fill in a questionnaire about PEED usability (Piórko et al., 1998). Pilots felt that PEED interrupted with flight operations but that it did not disturb concentration. The PEED buttons were considered difficult to operate, and too many flight phases or operational procedures were defined. The size and place of PEED (on the thigh) was considered convenient, and the flashes and beeps were not disturbing. In general, pilots felt that PEED was usable, but that improvement is mandatory if it is to be used in-flight.

The multilevel analysis of the mockup data revealed that PEED mental effort was not associated with increased physiological arousal. During flight however, it was, which is the opposite of the relation between RSME and physiological arousal. The in-flight results show that PEED and RSME measure different dimensions of mental effort. This multidimensionality makes sense from the perspective provided by the theory of Henry and Meehan (1981). This theory states that mental effort has two components, a "*euphoric*" component and a "*depression*" component. PEED mental effort seems to reflect the euphoric component, whilst the RSME seems to reflect the depression component (Moroney et al., 1995). Other authors have also acknowledged the multidimensionality of mental effort. Two well known examples are the NASA Task Load Index (NASA TLX by Hart & Staveland, 1988) and the

Subjective workload Index (by Reid & Nygren, 1988). To confirm this distinction, future research should involve measurements of adrenaline and cortisol, reflecting the euphoric and fatigue components respectively.

Regarding the hierarchical structure of the data, it was established that PEED mental effort assessments are more sensitive to individual differences between pilots, in comparison to RSME. This conclusion is based on the fixed base simulator data since the numbers of samples collected in flight are too few to allow multilevel analysis. Considering the observation that mental effort may be related to individual differences in euphoria and depression, it is important to have an instrument that is sensitive to the differences at the individual level. This propagates the use of PEED for in-flight measurements, and multilevel analyses for determining the hierarchies in the data. If such an endeavor is undertaken, enough data should be sampled (for example, flights, flight phases or subjects) to ensure sufficient data points to allow multilevel analysis.

Acknowledgements

The Flight Data Measurement and Recording System was installed by the EI department of NLR. We thank Tomasso Buti, Hans Brugman and Martin Joosse for their help with the data recording and analyses.

References

Amalberti, R. & Wioland, L. (1997). Human error in aviation. *Aviation Safety*, *17*, 91–108.

Backs, R.W. & Boucsein, W. (2000). *Engineering psychophysiology: issues and applications.* Hillsdale: Lauwrence Erlbaum Associates.

Berry, C.C. (1997). Multilevel statistical models for psychosomatic research. *Psychosomatic Medicine*, *59,* 350–351.

Bryk, A.S. & Raudenbusch, S.W. (1992). *Hierarchical linear models: Applications and data analysis methods.* London: Sage Publications.

Csikszentmihalyi, M. & Larson, R. (1987). Validity and reliability of the Experience-Sampling Method. *Journal of Nervous and Mental Disease*, *175,* 526–536.

Delespaul, P.A.E. G. (1995). *Assessing schizophrenia in daily life: the Experience Sampling Method.* Maastricht: University Press IPSER.

Goldstein, H. (1995). *Multilevel statistical models.* (2nd ed.). New York: John Wiley & Sons.

Hankins, T.C. & Wilson, G.F. (1998). A comparison of heart rate, eye activity, EEG and subjective measures of pilot mental workload during flight. *Aviation, Space, and Environmental Medicine*, *69*, 360–367.

Hart, S.G. & Wickens, C.D. (1990). Workload assessment and prediction. In: H.R. Booher. *MANPRINT: An approach to systems integration.* (pp. 257–296). New York: Van Nostrand.

Hanson, E.K.S. & Galinska, A. (1999). The effects of positive vertical acceleration on mental effort and performance during simulated aerobatics in a centrifuge. In: D. Harris *Engineering psycho-*

logy and cognitive ergonomics. (pp. 259–266). Aldershot: Ashgate.

Hanson, E.K.S. (1998). Feedback of Pilot Training Performance. Part 3: *Supplementing instructor debriefing with parameter feedback: Lessons learnt from an in-flight experiment*; phase II – 1998. Amsterdam: NLR. CR-98116-PT-3

Hart, S.G. & Staveland, L. E. (1988). Development of NASA TLX (Task Load Index): Results of empirical and theoretical research. In: P.A. Hancock and N. Meshkati *Human mental workload.* Amsterdam: Elsevier.

Henry, J.P. & Meehan, J.P. (1981). Psychosocial stimuli, physiological specificity, and cardiovascular disease. In: M.A. Hofer. and A.J. Stunkard *Brain, behavior, and bodily disease.* New York: Raven Press.

Jaccard, J. & Wan, C.K. (1993). Statistical analysis of temporal data with many observations: issues for behavioral medicine data. *Annals of Behavioral Medicine, 15*, 41–50.

Jorna, P.G.M. (1997). Context simulation: An interactive methodology for user centered system design and future operator behavior validation. In: N.B. Sarter and R. Amalberti *Coginitive Engineering in the Aviation Domain.* Lauwrence Erlbaum inc. Publishers.

Meijman, T.F., Zijlstra, F.R.M., Kompier, M., Mulders, H.P.G. & Broersen, J.P. (1986). The measurement of perceived effort. In: D.J. Oborne *Contemporary ergonomics.* London: Taylor & Francis.

Moroney, W.F., Biers, D. W. & Eggemeier, T.F. (1995). Some measurement and methodological considerations in the application of subjective workload measurement techniques. *The International Journal of Aviation Psychology, 5*, 87–106.

Mulder, L.J.M. & Mulder, G. (1987). Cardiovascular reactivity and mental workload. In: O. Rompelman and R.I. Kitney. *The beat-by-beat investigation of cardiovascular function.* Oxford: Oxford University Press.

Meijman, T.F., de Vries-Griever, A., de Vries, G.M. & Kampman, R. (1985). *The construction and evaluation of a onedimensial scale measuring subjective sleep quality.* Groningen: RUG.

van der Pal, J., Hanson, E.K.S. & Bohnen, H.G.M. (1999). If your mission is to enhance war fighter skills... pod the pilot. *Modern Simulation and Training, 5*, 36–40.

Piórko, A., Bazański, J., Galińska, A., Pich, J., Różanowski, K., Saganiak, R. & Knociński, D. (1998). *Feedback of pilot training performance. Phase II: Mental effort assessment, detecting workload chokepoints.* Warsaw: PAFIAM.

Reid, G.B. & Nygren, T.E. (1988). The Subjective Workload Assessment Technique: A scaling procedure for measuring mental workload. In: P.A. Hancock and N. Meshkati *Human mental workload.* Amsterdam: Elsevier.

Schwartz, J.E. & Stone, A.A. (1998). Strategies for analyzing ecological momentary assessment data. *Health Psychology, 17*, 6–16.

Smets, E.M.A., Garssen, B., Bonke, B. & Haes, J.C.J.M. d. (1995). The multidimensional fatigue inventory (MFI); Psychometric qualities of an instrument to assess fatigue. *Journal of Psychosomatic Research, 39,* 315–325.

Stokes, A. & Kite, K. (1994). *Flight stress: Stress, fatigue, and performance in aviation.* Cambridge: University Press.

Woodhouse, G., Rasbash, H., Goldstein, H., Yang, M. & Plewis, I. (1996). In: G. Woodhouse (Ed). *Multilevel modelling applications: A guide for users of MLn. London: Institute of Education.* University of London.

Chapter 28
Ambulatory Monitoring of Menopausal Hot Flashes

Robert R. Freedman
Departments of Psychiatry and Behavioral Neurosciences, and Obstetrics and Gynecology, Behavioral Medicine Division, Wayne State University School of Medicine, Detroit, USA

Introduction

Hot flashes (HFs) are the most common symptom of menopause and occur in the vast majority of women in the Western world. A hot flash is similar to a heat dissipation response because both comprise sweating and cutaneous vasodilation and can be provoked by external heating (Freedman, 1989).

Core body temperature (T_C) in homeotherms is regulated between upper thresholds for vasodilation and sweating and lower thresholds for shivering and peripheral vasoconstriction (Brück and Zersberger, 1990). Between these thresholds is a thermoneutral or null zone, within which major thermoregulatory responses do not occur.

Therefore, the obvious HF trigger would be an increase in T_C. Early workers in the field failed to find such T_C increases because their measurement methods (rectal and esophageal temperatures) were too slow (Kronenberg et al., 1984; Molnar, 1975). Using a more rapidly responding ingested telemetry pill, we did find small but significant T_C elevations preceding most HFs (Freedman et al., 1995; Freedman and Woodward, 1996; Freedman, 1998). If these T_C elevations occurred within a sufficiently narrow thermoneutral zone, the HF trigger could be explained. We measured this zone in postmenopausal women with and without HFs and found it to be zero in the former group and 0.4°C in the latter. This was primarily due to a lowering of the sweating threshold in the symptomatic women (Freedman and Krell, 1999).

Descriptive Physiology

The median age of HF onset is about 51 years (Kronenberg, 1990). Most women report daily HFs, with about 1/3 reporting > 10/day. HFs generally last 1-5 minutes and are described as sensations of heat, sweating, flushing, chills, and clamminess. Sweating is reported most often in the face, head, neck, and chest.

Peripheral vasodilation, as measured by skin temperature and blood flow occurs in all areas that have been measured (Figure 1). These include the fingers, toes,

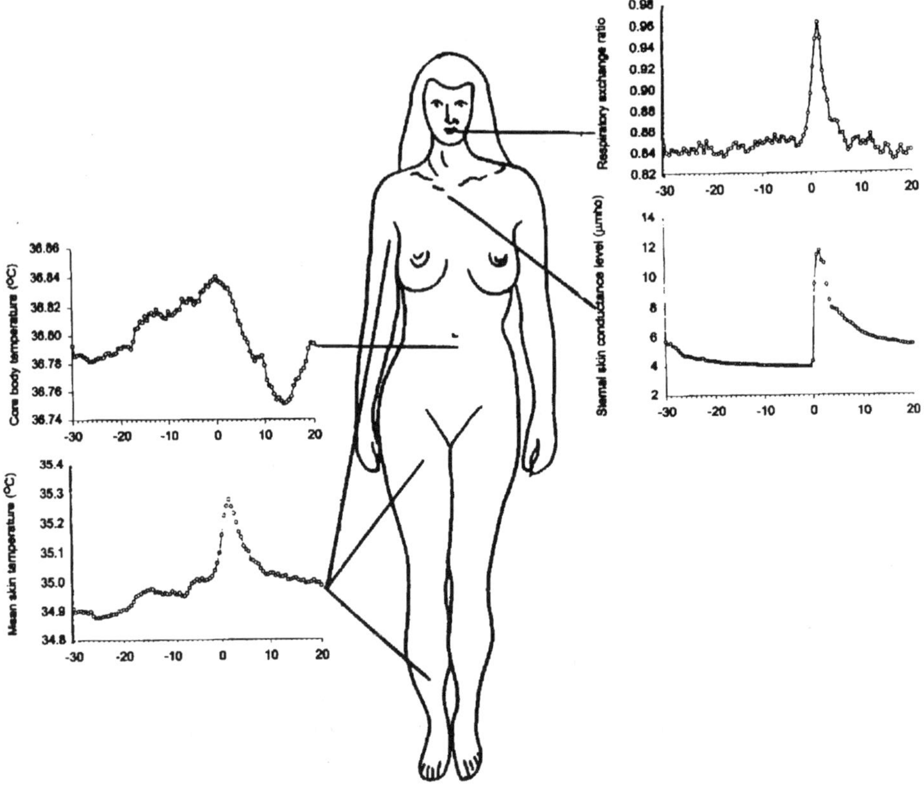

Figure 1. Peripheral physiological events of the hot flash. Data from Freedman (1998). Drawing by Jeri Pajor.

cheek, forehead, arm, chest, abdomen, back, calf, and thigh (Freedman, 1989, 1998; Molnar, 1975; Kronenberg, et al., 1984; Tataryn et al., 1980).

Sweating and skin conductance, an electrical measure of sweating, also increase during hot flashes. Molnar (1975) estimated total body sweat rate during HFs to be about 1.3 g/min. In our laboratory, we measured sweat rate and skin conductance level simultaneously from the sternum. Both measures increased significantly during 29 HFs recorded in 14 women (Freedman, 1998). Measurable sweating occurred during 90% of the HFs and there was a close temporal correspondence between both measures.

Significant elevations in metabolic rate (respiratory exchange ratio, Figure 1) and modest increases in heart rate (7-15 beats/min.) also occur, concomitant with the peripheral vasodilation and sweating (Freedman, 1989; 1998).

Objective Measurement of Hot Flashes

Towards the end of objectively evaluating treatment outcome, it would be useful to have an objective physiological measure that could be employed without the subject's self-report. This would be especially useful during sleep.

Temperature from the dorsum of one finger was proposed as the first physiological marker for menopausal hot flashes (Meldrum et al., 1979). In 7 symptomatic women, 41 skin temperature elevations > 1°C occurred within approximately 1 minute of the subjective hot flash. However, the duration of the temperature elevations averaged 31 minutes, whereas the duration of the subjective flushing was 2.3 minutes. Also, precise definitions of the onset of the temperature elevations were not reported.

Subsequently, skin conductance recorded from the sternum was investigated as a hot flash marker. Tataryn et al. (1981) found that 90% of 128 subjective flashes in 8 postmenopausal women were accompanied by elevations in sternal skin conductance compared to 82% for finger temperature and 81% for decreased tympanic temperature.

All of these changes were significantly reduced by estrogen administration in 4 of the women. However, the precise characteristics of the skin conductance responses were not defined.

Our laboratory subsequently sought to determine these characteristics (Freedman, 1989). Sternal skin conductance level, finger temperature, and heart rate were recorded for 4 hours in 11 postmenopausal and 8 premenopausal women. Twenty-nine subjective hot flashes were indicated by pushbutton in the first group. All of these were accompanied by an increase in sternal skin conductance 2 μmho/30 seconds. One skin conductance elevation occurred without a button press. No skin conductance elevations occurred in the premenopausal women. Thus, there was a concordance of 95% between the skin conductance criterion and the subjects' reports. Significant elevations in skin temperature and heart rate occurred during the flashes but were not as sensitive or specific as the skin conductance elevations.

We replicated these findings in 18 symptomatic and 8 asymptomatic postmenopausal women (Freedman et al., 1992). There was a concordance of 80% between the sternal skin conductance criterion (2 μmho/30 seconds) and the subjective reports (button press) in 15 flashes recorded in the symptomatic women. No events occurred in the asymptomatic women.

Our findings were then independently replicated by another laboratory (deBakker & Everaerd, 1996). In 2 separate studies of 20 symptomatic women, a concordance of 90% was obtained between the sternal skin conductance criterion and subjective reports. Measurements of finger temperature and blood flow were less predictive and did not improve the concordance rate when added to the skin conductance measure.

Ambulatory Monitoring

Skin Conductance

To evaluate treatment studies and to observe subjects in their natural environments, it would be useful to have a method that could be used outside the laboratory over extended time periods. We therefore developed methods for recording sternal skin conductance on ambulatory monitors for 24 hours.

Initial studies employed Oxford Medilog 4-channel recorders and an Oxford PB-2 playback system. Skin conductance level (SCL) was recorded using a 0.5 volt constant voltage circuit built into the recorder and an Oxford AM-3 DC pulse width modulation amplifier. Two Meditrace Ag/AgCl ambulatory monitoring electrodes were attached over the sternum. The existing gel was washed from the electrodes and replaced with 0.05 M KCl Unibase/glycol paste. Excess lead lengths were taped to the body to reduce artifacts. A subject-activated event marker was attached to the side of the recorder.

Medilog tapes were replayed at 60 x real time into an Analog Devices A/D board and IBM computer, and sampled at the real time equivalent of once every 15 sec. Simultaneous chart recordings were made using a Siemens Mingograph high-speed ink jet recorder. The computer was programmed to detect any increase in skin conductance level of at least 2 μmho in 30 sec. and to score all variables in 15 sec. epochs for 4 min. before and 2 min. after the peak of the SCL response.

Eight premenopausal women reporting regular menstrual cycles and 11 postmenopausal women reporting regular hot flashes were studied. They first received a 4 hour resting laboratory recording described in section below.

They then wore a Medilog recorder for a single 12 hour period from 10.00 to 22.00h while engaging in normal daily activities. They were instructed to press the event marker button each time a hot flash occurred.

Forty-three SCL increases $\geq$ 2 μmho/30 sec. occurred in the postmenopausal women; all were verified by inspection of the high speed ink jet chart recordings. Thirty-seven of the SCL elevations (86%) were accompanied by event marks. No event marks occurred in the absence of the criterion SCL change. No criterion SCL changes were detected by computer or by visual analysis in the recordings from the premenopausal women. Figure 2 shows the SCL data, compressed in time from recordings of one postmenopausal and one premenopausal woman. The former tracing (patient) shows 10 SCL increases meeting the criterion; the latter tracing (normal) shows none.

In a subsequent laboratory session, all subjects received a peripheral heating test in which two 40 x 60 cm circulating water pads maintained at 42°C were placed on the torso while supine in a 23°C room for 30 min. Eight of the eleven postmenopausal (72.7%) women had SCL increases meeting the 2 μmho/30 sec. criterion; all were accompanied by an event mark within 69 sec. One woman activated the event marker but had no demonstrable SCL change. Inspection of the SCL data from the eight premenopausal women showed that no criterion SCL changes occurred.

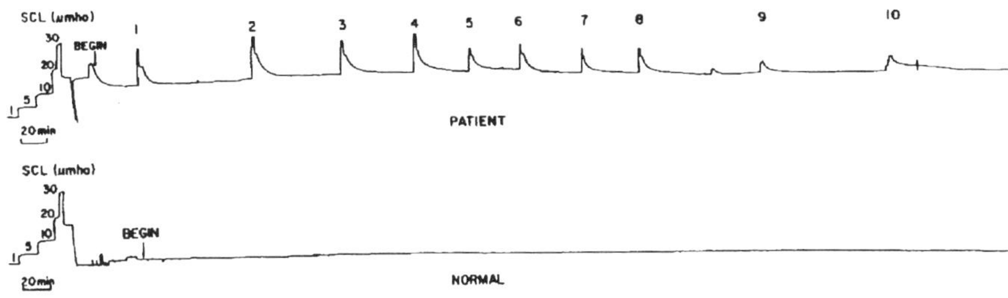

Figure 2. Two - 12 hour ambulatory sternal skin conductance recordings postmenopausal (patient) and a premenopausal (normal) woman. (From Freedman, 1989).

We then compared the SCL data from spontaneous, ambulatory, and heat-induced hot flashes for the 4 min. before and 2 min. after the peak of the SCL response. An analysis of variance of these data showed only a significant time main effect; there were no significant effects for type of hot flash or for the interaction between these two factors (Figure 3).

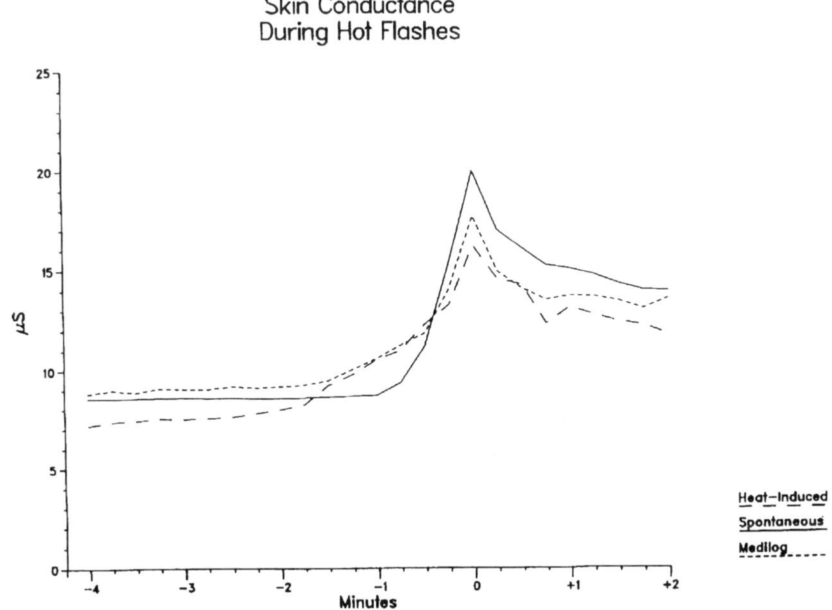

Figure 3. Sternal skin conductance mean data for spontaneous, ambulatory (Medilog), and heat-induced hot flashes. (From Freedman, 1989).

Thus, a sternal SCL increase of 2 μmho in 30 sec. was shown to have good agreement with patient self-reports (event marks). The agreement between SCL increases and event marks was 95% for spontaneous hot flashes recorded in the laboratory, 86% for those recorded during ambulatory monitoring, and 89% for heat-induced hot flashes. The temporal relationship between event marks and SCL increases was similar for spontaneous and heat-induced hot flashes. The SCL increases during spontaneous, heat-induced, and ambulatory hot flashes were similar in magnitude and time course. These changes did not occur in premenopausal women, during heat stress or ambulatory monitoring.

Core Body Temperature

We conducted several studies in which we measured core body temperature using an ingested radiotelemetry pill, which has a faster response time than the esophageal and rectal methods. The pill is swallowed 90 minutes before an experiment, to allow its egress from the stomach, and the signals are detected by a wire antenna and stored in a small digital recorder. The typical transit time through the gut is about 24 hours, during which the recorder samples the data every 30 seconds.

The circadian rhythm of T_C is well known, and similar variations in other thermoregulatory parameters, such as heat conductance and sweating, have also been shown. These patterns suggest that the thermoregulatory effector responses of hot flashes might also demonstrate temporal variations. A previous study showed circadian rhythmicity of self-reported hot flashes in some menopausal women, but no physiological data were collected (Albright et al., 1989). We therefore conducted a study to determine if HF occurrence was related to the circadian rhythm of T_C.

We recruited and screened ten symptomatic and 6 asymptomatic postmenopausal women (Freedman et al., 1995). Each received 24-hour ambulatory monitoring of sternal skin conductance level to detect hot flashes as well as ambient temperature, skin temperature, and T_C. Skin temperature was recorded using a thermistor taped to one finger and ambient temperature was recorded with a thermistor in a plastic holder on the wrist. SCL was recorded as described above. These measures were recorded on a Medilog recorder. T_C was recorded using the ingested radiotelemetry pill.

Cosinor analysis demonstrated a circadian rhythm ($p<.02$) of hot flashes with a peak around 1825 hours (Figure 4). This rhythm lagged the circadian rhythm of T_C in symptomatic women by about 3 hours. T_C values of the symptomatic women were lower than those of the asymptomatic women ($p<.05$) from 0000–0400 and at 1500 and 2200h. The majority of hot flashes were preceded by elevations in T_C, a statistically significant effect ($p<.05$). Hot flashes began at significantly ($p<.02$) higher levels of T_C (36.82 ± 0.04°C) compared to all non-flash periods (36.70 ± 0.005°C). These data are consistent with the hypothesis that elevated T_C serves as part of the hot flash triggering mechanism.

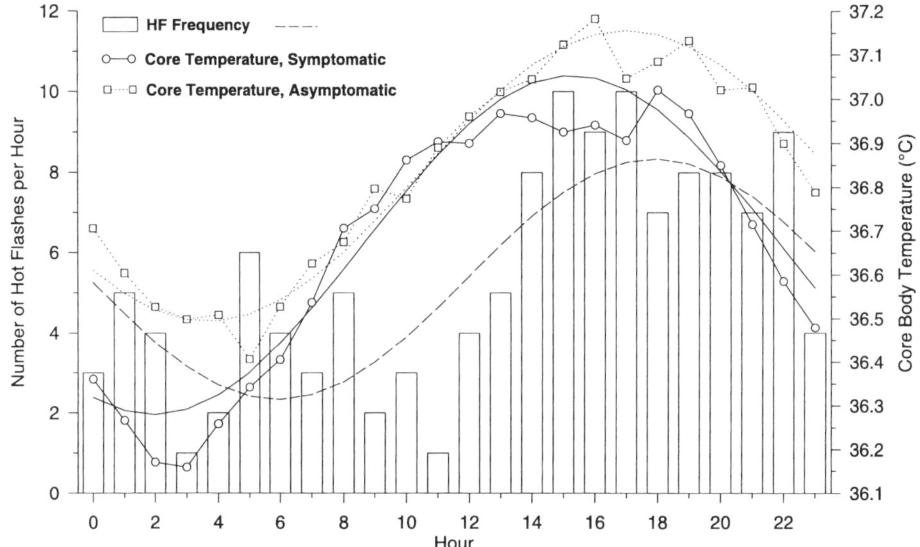

Figure 4. Hot flash frequency and core body temperature over 24 hours. Hot flash frequency in 10 symptomatic women shown as bars. Best-fit cosine curve for hot flush frequency as a dashed line (-----). 24-hour core temperature data for 10 symptomatic women as a solid line (o_____o) with best-fit cosine curve (_____). 24 hour core temperature data in 6 asymptomatic women as a dotted line (....) with best-fit cosine curve (....). From Freedman et al., 1995.

Sleep

Sleep disturbance is the second most common symptom of menopause and we were interested in comparing postmenopausal women with and without hot flashes. Ambulatory monitoring enabled us to do this in the subject's own home (Woodward and Freedman, 1994). Twelve postmenopausal women with hot flashes (mean age 52.6 $\pm$ 5.3 years) and seven postmenopausal women without hot flashes (mean age 57.4 $\pm$ 5.1 years) participated in our study. The symptomatic women reported at least five hot flashes per day and the asymptomatic women reported never having had a flash.

Twenty-four hour ambulatory monitoring was performed using an Oxford Medilog 8-channel cassette recorder and an Oxford 9000 playback system. Recorders were attached and started in our laboratory during the afternoon and ran continuously until subjects returned the following day. Subjects slept ad libitum in their own beds. Skin conductance level (SCL) was recorded from the sternum using a 0.5-V constant voltage circuit and Meditrace silver/silver chloride ambulatory monitoring electrodes, 1.5 cm in diameter , filled with 0.05 M KCl, Unibase/glycol paste. ECG was recorded with Meditrace ambulatory monitoring electrodes in a lead II configuration. EEG was recorded from C_4-A_1, using gold-cup electrodes applied with collodion. The EOG was recorded from the outer canthus of each eye, referred to each other using Ag/AgCl electrodes attached with adhesive collars. The EMG was recorded from submental muscle beneath the chin, also using Ag/AgCl electrodes. Excess lead lengths were taped to the body to reduce artifacts.

In order to detect hot flashes, the Medilog tapes were replayed at 20 x real time into an Analog Devices A/D board and IBM computer and sampled at the real time equivalent of 100 Hz. The computer was programmed to detect any SCL increase of at least 2 μmho within 30 seconds and to score the surrounding 4-6 minute period before and after the peak of the SCL response.

Sleep portions of the tapes were transferred onto standard chart recordings at real-time speed. These records were scored (blind to flashing or nonflashing status) in 30-second epochs by conventional criteria.

Results showed that women with hot flashes had significantly more time awake, more stage changes, lower sleep efficiency, and more stage 4 (slow wave) sleep compared to women without hot flashes. These findings are consistent with clinical reports of disturbed sleep in postmenopausal women.

Respiration

Several studies conducted in our laboratory demonstrated that training in slow, deep, abdominal breathing significantly reduces HF frequency (Freedman & Woodward, 1992; Germaine & Freedman, 1984). In the present study, we sought to determine whether this procedure affected HF frequency and/or ventilation recorded in the natural environment (Freedman et al., 1995).

Twenty-four postmenopausal women reporting frequent HFs were randomly assigned to receive 8 one hour biweekly treatment sessions of paced respiration or alpha-EEG biofeedback (placebo control).

Before treatment, all women received ambulatory monitoring of sternal skin conductance level (SCL) and abdominal and thoracic ventilation. Two Meditrace disposable Ag/AgCl electrodes, 1.5 cm in diameter, were filled with 0.05 *M* KCl paste and attached over the sternum. SCL signals were recorded on an Oxford Medilog 9000 recorder (Oxford, U.K.), using a constant-voltage circuit. The Medilog tapes were replayed at 20 x real time using an Oxford Medilog playback unit, an A/D converter, and an IBM computer. The computer was programmed to detect an SCL increase 2 μmho in 30 sec., which served as the objective definition of a HF.

Thoracic and abdominal ventilation were recorded on two additional channels of the Medilog using inductance plethysmography (Respitrace). Two insulated wire bands within elastic fabric were attached around the chest and just beneath the rib cage. The inductance changes from each band were calibrated with a laboratory spirometer to yield measurements of thoracic and abdominal tidal volume, respectively.

The Medilog recordings were repeated after the completion of treatment. Results showed that paced respiration subjects significantly (p<.001) reduced their HF frequency from 9.5/day ± 1.4 pre-treatment to 5.5 ± 1.5 post-treatment, whereas the alpha EEG biofeedback group did not significantly change, 6.1 ± 1.3 vs. 5.9 ± 1.1. There were no significant changes in abdominal or thoracic ventilation for either group in the natural environment. However, after training, when instructed to relax in the laboratory, the paced respiration group significantly (p<.001) increased abdominal and thoracic tidal volume and reduced respiration rate. The alpha EEG group showed no significant changes on any measure.

Solid State Equipment

Recently a solid-state recorder using RAM rather than cassette tape as the storage device has become available. The obvious advantage of this system is its lower failure rate due to the absence of moving parts. Also, playback is done on a standard PC computer, rather than a dedicated playback unit.

We evaluated the effectiveness of such a system in 19 postmenopausal women receiving tamoxifen for breast cancer who reported frequent HFs (Carpenter et al., 1999).

Participants' sternal skin conductance was recorded for a single 24 hour session starting at approximately 10:00 a.m. All participants were monitored between February and June 1998. Skin conductance levels were recorded using Meditrace silver/silver chloride electrodes (Graphic Controls; Buffalo, NY) and a 0.5 constant voltage circuit built in to the front end of a single DC channel of a Biolog ambulatory recorder (UFI, Model 3992/1 SCL; Morro Bay, CA). Electrodes were 1.5 cm in diameter and filled with 0.05 M potassium chloride Unibase/glycol paste which does not hydrate over the 24 hour period. The Biolog monitor is a solid-state device containing a microprocessor and 2 megabytes of memory. It is powered by a standard 9-volt battery and was programmed to sample 12-bit skin conductance data at 1 Hz. Participants were instructed to press an event marker on the Biolog when they felt a HF occurring. This event marker time-stamped the data with the exact time the HF was recorded and was considered the gold standard for comparisons. Data were recorded onto a random-access memory card, which was downloaded into a personal computer at the conclusion of the monitoring session using customized software (DPS v. 1.5, UFI).

Data from the Biolog were graphically displayed during analysis using the customized software (DPS v. 1.5). Analysis of each participant's 24-h-long data was performed by sequentially scanning 10-min data intervals for possible HF events. Any rapid increase in skin conductance was flagged by the data analyst as a possible HF event to ensure accurate coding of both HF and non-HF events. Each potential HF event was then further evaluated and either accepted or rejected by a trained data analyst in the context of activity (diary entries) and, when necessary, in the context of smaller (30-s) or larger (30-min) data windows. A zoom feature on the software allowed for both smaller and larger periods of skin conductance data to be graphically examined. HFs were defined as an increase in sternal skin conductance of at least 2 μmho during a 30-s period. If a HF was detected, a 20-min lockout period was applied during which no additonal HF events were scored.

A total of 356 possible HF events were flagged and scored by the data analyst. Each event was also scored by a blind independent rater using the same HF criterion. Agreement regarding HF status was reached on 332 of the 356 events (93%). Of these 356 possible HF events, 243 (68%) met our criterion for HFs, indicating successful oversampling of non-HF events. Oversampling of non-HF events was desired to reduce the likelihood the potential HF events were overlooked and not scored.

Analysis of data from the 181 waking HFs showed a concordance of 70% between computer-scored HFs and subjective recording by the event marker. These findings are similar to those obtained by our laboratory using Medilog tape recorders. There were no technical problems in the present study.

Summary

Hot flashes are the most common symptom of menopause and are characterized by sweating on the chest, neck, and face, and by cutaneous vasodilation. HFs can be reliably demarcated by criterion increases in sternal skin conductance, recorded in the laboratory or during ambulatory monitoring. We have used this measurement to objectively evaluate treatment studies, and to observe subjects over prolonged time periods in their natural environments.

Using an ingested radiotelemetry pill we found that there is a circadian rhythm of HFs, which is related to the circadian rhythm of core body temperature. By recording sleep EEG measures, we determined that postmenopausal women with HFs have significantly more disturbed sleep than those without HFs. Newer solid-state recorders have similar capabilities, without the disadvantages of cassette tapes and separate playback units.

In conclusion, ambulatory monitoring has much to offer researchers in thermoregulatory physiology. Obviously, the additional convenience to the subject and added value of naturalistic observations must be balanced against the loss of control of some elements of the experimental situation. In our experience, the advantages have generally outweighed the disadvantages.

Acknowlegement

Research conducted by the author was supported by NIH MERIT Award, R37-Ag05233.

References

Albright, D.L., Voda, A.M., Smolensky, M.H., Hsi, B. & Decker, M.(1989). Circadian rhythms in hot flashes in natural and surgically-induced menopause. *Chronobiology International, 6(3),* 279–284.

Brück, K. & Zeisberger, E. (1990). Adaptive changes in thermoregulation and their neuropharmacological basis. In: E. Schönbaum. & P. Lomax (Eds.) *Thermoregulation: Physiology and Biochemistry* (pp. 255–307). Pergamon Press: New York.

Carpenter, J.S., Andrykowski, M.A., Freedman, R.R. & Munn, R. (1999). Feasibility and psychometrics of an ambulatory hot flash monitoring device. *Menopause, 6(3),* 209–215.

deBakker, I.P.M. & Everaerd, W. (1996). Measurement of menopausal hot flushes: validation and cross validation. *Maturitas, 25,* 87–98.

Freedman, R.R. (1989). Laboratory and ambulatory monitoring of menopausal hot flashes. *Psychophysiology, 26(5),* 573–579.

Freedman, R.R. (1998). Biochemical, metabolic, and vascular mechanisms in menopausal hot flushes. *Fertility and Sterility, 70(2),* 1–6.

Freedman, R.R., Norton, D., Woodward, S. & Cornelissen, G. (1995). Core body temperature and circadian rhythm of hot flashes in menopausal women. *The Journal of Clinical Endocrinology & Metabolism, 80(8),* 2354–2358.

Freedman, R.R. & Krell, W. (1999). Reduced thermoregulatory null zone in postmenopausal women with hot flashes. *American Journal of Obstetrics and Gynecology, 181(1),* 66–70.

Freedman, R.R. & Woodward, S. (1996). Core body temperature during menopausal hot flushes. *Menopause, 65(6),* 1141–1144.

Freedman, R.R. & Woodward, S. (1992). Behavioral treatment of menopausal hot flushes: Evaluation by ambulatory monitoring. *American Journal of Obstetrics and Gynecology, 167(2),* 436–439.

Freedman, R.R., Woodward, S., Brown, B., Javaid, J.I. & Pandey, G.N. (1995). Biochemical and thermoregulatory effects of behavioral treatment for menopausal hot flashes. *Menopause, 2(4),* 211–218.

Freedman, R.R., Woodward, S. & Norton, D. (1992). Laboratory and ambulatory monitoring of menopausal hot flushes: Comparison of symptomatic and asymptomatic women. *Journal of Psychophysiology, 6,* 162–166.

Germaine, L.M. & Freedman, R.R. (1984). Behavioral treatment of menopausal hot flashes: Evaluation by objective methods. *Journal of Consulting and Clinical Psychology, 52(6),* 1072–1079.

Kronenberg, F. (1990). Hot flashes: Epidemiology and physiology. *Annals of the New York Academy of Science, 592,* 52–86.

Kronenberg, F., Cote, L.J., Linkie, D.M., Dyrenfurth, I. & Downey, J.A. (1984). Menopausal hot flashes: Thermoregulatory, cardiovascular, and circulating catecholamine and LH changes. *Maturitas, 6,* 31–43.

Meldrum, D.R., Shamonki, I.M., Frumar, A.M., Tataryn, I.V., Chang, R.J. & Judd, H.L. (1979). Elevations in skin temperature of the finger as an objective index of postmenopausal hot flashes: Standardization of the technique. *American Journal of Obstetrics and Gynecology, 135(6),* 713–717.

Molnar, G.W. (1975). Body temperature during menopausal hot flashes. *Journal of Applied Physiology: Respiration, Environmental and Excercise Physiology, 38,* 499–503.

Tataryn, I.V., Lomax, P., Bajorek, J.G., Chesarek, W., Meldrum, D.R. & Judd, H.L. (1980). Postmenopausal hot flushes: A disorder of thermoregulation. *Maturitas,* 2, 101–107.

Tataryn, I.V., Lomax, P., Meldrum, D.R., Bajorek, J.G., Chesarek, W. & Judd, H.L. (1981). Objective techniques for the assessment of postmenopausal hot flashes. *American Journal of Obstetrics and Gynecology, 57(3),* 340–344.

Woodward, S. & Freedman, R.R. (1994). The thermoregulatory effects of menopausal hot flashes on sleep. *Sleep, 17(6),* 497–501.

Chapter 29
Giving Feedback to Asthma Patients Ambulatory Monitoring in Patient Education

Christian Leopold[1] and Rainer Schandry[2]
[1]*Nets Healthcare GmbH, Munich*
[2]*Institute of Psychology, University of Munich, Germany*

Introduction

The keys to success in disease-state management include the accurate clinical data for the condition under assessment and the possibility of an early intervention in cooperation with the patient. Integrating the home monitoring of disease parameters into disease-state management enables physicians to decide on an extensive and patient-related data bases and offers patients the chance to benefit from an immediate intervention should their disease state be worsening. Examples for the application of home monitoring with hand-held computers are the treatment of obesity (Agras et al., 1990), diabetes (Ryff-De Lèche, 1992), asthma (Lefkowitz, Klimas & Ross, 1996), hypertension (Asmar et al., 1996), or chronic pain (Sorbi, Honkoop & Godaert, 1996).

Computer-tailored interventions (CTI)

The use of computers in patient education aims at combining the advantages of (a) economically favourable high participation rates and (b) elevated efficacy through interactive, individualized interventions. "Computer tailoring in health education can be defined as the adaptation of health education materials to one specific person through a largely computerised process. Computer-tailoring is more than personalisation. Personalisation means that a person's name is listed (once or several times) on the information that he or she receives. However, the information is not adapted to the individual's diagnostic, behavioral or motivational characteristics" (de Vries & Brug, 1999, p. 100).

Computer-based patient education allows a differentiated and economic contact with a large number of persons. In the past, most of the patient education programs used (non-computer-aided) paper-mailings or telephone calls, because of the omnipresence of these technologies, instead of the Internet or personal computers (Friedman et al., 1996; Friedman et al., 1997; Marks et al., 1998).

Certainly, the medium "computer" by itself is not generally more convincing and therefore superior to the traditional paper or face-to-face interventions (Coiera, 2000; Fishbein et al., 2000). As Detweiler et al. (1999) could demonstrate factors like the framing (positive – negative, gain – loss) of health information, it seems to be most relevant for people's preventative behavior.

However, on the diagnostic or input side of the interaction process, patients may prefer interactive computer programs to human interrogation on sensitive topics such as substance abuse, contraceptive use, or HIV. Paperny showed that, out of more than 4000 adolescents, the vast majority preferred a computer interview (89%) over a face-to-face personal interview or a questionnaire (6%). Most of the participants chose the computer when asked whether talking honestly about these kinds of questions was easier with a person or a computer (Paperny, 1997).

Large-scale experience with computerised, interactive patient encounters exists today in areas with a need for financial efficacy, that is, primary and secondary prevention programs. Examples for this are smoking cessation (Strecher, 1999), weight reduction (Brug, Campbell & Assema, 1999), asthma (Osman et al., 1994), diabetes (Binsted, Cawsey & Jones, 1995), and migraines (Buchanan et al., 1992).

Computer-tailored interventions and ambulatory assessment

Up to now, patient input to computer-tailored health-care programs primarily refers to data being more or less stable in time, like questionnaires. Repeated questionnaire assessment within weeks or months may outline a participant's dynamic development to a certain degree, but may never uncover real-life behavior on a short time scale. Therefore, the next logical step in individualising education programs is to integrate a diagnosis of behavior through ambulatory assessment. This has already been put into effect in clinic situations (for example, Mussgay & Rüddel, 1996), although experience is lacking with outpatient programs supporting computer-tailored patient education through ambulatory diagnostic assessment.

Unlike ambulatory assessment, patients' computer contact during computer-tailored intervention does not end after a phase of mere data recording. The collected data serve as the basis for individualising (pre-defined) education material. Usually, the repeated interactions of patients' data input and individualized education material output to the patient extend over a couple of input-output cycles.

Patient education

The main area of CTI is patient education. To date, patient education applied to patient groups, especially in the form of standardized patient education programs, is seen as a central element of diabetes and asthma therapy (Sheffer & Taggart,

1993). Its contents are defined in accordance with the consensus guidelines from different national and international boards (Crim, 2000; Dahl & Bjermer, 2000; Lalloo & Motala, 2000).

Although the vast majority of patients is treated in outpatient settings, patient education is most frequently realised in inpatient rehabilitation units. Aside from the better availability of outpatient institutions, outpatient patient education is able to control the newly learnt behavior in everyday life and in commonplace environments.

For economic reasons, patient education is most frequently implemented in group settings. In order to individualize group programs, it is necessary to specify certain modules for such patient subgroups as – in the case of asthma-allergic patients, chronic obstructive patients and self-management patients (Schultz, Stark & Petro, 1996). This approach, however, still comprises only subgroups and disregards the skills and needs of the individual patient. Targeting patient education to the individual patient without losing the economic advantage of standardized group training is difficult to achieve. Here the necessity to measure, document and interpret (1) a disease-related medical parameter (for example, peak flow, blood glucose), (2) severity of subjective symptoms and (3) the use of medication exists. Ambulatory recordings of these parameters offers the chance to realise computer-tailored interventions within group patient education.

In the following, we shall focus on asthma as an example for a disease where the advantages of a computer-tailored intervention program are quite easy to elucidate.

Asthma

Asthma is a lifelong, chronic illness with a high worldwide prevalence (Chinn et al., 1997; Murray & Lopez, 1997) that in most cases requires continuous pharmaceutical treatment. To date, no treatment healing asthma exists, although symptom reduction or even asymptomatology may be achieved (van Essen-Zandvliet et al., 1992). Major deficits in asthma therapy on the side of the patient are the lack of knowledge about a development of exacerbations and adequate therapy (Boulet, 1998; Chambers et al., 1999; Woeller et al, 1993), the lack of skills for practical handling of drug application systems (Gibson et al., 1993; Petro, 1994), a reduced compliance to therapy (Cochrane et al., 2000), and an underestimation of acute illness severity (Yoos & McMullen, 1997).

As the underlying pathological situation in the bronchii fluctuates, asthma severity may increase or decrease within days or even hours. Ideally, the treatment should be adapted immediately to the patient's momentary disease state. However, adaptive therapy requires permanent diagnostic monitoring in order to detect sudden changes. Monitoring should pertain to two main variables: (1) Peak-expiratory air-flow

(PEF) as a measure of airway obstruction, obtainable through a simple and inexpensive device, and (2) subjective symptoms. The frequency and intensity of subjective symptoms like breathlessness/dyspnea, coughing, wheezing, difficulties in breathing, exercise-induced breathlessness or night-time symptoms are important cues for changes in the disease state.

Insufficient symptom perception in asthma

Several reports do exist on insufficient symptom perception for a considerable number of asthma patients. Thus, in the case of an exacerbation, countermeasures like the intake of emergency medication or visits to the physician's office are frequently initiated too late (Yoos & McMullen, 1999). However, research on symptom perception in asthmatics does not unequivocally support a generally reduced symptom perception in asthma patients in contrast to healthy control persons (Dahme et al., 1991; James et al., 1998). Regardless of these inconsistencies in the literature, the Global Initiative For Asthma (GINA) of the NHLBBI/WHO states that "patients and health care professionals are often *unable to recognize the severity of an asthma exacerbation*, and studies in which the causes of deaths have been retrospectively examined show that, except in the United States, almost all the deaths occur outside the hospital." (GINA, 1995, p. 15). This implies the need for improving symptom awareness in asthma patients in order to reduce their risk of severe complications.

Undoubtedly, symptom perception is improved most effectively on the behavioral level (Harver, 1994; Szczepanski et al., 1994; van Wjk & Kolk, 1997). Nevertheless, symptom perception plays only a minor role in widely applied asthma education programs. In contrast to this, hypoglycaemic unawareness in diabetes has been successfully implemented by a U.S. research group (Cox et al., 1991) in an internationally applied training program.

A system for assessing and training symptom perception and disease-related behavior in asthma patients

In the following, a computer tailored intervention program integrating electronic ambulatory assessment, an analysis of ambulatory data, computer-based individualized written education material and a group training setting will be described for the area of asthma. This outpatient program was evaluated by comparing it to a conventional program. Both programs were run at the Institute of Psychology of the University of Munich.

Study design

Sixty-four patients participated. Half of the patients were each randomly assigned to either the control group or the experimental group. Patients of the experimental group were supplied (1) with an electronic ambulatory device for the registration of subjective symptoms and peak flow measurement, and (2) an electronic MDI (metered-dose inhaler) for recording the short-term asthma inhalations (also see section "ambulatory assessment"). The control group received an established, standardized, asthma patient, education program together with a detailed ambulatory monitoring plan. They used the same electronic devices, but with none or much simpler assessment tasks. Both groups took part in six training sessions over a period of two months. Questionnaires were given one day before, during and at the end of the intervention period.

At the first training session, patients received their ambulatory devices, were taught how to use the new technology and learned about their monitoring plan. Patients had to measure peak-flow at least twice daily: before 9:30 a.m. and after 5:00 p.m., but were free to do this more often. Furthermore, the plastic fixture of their regular short-term beta-mimetic (quickly active beta-agonist) canister was exchanged with an electronic sensor frame. In addition to peak flow measurement, participants in the experimental group rated ten disease-specific symptoms and entered the scores into the instrument (see below). Before peak flow measurement, these patients keyed in their own estimation of their current peak flow values.

After the first training session, both groups followed their monitoring plans for four weeks and then returned for the second training session with all their monitoring devices. The following five meetings were held weekly, and patient education and ambulatory recording were continued. Ambulatory data of the experimental group were immediately analyzed electronically during the training sessions, results were printed, given to the participants and discussed within a group setting. The control group continued with their monitoring plan without the collected data being addressed in any way. After two months of ambulatory assessment, patients returned all electronic devices during the last training session.

Subjects

Patients were recruited through newspaper articles, health insurances, pharmacies, hospitals, doctor's offices, radio and TV reports, and talks given to patient organisations. All patients suffered from moderate to severe asthma. Thus, they experienced disease-related symptoms several times a week, used their medication permanently during the whole year, and additionally used a short-term beta-2-agonist several times a month. Because of technical limitations, the powder-based short-term beta-2-agonist inhaler could not be replaced by an electronic unit. Thus, these persons had to be excluded from participating in order to avoid having to change their medication plan. The 64 patients were assigned to a total of 12 training groups consisting of five to six persons each. One participant decided to quit because his expectations were not fulfilled. Another eight patients had to cancel their participation before finishing the full program because of acute exacerbations or hospital stays. The remaining 55 patients (29 in the experimental group, 26 in the control group) had a mean age of 52 years (range 28 – 73 years), 34 of them were women, 21 were men.

Ambulatory assessment

Two devices (electronic peak-flow meter and electronic metered-dose inhaler) were given to the patients in order to record peak flow, symptom intensity, and frequency of medication use.

The electronic peak-flow meter ("AsthmaMonitor AM2", manufactured by Erich Jaeger GmbH, Höchberg, Germany) automatically stored and displayed all peak flow measurements made after the patient had blown rapidly into the peak-flow meter's tube. For detailed diagnosis, the spirometric parameters FEV1, FVC, MEF25, MEF50, MEF75, MMEF were also measured and stored, but not displayed. Furthermore, patients could navigate with four buttons (⇓, ⇑, ok, back/escape) through a symptom list of 10 items. On a three-line display of 20 characters length each, the questions were presented to the patients. On the bottom line, one possible answer category could be selected for the respective question. By pressing one of the arrow buttons, the answer category flipped to the next category and so forth. The highest category was "extremely"; the other categories were "very much", "rather", "little" and "none". The choice was accepted by activating the "o.k."-button. The subsequent question was displayed automatically. After the symptom rating and before measuring the peak flow, the participants were instructed to estimate their current peak flow value. Starting with the default value of 430 ml/min they could reduce or increase the value in steps of 5 ml/min.

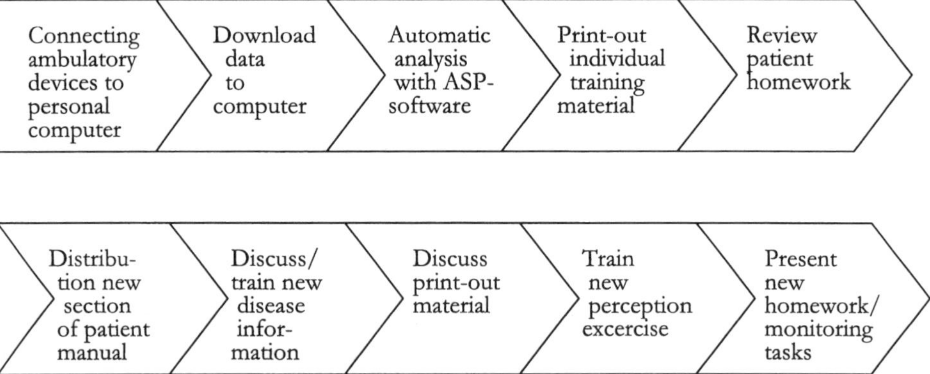

Figure 1. Flow chart of relevant segments during a training session of the experimental group.

Data could be downloaded to a PC with a serial interface and the proprietary software.

The electronic metered-dose inhaler "MDI Chronolog MC-311" (Medtrac Technologies, Inc. Lakewood, USA) detected the spraying of medication from the attached medication canister. All events (medication spraying) were time-stamped with "hh:mm:ss" and the actual date. The device had the size of the original metered-dose inhaler and no display. Data could be downloaded to a PC with a serial interface and the proprietary software.

"ASP" feedback software

The newly developed software "ASP" (AsthmaSchulungsProgramm) was programd in Java Vers. 1.71, which makes it compatible to all operating systems. The software structure covers a data bank system, decision-making algorithms, a graphical display module, and a set of text modules compromising the general and individualized patient education materials (see Figure 2). The data input into the data base was adopted to the data output format of the ambulatory devices.

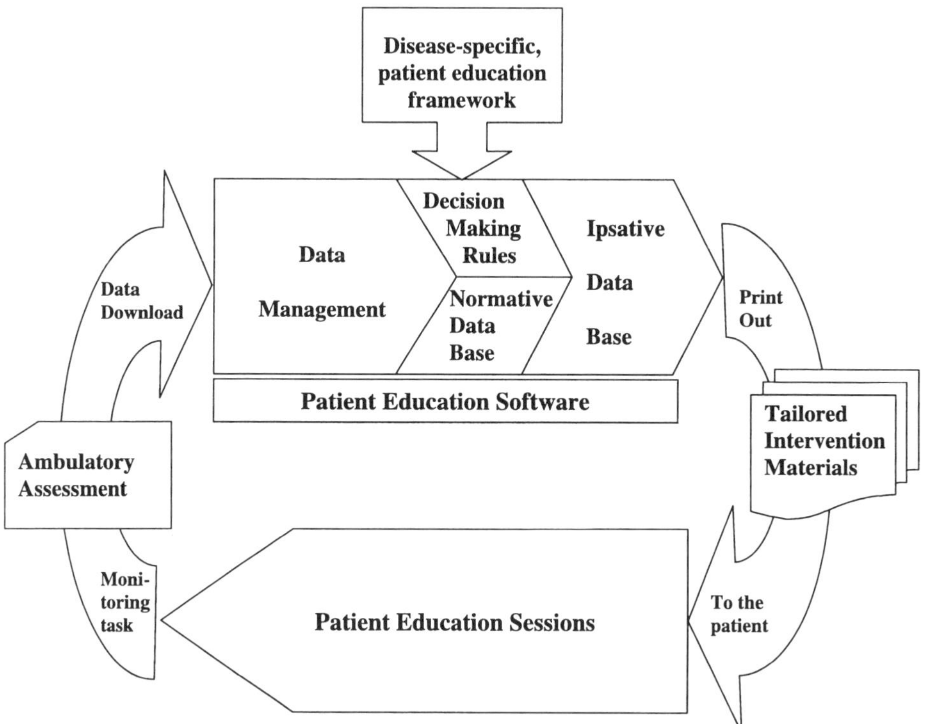

Figure 2. Concept and software architecture of computer-tailored patient education with ambulatory assessment.

Table 1. Categorisation algorithms and mode of patient presentation for ambulatory assessment data

Compliance	Peak flow	Medication	Symptoms	Interoception
• Percentage of peak flow measurements before 9:30 a.m. • Mean frequency of daily peak flow measurements • Mean frequency of daily symptom list input	• Time course highest/lowest daily peak-flow: Graphical display • Classification of data according to traffic light system (red, yellow, green): Graphical display • Frequency of values in the red, yellow, green area: Graphical display (bar chart) • Mean diurnal PEF variability: Mean value • Average peak-flow of time period A compared to average peak flow of time period B: Graphical display (bar chart)	• Frequency of daily use over time: Graphical display • Distribution of uses during day and night time over time: Graphical display	• Mean symptom intensity: Graphical display (bar chart) and absolute numbers • Time course of daily symptom intensity: Graphical display	• Comparison of a subjective general postulation of estimation precision and calculated estimation precision: Graphical display and numbers • Number of calculated accurate, over and under-estimations: Graphical display and numbers • Comparison of percentage of accurate estimations among all group members: Graphical display and numbers • Day-by-day time course of "absolute difference between measured and estimated peak flow": Graphical display • Average difference between peak flow measurements and estimations of time period A compared to time period B: Graphical display • Correlation between daily average symptom intensity and peak-flow values: Graphical display • Correlation between frequency of daily medication use and average daily symptom intensity

The ASP software categorizes the incoming patient data according to the decision-making algorithms, classifies them with respect to the education materials, produces the graphs and automatically sends the selected results to a printer. All graphs and numerical results are accompanied by a text element generally explaining the respective presentation and an individualized explanatory text. The education material addresses the five topics (1) compliance, (2) peak-flow measurement, (3) medication use, (4) symptoms and (5) interoception. Table 1 provides details for the decision criteria.

The "ASP" education program

A couple of validated asthma education programs are available for the German speaking countries (Petro, 1997). We chose the "Bad Reichenhaller Asthmaschulungsprogramm" (Prittwitz et al, 1989) as the informational core element of our patient education program. Reasons for this choice were, for example, it's high degree of structured information, the complete availability of transparencies, its widespread use among pneumologists and it's royalty-free application. For our training purposes, we abridged the original program in order to insert our new components.

We supplied the printed, individualized feedback material in an accompanying patient manual. The additional topics of this manual focused in more detail on the patients' compliance with peak flow measurements, symptom rating and medication use. Furthermore, the program concentrated on an in-depth analysis of peak flow values (see Table 1).

The patient's awareness of his bronchoconstriction and improvement of this awareness was the program's central training focus. Changing the home monitoring tasks, daily exercises to improve symptom awareness, apprehension of three relaxation techniques and discussion of the symptom-related, individualized print-outs were all carried out with the goal of improving the patients' symptom awareness.

On the basis of the correlations between peak flow values and subjective symptoms, we identified "lead-symptoms" for the subjective experience of bronchoconstriction for each patient. Calculating correlations between medication use and symptoms disclosed whether medication was used depending on symptomatology or not. Analysis of the differences between measured and estimated peak flow values reflected the participants' ability to perceive bronchoconstriction.

Methods of data assessment and analysis

For each patient, approximately 120 daily peak flow measurements, 120 symptom ratings of 10 symptoms and the 120 daily peak flow estimations were obtained. Asthma specific quality of life was assessed by a questionnaire (1 week before and three weeks after the end of the education program). This questionnaire (FAP, Schandry, 1995) encompasses disease-related areas of emotion, physical asthma symptoms, limitations in individual and social situations, asthma-specific avoidance behavior, and well-being (68 items).

During the first four weeks, all participants recorded data without training. These data were averaged across time and taken as a baseline period. The following four weeks (intervention period), data were also averaged across time. Since symptom reporting and PEF estimation was only done by the experimental group, no intra-group comparisons could be carried out for these variables.

Peak flow estimation was considered correct if the estimated value was within a range of plus/minus 10 % of the corresponding measured peak flow value. For data presentation to the patients, the mean ambulatory symptom values of the 10 symptoms were again aggregated to an average symptom intensity in the respective interval. Peak flow variability (as the diurnal variation in peak flow) was expressed as the formula:

$$\text{Variability} = (\text{maximum PEF}_{\text{Day n}} - \text{minimum PEF}_{\text{Day n}} / (0.5^* \text{ maximum PEF}_{\text{Day n}} - \text{minimum PEF}_{\text{Day n}}))^*100$$

On the basis of this data set, the following questions were investigated:

(1) Feasibility of the program; (2) compliance with the monitoring protocol; (3) changes in quality of life of the participants; (4) improvement of lung functions; and (5) improvement of the ability to correctly rate the actual degree of bronchoconstriction

Results

Peak expiratory flow

No significant difference in mean peak flow level occurred between groups at the beginning or at the end of the program (see Figure 3). The intra-group differences between these two time points were insignificant as well.

The mean diurnal peak flow variability for all groups was above 20 percent at the beginning. This confirmed the diagnosis of moderate asthma (Lebowitz, 1991, Quackenboss, Lebowitz & Krzyzanowski, 1991). At the start of the program both groups did not differ significantly. However, patients of the experimental group showed a significantly reduced peak flow variability at the end of the program (26% – 22%).

Quality of life: The FAP

Statistical analysis for the baseline period of intragroup differences of the quality of life questionnaire score did not reveal relevant differences at the beginning (see Figure 3). In the experimental group, a significant reduction in the FAP score was

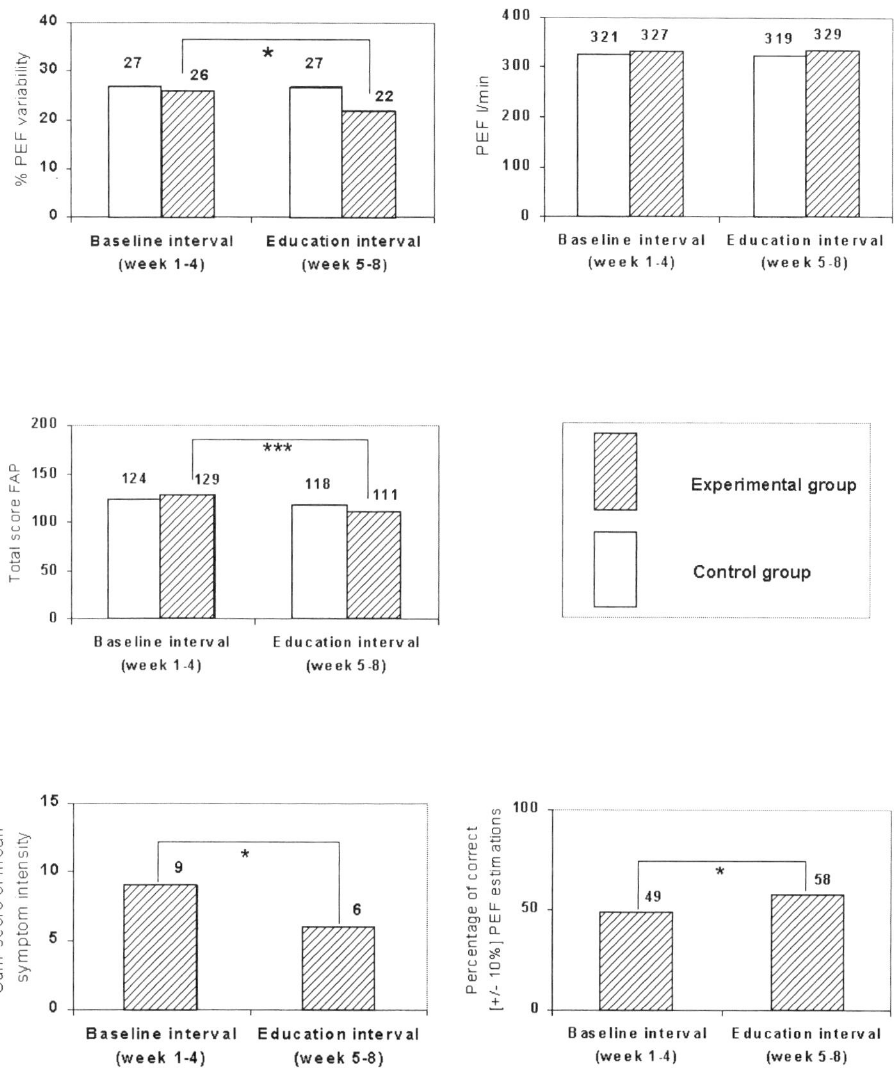

Figure 3. Summary of study results.
Upper right panel. Peak expiratory flow during baseline and education interval for experimental and control group. Upper left panel. Peak expiratory flow variability during baseline and education interval for experimental and control group. Middle panel. Quality of life (FAP, Questionnaire for asthma patients) before and after the education programme for experimental and control group. Lower right panel. Difference between estimation and measurement of Peak expiratory flow during baseline and education interval for experimental group. Lower left panel. Symptom intensity for experimental group during baseline and education interval.
Low quality of life scores are representing high quality of life. (* $p < 0.05$, ** $p < 0.01$, *** $p < 0.001$)

observed (that is, improvement in the quality of life). The FAP score of the control group was also reduced over time; the difference, however, did not reach statistical significance.

Precision of peak flow estimation

One task of the experimental group consisted in the estimation of peak flow before performing a peak flow measurement. At the beginning, 49 percent of all paired estimation measurements were correct according to the definition of +/- 10% of the measured peak flow value. During the course of the treatment, participants significantly increased their estimation capability to 58 percent correctly estimated peak flow values.

Symptom ratings

The mean symptom ratings of the 10 monitored symptoms were added up to a sum score of mean symptom intensity. From baseline interval to education interval, reported mean symptom intensity significantly decreased from 9 to 6 points.

Discussion

In the present study, modern ambulatory assessment technologies were employed in a newly developed outpatient asthma education program in order to individually tailor training interventions. The data analysis software and the training elements, such as patient manual, monitoring plans, and interoceptive exercises, were newly designed. For program evaluation, this program was compared to a conventional asthma management program.

Feasibility

The conception of the software, program logics, and the selection and application of the electronic monitoring devices resulted in a homogenous education program which was regularly attended by asthma patients.

The aim of the software development was the optimal translation of objective figures into easy-to-understand, individualized, subjectively meaningful graphics. Up to now, no such systematic effort has been undertaken to develop a patient-friendly illustration of disease progress and disease state.

To our knowledge, there is only one report dealing with new methods of depicting peak-flow. Boggs et al. (1999) enriched the pure peak-flow chart information through the use of statistics and demonstrated its usefulness in four cases. More knowledge is already accumulated in diabetes and hypertension research, for example, Kahn et al. (1991); Mansoor et al. (1996).

Compliance with the monitoring protocol

The majority of education programs aiming at chronic diseases focuses on an improvement of compliance (Cochrane et al., 2000). In a study from van der Palen, Klein and Rovers (1997), patients underwent a complex electronic monitoring and self-management plan in order to correctly apply their self-treatment guidelines. However, the patients were not able to integrate all complex self-management rules into their lives within six weeks.

Studies assessing adherence to electronic peak-flow measuring twice a day reported a decrease from nearly 100% percent at the beginning to 50% or even less after four weeks (Cote et al., 1998; Redline et al., 1996).

Compliance with electronic devices is essential for an ambulatory monitoring program. Therefore, we integrated detailed feedback on the individual adherence to electronic peak flow measurement and symptom rating. Furthermore, the first chapter in the patient's manual dealt with compliance. This part of the program could be dropped after a short time, because compliance was satisfactory from the beginning. All patients demonstrated a compliance above 50%. Obviously, repeated inspection of the graphical output was a sufficient reminder.

Spirometry

The primary medical outcome parameter was the peak expiratory flow level. However, neither intervention program succeeded in improving the mean peak flow level. In their review, Gibson et al. (2000) evaluated the effectiveness of asthma self-management programs. Although many programs were able to improve negative disease consequences like hospitalisation, days off work, and emergency room visits, lung function did not usually change.

Although we were able to show a significant reduction in symptom intensity over time, we were not able to document a parallel increase in PEF level. This effect has been reported repeatedly. Teeter and Bleeker (1998), for example, compared symptom intensity and PEF level in the hospital and during an eight-week follow-up. They found no correlation between changes in either parameters. Only the subjective symptoms improved, while the level of airway obstruction remained the same.

An important result pertaining to peak flow was that diurnal peak flow variability was reduced significantly in the experimental group. As we recorded patients' use of short acting beta-mimetics, we witnessed an overdosing in a few patients (Legoretta et al., 1998). During the education program, patients learned that medicaments for asthmatics are primarily inhalative corticosteroids at the present. After visiting a specialist, several patients changed their focus of asthma therapy from a short-acting beta-2-agonist, to inhalative corticosteroids for relaxing the bronchial muscles, and reducing the inflammation and hyper-responsiveness of their airways (Jans et al,

1998). A reduction in the inflammation of the airways leads to a diminished hyperresponsiveness and thus to a reduced variability in airway obstruction.

Quality of life

The experimental program yielded a significant improvement of quality of life over time. As the questionnaire includes the most important disease-related domains in the patients' daily living, it underlines the clinical relevance of individualized, monitoring-based patient education.

We assume that the individualized and personal problem-solving elements were most effective for making an improvement in the quality of life. Sommaruga et al. (1996) introduced cognitive behavioral elements in their asthma education. Although not measuring quality of life, they observed a reduction of the score of "external control", indicating an increase in the competence to influence the disease. Furthermore, we tried to strengthen the patients' capabilities in the doctor-patient communication during the course of our experimental group. Worstell (2000) presents the results of an interactive seminar for physicians on how to communicate better with their patients. This intervention led to significant improvement in medical and psychosocial parameters.

As a consequence of the psychological interventions, patients were able to change inadequate disease behavior with the aid of the security provided by daily monitoring and regular screening.

Symptoms

"Always looking into yourself makes you even sicker" is an accusation which is related to the question of an aggravation of symptoms through excessive self-monitoring.

In most cases, this mechanism is only activated under the participation of negative affectivity (Costa & McCrae, 1987). Stegen et al. (1998) carried out a study with a negative affectivity questionnaire and an experimental trial. In the questionnaire, subjects with high scores in negative affectivity reported significantly more symptoms than did subjects with low scores. However, if the CO_2 concentration of the air was increased experimentally, this difference disappeared. However, Watten and Batt (1996) found a positive correlation between negative affectivity and work-related symptom reporting. In their experimental study, Wiebe et al. (1994) supported the notion that there are different reporting patterns for diabetic complaints in people scoring differently in negative affectivity-related concepts like focus of attention and trait anxiety. As long as reinforced symptom perception is embedded in a positive frame like "While doing this, I am going to improve my therapy", attention driven symptom aggravation is unlikely. This framing suggests the controllability of a situation. Controllability is the positive influence to a symptom report (Thompson, 1981).

Our study documents a reduction of daily symptom reporting over time. On the symptom list of the electronic AM2, the answer category was the highest symptom intensity by default. Therefore, it may be assumed that the patients willingly decided in favour of weaker symptom intensities. This symptom reduction is in line with the other study results which suggest an improvement in the patients' disease.

Awareness of bronchoconstriction

A significant training effect was observed for the ability to perceive actual bronchoconstriction. Relevant training elements were the permanent feedback of symptoms and lung function, and the discussion and training of symptom perception. Recent publications stressed the strong relationship between asthma severity and symptom awareness, or perception of the actual lung function (Bijl-Hofland et al., 1999; Kikuchi et al., 1994; Laprise & Boulet, 1997). It is still under discussion whether the severity is followed by the unawareness or vice versa.

Conclusions and outlook

We based an individualized asthma patient education program on symptom perception and electronic ambulatory assessments. The program evaluation demonstrated a superiority of the new program in several medical and psychological parameters over a well-standardized group education program.

What may be the future developments for the area of computer-tailored programs and ambulatory assessment?

The present situation may go in two directions: firstly, strengthening of the patients' autonomy through home-based patient education programs and secondly, integrating diagnostic and therapeutic benefits of programs supported by ambulatory assessment in medical practice. Electronic diagnostic elements within ambulatory assessment of physiology and behavior shall become more sophisticated, for example, by using multiple sensors and/or more refined (bio)mathematical algorithms. Thus, more individualization will be possible in education programs. The general trend to patient empowerment, that is, integrating patients' will and health care activities into diagnostic and therapeutic processes, should be supported by this approach.

Acknowledgements

This research was supported by a grant of the German Research Foundation (DFG) awarded to the second author (Scha/308–11). We thank Andrea Sadorf and Evelyn Poth for their help in preparing and executing the patient education program.

References

Agras, W.S., Taylor, C.B., Feldman, D.E., Losch, M. et al. (1990). Developing computer-assisted therapy for the treatment of obesity. *Behavior Therapy, 21,* 99–109.

Asmar, R., Boutelant, S., Chaigon, M., Guedon, J., Topouchian, J., Mallion, J.-M. & Safar, M. (1996). Repeated measurements of non-invasive ambulatory blood pressure: Distinction between reproducibility and the proper effect of placebo. *Blood Pressure Monitoring, 1,* 283–288.

Bijl-Hofland, I.D. et al. (1999). Relation of the perception of airway obstruction to the severity of asthma. *Thorax, 54*, 15–19.

Binsted, K., Cawsey, A. & Jones, R.B. (1995). Generating personalised information using the medical record. In: *Artifical intelligence in medicine: Proceedings of AIME 95*, (pp. 29–41). New York: Springer Verlag.

Boggs, P.B., Hayati, F., Washburne, W.F. & Wheeler, D.A. (1999). Using statistical process control charts for the continual improvement of asthma care. *Joint Commission Journal on Quality Improvement, 25,* 163–81.

Boulet, L.P. (1998). Perception of the role and potential side effects of inhaled corticosteroids among asthmatic patients. *Chest, 113,* 587–92.

Brug, J., Campbell, M. & van Assema, P. (1999). The application and impact of computer-generated personalized nutrition education: A review of the literature. *Patient Education and Counseling, 36,* 145–156.

Buchanan, B.G., Moore, J., Forsythe, D., Banks, G. & Ohlsson, S. (1992). Involving patients in health care: Using medical informatics for explanation in the clinic. In: *Proceedings of the Symposium on Computer Applications in Medical Care,* (pp. 510–514).

Chambers, C.V., Markson, L., Diamond, J.J., Lasch, L. & Berger, M. (1999). Health beliefs and compliance with inhaled corticosteroids by asthmatic patients in primary care practices. *Respiratory Medicine, 93,* 88–94.

Chinn, S., Burney, P.G., Britton, J.R., Tattersfield, A.E. & Higgins, B.G. (1993). Comparison of PD20 with two alternative measures of response to histamine challenge in epidemiologic studies. *European Respiratory Journal, 6*, 670–679.

Chinn, S., Burney, P.G., Jarvis, D. & Lucynska, C. (1997). Variation in bronchial responsiveness in the European Community Respiratory Health Survey (ECRHS). *European Respiratory Journal, 10,* 2495–2501.

Cochrane, M.G., Bala, M.V., Downs, K.E., Mauskopf, J. & Ben Joseph, R.H. (2000). Inhaled corticosteroids for asthma therapy: patient compliance, devices, and inhalation technique. *Chest, 117,* 542–550.

Coiera, E. (2000). When conversation is better than computation. *Journal of the American Medical Informatics Association, 7*, 277–286.

Costa, P.T. Jr. & Mc Crae, R.R. (1987). Neuroticism, somatic complaints, and disease: Is the bark worse than the bite? *Journal of Personality, 55,* 299–316.

Cote, J., Cartier, A., Malo, J.L., Rouleau, M. & Boulet, L.P. (1998). Compliance with peak expiratory flow monitoring in home management of asthma. *Chest, 113,* 968–72.

Cox, D.J., Gonder-Frederick, L., Julian, D. & Cryer, P. (1991). Intensive versus standard blood glucose awareness training (BGAT) with insulin-dependent diabetes: Mechanisms and ancillary effects. *Psychosomatic Medicine, 53,* 453–462.

Crim, C. (2000). Clinical practice guidelines vs. actual clinical practice: The asthma paradigm. *Chest, 118*, 2 Suppl, 62S–64S.

Dahl, R. & Bjermer, L. (2000). Nordic consensus report on asthma management. Nordic Asthma Consensus Group. *Respiratory Medicine, 94*, 299–327.

Dahme, B., König, R., Nussbaum, B. & Richter, R. (1991). Haben Asthmatiker Defizite in der Symptomwahrnehmung? Quasi-experimentelle und experimentelle Befunde zur Interozeption der Atemwegsobstruktion. *Psychotherapie, Psychosomatik und Medizinische Psychologie, 41*, 490–499.

Detweiler, J.B., Bedell, B.T., Pronin, E. & Rothman, A.J. (1999). Message framing and sunscreen use: Gain-framed messages motivate beach-goers. *Health Psychology, 18,* 189–196.

de Vries, H. & Brug, J. (1999). Computer-tailored interventions motivating people to adopt health promoting behaviors: Introduction to a new approach. *Patient Education and Counseling, 36,* 99–105.

Fishbein, M., von Haeften, I., Hall-Jamieson, K., Johnson, B. & Kirkland Ahern, R. (2000). Evaluation of anti-drug public service announcements (PSAs): Comparison of computer-assisted and paper and pencil methodologies in a sample of adolescents from the boys and girls clubs of metropolitan Philadelphia. *Psychology, Health & Medicine, 5,* 259–270.

Friedman, R.H., Kazis, L.E., Jette, A., Smith, M.B., Stollerman, J., Torgerson, J. & Carey, K. (1996). A telecommunications system for monitoring and counseling patients with hypertension. Impact on medication adherence and blood pressure control. *American Journal of Hypertension, 9,* 285–92.

Friedman, R.H., Stollerman, J.E., Mahoney, D.M. & Rozenblyum, L. (1997). The virtual visit: Using telecommunications technology to take care of patients. *Journal of the American Medical Informatics Association, 4,* 413–25.

Gibson, P.G., Talbot, P.I., Hancock, J. & Hensley, M.J. (1993). A prospective audit of asthma management following emergency asthma treatment at a teaching hospital. *Medical Journal of Australia, 158,* 775–8.

Gibson, P.G., Coughlan, J., Wilson, A.J., Abramson, M., Bauman, A., Hensley, M.J. & Walters (2000) Self-management education and regular practitioner review for adults with asthma. *Cochrane database systematic review, 2,* CD001117.

GINA. Global Initiative For Asthma (1996). *Global strategy for asthma management and prevention NHLBI/WHO workshop report.* National Institutes of Health. National Heart, Lung, and Blood Institute. Publication Number 95–3659.

Harver, A. (1994). Effects of feedback on the ability of asthmatic subjects to detect increases in the flow-resistive component to breathing. *Health Psychology, 13,* 52.62.

James, L., Carroll, N., De Klerk, N., Elliott, J., Musk, A.W. & Ryan, G. (1998). Increased perception of airway narrowing in patients with mild asthma. *Respirology, 3,* 241–245.

Jans, M.P., Schellevis, F.G., van Hensbergen, W., Dukkers van Emden, T. & van Eijk, J.T. (1998). Management of asthma and COPD patients: Feasibility of the application of guidelines in general practice. *International Journal for Quality in Health Care, 10,* 27–34.

Kahn, M.G., Abrams, C.A., Orland, M.J. et al. (1991). Intelligent computer-based interpretation and graphical presentation of self-monitored blood glucose and insulin data. *Diabetes, Nutrition and Metabolism, 4,* 99–107.

Kikuchi, Y., Okabe, S., Tamura, G., Hida, W., Homma, M., Shirato, K. & Takishima, T. (1994). Chemosensitivity and perception of dyspnea in patients with a history of near-fatal asthma. *New England Journal of Medicine, 330,* 1329–1334.

Lalloo, U.G. & Motala, C. (2000). Guidelines for the management of chronic asthma in children and adults (editorial). *South African Medical Journal, 90,* 488.

Laprise, C. & Boulet, L.P. (1997). Asymptomatic airway hyperresponsiveness: A three-year follow-up. *American Journal of Respiratory and Critical Care Medicine, 156,* 403–409.

Lebowitz, M.J. (1991). The use of peak expiratory flow rate measurements in respiratory disease. *Pediatric Pulmonology, 11,* 166–174.

Lefkowitz, D, Klimas, J.T. & Ross, R.N. (1996). Comparison of a new hand-held interactive airway monitoring system and a conventional peak expiratory flow meter in the management of asthma. *American Journal of Managed Care, 2,* 1227–1235.

Legorreta, A.P., Christian-Herman, J., O'Connorm, R.D., Hasan, M.M., Evans, R. & Leung, K.M. (1998). Compliance with national asthma management guidelines and specialty care: A health maintenance organization experience. *Archives of Internal Medicine, 158,* 457–64.

Lewis, C.E. et al. (1984). A randomized trial of A.C.T. (asthma care training) for kids. *Pediatrics, 74,* 478–486.

Mansoor, G.A., Filho, A.J. P. & White, W.B. (1996). Effects of three methods of analysis on ambulatory blood pressure indices and the early morning rise in blood pressure. *Blood Pressure*

Monitoring, 1, 355–360.

Marks, I.M., Baer, L., Greist, J.H., et al. (1998). Home self-assessment of obsessive-compulsive disorder: Use of a manual and a computer-conducted telephone call. *British Journal of Psychiatry, 172,* 406–412.

Murray, C.J.L. & Lopez, A. D. (1997). Mortality by cause for eight regions of the world: Global burden of Disease Study. *Lancet, 349,* 1269.

Mussgay, L & Rüddel, H. (1996). Ambulatory blood pressure monitoring: Promises and limitations in behavioral medicine. In J. Fahrenberg. & M. Myrtek. (Eds.). *Ambulatory Assessment: Computer-assisted psychological and psychophysiological methods in monitoring and field studies,* (pp. 365–374). Göttingen: Hogrefe & Huber.

Osman, L.M., Abdulla, M.I., Beattie, J.A. G., Ross, S., Russell, I.T., Friend, J.A. et al. (1994). Reducing hospital admission through computer-supported education for asthma patients. *British Medical Journal, 308,* 568–71.

Paperny, D.M.N. (1997). Computerized health assessment and education for adolescent HIV and STD prevention in health care settings and schools. *Health Education and Behavior, 24,* 54–70.

Petro, W. (1997) (Ed.). *Patientenverhaltenstraining bei obstruktiven Atemwegserkrankungen.* München: Dustri Verlag.

Prittwitz, M., Betz, H.P., Lauber, B., Härtl, W., Selke, J., Kaspar, P., Morawa, R., Fleischer, M. & Petro, W. (1989). Bad Reichenhaller Modell der Patientenschulung Asthma, Bronchitis, Emphysem. In W. Petro (Ed.). *Patientenschulung für Atemwegserkrankte* (pp. 217–230). München: Dustri.

Quackenboss, J.J., Lebowitz, M.J. & Krzyzanowski, M. (1991). The normal range of diurnal changes in peak expiratory flow rates. Relationship to symptoms and respiratory disease. *American Review of Respiratory Diseases, 143,* 323–330.

Redline, S., Wright, E.C., Kattan, M., Kercsmar, C. & Weiss, K. (1996). Short-term compliance with peak flow monitoring: results from a study of inner city children with asthma. *Pediatric Pulmonology, 21,* 203–10.

Ryff-De Lèche, A., Engler, H., Nützi, E., Berger, M. & Berger, W. (1992). Clinical application of two computerized diabetes management systems: Comparison with the log-book method. *Diabetes Research, 19,* 97–105.

Schandry, R. (1995). *Fragebogen für Asthmapatienten. Handanweisung und Fragebogen.* Frankfurt a.M.: Swets.

Schultz, K., Stark, H.J. & Petro, W. (1996). Standardisiertes Trainingsprogramm für Hausstaubmilbenallergiker. *Pneumologie, 50,* 158.

Sheffer, A.L. & Taggart, V.S. (1993). The National Asthma Education Program. Expert panel report guidelines for the diagnosis and management of asthma. National Heart, Lung, and Blood Institute. *Medical Care, 31,* MS20–28.

Sommaruga, M., Spanevello, A., Migliori, G.B., Neri, M., Callegari, S. & Majani, G. (1995). The effects of a cognitive behavioral intervention in asthmatic patients. *Monaldi Archives for Chest Disease, 50,* 398–402.

Sorbi, M.J., Honkoop, P.C. & Godaert, G.L.R. (1996). A signal-contingent computer diary for the assessment of psychological precedents of the migraine attack. In J. Fahrenberg & M. Myrtek (Eds.), *Ambulatory assessment: Computer-assisted psychological and psychophysiological methods in monitoring and field studies* (pp. 403–412). Göttingen: Hogrefe & Huber.

Stegen, K., Neujens, A., Crombez, G., Hermans, D., Van de Woestijne, K.P. & Van den Bergh, O. (1998). Negative affect, respiratory reactivity, and somatic complaints in a CO2 enriched air inhalation paradigm. *Biological Psychology, 49,* 109–22.

Strecher, V.J. (1999). Computer-tailored smoking cessation materials: A review and discussion. *Patient Education and Counseling, 36,* 107–17.

Szczepanski, R., Brockmann, G., Könning, J., Schmidt, S. & Wegner, R.E. (1994). Zur Lebensqualität von Kindern mit Asthma bronchiale. In F. Petermann & K.-C. Bergmann (Eds.). Lebensqualität und Asthma (pp. 123–132). München: Quintessenz

Taylor, D.M., Auble, T.E., Calhoun, W.J., Mosesso, V.N., Jr. (1999). Current outpatient management of asthma shows poor compliance with International Consensus Guidelines. *Chest, 116*, 1638–45.

Teeter, J.G. & Bleeker, E.R. (1998). Relationship between airway obstruction and respiratory symptoms in adult asthmatics. *Chest, 113,* 272–77.

Thompson, S.C. (1981). Will it hurt less if I can control it? A complex answer to a simple question. *Psychological Bulletin, 90*, 89–101.

van der Palen, J., Klein, J.J. & Rovers, M.M. (1997). Compliance with inhaled medication and self-treatment guidelines following a self-management program in adult asthmatics. *European Respiratory Journal, 10*, 652–57

van Essen-Zandvliet, E.E. et al. (1992). Effects of 22 months of treatment with inhaled corticosteroids and/or beta2-agonists on lung function, airway responsiveness, and symptoms in children with asthma. The Dutch Chronic Nonspecific Lung Disease Study Group. *American Review of Respiratory Diseases, 146,* 547–554.

van Wijk, C.M. & Kolk A.M. (1997). Sex differences in physical symptoms: The contribution of symptom perception theory. *Social Science and Medicine, 45*, 231–46.

Watten, R.G. & Batt, B. (1996). Negative affectivity influences report of work-related symptoms. *Journal of Human Ergology, 25,* 131–44.

Wiebe, D.J., Alderfer, M.A., Palmer, S.C., Lindsay, R. & Jarrett, L. (1994). Behavioral self-regulation in adolescents with type I diabetes: negative affectivity and blood glucose symptom perception. *Journal of Consulting and Clinical Psychology, 62*, 1204–212.

Woeller, W., Kruse, J., Winter, P., Mans, E.J. & Alberti L.T.I. (1993). Cortisone image and emotional support by key figures in patients with bronchial asthma. An empirical study. *Psychotherapy and Psychosomatics, 59*, 190–6.

Worstell, M. (2000). Asthma: Individual patient perspective and current unmet needs. *Clinical and Experimental Allergy, 30*, 11–5.

Yoos, H.L. & McMullen, A. (1999). Symptom perception and evaluation in childhood asthma. *Nursing Research, 48,* 2–8.

Chapter 30
Ambulatory Assessment of Hypoglycemia Unawareness in Type 1 Diabetes

Thomas Kubiak and Norbert Hermanns
Research Institute of the Diabetes Academy Mergentheim, Diabetes Center Mergentheim, Bad Mergentheim, Germany

Introduction

In type 1 diabetes, a disorder in carbohydrate metabolism caused by an absolute insulin deficiency necessitates the patient to substitute insulin. This includes subcutaneous administration of insulin several times a day and adapting the dosages to exercise and carbohydrate intake, as well as performing blood glucose (BG) self-measurements (cf. Davidson, 2000). Primary goal is to avoid prolonged elevated BG values (hyperglycemia; BG > ~160 mg $\times$ dl^{-1}) in order to prevent severe long-term diabetic complications (for example, blindness, renal failure, polyneuropathy) the development and progression of which are largely determined by chronic hyperglycemia (cf. The DCCT Research Group, 1993; American Diabetes Association, 2001). To assess achieved metabolic control, glycated hemoglobin values (HbA_1, HbA_{1c}) are referred to reflecting average BG levels of the past two to three months.

Hypoglycemia (low BG levels, BG < ~ 60 mg $\times$ dl^{-1}) is a major limiting factor in achieving good glycemic control (Cryer, 1997). Hypoglycemia occurs whenever there is a mismatch between administered amount of insulin and required dose (for example, in case of non-routine exercise) that lets BG levels drop (Amiel, 1993). At certain glycemic thresholds, low BG normally triggers a cascade of mostly hormonal counterregulatory mechanisms in order to autonomously prevent or correct hypoglycemia (Cryer, 1997). Part of this cascade is an intense sympathoadrenergic activation with concurrent increased secernation of epinephrine from the adrenal medullae. Besides autonomic activation, hypoglycemia leads to acute cerebral glucose deprivation (neuroglycopenia) which results in initially mild cognitive dysfunction progressing as BG drops.

Usually, patients detect hypoglycemia because of typical hypoglycemia warning symptoms (Hepburn et al., 1991; Deary, 1999). Thus, if hypoglycemia is detected, adequate self-treatment can be initiated (intake of fast-acting carbohydrates to elevate BG to normal; cf. Gonder-Frederick, Cox, Kovatchev, Schlundt & Clarke,

1997). Sympathoadrenergic counterregulation is associated with autonomic symptoms (for example, pounding heart, sweating, trembling), cerebral glucose deprivation with neuroglycopenic symptoms (for example, difficulty in speaking, emotional changes, lapses of attention; Deary, 1999). Although it is difficult to classify patients' subjective symptom reports concerning their symptoms' neuroglycopenic or autonomic nature, there is evidence that initially neuroglycopenic symptoms are subtle and harder to perceive than autonomic symptoms associated with intense sympathoadrenergic activation (Towler, Havlin, Craft & Cryer, 1993; Frier, 1999).

Symptomatic mild hypoglycemia, as described above, can be detected and treated by the patient himself. *Severe hypoglycemia*, however, results from BG levels dropping that low that the patient is unable to take action anymore (due to advanced neuroglycopenia), finally leading to helplessness or even hypoglycemic coma. Severe hypoglycemia poses a significant threat and may cause bodily damage (for example, accident hazard, permanent brain damage, acute cardiovascular dysfunction; Deary, 1999; Fisher & Heller, 1999; Perros & Deary, 1999). Whereas symptomatic mild hypoglycemia cannot be avoided in insulin therapy optimized to reduce risk for development of diabetic complications, the occurrence of recurrent severe hypoglycemia has to be minimized (Bolli, 1999).

Hypoglycemia Unawareness Syndrome

A common adverse effect of near-normal glycemic control is the development of so called hypoglycemia unawareness with an estimated prevalence of approximately 25% (Hepburn et al., 1990; Pramming, Thornsteinsson, Bendtson & Binder, 1991). Hypoglycemia unawareness syndrome (HU-syndrome) consists of partial or complete loss of hypoglycemia warning symptoms resulting in a reduced ability to perceive hypoglycemia and to initiate self-treatment in time (Frier, 1999). In its typical clinical presentation, patients report of hardly sensing any symptoms of developing hypoglycemia, at worst leading to recurrent sudden severe hypoglycemic episodes. HU-syndrome is one of the most important risk factors for occurrence of severe hypoglycemia (Gold, MacLeod & Frier, 1994; Gold, Frier, MacLeod & Deary, 1997). Etiology of the presumably heterogenous HU-syndrome is unknown in detail, a multifactorial origin can be assumed. However, some crucial etiological factors have already been identified (Frier, 1999). One major etiological factor for HU-syndrome development is the frequent exposure to low BG levels (mild hypoglycemia), which is largely determined by the individual's diabetes-related self-care behavior. Frequent exposure to mild hypoglycemia induces a reversible central nervous adaptation process which leads to shifting of glycemic thresholds for the protective physiological responses to hypoglycemia (lower BG levels necessary to trigger responses) resulting in loss or delay of autonomic symptoms and impaired perception of hypoglycemia ("hypoglycemia-associated autonomic failure"; Cryer, 1997).

Due to loss/delay of autonomic symptoms, patients with HU-syndrome have to rely more on initially subtle neuroglycopenic effects as symptoms to detect (Frier, 1999). Due to shift of glycemic thresholds the patient's "time window" for action to take is narrowed (from onset of symptoms/detection of hypoglycemia until helplessness because of severe neuroglycopenia).

Commonly Used Diagnostic Procedures

In clinical settings, the diagnosis of HU-syndrome often relies on the patient's or practitioner's overall retrospective judgment of exposure to mild hypoglycemic episodes, occurrence of severe hypoglycemia, and quality symptom perception. In research, experimentally induced hypoglycemia is usually investigated to assess glycemic thresholds of hypoglycemia-related physiological responses and reported symptoms (Heine, 1993). While the latter method is highly invasive (requiring i. v. cannulae to be placed), very costly, time-consuming and, for clinical purposes, lakking ecological validity (for example, concerning reactivity of symptom assessment in laboratory settings), the former method based on overall judgments is susceptible of retrospection bias and far away from actual self-care behavior making its reliability and validity questionable.

Finally, in clinical practice as well as epidemiological research, several easily obtainable parameters are used to assess risk of future severe hypoglycemia and HU-syndrome, among others HbA_{1c} ("low" near-normal glycated hemoglobin strongly associated with higher risk for severe hypoglycemia; The DCCT Research Group, 1993), diagnosis of neuropathy (a putative cause for irreversible loss of autonomic reactions to hypoglycemia; cf. Bottini et al., 1997), C-peptide (as a measure for remaining endogenous insulin production considered a protective factor; Bott, Bott, Berger & Mühlhauser, 1997), and duration of disease (as a descriptive marker as, for example, disease duration is associated with occurrence of neuropathy and low C-peptide). Main advantage of these parameters lies in their ready availability, the low specifity with regard to HU-syndrome being a major drawback, though.

In the next two sections, practicable techniques for ambulatory assessment of two key factors of HU-syndrome that offer the possibility to overcome the shortcoming of the commonly used methods described will be outlined from a clinical perspective: (1) self-care behavior (exposure to low BG), and (2) quality of symptom perception.

Assessment of Relevant Self-Care Behavior

Blood Glucose Memory Meters

As described, the development of a HU-syndrome is largely determined by the frequency of exposure to low BG levels, which, in turn, is determined by the individual's self-care behavior, that is, how low his individual BG target values are and how low BG has to drop for the patient to initiate self-treatment. Insulin therapy requires frequent BG self-measurements on a regular basis. Nowadays, most people with diabetes use BG meters with memory function, that store from 100 up to ~900 values depending on the model used. The data gathered via patients' memory meters provide an objective measure reflecting "every day" self-care behavior, for example, in terms of how low and how often does a patient allow his BG to drop (cf. Cox, Kovatchev & Julian, 1994; Kovatchev et al., 1997).

Table 1 depicts correlations between number of severe hypoglycemic episodes (past 12 months), common risk markers for severe hypoglycemia (HbA_{1c}, diabetes duration, polyneuropathy , C-peptide, disease duration), and the proportion of BG values in hypoglycemic range (< 60 mg $\times$ dl^{-1}) computed from memory meter data that were obtained from 61 type 1 diabetics prior to inpatient treatment[1] (M ± SD: age [yrs.] 37.7 ± 11.4, duration of diabetes [yrs.] 17.3 ± 9.5; number of BG measurements 316.4 ± 377.6). A significant correlation between proportion of low BG readings and number of severe hypoglycemic episodes is observable. Note, that all of the commonly used risk factors fail to correlate significantly with severe hypoglycemia. Despite the expectable high intercorrelation between HbA_{1c} and low BG readings, a gain in variance explanation is reached if relying on BG data (partial correlation controlling for HbA_{1c}: $r=.30$; $p<.05$).

Table 1. Correlations between number of severe hypoglycemic episodes (past 12 months), conventional biomedical risk factors (HbA1c, peripheral neuropathy, C-peptide) and proportion of low blood glucose values (<60 mg x dl-1) as computed from blood glucose data (N=61).

	SH episodes	HbA_{1c}[a]	Low BG	PNP[b]	C-peptide[c]	DD
SH episodes	-					
HbA_{1c}	-.24[d]	-				
Low BG	.37**	-.41**	-			
PNP	-.06	.24	-.06	-		
C-peptide	-.09	.06	-.17	-.08	-	
DD	.21	-.13	.14	.27*	-.27*	-

Notes. SH episodes: number of severe hypoglycemic episodes (requiring i. v. glucose or i. m. glucagon treatment). Low BG: proportion of low blood glucose values (< 60 mg $\times dl^{-1}$). PNP: peripheral neuropathy. DD: duration of diabetes (yrs.). Coefficients displayed are Pearson coefficients. For correlations with PNP, Spearman's rank correlations were computed.

[a] Range in non-diabetics (%): 4.3–6.1

[b] Diagnosis of neuropathy according to 128 Hz tuning fork probe (5/8 criterion).

[c] C-peptide (nmol×L^{-1}; sulphonylurea stimulated) as measure for remaining endogenous insulin secretion.

**p<.01; [d] p=.059

These descriptive results based on retrospective number of severe hypoglycemia are substantiated by trying to predict future severe hypoglycemia (6.1 ± 2.8 months follow-up) via backward stepwise logistic regression (probability to remove p=.15). On the first three steps C-peptide, diabetes duration, and polyneuropathy are eliminated leading to the final model containing low BG readings and HbA_{1c} as predictors achieving an explanation of variance of 24% (MacFadden's Rho^2=.234; Table 2).

Table 2. Logistic regression for prediction of occurrence of severe hypoglycemia (N=61, follow-up: 6.1 ± 2.8 months).

	coefficient	SE	t	odds ratio
constant	-9.61	3.26	-2.95^{**}	
proportion low BG (< 60 mg × dl^{-1})	0.19	0.07	2.69^{**}	1.20
HbA_{1c} [a]	0.69	0.35	1.99^{*}	1.99

Notes. Log likelihood: -21.74^{**}; MacFadden's Rho^2=.234; BG: blood glucose. Bounds for odds ratios (95%), low BG: 1.378 (upper), 1.052 (lower); HbA_{1c}: 3.948 (upper), 1.01 (lower)

[a] Range in non-diabetics (%): 4.3-6.1

* p<.05

** p<.01

Results of retrospective correlations and prospective logistic regression analysis point to a possible advantage of BG data to determine patients' risk for occurrence of severe hypoglycemia compared with conventional risk markers, even possibly being of higher predictive value than glycated hemoglobin. This potential advantage could justify the higher amount of time and effort needed for BG data analysis.

Continuous Blood Glucose Monitoring

Portable continuous BG monitor systems have become available recently (Continuous Glucose Measurement System®, CGMS®, MiniMed™, Sylmar CA, USA; Bode, Gross, Thornton & Mastrototaro, 1999; Mastrototaro, 1999), that allow for ambulatory monitoring BG levels for up to 72 hours. The use of the device is invasive, requiring a subcutaneous catheter to be inserted. The major advantage of the CGMS for assessing hypoglycemia awareness is the opportunity to *continuously* register BG levels in a non-reactive way (the device does not support online display of BG values), whereas BG data drawn from meters is based on point measurements relying on the frequency the patients measure their BG (cf. Bolinder, Hagstroem-Toft, Ungerstedt & Arner, 1997). Furthermore, the CGMS allows for entering events comparable to similar features in 24h-blood pressure-measurement. For example patients can enter an event if they feel hypoglycemia symptoms and suspect hypoglycemia allowing to compute a rate of hypoglycemia detection. Table 3 illustrates results of a pilot study with 12 type 1 diabetics using the CGMS. Patients were classified as hypoglycemia unaware (N=6; M ± SD: age [yrs.] 38.5 ± 12.7, duration of diabetes [yrs.] 21.0 ± 10.9) vs. aware(N=6; M ± SD: age [yrs.] 37.0 ± 11.6, duration of diabetes [yrs.] 19.0 ± 11.4) on the basis of self-assessment and past severe hypoglycemia. Continuous BG monitoring was performed for 56 ± 11.9 hours (M ± SD). Note, that hypoglycemia unaware patients fail to detect hypoglycemia more often. Unfortunately, in clinical practice, CGMS use is limited by the maximal duration of 72 hours (compared to several months of BG data one is able to collect using meters) and the currently high costs associated with its use (momentarily, in Germany, approx. $3,000 per device, $50 per use).

Table 3. Results of pilot study on use of continuous blood glucose monitoring in hypoglycemia aware vs. unaware type 1 diabetics.

	aware[a] (N=6)	unaware (N=6)
mean BG (mg x dl^{-1})	128.9 ± 22.4	108.5 ± 18.6
hypoglycemic episodes (< 60 mg × dl^{-1}, episodes/24h)	2.3 ± 1.6	5.2 ± 2.5*
detected episodes[b] (%)	61.7 ± 44.9	6.8 ± 10.7*

Notes. All values M±SD. BG: blood glucose.
[a] Operationalization of unawareness based on criterion of impaired hypoglycemia awareness in self-assessment plus at least one severe hypoglycemic episode in the past 12 months (as opposed to none in aware group).
[b] Detected episodes as entered via event function directly into the monitoring system.
* p<.05

Assessment of Symptom Perception

Quality of hypoglycemia symptom perception can be assessed using hand-held computers (HHC; Clarke et al., 1995; Schandry & Leopold, 1996) giving the opportunity of in-field symptom assessment instead of relying on an overall retrospective judgment of symptom perception quality and, compared with conventional diary techniques, the possibility of exact time measurements and administration of cognitive performance tests.

To address the issue of quality of symptom perception in diabetics, HHC (PSION™ Series 3a®, PLC London, Great Britain) were handed out to 68 type 1 patients for one week during inpatient treatment (M ± SD, age [yrs.] 30.8 ± 12.1; duration of disease [yrs.] 14.9 ± 8.6). Autonomic (trembling, pounding heart, sweating) and neuroglycopenic (difficulty concentrating, tiredness) symptom report data were acquired and a reaction choice test administered via HHC. Furthermore, patients entered BG estimations prior to entering their BG measurements Patients were not prompted to perform a HHC protocol, but were to trigger protocols themselves (number of trials performed M ± SD, 36.0 ± 21.1). Out of 68 patients, 49 (N=37 hypoglycemia aware vs. N=12 unaware patients) experienced mild hypoglycemic episodes while using the HHC (Table 4). Aware and unaware patients differ significantly in autonomic and neuroglycopenic symptom increase during hypoglycemia (computed as z-scores from individual euglycemic baselines) with the unaware group showing hardly any increase. On group level, neuroglycopenic effects regarding errors in choice reaction task are clearly observable. Effects on reaction time, however, fail to reach significance with the unaware patients experience no substantial deterioration on group level. Results suggest that some unaware patients actually experience neuroglycopenic effects (errors) they do not, for some reason, perceive as symptoms. Detection rate of hypoglycemia differs notably between groups. Note the difference between detection rates as observed in the CGMS pilot study described. One possible explanation – besides the small sample of the CGMS study – may lie in the longer period of time of HHC use (7 days vs. 2-3 days).

Table 4. Symptom report, choice reaction test, and hypoglycemia detection rates in hypoglycemia aware vs. unaware patients (hand-held computer data; N=49).

	aware[a] (N=37)	unaware (N=12)
Proportion hypoglycemic readings (< 60 mg × dl^{-1})	21.54 ± 32.2	35.64 ± 27.5
Symptom increase[b]		
- autonomic	2.17 ± 2.5	0.90 ± 0.4**
- neuroglycopenic	0.98 ± 1.5	-0.01 ± 0.01**
Cognitive deterioration[b]		
- reaction time (ms)	0.45 ± 1.7	0.07 ± 1.5
- errors (number)	1.83 ± 5.3	1.63 ± 4.2
Detection rates		
- overall hypoglycemia detection[c] (%)	34.39 ± 34.1	12.96 ± 18.8**
- detection with symptom increase[d] (%)	18.22 ± 20.1	6.8 ± 15.4[e]
- detection without symptom increase (%)	16.17 ± 30.0	6.1 ± 14.3

Notes. All values M±SD.

[a] Operationalization of unawareness based on criterion of impaired hypoglycemia awareness in self-assessment plus at least one severe hypoglycemic episode in the past 12 months (as opposed to none in aware group).

[b] Symptom increase and cognitive deterioration calculated as z-scores based on individual euglycemic baselines.

[c] Detection rates based on individual differences in measured blood glucose vs. prior estimation of blood glucose level.

[d] Significant symptom increase defined via one SD criterion based on individual euglycemic baselines.

** $p<.01$; [e] $p=.092$

Interestingly, on group level not all detected episodes are accompanied with significant symptom increase (one SD criterion based on euglycemic baseline), neither in aware nor unaware patients. These results suggest a possible role not only of internal symptoms, but also of external cues (for example, situational, social context, knowledge about time course of insulin action; cf. Frier, 1999) or potential distractions, for example leading to wrong interpretation of symptoms as not hypoglycemia-associated (cf. Gonder-Frederick et al., 1997).

Conclusions

Presently used methods for assessment of hypoglycemia unawareness are retrospective overall judgments far away from actual self-care behavior or laboratory studies with questionable results regarding external validity and transfer to every-day settings. Furthermore, most often biomedical risk markers (for example, HbA_{1c}, neuropathy) are referred to. These parameters are usually readily available and, at least glycated hemoglobin, a strong predictor of future hypoglycemia. However, these markers lack specifity regarding hypoglycemia unawareness and relevant etiological factors, like self-care behavior and symptom perception.

Ambulatory assessment techniques as outlined in this chapter can make a significant contribution to clinical management of hypoglycemia unawareness in type 1 diabetes. Using ambulatory assessment, exposure to low BG as assessed by memory meter data provide a valid and realistic operationalization of HU-syndrome relevant self-care behavior. Thus, by means of BG data assessment, intraindividual evaluation of treatment efforts and, enhancing prognostic validity based on common biomedical markers, prediction of future risk for HU-syndrome development could be made feasible in clinical settings. Use of continuous BG measurement, though still expensive, can provide a way of assessing exposure to low BG without having to rely on patients' adherence to self-testing. Furthermore, continuous BG monitoring would allow for obtaining data concerning the duration of exposure to low BG as well (as opposed to merely quantifying the number of low BG episodes). Duration of low BG can be assumed to be an important etiological factor for hypoglycemia unawareness not studied yet in the field. Furthermore, use of hand-held computers provides a means for valid assessment of hypoglycemia warning symptoms and offers possibilities to reveal interoception characteristics remaining unknown if assessed retrospectively.

References

American Diabetes Association (2001). Clinical Practice Recommendation 2001. *Diabetes Care, 24* (Suppl. 1).

Amiel, S.A. (1993). The risks of hypoglycaemia with insulin therapy. In B.M. Frier & B.M. Fisher (Eds.), *Hypoglycaemia and diabetes. Clinical and physiological aspects* (pp. 302–327). London: Edward Arnold.

Bode, B., Gross, T., Thornton, K. & Mastrototaro, J. (1999). Continuous glucose monitoring used to adjust diabetes improves glycosylated hemoglobin: a pilot study. *Diabetes Research and Clinical Practice, 46*, 183–190.

Bolinder, J., Hagstroem-Toft, E., Ungerstedt, U. & Arner, P. (1997). Self-monitoring of blood-glucose in type I diabetic patients: comparison with continuous microdialysis measurements of glucose in subcutaneous adipose tissue during ordinary life conditions. *Diabetes Care, 20*, 64–70.

Bolli, G.B. (1999). How to ameliorate the problem of hypoglycemia in intensive as well as non-intensive treatment of type1 diabetes. *Diabetes Care, 22* (Suppl. 2), 843–852.

Bott, S., Bott, M., Berger, M. & Mühlhauser, I. (1997). Intensified insulin therapy and the risk of severe hypoglycaemia. *Diabetologia, 40*, 926–932.

Bottini, P., Boschetti, E., Campanelli, S., Ciofetta, M., Del Sindaco, P., Scionti, P., Brunetti, P. & Bolli, G.B. (1997). Contribution of autonomic neuropathy to reduced plasma adrenaline responses to hypoglycemia in IDDM. Evidence for an non-selective defect. *Diabetes, 46*, 814–823.

Clarke, W.L., Cox, D.J., Gonder-Frederick, L.A. & Julian, D. (1995). Reduced awareness of hypoglycemia in adults with IDDM. A prospective study of hypoglycemic frequency and associated symptoms. *Diabetes Care, 18*, 517–522.

Cox, D.J., Kovatchev, B.P. & Julian, D.M. (1994). Frequency of severe hypoglycemia in insulin-dependent diabetes mellitus can be predicted from self-monitoring blood glucose data. *Journal of Clinical Endocrinology and Metabolism, 79*, 1659–1662.

Cryer, P. (1997). *Hypoglycemia. Pathophysiology, diagnosis, and treatment.* Oxford: Oxford University Press.

Davidson, J.K (2000). *Clinical Diabetes. A problem-oriented approach.* Stuttgart: Thieme.

Deary, I.J. (1999). Symptoms of hypoglycaemia and effects on mental performance and emotions. In B.M. Frier & B.M. Fisher (Eds.), *Hypoglycaemia in Clinical Diabetes* (pp. 29–54). New York: Wiley.

Fisher, B.M. & Heller, S.R. (1999). Mortality, cardiovascular morbidity and possible effects of hypoglycaemia on diabetic complications. In B.M. Frier & B.M. Fisher (Eds.), *Hypoglycaemia in Clinical Diabetes* (pp. 167–186). New York: Wiley.

Frier, B.M. (1999). Impaired hypoglycaemia awareness. In B.M. Frier & B.M. Fisher (Eds.), *Hypoglycaemia in Clinical Diabetes* (pp. 111–146). New York: Wiley.

Gold, A.E., MacLeod, K.M. & Frier, B.M. (1994). Frequency of severe hypoglycemia in patients with type 1 diabetes with impaired awareness of hypoglycemia. *Diabetes Care, 17*, 697–703.

Gold, A.E., Frier, B.M., MacLeod, K.M. & Deary, I.J. (1997). A structural equation model for predictors of severe hypoglycaemia in patients with insulin-dependent diabetes mellitus. *Diabetic Medicine, 14*, 309–315.

Gonder-Frederick, L., Cox, D.J., Kovatchev, B., Schlundt, D. & Clarke, W.L. (1997). A biopsychobehavioral model of risk of severe hypoglycemia. *Diabetes Care, 20*, 661–669.

Heine, R.J. (1993). Methods of investigation of insulin-induced hypoglycaemia. In B.M. Frier & B.M. Fisher (Eds.), *Hypoglycaemia and diabetes. Clinical and physiological aspects* (pp. 165–175). London: Edward Arnold.

Hepburn, D.A., Patrick, A.W., Eadington, D.W., Ewing, D.J. & Frier, B.M. (1990). Unawareness of hypoglycaemia in insulin-treated diabetic patients: prevalence and relationship to autonomic neuropathy. *Diabetic Medicine*, *7*, 711–717.

Hepburn, D.A., Deary, I.J., Frier, B.M., Patrick, A.W., Quinn, J.D. & Fisher, B.M. (1991). Symptoms of acute insulin-induced hypoglycemia in humans with and without IDDM, Factor-analysis approach. *Diabetes Care*, *14*, 949–957.

Kovatchev, B.P., Cox, D.J., Gonder-Frederick, L.A., Young-Hyman, D., Schlundt, D. & Clarke, W. (1998). Assessment of risk of severe hypoglycemia among adults with IDDM. Validation of the low blood glucose index. *Diabetes Care*, *21*, 1870–1875.

Mastrototaro, J. (1999). The MiniMed continuous glucose monitoring system (CGMS). *Journal of Pediatric Endocrinology and Metabolism*, *12* (Suppl. 3), 751–758.

Perros, P. & Deary, I.J. (1999). Long-term effects of hypoglycaemia on cognitive function and the brain in diabetes. In B.M. Frier & B.M. Fisher (Eds.), *Hypoglycaemia in Clinical Diabetes* (pp. 187–210). New York: Wiley.

Pramming, S., Thornsteinsson, B., Bendtson, I. & Binder, C. (1991). Symptomatic hypoglycaemia in 411 type I diabetic patients. *Diabetic Medicine*, *8*, 217–222.

Schandry, R. & Leopold, C. (1996). Ambulatory assessment of self-monitored subjective and objective symptoms in diabetic patients. In J. Fahrenberg & M. Myrtek (Eds.), *Ambulatory assessment. Computer-assisted psychological and psychophysiological methods in monitoring and field studies* (pp. 393–402). Seattle, WA: Hogrefe.

The DCCT Research Group (1993). The effect of intensive treatment of diabetes on the development and progression of long-term complications in insulin-dependent diabetes mellitus. *New England Journal of Medicine*, *329*, 977–986.

Towler, D.A., Havlin, C.E., Craft, S. & Cryer, P. (1993), Mechanisms of awareness of hypoglycaemia. Perception of neurogenic (predominantly cholinergic) rather than neuroglycopenic symptoms. *Diabetes*, *42*, 1791–1798.

Chapter 31
Feasibility of Ambulatory Sleep Diagnosis

Egon Stephan, Dirk Alfer, Ansgar Feist, Leonie Fricke, Markus Mühlensiep, Rolf K. Weiss, and Jörn P. Sieb
Department of Psychology, University of Cologne, Germany

Introduction

Sleep disorders, such as difficulties in sleep onset and maintenance, are amongst the most frequent complaints in medical practice. In western industrialized nations, the prevalence of sleep disorders amounts to approx. 20 – 30 % of the population. About half of the affected persons are in need of treatment (Hajak & Rüther, 1995).

Generally, there are three classification schemes currently used for sleep disorders: The Diagnostic and Statistical Manual of Mental Disorders, the DSM IV (American Psychiatric Association, 1994); the International Classification of Sleep Disorders ICSD (American Sleep Disorders Association, 1990); and the International Classification of Diseases ICD 10 (World Health Organisation, 1991). The DSM IV as well as the ICD 10 offer simple and clear structures, however, more interesting for scientific purposes is the ICSD with more than 80 diagnostic categories. The ICSD suggests a subdivision into four major groups. The first group includes the so-called dyssomnia. These are sleep disorders, which prevent either the onset or maintenance of sleep or cause excessive sleepiness, for example, psychophysiological insomnia. This sleeplessness is caused and perpetuated by physical stress and conditioned sleep-preventing associations. The second group, the so-called parasomnia, include sleep disorders, like somnambulism, that interrupt the normal sleep process. The third group includes sleep disorders associated with medical and psychiatric conditions such as depression. The fourth group embraces all the other proposed sleep disorders on which sufficient research has yet to be conducted, without which their status as sleep disorders cannot be firmly established.

Basically, all sleep disturbances, that do not require constant medical monitoring, are suitable for ambulatory sleep diagnosis. An ambulatory polysomnography is possible when psychophysiological insomnia is suspected, whereas a high degree of sleepwalking where the patient can be injured seriously, necessitates an in-patient polysomnography.

Although there are advantages of stationary polysomnography (e.g., the direct sleep observation by specialist staff and the possibility of control and correction of the recording quality during measurement), there are a number of disadvantages, too. With the growing interest in sleep research and sleep medicine, an increasing number of sleep laboratories have been established in Germany in recent years. Nevertheless, the demands for diagnosis and treatment of sleep disorders can not be currently met. Long waiting times for the patients show the strain on the sleep medical centers; furthermore, considerable journey time and expense incurred by the patients. Regarding the diagnosis, it is important to note that the accommodation in a laboratory is an exceptional situation for the patient, at least on a subjective level. Thus, the external validity of the diagnosis should be scrutinized, at least on the first night.

As a result of the stationary examination, substantially higher costs incur for the patient or the health insurances, compared to an out-patient examination. A special advantage of ambulatory sleep diagnosis lies in the flexibility of the application of its step-by-step approach. Thus, a patient with a suspected sleep apnea syndrome can sleep at home overnight with a device that measures thoracic breathing, the flow of breath through the nose and mouth as well as the oxygen saturation of the blood. The evaluation of these parameters can normally be done quickly, even a computer-based analysis is possible. If the suspicion is confirmed, then an extensive polysomnography can be done, even on an in-patient basis, if necessary. The consistent use of ambulatory measuring instruments would relieve the existing sleep laboratories measurably. This has the advantage that the therapeutic procedure (e.g., reduction of morbidity and mortality) could be greatly accelerated even for patients who cannot be examined on an out-patient basis.

The ambulatory measurement has conceivable advantages because the patients do not have to make time and have lesser expenses for the examination itself. This can only speak in favor of the ambulatory assessment, if the quality of measurement is comparable to the registration in the laboratory. Exactly this, ambulatory measurement with the quality of the laboratory, can be achieved with the Varioport system and the additional module developed for polysomnography (see "Some new developments in ambulatory assessment devices", this Volume).

Integration of ambulatory measuring methods in step-by-step diagnosis

In which cases is it really necessary to transfer a patient to a sleep laboratory or a medical sleep center? The "Insomnia-Group" of the German Sleep Society (DGSM) (Müller & Paterok, 1999) has set up guidelines summarizing the most important indications for a transfer:

First, patients with severe sleep disorders accompanied by a significant reduction of well-being and/or a strong decrease in efficiency should go to a sleep laboratory. Persons with chronic and therapy-resistant sleep disorders, who have not shown any kind of improvement after a year of treatment, should contact a sleep laboratory. A sleep laboratory examination is inevitable for patients with a sleep disorder suspected as organically caused, and patients, who are stressed by the diagnostic and/or therapeutic procedures aimed at their illnesses. Sleep disorders that are hard to treat and show a co-morbidity to physical or psychological illnesses (which presumably interact with the sleep disturbance) as well as conspicuous sleep behavior of unknown etiology, for example, parasomnia, should be examined in a sleep center. Because of the discrepancy between those with severe sleep disturbances seeking help and the availability of in-patient polysomnography places, the ambulatory pre-diagnosis achieves an important status regarding the indication of the appropriate subsequent therapy (Hajak & Rüther, 1995). The advantages of ambulatory measurement instruments are particularly evident in stepwise testing. These present new opportunities for sleep medicine and sleep research.

Schönhofer (1997) for instance, recommends a four-step plan for the diagnosis of sleep apnea. The first step consists of applying standardized questionnaires for specific symptoms and the consequences of "sleep-related breathing disorders" (Schlafbezogene Atemstörung, SBAS). The second step involves conducting a clinical examination that justifies an ambulatory examination with a screening-device that follows in the third step, that is, the continuous monitoring of respiration, the oxygen saturation as well as the heart rate and other parameters. The aim of this ambulatory examination is the detection of oxygen desaturation and repetitive changes in the heart rate (variability) as well as breath stoppages and/or snoring. In the last step, further polysomnographic diagnoses are carried out and controlled on an in-patient basis in a sleep laboratory.

The use of such strategies for other sleep disorders is also conceivable. In the cases of restless-leg syndrome (RLS), or the periodic-leg-movement syndrome (PLMS), respectively, a questionnaire could give first indications as well. As one of the further steps, the measurement of leg movements during sleep would be possible with the help of two actometers. Another possibility is the recording of an electroencephalogram (EEG), electroocculogram (EOG), and electromyogram (EMG) together with the corresponding EMG recording leads on the leg, so that the leg movements may be examined in relation to a sleep profile made according to Rechtschaffen and Kales' evaluation rules (1968). The effects of possible leg movement on the sleep architecture can be observed directly, too. As a last step the ambulatory measurement of respiratory parameters is conceivable, which would exclude snoring and breath stoppage. This would mean, executing a complete polysomnography under field conditions.

These examples clearly show the decisive advantages of ambulatory measurement devices to be found in the combination of these options. The psychological and medical diagnostic alternatives can be used optimally that way. Above all, a detailed case history can be substantiated by various disorder-specific questionnaires (based on observation and introspection) as well as a sleep diary offers the opportunity to select the optimal screening. Through ambulatory measuring it is possible to arrive at a differential diagnosis, to take further diagnostic steps or begin with the treatment of the sleep disorder.

The diagnosed type of sleep disorder offers indications for therapy. Here a rough distinction between the medical and psychological treatment options is possible, however, it is important to note that combined therapies are often the most effective, since most sleep disorders do not occur in a "pure form", and adaptation of the therapy to the needs of the individual is required. Of course, medical forms of treatment are essential for organic sleep disorders. For instance, the treatment of choice for "obstructive sleep apnea" is a nocturnal mechanical ventilation system offering continuous positive airway pressure ("CPAP-therapy").

Regarding the psychological treatment, there is still a substantial deficit in available treatment for patients with sleep disorders, although insomnia (non-organic difficulties in sleep onset and maintenance) is one of the most frequent health problems in the general population (Hohagen, 1997). At the moment, only two group-therapy manuals have been published. They were especially developed for the treatment of this kind of sleep disorder. Although there are many sleep laboratories, only few offer group therapy, so that patients who want to participate in them have to endure long journeys. The group programs are based on sleep education (information about the nature of sleep and the rules for sleep hygiene) and cognitive techniques (e.g., pictures of rest, train-of-thought stopping, and cognitive restructuring). The group program by Riemann and Backhaus (1996) puts major emphasis on relaxation, whereas sleep restriction is the most important element in Müller and Paterok's sleep training (1999).

The results of the ambulatory polysomnography can also be included in the therapy for certain patients. Rüther and Hajak (1995) suggest a sleep-state misperception as a major indicaton for the polysomnography in insomnia. This proposal could be included in the therapy for this type of insomnia by discussing the difference between objective and subjective sleep quality. Attention should be paid to maintaining a sensitive approach. The patients' complaints should be taken seriously, in order to maintain access to him or her.

Ambulatory polysomnography and its variants offer a reasonably priced option for measuring therapy success in many sleep disorders, for example, restless-leg syndrome (RLS), periodic-leg movement (PLMS), or insomnia.

Laboratory and ambulatory polysomnography - some empirical findings

The aim of a polysomnographic examination is to determine the individual's current, typical sleep pattern. The fact that polysomnographic procedures cause subject's reactivity poses a problem. Sensors, cables, and so forth inevitably disturb sleep. In in-patient sleep examinations in a sleep laboratory, the unusual surroundings also interfere with sleep. The resulting problems in interpretation and generalization of the sleep laboratory data are well known. The most intensively researched were the adaptation effects and the relationship between certain patient groups and findings achieved with different technological approaches.

Agnew, Webb and Williams (1966) were the first to describe an adaptation effect. They labeled it the "First-Night Effect" (FNE). After registering the sleep of 43 persons on four consecutive nights in the sleep laboratory, they found that in each case more arousal and less REM sleep occurred in the first night. Furthermore, a delayed occurrence of stage 4 sleep and REM appeared as well as more stage changes. However, on the second night the patients appeared to have adapted. As a result, at least two subsequent examinations are necessary and the first night is only evaluated as the "adaptation night", in order to gain interpretable data in the sleep laboratory.

The development of portable measuring devices has opened new possibilities in sleep study. Portable polysomnography systems have reached a high technical level of data recording (Broughton, Fleming & Fleetham, 1996; Fry, DiPhilippo, Curran, Goldberg & Baran, 1998; Jain, Martens, Mutz, Weiss & Stephan, 1996; White, 1996).

Regarding adaptation or generalization, the difference in the surroundings in which sleep recording is done makes the use of portable measuring devices all the more important. According to Hemmeter (1997), the adaptation in the assessment of patients in their usual environment is not as important as it is in the sleep laboratory. However, it stands to reason that the stress resulting from the ambulatory conditions of the examination (e.g., caused by the technology and the awareness of being examined) can falsify the usual sleep patterns and adaptation will occur with repeated measurement.

"Do our methods lead to insomniacs' madness?" Edinger et al. (1997) asked this provocative question to point out that sleep laboratory tests on patients with insomnia can lead to systematically biased results. Several studies have shown that only minimal differences exist between the sleep of patients and healthy subjects in the results of sleep laboratory examinations. Edinger et al. (1997) demonstrated that sleep examinations under domestic conditions show differences between patients and healthy subjects. They concluded that sleep examinations under domestic conditions have a higher sensitivity for insomnia.

The following studies present results focusing on the question of the differences between sleep exams under laboratory and field conditions.

Study I

Fricke (1997) presented an extensive study, which was conducted at the Psychological Institute of the University of Cologne. In this study the phenomenon of the "First Night Effect" and its dependency on sleep surroundings and the personal characteristics of the sleeper were examined.

Methods

A total of 20 subjects (16 female and 4 male psychology students, average age: 25.5 years) were examined in each case with a portable polysomnography device (Vitaport 2) for four nights, two nights in the laboratory and two nights at home. The two nights in the same location were consecutive, the assessments in the other location took place a week later. In order to control for sequence effects, the sequence of the conditions (first laboratory or first at home) was varied systematically. However, the laboratory conditions in this study deviated from the typical sleep laboratory conditions as the room used for this assessment was at the Institute and was furnished to create a particularly pleasant atmosphere. Monitoring by a person or camera did not take place. Also, due to the portable assessment devices, the subjects remained mobile and could therefore determine when they went to bed as well as choosing their evening activities freely.

All subjects filled out sleep diaries for several weeks, mood questionnaires, and special sleep questionnaires as well as the Freiburg Personality Inventory (Freiburger Persönlichkeitsinventar FPI-R) by Fahrenberg, Hampel and Selg (1984). The hypothesis was that the comparably greater strangeness of the sleep environment in the laboratory would lead to a more pronounced first night effect. Furthermore, relationships between the first night effect and different personality measures were examined.

Results

The results showed a first night effect for the laboratory conditions, as well as the field conditions (Table 1). Significant differences between the first and the second night could be demonstrated in sleep parameters, including: time of arousal, rate of light sleep and rate of slow-wave sleep. In terms of adaptation, the field measurements did not differ significantly from the laboratory measurements. However, one significant difference between the laboratory and the field appeared in slow-wave sleep: the subjects spent more time in slow-wave sleep in the sleep laboratory than at home. No significant results were found in the correlations between personality characteristics and the first night effect.

Discussion

The data obtained could not confirm the hypothesis that smaller adaptation effects

Table 1. Overview of sleep parameters

	Field		Laboratory		Adaptation Effect	Situation Effect
Sleep Statistics	Night 1 n=20	Night 2 n=20	Night 1 n=20	Night 2 n=20	p	p
Arousals to wake (count)	23.4	23.0	26.5	22.3	.047 *	.540
Sleep-onset latency (minutes)	21.7	27.5	25.6	17.3	.777	.485
Latency of slow-wave sleep (minutes)	16.8	21.1	28.1	18.0	.313	.218
Latency of REM sleep (minutes)	111.4	96.1	107.6	85.6	.059	.557
Light sleep (% of total sleep time)	70.4	65.5	69.4	67.7	.002 **	.567
Slow-wave sleep (minutes of time in bed)	48.9	55.1	42.2	47.2	.046 *	.008 **
* p < .05 (significant effect), ** p < .01 (highly significant effect)						

appear in the field than in the laboratory. The characteristic features of the test situation which disturbed the sleep and to which the test person could have adapted to during the first night do not appear to be more pronounced in the laboratory than in the field. The different rates of slow-wave sleep point to qualitatively better sleep in the laboratory. The results make sense when we consider that the laboratory conditions provided a very pleasant atmosphere (see above). The subjects were undisturbed and almost alone in a big building. However, peculiarities of the subject sample (students) has to be taken into consideration. It is noteworthy that some characteristics of the domestic sleep environment, gained from the questionnaires and sleep diaries of these subjects, do not appear "typical" for the whole population. The laboratory conditions are quite familiar for the students of the institute, who were the subjects in this study. The findings of this study can only be generalized in a limited fashion. They may be applicable to studies of different patient groups for clinical purposes (in a clinical atmosphere).

Study II

The characteristic features of the examination situation and the sample seem to have an influence on the extent of the reactivity of the subjects of polysomnographic measurements. This is confirmed by a study by Alfer (2000), which was executed in a co-operation between the Psychological Institute of the University of Cologne and the Neurological University Clinic in Bonn. In extension to the questions and methods of the study by Fricke (1997), the following questions were examined: (1) Is sleep quality better with polysomnographic assessments under field or sleep-laboratory conditions? (2) What role do the adaptation effects play? (3) Are there differences in the subjects' acceptance of the measurement methods?

Methods

The participants included 10 male patients (mean 53.9 years), who were to be examined in the Neurological University Clinic in Bonn because of sleep-related breathing problem. In addition to the regular two assessment nights in the laboratory, two additional assessment nights were conducted for each patient under field conditions with the aid of portable measuring devices (Varioport). There was at least one week between the two laboratory and the two field assessments, respectively, whereby the order (laboratory or field first) was balanced. As two different polysomnography systems were used, controls for unwanted effects of the two systems on the comparison of the laboratory or field data had to applied. For this purpose, parallel sleep measurement with both systems was used. The findings pointed out system differences, that have to be considered in the comparison of other laboratory and field data.

The laboratory situation was a room in the Neurological Clinic in Bonn. This room is windowless, has its own ventilation and sink and is monitored by a camera. The surveillance room is nearby, from which the study was supervised at night. In case the subject needed to leave the bed or the room, for example, for going to the toilet, he or she had to contact the night watch, so that the electrodes could be removed temporarily. The field situation corresponded to the domestic environment of the patient. For the fastening of the sensors and the start of the recording the patient was visited at home. The choices related to activities before going to bed, bed time, as well as getting up in the morning, etc., were left to the patients, as was the removal of the electrodes and sensors the next morning.

The dependent variables were sleep parameters resulting from the polysomnography, as well as data from questionnaires, which were completed by the subjects after each of the four assessments. The subjects rated 11 statements about the disturbing aspects of the polysomnography. Another questionnaire was filled out by the participnats after the last assessment, registering the subjective differences between laboratory and field measurements. The testing of the hypotheses was done with the aid of a two-factorial variance analysis with repeated measurements of both factors (2 within, 0 between).

Results

The analysis included 19 laboratory and 20 field records. An invalid laboratory recording lead to the exclusion of the entire record of one subject. None of the field measurements showed any kind of evaluation problems. In retrospect, a comparison of all nine subjects showed that the field situation had greater similarities with their usual sleep situation. The field variant was preferred by all subjects. The sleep environment and freedom of movement was of particular importance to all the subjects. The analysis of the polysomnography itself and the questionnaire assessments showed a much more differentiated picture (Table 2).

Table 2. PSG and questionnaire results

	Laboratory			Field			Situation Effect
	Night 1 n=9	Night 2 n=9	Mean n=18	Night 1 n=9	Night 2 n=9	Mean n=18	p
Sleep Parameter							
Sleep-efficiency index (%)	77.4	74.1	75.8	89.3	91.3	90.3	.0150 *
Arousals to wake (count)	15.9	22.2	19.1	19.2	21.8	20.5	.7075
Sleep-onset latency (minutes)	23.4	35.4	29.4	11.4	8.5	9.9	.0470
Slow-wave sleep latency (minutes)	30.4	57.2	43.8	20.2	17.6	18.9	.0363 *
REM-sleep latency (minutes)	85	86.8	85.9	76.1	65.6	70.8	.0161 *
Wake after sleep onset (minutes)	20.6	22	21.3	6.9	6.8	6.9	.0154 *
Light sleep (% of sleep period time)	63.2	63.8	63.5	62.4	64	63.2	.9290
Slow-wave sleep (% of sleep period time)	11.8	8.4	10.1	10.2	7.9	9.1	.5488
REM sleep (% of sleep period time)	12.1	13	12.6	19.6	21.2	20.4	.0119 *
Ratings (high rate: agreement)							
"I slept badly" (Ich habe schlecht geschlafen)	3	3.1	3.1	3	2.7	2.8	.5121
"My sleep was different from my normal sleep due to the assessment" (Mein Schlaf war wegen der Untersuchung anders, als ich es gewohnt bin)	3.33	3.11	3.22	2.44	1.89	2.17	.0308 *
"My sleep was different from my normal sleep, but for other reasons than the assessment" (Mein Schlaf war aus anderen Gründen als der Untersuchung anders, als ich es gewohnt bin)	2.89	2.22	2.56	1.56	1.33	1.44	.0304 *
"The device was tiresome" (Die Apparatur war lästig)	3.00	3.44	3.22	3.11	2.44	2.78	.1981
"The device was strange, it was eerie" (Die Apparatur hat mich befremdet, war mir unheimlich)	1.67	1.78	1.72	1.78	1.44	1.61	.7078
"I felt restricted in my movements" (Ich fühlte mich in meiner Bewegungsfreiheit eingeschränkt)	3.00	3.44	3.22	3.11	2.67	2.89	.3319
"The sleep environment bothered me" (Die Schlafumgebung hat mich gestört)	2.67	2.89	2.78	1.11	1.11	1.11	.0158 *
"Habits relating to my sleep were influenced by the assessment" (Gewohnheiten, die mit meinem Schlaf zu tun haben, wurden durch die Untersuchung beeinflusst)	2.33	2.33	2.33	1.11	1.33	1.22	.0257 *
"While the assessment was being conducted I was thinking about the fact that I was being examined now" (Während der Untersuchung hat es mich gedanklich beschäftigt, dass ich gerade untersucht werde)	1.56	2.00	1.78	1.89	1.33	1.61	.1950
"I felt uncomfortable being 'watched'" (Ich fühlte mich unangenehm "beobachtet")	1.22	1.67	1.44	1.44	1.22	1.33	.4468
"To have my usual sleep recorded has put me under pressure" (Meinen gewohnten Schlaf vorzuführen hat mich unter Druck gesetzt)	1.44	1.44	1.44	1.44	1.33	1.39	.5943
*: p < .05 (significant effect)							

Significant differences were found between laboratory and field measurements. In the domestic environment, the subjects achieved higher sleep-efficiency values (share of total sleep time of the time spent in bed) and fell asleep faster (sleep-onset latency). They reached slow-wave and REM sleep (slow-wave sleep latency and REM-sleep latency) faster, spent less time awake after sleep onset and more time in REM sleep in the field setting than in the sleep laboratory.

Ratings conducted after each assessment night concerning the factors, that disturbed sleep, also showed differences between the assessment conditions. Compared to sleep in the field, the sleep in the laboratory was clearly different from what the subjects were used to. In the laboratory, the sleep environment interfered significantly and sleep-related habits were more strongly affected than in the field. However, contrary to expectations, differences related to restriction of movement were not found in the ratings. Adaptation effects were not evident under laboratory or field conditions.

Discussion

The data obtained can contribute to answering the hypotheses. On the basis of the polysomnography and questionnaire data it was possible to show that the sleep registered in these studies showed differences between laboratory and field conditions. The sleep quality revealed by the polysomnographic data was better under field conditions than in the laboratory. Questionnaire data showed that the sleep-disturbing aspects were indeed weaker in the field than in the laboratory. All subjects preferred the field variant and considered the sleep examined in the field to be more like their habitual sleep. However, adaptation effects like the first night effect could not be proven in either the laboratory or the field. The results obtained can be seen as evidence that the results of the measurements taken under field conditions are more externally valid than those under laboratory conditions.

Conclusions

The results of the two studies clearly differ. It may be that the differences between the examination conditions and the samples are of decisive importance here. The clinical laboratory conditions in the second study were clearly more uncomfortable than the laboratory conditions in the first study. The subjects' statements confirmed that the windowless, monitored clinic room (in study II) definitely represented a disturbing sleep environment, whereas the cozily furnished institute room (in study I) was unfamiliar, but not very disturbing. The field conditions differed, too. The field measurement instruments in the first study were applied in the laboratory (placement of sensors and starting the recording), whereupon the subjects went home to sleep. In the second study, the preparation for measurement took place directly in the subjects' domestic surroundings, where they were already "ready for bed".

These differences in the laboratory and field conditions could have led to the different results in the studies. Also, the subjects in study I (80 % female, average age 25.5 years) were healthy psychology students and younger than the subjects in study II (100 % male, average age 53.9 years). These differences could also have contributed to the discrepancies in the results.

One can conclude from these studies that polysomnographic measurements are clearly influenced by environmental factors. In order to be as representative as possible, that is, to obtain externally valid results, the examination conditions should correspond as closely as possible to the subjects' usual environment. Disturbing aspects of the measuring methods, such as movement restrictions, should be minimized. According to Edinger et al. (1997) this might be import for examinations of patients with insomnia (see above). The polysomnographic assessment of patients' sleep characteristics apparently requires a sensitivity, that very likely can be best achieved with ambulatory measurement procedures.

Problems and solutions achieved

Many of the problems with ambulatory measurements arise from the fact that the measurement is not continually supervised by a control person, who could ease smaller disturbances immediately. Therefore, the focus has been primarily on preventing such problems before they occur in the first place.

Cable Safety

One problem for ambulatory measurement is the safety of the cables. While performing a polysomnography on an in-patient basis, an electrode, that becomes loose, can be replaced without endangering the whole measurement procedure. This is not possible on an out-patient basis. Therefore, special care is taken in fitting the electrodes. In addition, the electrodes attached to the head are "braided" so that a sudden movements straining the better fastened facial electrodes and the EEG electrodes (C 3, C 4 and 0 1) are minimized. A "cable collar" offers additional safety. All cables are supposed to have little extra length and should lead to the polysomnography module (PSG module) in the shortest way possible. Where the cables are outside the collar (e.g., the leg electrodes), they are fixed with tape. At the knee and elbow the cables are fastened with tape above or below the joint.

Signal Quality

The signal quality has also been a problem for the development of the PSG module. To a great extent this is due to the choice of the pool electrodes (C 3, C 4, 0 1). At first relatively expensive gold electrodes were used, because they are supposed to be less maintenance intensive. Unfortunately, it turned out that the gold layer on these electrodes came off after a few uses. The signals from the electrodes were very susceptible to stray effects of the ECG and rarely showed satisfactory impedances. Therefore, a switch was made to silver-chloride electrodes. They are more maintenance intensive, since they have to be chlorinated regularly, but they are more durable, less prone to disruptive influences and produce outstanding impedances (often < 5 kOhm). Another unwanted influence stems from what is called net humming (in Germany 50 hertz), which shows up in the channels when the patient is in the vicinity of electrical equipment or an electrical cable, that are in use. This problem can be solved with the aid of a filter program, which filters out the majority of interferences after scanning the data. This filter program was developed at the Psychological Institute in SPIL (Signal Processing and Inferencing Language, Jain et al., 1996).

The quality of the signals is highly dependent on the quality of the mass. Despite careful wiring it is possible that the mass electrode which is part of the ECG channel gets detached or shows an impedance, that is too high. For this reason two mass electrodes are always used in the new PSG modules, which reduces the risk of data loss.

Furthermore, particular attention must be paid when attaching the electrodes; all points, where they are to be fastened, should be carefully pre-treated. The preparation of the skin with an abrasive paste and the follow-up remove of skin oils and disinfection with alcohol reduces resistance, and thereby substantially increases the quality of the signals.

Technical Solutions

Since the ambulatory measurement system should ideally be independent of the local power grid, low power consumption is required. This was the case with the Varioport recorders used in the second study. Also, a sufficient storage capacity is essential. A complete polysomnography can easily require storage space of 80 to 90 MB, which fits on the compact flash cards used. (For further technical specifications refer to the Chapter "Some new developments in the ambulatory assessment devices", this Volume).

Unsolved Problems

In spite of intense efforts, there are always problems, for which solutions are not yet available or which have not yet been put into practice. These problems in our experience occur, because there is no supervisor present during measurement.

Subject Safety

Certain diseases require constant monitoring of the test subject. Among them are epilepsy or Schenck syndrome, in which the usual relaxation of the musculature is disturbed during REM phases, that is, dreams are acted out physically. Only these two disorders carry the risk of injury to the person while sleeping. During an ambulatory polysomnography there is the additional risk of strangulation by the cables, and of skin injuries when the electrodes are torn off, especially in the head region.

Diagnosis of Respiratory Disruptions

Under certain conditions there are serious limitations on the measurement of breathing function by the PSG module. This is true when measuring people with Continuous Positive Airway Pressure (CPAP) devices or similar respiration aids. The use of a Flow sensor, that is essential to the differential diagnosis of breathing difficulties, is not possible under those circumstances. The situation is similar when patients have a stuffy nose due to colds or allergies.

Outlook: Movement detection video recording of sleep and the possibilities of data compression

Sleep videos are a standard part of polysomnographic examinations. These videos are indispensable for the diagnoses of nocturnal epileptic seizures, parasomnia, disturbed REM sleep, etc. They also provide impressive pictures of sleep apnea. For the evaluation of sleep quality the movement of the sleeper during the night is very informative. However, because of the excessive time involved, these tapes are often not evaluated – or only selectively. These videos would be particularly useful in ambulatory sleep diagnosis to fill in for the missing experiment supervisor.

We have developed a procedure, which allows the digital video recorder to record when the sleeper moves and thus we reduce the recording to approximately five minutes (depending on the level of sensitivity). This recording method allows a routine evaluation of sleep behavior. We use a black-and-white video camera with a sensitivity of 0.1 lux and an infrared light source. The video signal is fed into the video input of a PC TV card. The data is recorded on the hard drive, when a frame differs from the previous one by an adjustable value and stops after an adjustable time after the last movement. The running time is displayed in the picture. Screen windows with interfering movement information (e.g., a running clock) can be disguised. The uncompressed picture data for a night takes up on the average less than 100 MB.

However, questions that require parallel video evaluation, often emerge in the evaluation of the physiological data. For this it would be preferable to have access to video data for the whole night. Also, the use of a video recorder can be unsatisfactory, due to the need to rewind to the interesting places on the tape. At the same time a substantial amount of space is required to archive the tapes. Through compression procedures like MPEG-4 it is possible to select a smaller picture format and reduce the picture-data rate. It is also possible to store a complete sleep video together with the physiological data with negligible quality loss on a CD-R. This allows the video data to be evaluated along with the physiological data.

References

Agnew, H.W., Webb, W.B. & Williams, R.L. (1966). The first night effect: An EEG study of sleep. *Psychophysiology, 2* (3), 263–266.

Alfer, D. (2000). *Polysomnographie in Labor und Feld – Formative Evaluation und vergleichende Validitätsuntersuchung. (Polysomnography in the Laboratory and Field – Formative Evaluation and Coimparative Validity Studies).* Unpublished graduate thesis, Psychology Department of the University of Cologne.

American Psychiatric Association (1994). *Diagnostic and statistical manual of mental disorders, 4th edition DSM-IV.* Washington, D.C.: American Psychiatric Association

American Sleep Disorders Association (1990). *The international classification of sleep disorders: diagnostic and coding manual.* Lawrence: Allen.

Broughton, R., Fleming, J. & Fleetham, J. (1996). Home Assessment of Sleep Disorders by Portable Monitoring. *Journal of Clinical Neurophysiology, 13* (4), 272–284.

Edinger, J.D., Fins, A.I., Sullivan, R.J., Marsh, G.R., Dailey, D.S., Hope, T.V., Young, M., Shaw, E., Carlson, D. & Vasilas, D. (1997). Do Our Methods Lead to Insomniacs' Madness?: Daytime Testing After Laboratory and Home-Based Polysomnographic Studies. *Sleep, 20* (12), 1127–1134.

Fahrenberg, J., Hampel, R. & Selg, H. (1984). *Das Freiburger Persönlichkeitsinventar FPI (The Freiburg Personality Inventory FPI)* (4. rev. edition). Göttingen: Hogrefe.

Fricke, L. (1997). *Untersuchung zum Schlafverhalten: Der First Night Effect in Labor und Feld und sein Zusammenhang mit Persönlichkeitsfaktoren. (Study of Sleep Behavior: The First Night Effect in the Laboratory and Field and the Relationship with Personality Factors),* Unpublished graduate thesis, Psychology Department of the University of Cologne.

Fry, J.M., DiPhillipo, M.A., Curran, K., Goldberg, R. & Baran, A.S. (1998). Full Polysomnography in the Home. *Sleep, 21* (6), 635–642.

Hajak, G. & Rüther, E. (1995). *Insomnie (Insomnia).* Berlin: Springer-Verlag.

Hemmeter, U. (1997). Ambulantes Monitoring. In H. Schulz, (Ed.), *Kompendium Schlafmedizin für Ausbildung, Klinik und Praxis* (Chapter I – 6.1.1) (pp. 1–2). Landsberg/Lech: Ecomed.

Hohagen, F. (1997). Epidemiologie. In: H. Schulz (Ed.), *Kompendium Schlafmedizin.* (Chapter IV – 1.1) (pp. 1–2). Landsberg/ Lech: Ecomed.

Jain, A., Martens, W.L.J., Mutz, G., Weiß, R.K. & Stephan, E. (1996). Towards a comprehensive technology for recording and analysis of multiple physiological parameters within their behavioral and environmental context. In J. Fahrenberg & M. Myrtek (Eds.), *Ambulatory Assessment* (pp. 215–235). Göttingen: Hogrefe.

Müller, T. & Paterok, B. (1999). *Schlaftraining – Ein Therapiemanual zur Behandlung von Schlafstörungen (Sleep Training – A Therapy Manual for the Treatment of Sleeping Disorders).* Göttingen: Hogrefe.

Rechtschaffen, A. & Kales, A. (Eds.) (1968). *A manual of standardized terminology, techniques, and scoring system for sleep stages of human subjects.* Washington, D.C.: U.S. Government printing Office.

Riemann, D. & Backhaus, J. (1996). *Behandlung von Schlafstörungen – Ein psychologisches Gruppenprogramm (Treating Sleep Disorders – A Psychological Group Program).* Weinheim: Psychologie Verlags Union.

Schönhofer, B. (1997). Ambulante Registrierung der Atmung im Schlaf. In: H. Schulz (Ed.), *Kompendium Schlafmedizin* (Chapter I – 6.2) (pp. 1–6). Landsberg/Lech: Ecomed.

White, D.P. (1996). Complex Home Monitoring. *Sleep, 19* (10), 248–250.

World Health Organisation (1991). *Tenth Revision of the International Classification of Diseases, Chapter V (F): Mental and behavioural disorders (including disorders of the psychological development). Clinical descriptions and diagnostic guidelines.* Geneva: World Health Organisation.

Chapter 32
Electrodermal Long-Term Monitoring in Everyday Life

Wolfram Boucsein, Florian Schaefer, and Thorsten Sommer
Physiological Psychology, University of Wuppertal, Germany

Introduction

Although electrodermal activity (EDA) has been widely applied in various areas of psychophysiological research (see Boucsein, 1992; Hugdahl, 1995, p. 129), it has been rather seldom used so far in ambulatory monitoring. The major reason is that long-term recording of EDA generates a number of problems (Boucsein, 1992, pp. 126–128) most of which origin in the change of the electrode-electrolyte-skin system if recording exceeds a couple of hours. In order to prevent the common electrode cream from drying out as a consequence of its moist penetrating into the skin surface, Edelberg (1963) proposed the use of a polyethylene glycol instead of a water based ointment. However, since the conductivity of a 0.05 Mol NaCl isotonic electrode cream based on polyethylene glycol is only 4 % of an isotonic cream based on a water containing ointment (Edelberg, 1967), such a solution is not practicable for ambulatory monitoring of EDA. However, Turpin, Shine and Lader (1983) could show in an ambulatory monitoring study over 6 hours that hydration effects were significantly lower for polyethylene glycol than for a methyl-cellulose based cream.

In the first part of the present study, a standard EDA electrode-electrolyte recording system was probed with respect to its usability for a 24-hour ambulatory monitoring. As an external validity criterion, parallel electrodermal recordings with a laboratory recording device (see Boucsein, 1992, Fig. 33) were obtained in a laboratory experiment prior to the 24-hour study.

In the second part of the study, reliability estimates were obtained for electrodermal responses in different habituation series after 24-hour ambulatory monitoring. In addition, a comparison between newly attached electrodes and the old ones was performed in order to estimate the strength of the possible electrode effect on reliability. Furthermore, the comparison with the laboratory recording device was repeated at the end of the 24-hour period. It was intended to repeat the estimated validity coefficient by comparing the results of the laboratory experiment performed in the first part of this study with the results of the laboratory experiment at the beginning of the 24-hour period.

The third part of the present study applied ambulatory EDA monitoring during a whole day and night period. In addition, a manipulation of the information uptake immediately before sleep onset was introduced, in order to check the amount of information processing during sleep that might be reflected in EDA. During the day, subjects (Ss) recorded their activities by means of a pocket-computer-based retrospective monitoring system (Käppler, Becker & Fahrenberg, 1993). This information was used to determine the amount of EDA during different settings that appear in everyday life. In addition to EDA, heart rate (HR), skin temperature, body posture and activity were recorded throughout the 24-hour period. All ambulatory measures were recorded by the Vitaport 2.

A total of 24 female students participated in the present study. They were all psychology students, receiving credit for their participation. Due to various problems described below the number of Ss for the data analyses was much lower.

Comparison of ambulatory and laboratory EDA recordings

Although the principles of EDA measurement used by the Vitaport 2 almost correspond to the EDA recording in stationary laboratory devices, intraindividual comparisons of both recording methods were performed. Two pairs of standard Ag/AgCl electrodes were fixed on the non-dominant hand, one of them at the standard thenar/hypothenar recording sites (Boucsein, 1992, Fig. 27) and another one in 2.0 – 2.5 cm distance (dependent on the hand size) distal from the first pair of electrodes. They were filled with a 0.9 % NaCl electrolyte made from Unibase (Boucsein, 1992, p. 106) and fixed with double-sided adhesive rings. The electrode positions were balanced between the Vitaport 2 and the laboratory system. In addition, a comparison between two identical stationary laboratory recording devices was performed.

Recordings were made during a 2 min baseline and a standard habituation series of 8 white noise stimuli (1 sec, 90 dBA) with a variable interstimulus interval (ISI) of 22.5 sec. In order to evoke dishabituation responses, these were followed by 16 different meaningful auditory stimuli (for example., breaking glass, barking dog, shriek, etc.), with a mean duration of 1 sec, an intensity of 90 dBA, and a variable ISI with a mean of 22.5 sec. The Ss were seated in an armchair in an air-conditioned IAC cabin (9 square meters, 23 ^{0}C, 50 % relative humidity). EDA was measured as skin conductance response (SCR) with 0.5 V constant voltage (DC) and a time constant of 10 sec. The sampling rate for A/D converting was 20 Hz in case of the laboratory device and 16 Hz in case of the Vitaport 2.

Together with the EDA recording, Ss were attached to four more recording channels to be used in the 24-hour ambulatory monitoring. Skin temperature was taken from the palm of the same hand as the EDA recordings, using a YSI thermistor (type 4499E). The thermistor was attached with Fixomull stretch (that allows for air circulation) shortly above the hypothenar electrode. The cable leading to the Vitaport 2 was also fixed with Fixomull stretch to the body. Heart rate was recorded from the chest (sternum vs. left short rib, ground electrode lateral right) with disposable electrodes (55 mm diameter, contact area 20 mm diameter, Becker Meditec). The clips of the electrode cables were additionally fixed with Transpore band, and the cables were fixed to the body with Fixomull stretch.

Movements of the arm having EDA electrodes attached were recorded by the movement detector for Vitaport 2 (Becker Meditec). The detector uses one piezo-electric sensor for vertical accelerations which can not be calibrated in g, thus allowing only for detecting the appearance of movements and their relative intensity. The detector was attached with Fixomull stretch to the outer aspect of the left lower arm on the extensor digitorum muscle. The cable was also fixed to the body with Fixomull stretch.

Body position was recorded with a sensor manufactured by Becker Meditec which detects whether the subject is standing, sitting, or lying down by means of pressure differences in a tube filled with liquid. The sensor was attached to the right body side between the 6th and 8th rib, its glycerine filled tube reaching down to the lower leg. The whole recording device was fixed to the body with Fixomull stretch. Table 1 shows the sampling rates and resolutions for all five physiological variables recorded by the Vitaport 2.

The Vitaport 2 settings were made using the Vitagraph program (Mutz, 1997). The settings used in the present study are shown in Table 1. Evaluations of SCRs were performed by the EDR_PARA program (author: F. Schaefer) and the statistical evaluation was performed with SPSS 9.0.

The mean product-moment-correlation between SCR amplitudes from parallel recordings with the Vitaport 2 and the laboratory device was $r = 0.953$ calculated over three Ss using Fisher's z-transformation. Figure 1 shows the respective scatter plots and the regression lines. When using another identical laboratory devices instead of Vitaport 2 at the same sites, the mean correlation over two Ss was $r = 0.988$.

As can be inferred from Figure 1, there is a highly sufficient comparability between the SCR amplitudes obtained by the ambulatory and the laboratory recording devices.

Reliability and validity of ambulatory EDA recording

The reliability data reported here were obtained as part of the 24-hour monitoring described in Section below. Unfortunately, due to the recording problems men-

Table 1. Definition data for Vitaport 2 used during the 24-hour-monitoring.

Signal Name/unit	Sensor	Pre-processing	scan/ store	Format	ext. U	MUL/ DIV	Offset	Resolution Range	Ampli-fication	HP (Hz) T (sec)	TP (Hz)	DyRange DyOffs	Others
Heart Rate HR / PM	Electrodes 2 + (GND)	Heart Rate	512 4	Byte	off	1 1	0000	1 256	500	- 0.150	100	200.0 0.0	Filter-Pars $0514 Filter: 64 Hz
Activity Akt / adc	Vitaport Sensor	none	16 16	Byte	off	1 1	127	1 256	100	0.48 0.33	10	200.0 0.0	
Position LAGE / adc	Vitaport Sensor	none	16 16	Word	on	1 1	2047	1 4096	20	DC-NRM	10	2000.0 0.0	Tube open!
Temperature Temp / gC	YSI 4499E-Sensor	SPIL	32 32	Word	on	1 100	0000	0.010	40	DC-NRM	20	20.0 20.0	
EDA EDA / µS Channel 67	Ag/AgCl-Electrodes 2	Skin Conductance	16 16	Word	-	1 300	0000	0.003	100 µS full scale	-	-	100.0 0.0	GSR-Mode Testmode off DC-MOD
Tone Trigger Trigg / mV		none	512 16	Byte	off	585 30000	127	0.020	500	DC-NRM	10	250.0	

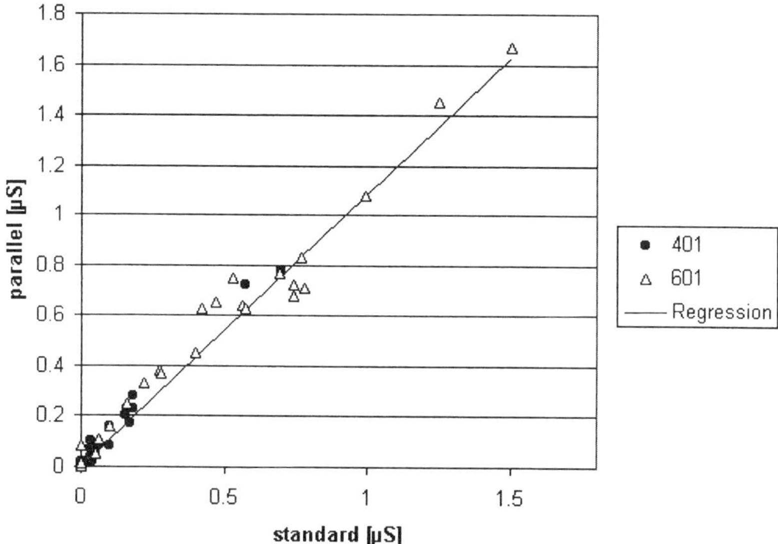

Figure 1. Comparison between the amplitudes (µS) of two laboratory recording devices used in parallel. Data from 2 Ss (No. 401 & 406); 24 acoustic stimuli for each subject. Position of the electrodes: thenar/hypothenar (standard) and 2.0 - 2.5 cm above the standard position (parallel).

tioned in below, only 12 out of the 24 Ss could be used for the reliability study performed during the first morning.

Three standard habituation series with 10 white noise stimuli each as described above were presented in sequence to allow a comparison between newly attached and old electrodes as well as ambulatory and laboratory EDA recording. The laboratory setting and the measurement techniques were the same as in the first part of the study.

The mean correlation between the Vitaport 2 and a standard laboratory device with freshly attached electrodes for both devices as obtained by Fisher´s z-transformation was r = 0.956. This high correlation dropped to r = 0.846 when using the Vitaport electrodes which had been remained on the sites for 24 hours (3 Ss, see Figure 2).

In order to control for the influence of changes in the electrode-electrolyte-skin system during the 24-hour recording period, the old electrodes used with the Vitaport 2 were removed from the standard recording site and replaced by new ones, while the electrodes for the laboratory recording stayed in position. Five Ss could be evaluated for this comparison. For each of them the intraindividual correlation between the SCR amplitudes obtained with both recording methods were calculated, subjected to Fisher's z-transformation and averaged. The mean correlation between Vitaport 2 and the laboratory recording device was r = 0.899, more resem-

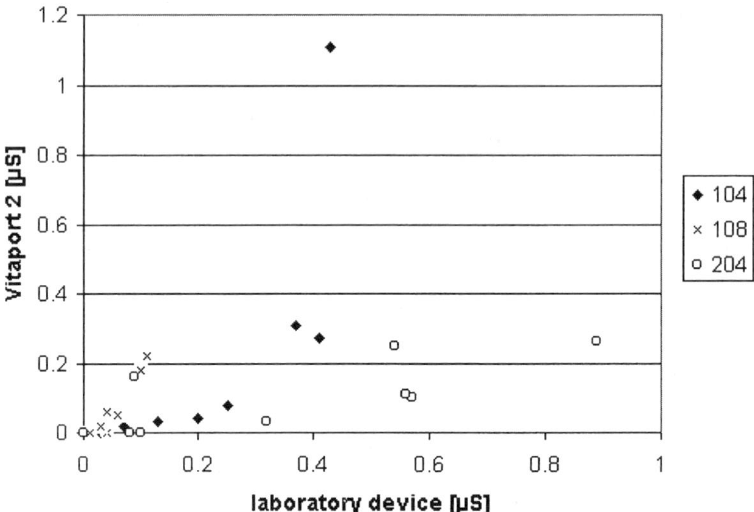

Figure 2. Comparison between the amplitudes (µS) of the Vitaport 2 and a laboratory devices used in parallel after a period of 24 hours. Data from 3 Ss (No. 104, 108, & 204); 10 acoustic stimuli for each subject. Position of the electrodes: thenar/hypothenar (Vitaport 2) and 2.0 - 2.5 cm above the standard position (laboratory device).

bling the coefficient obtained on the first day than the results with the old electrodes used for Vitaport 2 as depicted in Figure 2. Therefore, changes in the electrode-electrolyte-skin system may be blamed for the apparent lack of both reliability and validity of the Vitaport 2 recordings after 24 hours. The major reason for this can be seen in a pronounced epidermal hydration so that the sweat glands could no longer form shunts to the skin surface.

Twenty-four-hour ambulatory monitoring

After the first laboratory session, Ss were released with the Vitaport 2 and a Psion 3c pocket computer in order to carry on with their everyday life activities. They were given a Sony walkman with one of two tapes to be listened to immediately before going to sleep.

The two tapes were prepared for an experimental manipulation of the type of information taken up before sleep. It has been found earlier that the amount of EDA is reduced during REM sleep as compared to slow wave sleep (SWS), although in most cases a clear cut separation of the sleep stages could not be performed (for summaries, see Freixa i Baqué, 1983, and Boucsein, 1992, pp. 273 f.). Only a few studies were performed on the influence of information processing during sleep on EDA. Kushniruk, Rustenburg and Ogilvie (1985) found a significant increase of

EDA in case of bizarre dream contents during the REM phase. As to the results of Lester, Burch and Dosset (1968), stressful experiences before going to sleep increase the so-called "GSR storm" (a considerable increase in spontaneous EDA) to be observed during the stages of deep sleep. Subjects being asked to get more involved in their own dreams as usual showed an increase in EDA during sleep (Pivik, 1978). Since the ambulatory monitoring performed in the present study did not include EEG and EOG measurements, a differentiation of sleep stages could not be performed. Therefore, a rather general hypothesis was formed stating that an uptake of exciting information prior to sleep would increase spontaneous EDA during sleep, especially while being in the SWS stages occurring during the first 90 minutes after sleep onset.

Half of the 24 Ss that participated in the present study was given a tape with a horror story taken from Sibylle Berg's (1999) short story collection "Sex II". Its length was 16 minutes and 29 seconds. The other half of Ss served as controls and received another tape with a rather boring description of different light conditions in an Italian village, written by Gianni Celati (1994), lasting 19 minutes and 46 seconds. Both tapes were produced in the audiovisual media center of the Wuppertal University and read by a semi-professional male reader (Udo Lutz). The Ss were not informed about the experimental manipulation nor pre-warned about the content of their bedtime story (marked A or D). Their assignment to the experimental conditions was quasi-random (odd vs. even Ss numbers).

From the participating 24 Ss, only 12 could be evaluated for this part of the study. Ten Ss had at least one of the EDA electrodes detached on the next morning, leading to data loss. One subject forgot to listen to her tape, and another subject did not go to sleep after listening to her tape but left her home for personal reasons. Out of the remaining 12 Ss, seven listened to the horror story while five served as controls. Their average age was 30.3 years (s = 5.6 years) and 27.0 years (s = 2.8 years), respectively, differing not significantly.

Two items of a questionnaire presented after the second laboratory session referred to the sleep study part. The first item (Likert scale from 1 through 7) asked for the excitement induced by the respective tape. The horror story yielded a mean of 5.4 (s = 0.53) and the control story a mean of 2.0 (s = 1.0), differing significantly from each other ($t = 7.746$, $df = 10$, $p < .001$). The second item asked for the estimated time elapsed between the termination of the tape and sleep onset, which averaged 17 minutes (s = 9 minutes) in the horror story group and 7 minutes (s = 12 minutes) in the control group, differing not significantly ($t = 1.603$, $df = 10$, $p = .14$).

For each 5 minute interval, three different EDA parameters were evaluated: The mean electrodermal level (EDL), the frequency of spontaneous electrodermal changes (non-specific electrodermal response frequency, NS.SCR freq.), and the mean amplitude of those changes (NS.SCR amplitudes). They were averaged for five minutes and the group comparisons were performed for the three hours before listening to the tape, for the listening period, and for the three hours after beginning to listen to the tape. The same evaluation periods were used for the other physiological measures recorded by the Vitaport 2. Mann-Whitney U-tests were applied for statistical comparisons.

No significant differences between the experimental groups were found in the EDL. There was a general decline of EDL during the whole evaluation period that was interrupted in both groups at the beginning of the tape, and also towards the end of the tape in the horror story condition. In the neutral group, there was a rise of the EDL 90 minutes after a starting to listen to the tape. Since the tapes lasted about 20 minutes, such a difference may be attributed to an enlargement of EDA prior to the first REM phase that would have been in line with results from the literature in case of significance.

Figure 3 shows the results for the NS.SCR freq. No significant group differences were found 150 minutes before listening to the tape. The spontaneous EDA in both

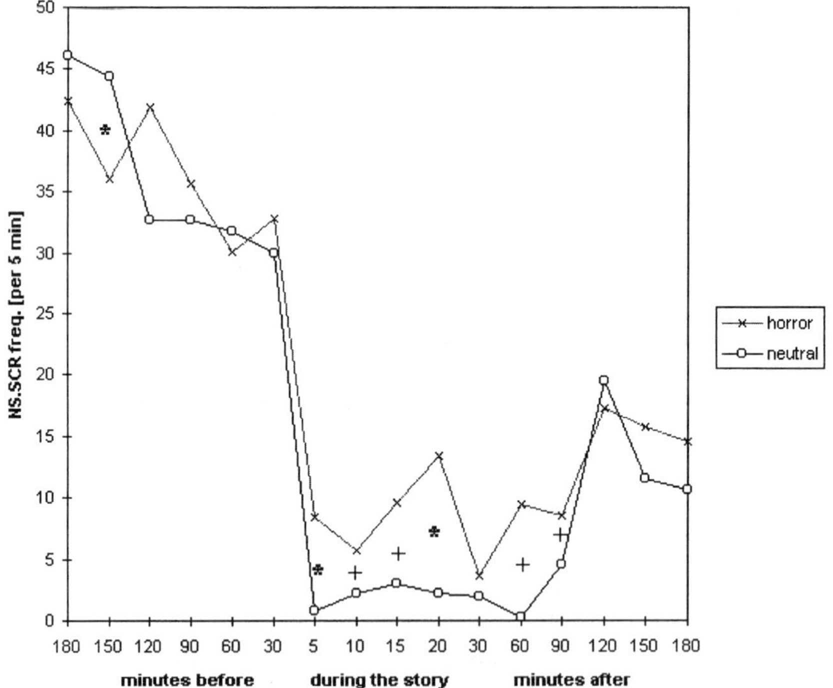

Figure 3. NS.SCR freq. (number of SCRs in 5 minutes) 3 hours before, 20 minutes during, and 3 hours after the bedtime story. Significant differences ($p < 0.05$) between the horror story and the neutral story are marked with an asterisk. A tendency towards significant differences ($p < 0.10$) is marked with a plus.

groups dropped markedly prior to the tape listening which may be attributed to the cessation of activities after laying down in order to hear the recording. During listening to the story, the horror group emerged a much higher NS.SCR freq. compared to the control group. The effect was significant in the first and last 5-minutes intervals ($U = 2$ and $U = 6.5$, $p < .05$) and almost significant in the second and third interval ($U = 8.5$, $p < .10$ in both instances). A tendency towards a significance increase in NS.SCR freq. after the horror story was found 60 and 90 minutes after the tape onset ($U = 8$ and $U = 9.5$, $p < .10$), pointing to an increase of EDA during the first SWS period when the horror story was listened before going to sleep. Afterwards, both groups showed a marked increase in the NS.SCR freq. which somehow parallels what was seen in the control group's EDL.

The respective results of the NS.SCR amplitudes are shown in Figure 4. Again, the control group's EDA was higher 150 minutes prior to listening to the tape and also 30 minutes before the tape was started but only as a tendency towards significance ($U = 8.5$, $p < .10$ in both instances). During the listening, the horror story group showed a significantly elevated NS.SCR amplitudes in the second, third, and fourth 5-minutes intervals ($U = 5$ for the second and third, and $U = 1$ for the fourth interval, $p < .05$ in all instances). The same difference remained significant 60 minutes after the tape onset ($U = 7.5$, $p < .05$), thus confirming the increase in EDA during the first SWS period as already seen in the NS.SCR freq.

No significant group differences in skin temperature emerged during the period before listening to the tape. During the first 15 minutes, skin temperature was significantly higher in Ss listening to the horror story as compared to the controls ($U = 6$, $p < .05$ for all 5-minute periods). This effect was reversed between 90 and 180 minutes after the start of the tape ($U = 8$, $p < .10$ at 60 minutes; $U = 7$, $p < .05$ at 120 and 150 minutes; $U = 4$, $p < .05$ at 180 minutes). The changes in skin temperature did not correspond with the EDL changes measured at the same hand as could have been expected.

Arm movements as recorded by the activity sensor appeared more frequently in the horror story group compared to the control group 90 minutes prior to listening to the tape ($U = 3.5$, $p < .05$). Tendencies for significant differences in the same direction showed up 120 minutes and 30 minutes before ($U = 9.5$, $p < .10$ in both instances) listening to the tape, and afterwards at 90 minutes ($U = 8$, $p < .10$), 120 minutes ($U = 9$, $p < .10$) as well as 150 minutes after starting the tape ($U = 8$, $p < .10$). Although these movements may have influenced the amount of non-specific EDA, a close correspondence cannot be seen, especially since the differences in EDA that emerged during listening to the tape do not correspond to the arm movements. No significant group differences were found in HR.

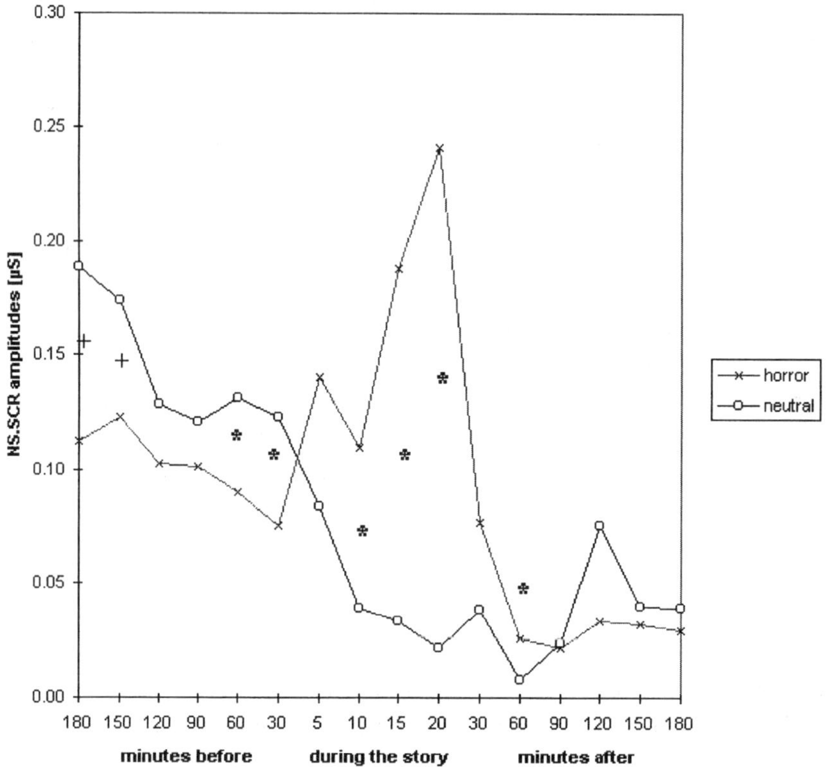

Figure 4. Mean NS.SCR amplitudes 3 hours before, 20 minutes during and 3 hours after the bed-time story. Significant differences ($p < 0.05$) between the horror story and the neutral story are marked with an asterisk. A tendency towards significant differences ($p < 0.10$) is marked with a plus.

General discussion and conclusions

The present study has revealed that long-term ambulatory recording of EDA in the field is restricted by some methodological problems. First, the standard electrode sites at the Ss' hands cause more problems during the daily acticivities compared that is, with chest electrodes for ECG. In addition, it is very likely that the skin hydration during the 24 hours of recording may have contributed to the drop in concurrent validity after that period (see Boucsein, 1992, p. 127). Therefore, it has to be concluded that standard methodology using Ag/AgCl electrodes together with 0.05 Mol NaCl isotonic electrode cream may not be the ideal solution for long-term EDA monitoring, which is in line with the results of Turpin et al. (1983) who found hydration effects on their EDA measure even after 6 hours.

Furthermore, using classical palmar recording sites for 24-hour ambulatory monitoring of EDA can not be recommended since the present study emerged drop outs of about 50 % of the Ss due to electrode detachment and cable problems. Other recording sites such as the inner aspect of the foot (see Boucsein, 1992, Fig. 28) should be considered in further studies instead (see also Boucsein & Thum, 1996). Maybe even less reactive sites at the arms or the trunk (see Edelberg, 1967, Tab. 1.1) could serve better for long-term electrodermal recording, since the danger of electrode detachment will be much less, thus possibly outweighing the disadvantage of a decreased electrodermal reactivity. In addition, other than the standard electrode/electrolyte combination should be probed in order to counteract skin hydration (Edelberg, 1967, pp. 39–42). The limit of the standard technology used here may be six or eight hours for both reasons, electrode fixation and skin hydration problems.

The sleep recording part of the present study clearly emerged that EDA was increased during the first sleep cycle after listening to a horror story as compared to a control story. As could be expected, EDA increased during listening to the horror story as well. In addition to EDA being a valid indicator for the emotional type of stress (Boucsein, 1992, pp. 277–291), it has been shown that processing such a stressful information during the first phase of SWS can also increase EDA, as found earlier by Johnson and Lubin (1966). No such differences were found in HR. The changes in EDA could neither be explained by skin temperature nor by arm movements, so that monitoring EDA during sleep may be recommended for probing the aftereffects of stressful information uptake prior to sleep.

A descriptive analysis of the Psion 3c data yielded that ambulatory EDA recordings during the day seem to be predominantly influenced by both physical activity and environmental factors such as ambient temperature. It has to be taken into account, however, that the method of evaluation of environmental settings used here was relatively rough and based on a retrospective classification of different settings.

Ambulatory monitoring per se was not a jeopardizing factor for the everyday activities of the participants and did not cause major problems with the social environment. However, sporting activities were reduced by several Ss. The use of an improved methodology as suggested earlier would certainly make ambulatory EDA recording a valuable tool even in 24-hour monitoring.

References

Berg, S. (1999). Sex II. Leipzig: Reclam-Verlag.

Boucsein, W. (1992). *Electrodermal activity*. New York: Plenum Press.

Boucsein W. & Thum, M. (1996). Multivariate psychophysiological analysis of stress-strain processes under different break schedules during computer work. In: Fahrenberg, J. & Myrtek, M. (Eds.). *Ambulatory Assessment: Computer-assisted psychological and psychophysiological methods in monitoring and field studies* (pp. 305–313). Göttingen: Hogrefe & Huber Publishers.

Celati, G. (1994). Der wahre Schein. Frankfurt: Fischer-Verlag

Edelberg, R. (1963). *Development of an electrode for long term application in biological recording*. Houston: unpublished research report.

Edelberg, R. (1967). Electrical properties of the skin. In: Brown, C. C. (Ed.). *Methods in psychophysiology* (pp. 1–53). Baltimore: The Williams & Wilkins Company.

Freixa i Baqué, E. (1983). Reliability of spontaneous electrodermal activity in humans as a function of sleep stages. *Biological Psychology, 17,* 137–143.

Hugdahl, K. (1995). *Psychophysiology. The mind-body perspective.* Cambridge, MA: Harvard University Press.

Johnson L. C. & Lubin A. (1966). Spontaneous electrodermal activity during waking and sleeping. *Psychophysiology, 3,* 8–17.

Käppler, C., Becker, H. U. & Fahrenberg, J. (1993). Ambulantes 24-Stunden-Monitoring als psychophysiologische Assessmentstrategie: Reproduzierbarkeit, Reaktivität, Retrospektionseffekt und Bewegungskonfundierung. *Zeitschrift für Differentielle und Diagnostische Psychologie, 14,* 235–251.

Kushniruk, A., Rustenburg J. & Ogilvie, R. (1985). Psychological correlates of electrodermal activity during REM sleep. *Sleep, 8,* 146–154.

Lester, B., Burch, N. & Dosset, R. (1968). Nocturnal EEG-GSR profiles. The influence of presleep stages. *Psychophysiology, 3,* 238–248.

Pivik, R. T. (1978). Tonic states and phasic events in relation to sleep mentation. In: A. M. Arkin, J. S. Antrobus & S. Ellman (Eds.). *The mind in sleep: Psychology and Psychophysiology* (pp. 245–271). New York: John Wiley & Sons.

SPSS (2000). Version 9.0. SPSS Software GmbH, 2000

Turpin, G., Shine, P. & Lader, M. (1983). Ambulatory electrodermal monitoring: Effects of ambient temperature, general activity, electrolyte media, and length of recording. *Psychophysiology, 20,* 219–224.

Chapter 33
Some New Developments in Ambulatory Assessment Devices

Egon Stephan, Gerhard Mutz, Ansgar Feist, and Rolf K. Weiss
Department of Psychology, University of Cologne, Germany

The History of the 'Cologne Vitaport Family' ("Kölner Vitaport Family")

Since 1988 psychophysiological research has been conducted in psychology and medicine at the University of Cologne Psychology Department. In order to react quickly and flexibly to the changing demands placed on our device, these recorders/analyzers have been developed and produced at this Department. Through this development a series of devices has evolved described by Jain, Martens, Mutz, Weiß, and Stephan (1996) as the "Kölner Vitaport System". The interest in these systems was so great that since 1989 the devices were also sold to other researchers.

In 1995 the Kölner Vitaport System with the brand name Vitaport, was licensed and then sold two years later to the Dutch company Temec. Meanwhile, a new series of devices with the name of "Varioport" was being developed and tested at our Department. These devices offer state-of-the-art technology and represent an improvement in performance in comparison to the original Vitaport devices.

The Varioport Family Concept

These devices were designed with a highly flexible number of parameters in order to fulfill the varied requirements of their application, ranging from one to 32 channels and more. The devices had to be small, light-weight and able to operate for several days or weeks on one set of batteries.

The Vitaport II was equipped with 8 channels, had a minimum weight of 700 grams and was 5.5 cm thick in its most basic form, that is, with only one module. Some subjects regarded its weight and size as a considerable burden.

The basic device of the Varioport System was produced using a standard industrial case with the dimensions of 12 x 6.5 x 2.2 cm and a weight of only 170 grams. This basic device contains 8 analog inputs for any pre-amplifier and a serial high-speed bus to allow the number of channels to be increased to 64.

This device allows measurements requiring only one channel or as many as 64 channels. If the user needs only a few channels, he can assemble an optimal, variable (hence "Varioport") system to meet his needs. The location of the extremely miniaturized pre-amplifiers close to the electrodes has improved the reliability and the quality of the data.

This new generation of Varioport devices is largely compatible with the Vitaport System. Also, a whole family of data-logging devices has been created, which is currently being tested at our and other institutes (see Figure 1).

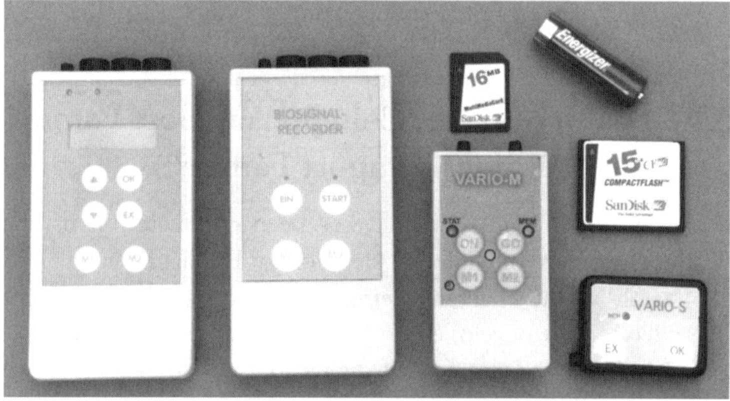

Figure 1. Overview of the Varioport Family. From left: Varioport A, Varioport B (OEM Recorder), Varioport M and Varioport S; for size comparison a Mignon battery is shown.

Varioport A

The Varioport A recorder uses the same 32-bit micro-controller as the Vitaport II (MC68331). In order to lower the power consumption, the supply voltage was reduced to 3 volts. Thus, the operating time has been nearly doubled although there are now only 2 batteries instead of the 4 used by the Vitaport II. Media compact flash cards (type I) are used as a storage medium, which are available up to 192 MB. The firmware was re-coded and equipped with even more efficient power management.

The device has an 8-channel power amplifier with a sensitivity of +/- 125 millivolts and a resolution of 12 bits. Pre-amplifiers and sensors are available in a multitude of varieties. The one-channel sensors are limited by their construction to one purpose only and cannot be modified by any currently available software. Most users focus on a particular mode of application and do not take advantage of the flexibility provided by a software-modifiable amplifier. In addition, the digital amplifiers can be connected to the serial bus (SPI-Amps), which increase the number of channels to 64. These amplifiers contain their own AD converters with 16-bit resolution and 8 channels. The amplification of each channel has two levels and can be switched from AC to DC. Each channel has a differential input with integrated electrode-impedance measurement. The pre-setting of the alias filter can be set using the hardware (default 100 hertz). The power consumption of the eight-channel module is approximately 3 – 4 milliamperes. The amplifiers are able to measure nearly all signals of interest in psychophysiology. A universal amplifier module for eight channels has the dimension 11 x 6 x 1 cm.

Polysomnography Module

A polysomnography module was especially developed for sleep research (Figure 2). It can be connected to the Varioport A as well as to the Varioport B via the serial bus. In total, 16 analog channels and three serially transferred channels for the oxygen sensor ("Nonin™") can be measured with this module. The oxygen sensor measures oxygen saturation, pulse plethysmogram, and heart rate. The 16 analog channels have a resolution of 16 bits. The polysomnography module allows the measurement of three EEG channels (C3-A2, C4-A1, O1-A2), two EOG channels, three EMG channels (submentalis, two tibialis), and an ECG channel. The thoracic and abdominal breath effort are recorded by an induction plethysmograph, while the flow of breath is registered by thermistors on nose and mouth. Additional channels serve to measure the ambient light, snoring sounds, and the body position (in two axes).

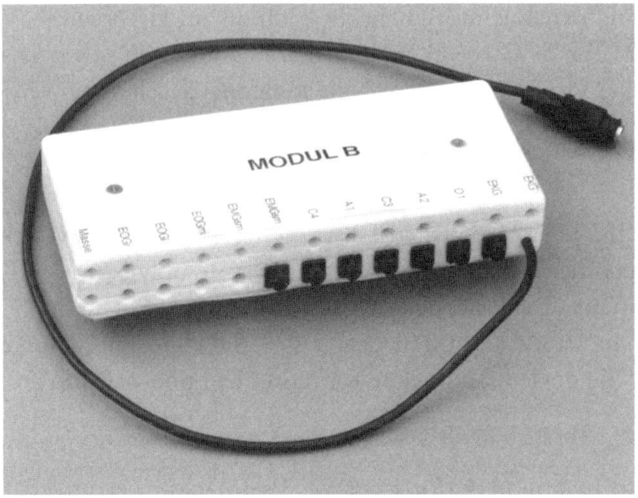

Figure 2. Polysomnography module for measuring 19 channels.

Varioport B (OEM recorder)

The availability of integrated processors makes possible the construction of a Varioport variant consisting of fewer construction elements, that is still efficient enough for the majority of usages. The eight-bit RISC processor also achieved lower power-consumption rate and contains the required program and data memory on the same chip. There is no display and there are only two operator keys and two marker keys. There are four 12-bit amplifiers with differential inputs, so that up to four channels can be used without a pre-amplifier. The digital Varioport A amplifiers are connectable and can be extended to up to 60 channels. A second serial interface allows the connection of an intelligent oxygen sensor (for example, "Nonin™").

This recorder is almost the equal of the Varioport A and requires no complex preprocessing. The device's software and data are completely compatible with the Varioport A. However, the structure of the micro-controller is basically different, so that large differences result in the "real-time SPIL" (Signal Processing and Inferencing Language, see below).

Varioport M

For special purposes, a still smaller and more inconspicuous device is required, that is still able to record as many environmental parameters as may be required, as well as some physiological data. This requirement led to the development of the Varioport M with the dimensions 8.5 x 4.5 x 1.7 cm and a weight of only 70 grams. The highly integrated RISC processor mentioned above made further miniaturization of the electronics possible. A multimedia card (currently up to 64 MB) is used as the storage medium.

The device registers the ambient temperature, sound and light, as well as all three axes of static and dynamic movement. In addition, an HF receiver is integrated in the Varioport M for ECG breast belts, that are common in sport, as well as inputs for three external signals (for example, an additional acceleration sensor). Powered by two LR1 batteries, the device can operate for longer than a week.

Varioport S

For measuring the physical activity of hyperactive children, an even more miniaturized activity recorder was developed. With a size of only 5.5 x 4 x 1.3 cm and its weight of 40 grams, the device records all three spacial axes statically and dynamically as well as the temperature. The data is stored on an eight MB integrated flash-memory card. The device can operate for more than one week on an LR3 battery.

Dialog Pad

Various palm-top computers (for example, Psion) have been used for recording psychological variables in the field. To simplify use, when no programming skills are available, we developed an instruction language for question lists, in order to program the computer with extensive, event-driven lists of questions. Unfortunately, this solution, which was developed using Psion equipment, has some disadvantages, such as the comparatively high energy consumption of the Psion. Also, this palmtop computer is fairly large and heavy. The advantages are that the Psion, however, is equipped with a user-friendly keyboard. Therefore, we developed a miniaturized dialog pad with an active serial interface which can run up to four weeks (Figure 3) using the above-mentioned RISC processor. It has the dimension 10.4 x 5.7 x 2 cm and weighs 95 grams. The display is a 2 x 16 character LCD screen. To assist the user under varying light condition, a photo sensor in the dialog pad continuously measures the ambient light and adjusts the background display illumination automatically.

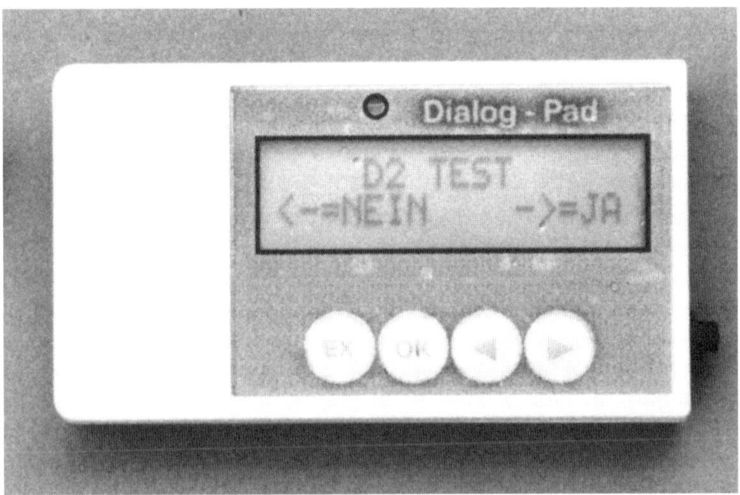

Figure 3. The dialog pad for recording psychological variables in the field.

The device can register several months of data using two AAA batteries (with a non-activated serial interface). Each recorder in the Varioport series is capable of responding to event-driven queries, for example, a question can be prompted by a sharp rise in the heart rate without any significant physical activity. The formulation of questions in the questionnaire's catalogue is very simple and can be done in any text editor for which no programming skills are required. Complex questionnaire structures, as well as two vigilance tests, can be pre-defined. However, the system is not designed for free-text inputs. The input is saved on an internal 1MB flash memory.

Variograf Software

The control software (formerly Vitagraf) is being constantly upgraded, especially the internal computer language SPIL (Signal Processing and Inferencing Language), which is available in both, an off-line and an on-line version (real-time SPIL).

Real-Time SPIL

Real-time SPIL is a subset of SPIL, which is implemented as an object code on the recorder. Vitaport II and Varioport A are based on 68020 machine code.

Universal Real-Time SPIL

Since the RISC processor used in the new variants of the Varioport uses "Harvard structure", it cannot execute machine code in RAM. Therefore, an option was installed in the SPIL compiler to put out an optimized "Token" code instead of machine code, which can be interpreted by the RISC processors. Unfortunately, this variant is much slower than the previous one. Also, the processor includes no hardware multiplier, however, it can emulate mathematical SPIL commands, but only comparatively slowly. For the development of extensive and efficient real-time preprocessing programs the Varioport A is to be preferred.

Outlook

Sleep Diagnosis and testing

Usual sleep diagnosis is very complex for the examiner because of the multiplicity of electrodes and sensors, and annoying for the patient because of the cables. This complicates the application particularly for ambulatory patients. We are therefore working on a concept which functions largely without the annoying cables and offers advantages to both examiners and patients alike. In order to give the subjects more freedom of movement, telemetric procedures have been used in the past. The disadvantages in previous systems, aside from the high sensitivity, were the equipment costs and the restriction of movement for the subject, who had to stay in the vicinity of the telemetric transceiver.

We have tried to find a way to amplify, optimally pre-process and store the data from each separate sensor near the electrodes and sensors. This requires very tiny, efficient data logs, which can be integrated in the casing, together with the sensors. The Vario S presented above, for instance, is such a device, that in its standard design includes temperature, position and acceleration sensors. However, the recording of electro-physiological parameters requires the use of the customary electrodes, if one wants to maintain the quality. In sleep diagnosis, most of the electrodes are taped to the head. The cables dangle freely over a relatively long distance before they lead into the amplifier. This does involve a higher level of interference, especially with weak EEG signals. To deal with this, we have developed a device, which allows amplifier and data recording to be contained in the smallest space possible and can be worn directly on the vertex. Thereby, the electrodes and sensor cables can be kept extremely short. The positioning of the EEG electrodes is done according to Rechtschaffen and Kales' (1968) Ten-Twenty System. This requires time-consuming measuring of the head surface.

Polysomnographic Hood

Together with Falk Minow in Munich, we have designed a polysomnographic hood, in which the electrodes are woven, so that the guidelines of the Ten-Twenty System are fulfilled. The submental EMG, the sensors for oronasal flow and the microphone to register snoring are also integrated: Disposable material is saved, which increases the comfort for the patient and shortens the set-up time.

With a reflex sensor pulse oximetry can be integrated into the polysomnographic hood. The remaining parameters are recorded in a chest box, which is clipped to a breast belt. Here, the ECG, body position, acceleration, thoracic breathing, abdo-

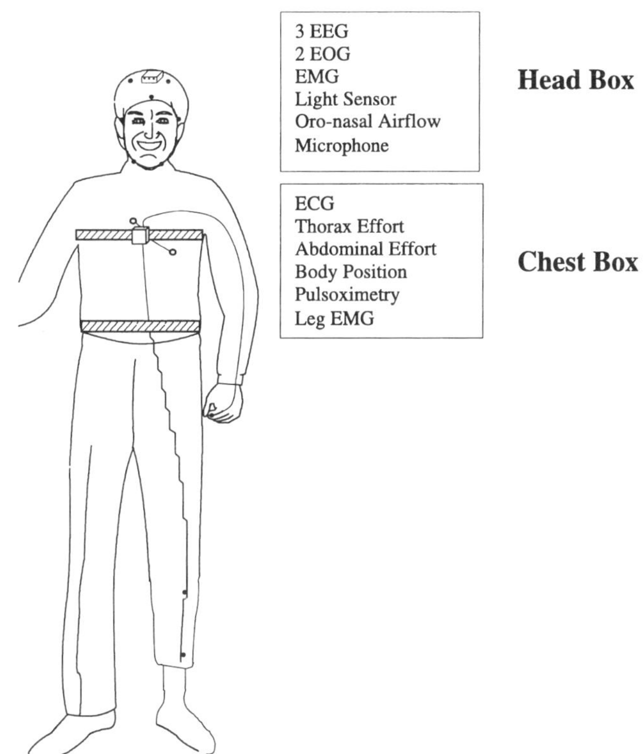

Figure 4. Polysomnography with Head- and Chestbox.

minal breathing, the tibialis EMG, and the pulse oximetry are registered (Figure 4).

The comfort for the patient can be further increased by using a Vario S with acceleration sensor carried on the ankle instead of the cable for the tibialis EMG measurement. Thus an entirely decentralized measurement with independent sensors is possible, which is also very comfortable for the patient. For the examiner, however, the system is laborious, since he has to ensure the power supply to all the devices as well as pay careful attention to the data assembly of the separate devices.

References

Jain, A., Martens, W.L.J., Mutz, G., Weiß, R.K. & Stephan, E. (1996). Towards a comprehensive technology for recording and analysis of multiple physiological parameters within their behavioral and environmental context. In J. Fahrenberg & M. Myrtek (Eds.), *Ambulatory Assessment* (pp. 215-235). Göttingen: Hogrefe.

Rechtschaffen, A. & Kales, A. (Eds.) (1968). *A manual of standardized terminology, techniques, and scoring system for sleep stages of human subjects.* Washington, D.C.: U.S. Government printing Office.

Chapter 34
From Ambulatory Assessment to Telemedicine. Conceptual, Technical and Political Aspects of Remote Data Assessment and Transfer

Christian Leopold
Nets Healthcare GmbH, München, Germany

Introduction

Ambulatory assessment, as defined in *Ambulatory Assessment. Computer-assisted psychological and psychophysiological methods in monitoring and field studies*, "involves the acquisition of psychological data and/or physiological measures in everyday life (that is, natural settings) according to an explicit assessment strategy which relates data, theoretical constructs, and empirical criteria specific to the given research issue" (Fahrenberg, 1996, p. 4.).

This definition concentrates on the assessment of data in real-life settings like at home, at work, during a longer clinic stay or under extreme conditions like parachuting or oral exams. Within this context, psychological assessment does not necessarily require the use of electronic data recording (Vogt & Schandry, 1995). However, complex psychological data assessment and realistic physiological recording lead to the application of computer technologies.

Still, the definition concentrates on research issues, implicitly excluding, for example, regular therapeutic situations like computer-tailored patient education, psychophysiologically supported behavior therapy (in both in patient or outpatient settings).

The method of ambulatory assessment helped to overcome several traditional shortcomings of psychology (for example, Baumann et al., 1996; Pawlik, 1996). Having overcome early technological hurdles, the next-step methodological problems also seem to be narrowed down to a practical level (Stemmler, 1996). Since we will be able to apply more and more sophisticated solutions to the methodological and technical problems within ambulatory assessment, future developments should permit the design of further therapeutic applications.

If, amongst others, one aim of ambulatory assessment is to be its integration into "experimental" or even routine health care, it might be useful to identify and discuss the elements relevant for this process. Taking a contrasting look into neighbouring areas of research might foster the future developments of ambulatory assessment. The employment of modern computer technology within therapy is already well known in medicine. The domain in medicine most comparable to ambulatory assessment is telemedicine. Before looking in depth at telemedicine, I will give some examples for already existing applications of ambulatory assessment in medicine.

Examples for ambulatory assessment in medicine

The following section will document some applications of ambulatory assessment within medicine. Integrating the ambulatory assessment approach instead of a doctor's practice measurements might disclose new diagnostic and therapeutic insights. There are for example, some references for clinically relevant reactivity effects (Mucha et al., 1996). The home-based multiparametric assessment would draw a much better picture for therapeutic interventions.

For a differentiated verification of pharmaceutical therapeutic success in Parkinson patients, it is helpful to record the patients´ tremor activity through accelerometry (Smeja et al., 1999).

The diabetic patient and his/her physician are already able to collect ambulatory monitoring data. An expert system analyses the data through a set of software tools, and suggests an adjustment in therapy in order to tackle the identified metabolic problems and to fit the patient's needs (Montani et al., 1999).

The assessment of blood pressure during treatment by measuring the casual blood pressure is potentially inaccurate. The introduction of ambulatory blood pressure monitoring in the care of hypertensive patients, however, has some potential advantages. The blood pressure values have proved to have a better correlation with end-organ damage in hypertensive patients than do those observed for casual blood pressure, and a better prognosis in terms of cardiovascular morbidity and mortality (Pickering & James, 1994). Moreover, circadian variability and variability between the half-hour blood pressure average are also prognostic in hypertensive patients (Frattola et al., 1993). In cardiologic practices, 24-h-ambulatory blood pressure recording is already prescribed to patients. This diagnostic intervention yields three advantages for the doctor: No distortion of results by unfamiliar assessment situations, dynamic information because of multiple measurements and recording under basic (nighttime) conditions. Research has proved that the relationship between daytime and nighttime blood pressure information can be more valid with respect to future cardiovascular problems than the daytime information (Frisina et al., 1996). The reimbursement of the ambulatory 24-hour-blood pressure measurement within the [German] healthcare system is a good example for the accepted usefulness of ambulatory assessment. Sleep medicine outside the doctor's laboratory is likely to follow soon.

Routine projects containing ambulatory assessment in medicine can also be found as patient diaries within clinical studies for therapy and drug evaluation. The compliance with drug intake instructions (Coutts, Gibson & Paton, 1992) and a reduction in diary failures, like forgetfulness or fraud (Tattersall & Ellis, 1989) are the main reasons here.

While improving the interactions of drug and patient's metabolism, the pharmaceutical industry and governmental institutions (for example, the U.S. Food and Drug administration; FDA) are concentrating on a more precise diagnosis and the (home) monitoring of patients' disease states. Because of inter-patient variation and concerns for safety, so called "theranostics" may be required to objectively quantify a drug's effects on cells in order to prescribe appropriate dosing for each patient (Theranostics: The influence of diagnostics on pharmaceutical therapy, report, 2000). The term "theranostics" (or predictive medicine) describes an evolving group of products that link diagnostics with pharmaceutical treatment. The theranostic might identify which patients would be most suited to a particular drug therapy or could be used to provide feedback on how well a drug is working in order to tailor the optimum treatment regimen. Many theranostics need to be point-of-care tests. In many cases, the results of the tests need to be available quickly and at the patient's side, in order to influence therapy. The potentials of classical ambulatory assessment, such as theranostics, have not yet been clarified.

Ambulatory assessment in psychology can have three aims: Diagnosing behavior, initiating new behavior or states, or maintaining newly learned behavior. The latter seems much easier for an automatic approach, because duration, frequency and the grade of personalisation plays no great role. Intensity and complexity, however, may be essentials for the phase of learning new health care patterns. As an diagnostic tool, ambulatory assessment of medication intake, for example, in psychiatric (Elixhauser et al., 1990) or in elderly patients (Kruse et al., 1992) may provide evidence that patients are less compliant, hence requiring more intense psychological care and observation. The documentation of therapeutic success and therapeutic intervention at the same time may be found in ambulatory computer-assisted behavior therapy for obesity. The frequency of self-monitoring behavior data was directly related to therapeutic success (Burnett et al., 1992). Similar to weight reduction, ambulatory assessment of disease behavior in a computer-administered self-assessment behavior program for obsessive-compulsive behavior may be documentation and intervention in one. Baer and Greist (1997) initiated their BT STEPS in order to primarily monitor and treat patients with a computer program. 71% of the 65 participants reported an improvement because of the program.

These examples already draw a picture, showing the usefulness of ambulatory assessment within medicine. In medicine, ambulatory monitoring like approaches in most cases are telemonitoring applications. For a comparison of telemedicine and ambulatory assessment see Table 1.

Table 1. Comparing basic aspects of telemedicine and ambulatory assessment.

Aspect	Telemedicine	Ambulatory Assessment
Content focus	Medical issues	1. Psychological and 2. Medical issues
Primary technology	Telecommunication of data, voice, pictures and video	Miniaturised sensor technology, data recording and storage
Application	Practical medicine	Research
Initial idea	Economically offering health care to people without near-by access	Research methodology for new insights in psychology / psychophysiology concepts
Frequent thematic issues	Teleconsulting, teleradiology, telemonitoring, telecare	Stress, patient diaries, workplace strain, psycho(physiological) diagnostics
Degree of technological progress	High	Moderate
Degree of practical employment	Moderate	Low
Number of participants per project	100 – 10.000	10-500
Public funding	high	low

Telemedia

Conceptual aspects

Already for about thirty years (Bashshur & Lovett, 1977) western countries have been elaborating on telemedicine technology and concepts. The need for telemedicine was born out of the financial burdens for the receipts of health care. The initial argumentation was that there are large segments of the (U.S.) population for whom equity of access to health care has not been fully attained. Telemedicine should be a technological response to such problems in the delivery of health services that result from the maldistribution of medical manpower and facilities towards the distribution of the client population.

The immediate benefit of telemedicine is to bring medical services to isolated, geographically dispersed, and physically confined persons unable to reach a physician within a reasonable time or distance. Indeed, its major promise was to bring health services to people wherever it is not possible or feasible to bring people to health services. Telemedicine does *not* focus on the data assessment, but on the healing and treatment of patients, while taking into consideration that this treatment is independent of the patient's site. This premise led the American "Telemedicine Research Centres" to define telemedicine as "the use of electronic signals to transfer medical information from one site to another" (see also http://tie.telemed.org /TIEmap.html or Hayes et al., 1996). Another frequently quoted definition is from Field (1997, p. 28): "Telemedicine is the use of information and telecommunication technologies to provide and support healthcare when distance separates the participants."

Summarizing the definitions, the term telemedicine describes the use of telecommunication technology to enhance the delivery of medical services.

Hence, this approach, by definition, demands a strong telecommunication technology. Compared to ambulatory assessment, for example, the electronic collection of medical data at home is not immediately considered to be a telemedical application. After data collection, electronic data transmission from one site to another is necessary for a valid use of the term "telemedicine".

Meanwhile telemedicine has widened up to a complex construction consisting of for example:

- tele-consultation: the integration of an external expert for therapy and diagnosis through electronic means, for example, the transfer of written, acoustic or graphical information (as in tele-radiology, tele-pathology) or
- tele-conferencing: visual online information exchange between medical experts in a video conference or
- tele-surgery: the provision of surgical care over a distance, with direct, real-time visualization of the operative field.

Telemedicine in home care can be distinguished between telecare, telemonitoring and the communication between care providers. The telemonitoring of vital signs and other physiological parameters, for example, blood pressure, temperature, and heart rate (see also Table 2), includes services where a patient stays at home but is under the supervision of one or more healthcare providers, and/or social workers, using remote-monitoring.

Of 167 investigated telemedicine projects in Europe, 62% were dealing with teleconsulting, 13% telecare, 11% tele-education and 8% telemonitoring (The Emerging European Health Telematics Industry, 2000).

As telecommunication is one defining element of telemedicine or telemonitoring, it may be useful for further understanding to first of all have a closer look at the technical prerequisites (Allen, 1996).

Technical aspects: telecommunication

The main issue in telecommunication is transporting as quickly as possible as much data as possible. This is of special importance if the data involves pictures or video signals (high bandwidth), of less importance (small bandwidth) if they are audio and voice signals and of almost no importance for biosignals (exception: high resolution EEG or MEG). The process of data transmission is basically determined by four elements: The principle of data transmission and its network, the standards behind it, the protocol for the standard, and the format of the data. These elements will be described in detail and examples are given.

Table 2. Sample selection of commercially available telemonitoring systems.

Signal/parameter	Wireless transmission	Analogue or ISDN transmission	Company/product
Blood glucose	No	Yes	Aerotel/Gluco-Tel
Blood pressure, pulse	No	Yes	American Medical Development/AMD 9200
Blood pressure, weight, pulse, pulse oximetry	No	Yes	AvidCare/AvidCare Monitor
Foetal heart rate, tocography, maternal blood pressure	No	Yes	Card Guard/Foetal monitor CG-900P
Real time ECG with pacemaker pulse	No	Yes	Card Guard/PMD® CG4000
Spirometry with PEF, FEV1, FVC, MEF25, MEF50, MEF75, MMEF	Yes	Yes	Erich Jaeger/AM2 with HC1
Medication compliance, patient reminders, disease information	No	Yes	InforMedix/MediMonitor®
Patient activated ECG event recorder	Yes	Yes	Micromedical Industries /Heart Tel
Subjective patient ratings, (physiological recordings), adaptive dialogs	Yes	Yes	Nets AG/CCM 2.0 with Dialog Solutions™
Continuous ECG monitoring, data transmission via integrated GSM module	Yes	No	Schiller AG/Microvit MT-120
Real-time levels of oxygen saturation, pulse rate	No	Yes	SHL TeleMedicine/HCC with Tele Pulse Oxymeter
ECG with place detection through GPS (Global Positioning System)	Yes	No	Vitaphone/Herz Handy®

Principles of data transmission. Telecommunication networks consist of a hardware system, being the backbone for data transmission, like copper cables, optical fibres, or over-the-air radio or satellite transmission. They determine the upper transmission rates. However, the so-called "last mile" of data transmission to the recipient in most cases determines the available data transmission speed.

The transmission standards. How the data transmission is basically organised at the sender and receiver hardware is determined by a corresponding standard like ISDN (Integrated Services Digital Network, for example, H.320) and its available services ADSL/DSL (Asymmetric / Digital Subscriber Line), or GSM (Group Special Mobile/Global System for Mobile Communications) for wireless transmission with the services of GPRS (General Packet Radio Service) or HSCSD (High Speed Circuit Switched Data). The new mobile communications standard UMTS (Universal Mobile Telecommunications System) starting in Europe about 2003 is the next known endpoint of wireless transmission technology.

Example: H.320 encompasses a set of standards for narrow-band, visual telephone systems and terminal equipment, commonly used in interactive, live video applications for telemedicine. It describes a generic system configuration consisting of a number of elements, a definition of communication modes and terminal types, call control arrangements, terminal aspects, and interfunctional requirements.

The transmission protocols. The action of transmission is controlled by a protocol which determines whether data are compressed, how files are segmented and how the correctness of signal transmission is guaranteed for the sender and receiver.

Example: There is an ongoing tendency in telemedicine to integrate the Internet into different technical solutions. TCP/IP (Transfer Control Protocol / Internet Protocol) as the Internet's networking protocol are the most complete and accepted networking protocols available. When a particular application sends data through TCP, TCP breaks the message into packets, sized appropriately to the network. The IP protocol basically addresses and sends these packets.

The data formats. Furthermore, the exchange between different software products needs unique and compatible data formats and standards like XML, HL7, DICOM, etc.

Examples: DICOM (Digital Imaging and Communications in Medicine) is the industry standard for the transferral of radiologic images and other medical information between computers.

HL7 (Health Level Seven) is a standard for the electronic interchange of clinical, financial and administrative information among independent health care oriented computer systems; for example, hospital information systems, clinical laboratory systems, enterprise systems and pharmacy systems.

XML (eXtended Markup Language) is a standard coming from outside the healthcare system. It uses the definition of style sheets, which allows data extraction from a file into an SQL-database. The document definition for medical purposes has only just begun. XML seems to become a generic standard for a wide range of data base applications. Modern HTML-Browsers are able to display XML-files.

Yet, there is no unique digital data standard for biosignals. All systems use their proprietary data format. No standard interfaces are defined.

Data privacy

In order to distinguish different data sets, to identify matching data, to support research data, or to enhance data processing and reimbursement, the patient's name or personal characteristics have to be transmitted. Although the trend suggests that the "de-personalising" of medical data files could be implemented, instead of relentlessly trying to protect personalised files, I will mention the most relevant aspects of data security and data privacy.

The processing of personalised health data is completely different to the processing of perfectly anonymous data. As soon as personalised health data are transmitted through a public network, the security of data is of major importance.

In most countries, data security and data privacy laws contain special regulations for health data. Accordingly, health data may usually be collected only if the subject has given his explicit consent. According to German data privacy laws, each patient has to give his informed consent to each single data transfer.

Of central importance is the duty to inform persons from whom data is collected of the purposes for which the data is to be used, in order to ensure that proper consent has been obtained and to enable the subjects to object to processing, on compelling legitimate grounds, if they so desire (Lloyd, 1996), (European Data Protection Directive, Art. 14). The subject must also be given access "without constraint at reasonable intervals and without excessive delay or expense" (Art. 12). The information to be provided concerns the confirmation of processing, purposes of processing, categories of data and recipients, or the categories of recipients. Patients will also have a right to information about the logic of any automated decision-making (Art. 15) which might, for instance, be concerned with the allocation of health care services. The subject may also require the rectification, erasure or blocking of data which does not comply with the Directive, "in particular because of the incomplete or inaccurate nature of the data" (Art. 12(b)).

Data security

Besides the fact that data should not be corrupted during transport, they should also be safe in the event of any willful data misuse. The security of networks and data communication can be directed through four main areas: cryptography, access control, authentication, and secure network protocols (Smith & Eloff, 1999).

Cryptography. Before data transport, a mathematical algorithm for all data is used to transform them into a new format. This algorithm or key is only known to authorised people. If encryption and decryption is performed using the same algorithm, it is called symmetric. If both parties are applying two different keys (a private key and a public key), the procedure is called asymmetric. In any case, it is important to keep the keys a secret.

Access control. Access control determines who is permitted access to the data stored or transmitted over the system. There may need to be multiple layers of security to control access, for example, persons having access to basic patient data, but not to confidential medical records or telemonitored data. Access authorisation to computer systems consists of more physical means, like locks, biometric devices (palm prints or retinal scans) or logical means like passwords.

Authentication. Authentication is dealing with the safe and provable recognition of sender and recipient of data. Main requirements are a) only specified individuals have access to the data b) the author/creator of the data/document shall be identified c) the documentation of all versions and revisions of data (including when and by whom). Amongst others passwords, digital signatures or "Health Professional Cards" (HPC) are able to participate to authentication solutions. Related to authentication is the integrity of data, meaning the characteristic of data and information being accurate and complete and the preservation of accuracy and completeness.

Secure networks. A common approach to help insure network security is to not connect it to the Internet or other public network. The problem with this approach is that while an isolated network may be more secure, it has limited functionality. The role of a network firewall is to insulate the users of a local private network from external threats. Generally the firewall works as a filter to incoming packets of information which are often commands issued to the local system server.
Further problems exist where the information is transmitted in the clear over the network. To protect web information from traveling in the clear there are a number of possible approaches available. The Secure Sockets Layer (SSL) protocol creates a secure connection between an internet client and a server. In two phases server and client authentication and a private key for data encryption are established.

Legal aspects. In most countries, health care data processing is protected by certain laws. However, the situation of international telemedicine is quite new to lawyers and some topics are still under discussion.

Depending on the national legal situation it may already be difficult to allow physicians to practice outside of their licensed geographical area (state, district). If data are even crossing national borders, liability still remains an open question. Who is responsible for damage and which judicial system can be applied. If data are transferred from a physician to another physician / person, is the recipient still liable to medical confidentiality? (Stanberry, 1998) In case of a trial, if the patient data are no longer in the house of the responsible physician, does he/she still has the right to refuse to testify? Some legal experts also consider the freedom to choose one's own physician and prohibition against advertising as a physician to be a critical issue in telemedicine. Especially in Germany, reimbursement regulatory agencies must take care that even unpaid telemonitoring services do not simultaneously increase the number of paid patient contacts. Up to now most health care systems only consider reimbursement as possible, if the patient was physically present at the doctor´s practice. These open questions indicate the need for national and international regulations in defined political structures.

Health policy aspects

Individual, island-pattern telemedical hardware solutions neglect the networking concept and reduce the potential of telemedicine to a remote data transfer.

Connecting different telemedical projects increases their effectiveness, although this requires the compatibility of technology, data acquisition plans, data analysis, and data banking. The standardisation of these areas brings with it a strong interference in solid organisational structures (Aas, 1999; Whitten & Allen, 1995). Modern electronic and telematic medicine accelerated the actual trend of cross-border, global interactions and collaborations. Telemedicine supports the need of standardisation, harmonisation, and guidelines. These are also the aims of international funding organisations sponsoring telemedicine. Along with international harmonisation, it is seen that the future of national health care systems is strongly related to the future developments in telemedicine and telematics (*tele*communications + infor*matics*). (Rigby, 1999). In 1989, the European Commission started a first systematic stimulation of telematic applications with the "Advanced Informatics in Medicine" (AIM) program, later on integrated into the telematics program. Up to now, the European Commission spent about 250 million EUROs for more than 150 telematics projects (Dietzel, 2001).

However, globally there is a discrepancy between governmental development funds, on the one hand, and the integration of telemedicine concepts in an official legal health policy framework, on the other. Easy pooling of large data bases from different sites offers new insights into current data, like better diagnostic results or the respective quality of health care structures. These issues are in line with the idea of national and international health reports. Nevertheless, this new data contains the potential for basic restructuring measures within the health care system. Because of its many conflicting interests, major changes are not intended by all institutional elements of the health care system. Hence, the integration of telemedicine concepts in legal health policies is very slow.

The first element of this regulatory framework is the development of an appropriate reimbursement process (Fields, 1999). In Europe and in the U.S., the reimbursement of telemedical health care services is still a matter of negotiations and profound improvements have not yet been achieved (DeParle, 2000). This open state is still hindering a directed development of telemedicine.

Aside from the matter of financing, a legal basis will have to be established in order to restructure the education of medical doctors and psychologists, or psychotherapists. Within the European harmonisation of academic education, telemedical approaches do not have to stop along a political border.

Telecare and telemonitoring intensively interfere with actual hospital plannings. All forecasts concerning the future development of healthcare claim that there will be a strong reduction of treatments in hospitals and predict the increased closure of hospitals (Arnold & Paffrath, 1998). This is the consequence of stronger savings in the healthcare systems and will be strengthened by any trend of health care privatisation. Outpatient systems like telecare and telemonitoring will replace many hospital services. A British study indicated that about 15% of home visits could be replaced by telecare because of the absence of hands-on procedures (Wootton et al, 1998). A retrospective U.S. analysis of 906 home nursing visits claims half of the visits could have been performed with telemonitoring technology (Allen et al., 1999).

The U.S. Military Health Care System investigated the clinical and business situation for telecare in Europe. They summarise that 31,000 conventional consultations per year in Europe could be replaced by telemedical applications. The potential savings amounted to $3.7 million in travel costs and 25,000 working days (Navein, Arose & Pietermich, 1999). Although theory and empirical data support an introduction of telemedicine into health care, governments and economic experts are reluctant towards telemedicine (Bashshur & Neuberger, 1995). A widespread evaluation of telemedicine is still lacking (Holle & Zahlmann, 1999).

Despite these burdens, it seems realistic that governmental institutions of western countries will regulate the introduction of telecare and telemonitoring within the next decade.

Integrating telecommunication technology into ambulatory assessment

Integrating telecommunication technology into ambulatory assessment means the long-distance transmission of data from the subject to a central site. It is then possible to combine the advantages of ambulatory assessment with those of telecommunications. Implicitly, it may also mean the networking of data recording and data management between researchers or health care institutions.

Combining ambulatory assessment with telecommunication has some potential advantages and disadvantages. In the following, I will concentrate on the wireless and continuous data transmission model for the transfer of recorded data from the patient to a central data management site. Subsequently, the pros and cons of an extension of ambulatory assessment with telecommunication technologies are discussed.

Transmission of data. Pros of wireless telemonitoring:

- A continuous back and forth of data streams between subject and research centre allows checking and correcting of the ongoing data assessment, for example, altering the configuration of data acquisition without calling the patient into the laboratory. The advantage of real-time data transmission and analysis is that the investigator or the computer system may immediately intervene during the recording process. This leads to less invalid data, less frustration, and fewer costs.
- Giving immediate feedback through the actual data analysis to the participant.

- Reaching populations who are unable to come to the laboratory frequently during long-term data recordings, for example, for storing or data checks.
- Shortening the duration of data recording through precise identification of the point in time for a sufficient amount of data.

Networking solutions of data recording and management. Pros of standardised technical recording solutions:

- A central data base allows for the computation of "meta-analyses" and benchmarking;
- Quality assurance for all members of the network;
- Central, automatic configuration/updating of new software versions is possible;
- Compatibility of data formats means an easy exchange of data;
- Encompassing databases offer a better standing within regulatory and financial negotiations with health care sponsors;
- Low individual costs (the system components are shared by a user community).

When ambulatory assessment is called telemonitoring. Some examplary scenarios.

As the functional and technical advantages of integrating telecommunication technology into ambulatory assessment were summarized in the section above, applications of this relatively new combination shall be outlined now.

The diagnostic process in medicine assesses actual data from one static point in time. Repeatedly retrieving data at the patient's home in order to describe a dynamic disease process over a long time period is a new concept within medicine. Appropriate analytic and diagnostic knowledge is still lacking. The in-depth observation and interpretation of multiple data points mostly exceeds the human capabilities. Digital computer processing may support this ongoing diagnostic approach by proposing certain actions to the physician or by reminding him/her of predefined measures. Some examples for treatment and diagnostics will be given below.

The transfer of telemedical elements into ambulatory assessment may also be fruitful for psychotherapy, psychiatry and patient education (see also Leopold & Schandry, this Volume). Psychophysiological diagnostics may become extremely important while referring the patient to his/her most effective treatment. New assessment instruments could be designed for psychological diagnostics. Future psychiatric or psychological treatment may integrate psychophysical ambulatory recording in order to support diagnostics and the therapy of psychological disorders. New models like telemedical provision of consultation-liaison services to the primary care setting will then be possible (Hilty et al., 2000). Generally, nine principal telemonitoring health care scenarios in medicine and psychology can be identified to date, being realised with actual available technology:

- Diagnostics. In order to clarify his/her diagnosis, a doctor / therapist provides his/her patient with a (psychological, psychophysiological or medical) ambulatory monitoring device. After some days or weeks, the patient returns the device to the doctor's practice. The data is analysed and integrated in his/her therapeutic plan.
- Diagnostics and intervention. A doctor/therapist has identified a patient for the useful employment of an ambulatory monitoring device within the context of his/her (behavioral medicine) therapeutic plan. The monitoring and feedback of psychological and psychophysiological data in the patient's natural environment are a substantial part of his/her therapy.
- Diagnostics and teleconsultation. Within a patient's more long-term diagnostic process, a primary care practice wishes to consult a medical expert who has experience in ambulatory monitoring. The recordings of the ambulatory monitoring device are transmitted to the expert via a telecommunication system ("centre of competence"). The expert's advice is then fed back to the primary care practice.
- Diagnostics and treatment optimisation. After diagnosis, a doctor/therapist has identified a number of therapeutic approaches for a patient's problem. After having given an ambulatory device to the patient for a certain length of time, he/she is able to verify the data, and to change the (electronically supported) therapy and diagnostic program accordingly. This iterative process of ambulatory diagnosis and therapy occurs until a predefined treatment goal has been reached.
- Physician-based, computer tailored training. After a consultation in his/her general practitioner's practice, the patient enrols for example, in a migraine training program. The medication, pain frequency and intensity registered at home trigger a computer-tailored patient education program. The recorded data is also available to the doctor for therapy adjustments.
- Call centre-based disease management. The patient is offered an education program for his/her chronic disease like diabetes or asthma by his/her health insurance or health maintenance organisation (HMO). The program is a combination of written education material, call-centre based training and an ambulatory assessment device which is connected with the call centre. Call-centre training integrates the ambulatory assessment data.
- Externally triggered diagnostics/interventions. The patient is equipped with a telemonitoring spirometer which also continuously receives information from an external data base, for example, pollen information. At a certain level of pollen concentration, the patient is prompted to assess his/her lung function with the spirometer. An analysis of the lung function parameter may confirm his/her allergy against pollen.

- Telemonitoring surveillance. A patient is under a severe drug treatment. He/she registers his/her daily medication use and a medical parameter, like blood coagulation. If parameters are beyond the range of a physiologic equilibrium, the telemedical system sends an alert message to a physician. He/She looks up the actual patient´s telemonitoring data, calls the patient and asks for his/her symptoms, etc.
- Individualised tele-rehabilitation. A patient with a cognitive disorder, like mild dementia or a situation following a head injury, etc. is send little cognitive and behavioral tasks. The results are keyed into the recording device and transmitted to a centre. Therapy progression is documented, task success is fed back to the patient and the difficulty of the tasks is adapted to the patient's responses.

One actual example for the interaction of ambulatory assessment and telemonitoring

Finally, using asthma and diabetes as an example, I will take out one scenario above and describe in depth the mutual exchanges between ambulatory assessment and telemedicine. After defining the relevant demands for such a case, a flexible technology system delivering these features will be presented.

Patients of both chronic diseases do benefit from a permanent registration of their primary disease parameters through the optimal adaptation of daily therapy or that required during exacerbations (see also Leopold & Schandry, this Volume).

According to the patient self-management theory, patients should be able to interpret their own patient diaries. The same diary information should also be easily accessible to the responsible doctor, or to other involved health care providers, for example, case manager, education nurse or researchers.

Recording peak-flow or blood glucose values documents the basic medical parameters. However, health psychology could show that a valid assessment of chronic health states has to include subjective measures also, like symptom lists or quality-of-life questions. Furthermore, patients of both diseases cited carry a potential risk of symptom unawareness, consisting of an overestimation of blood glucose or peak-flow. Studies proved that diary methods are effective for assessing the patients' capabilities of symptom perception (Cox et al, 1991; Leopold, Poth & Schandry, 1999). All data should then be analysed according to the strategies of ecological momentary assessment data (EMA) which involve new statistical procedures that include the potential for individual diagnostic evidence (Litt, Cooney & Morse, 1998; Schwarz & Stone, 1998).

Within an sophisticated, standardised ambulatory monitoring plan, the assessment of physiological parameters, subjective measures of well-being and of interoceptive ability may only be allowed within certain time intervals, for example, in the morning from 7 a.m. – 9:30 a.m. A reminder system also might inform patients about data input before this interval or after the interval should data input be missing.

Improving the patients' compliance the monitoring protocol should consist of an adaptive survey structure not bothering the patients with unnecessary questions. An individualised alert system should provide patients with the actual security of knowing whether they are within or beyond certain therapeutic limits. Furthermore, sending short messages with study or disease education information to the patients should also increase the data quality and the patients' compliance. Sophisticated assessment plans and analyses should be able to reduce or detect accidental or intentional misuse during data input (online range checks, offline data mining for pattern detection).

In conclusion, all collected data has to be statistically analysed, and the results must be depicted clearly and graphically in real-time. Relevant results like trends should individually be fed back to patients and health care providers simultaneously in real-time. Researchers or a healthcare provider should be able to electronically change the monitoring protocol easily from his desk, even for a larger patient population.

All listed points belong into the field of ambulatory assessment. On the other hand, taken together, this setting describes typical elements of telemedicine, like telemonitoring, telecare or teleconsultation.

Meanwhile, modern telecommunication technologies offer ambulatory systems which are able to realise these complex assessment situations for ambulatory assessment and/or telemedicine.

To date, the Nets AG (Munich), a German technology provider, markets a unique solution for ambulatory assessment applications mainly based on mobile phones and internet (Kapsner & Sangha, 2000). Meanwhile the system has successfully been used in a series of projects. As an Application Service Provider-model (ASP), without the installation of a special software, the Communication Chain Management™ platform (CCM™ 2.0) allows the construction of complex, adaptive, individualised, monitoring dialogs with patients or subjects (as cited in the asthma/diabetes example above).

The user interface may be a mobile phone, an Internet PC with the usual Internet browser (for example, Microsoft Internet Explorer), a pager, PDA (Personal Digital Assistant) or any other digital device. Communication features can be defined freely according to the respective monitoring design. Data input, data analyses and data output work in real-time, thus enabling patients and researchers an online look at their actual data. Physiological sensor systems like ECG, blood glucose, peak-flow, etc. can be connected with the mobile phone, for example, through a cable, an infrared interface or, in the future, through BlueTooth, a technology standard for wireless, network-like communication between any electronic device within the range of 10 – 100 metres technology. Right now, the system's transfer rates are limited to the actual Wireless Application Protocol (WAP), although future services like GPRS and ultimately UMTS will increase the transmission potentials for sound, digital pictures or digital video signals. Ambulatory assessment based on modern telecommunication will then be open for perfectly new possibilities.

Conclusions

Up to now, ambulatory assessment was guided by the developing technology and the progress in research. Certainly, telemedicine involved the same basic principles, but it is now directed internationally by legal and political opinions indicating a major public interest. If modern ambulatory assessment were to employ the possibilities of telecommunication for the central pooling of data, national and international multicentre studies, or the support of therapy, it might initiate a similar trend within the fields of psychology and medicine.

References

Aas, I.H. (1999). Telemedicine and the organization of the health sector. *Journal of Telemedicine and Telecare, 5,* S26–28

Allen, A. (1996). Introduction to telecom strategies; telecom services for the health care industry: predicting the future. *Telemedicine Today, 4,* 15–16.

Allen, A., Doolittle, G.C., Boysen, C.D., Komorowski, K., Wolf, M., Collins, B. & Patterson, J.D. (1999). An analysis of the suitability of home health visits for telemedicine. Journal of Telemedicine and Telecare, 5, 90–96.

Arnold, M. & Paffrath, D. (1998). *Krankenhaus-Report '98. Schwerpunkt Überkapazitäten im Krankenhaus.* München: Urban & Fischer

Baer, L. & Greist, J.H. (1997). An interactive computer-administered self-assessment and self-help program for behavior therapy. *Journal of Clinical Psychiatry, 58,* 23–28.

Bashshur, R. & Lovett, J. (1977). Assessment of telemedicine: Results of the initial experience. *Aviation Space and Environmental Medicine, 48,* 65–70.

Bashshur, R.L. & Neuberger, N. (1995). Telemedicine and health policy: is there life after the recissions? *Telemedicine Journal, 1,* 151–154.

Baumann, U., Thiele, C., Laireiter, A.R. & Krebs, A. (1996). Computer-assisted interaction diary on social networks, social support and interpersonal stress. In J. Fahrenberg & M. Myrtek (Eds.), *Ambulatory assessment: Computer-assisted psychological and psychophysiological methods in monitoring and field studies* (p. 69–84). Göttingen: Hogrefe & Huber.

Burnett, K.F., Taylor, C.B. & Agras, W.S. (1992). Ambulatory computer-assisted behavior therapy for obesity: An empirical model for examining behavioral correlates of treatment outcome. *Computers in Human Behavior, 8,* 239–248

Coutts, J.A.P., Gibson, N.A. & Paton, J.Y. (1992). Measuring compliance with inhaled medication in asthma. *Archives of Diseases in Childhood, 67,* 332–333.

Cox, D.J., Gonder-Frederick, L., Julian, D. & Cryer, P. (1991). Intensive versus standard blood glucose awareness training (BGAT) with insulin-dependent diabetes: Mechanisms and ancillary effects. *Psychosomatic Medicine, 53,* 453–462.

DeParle, N.A. (2000). From the Health Care Financing Administration. *Journal of the American Medical Association, 284,* 1372.

Dietzel, G.T.W. (2001). E-Health und Gesundheitstelematik. Herausforderungen und Chancen. *Deutsches Ärzteblatt, 98,* 158–161.

Elixhauser, A., Eisen, S.A., Romeis, J.C. & Homan, S.M. (1990). The effects of monitoring and feedback on compliance. *Medical Care, 28,* 882–893.

Fahrenberg, J. (1996). Ambulatory assessment: Issues and perspectives. In J. Fahrenberg & M. Myrtek (Eds.), *Ambulatory assessment: Computer-assisted psychological and psychophysiological methods in monitoring and field studies* (p. 3–20). Göttingen: Hogrefe & Huber.

Field, M.J. (1997). Telemedicine: a guide to assessing telecommunications in healthcare. *Journal of Digital Imaging, 10,* 28.

Fields, F. (1999). A "what if" scenario for telemedicine reimbursement based on ATSP/IT survey findings. *Telemedicine Today, 7,* 32.

Frattola, A., Parati, G., Cuspidi, C., Albini, F. & Mancia, G. (1993). Prognostic value of 24-hour blood pressure variability. *Journal of Hypertension, 11,* 1133–1137.

Frisina, N., Pedullà, M., Mento, G. & Lanuzza, B. (1996). Frequency domain of heart rate and blood pressure variability in essential hypertensive patients during sleep: Differences between dippers and non-dippers. *Blood Pressure Monitoring, 1,* 425–431.

Hayes, T., Kinsella, A., Brown, N.A. & Perednia, D.A. (1996). The Telemedicine Information Exchange (TIE). *Journal of Telemedicine and Telecare, 2,* 20–27.

Hilty, D.M., Sison, J.I., Nesbitt, T.S. & Hales, R.E. (2000). Telepsychiatric consultation for ADHD in the primary care setting. *Journal of the American Academy of Children and Adolescents Psychiatry, 39,* 15–16.

Holle, R. & Zahlmann, G. (1999). Evaluation of telemedical services. *IEEE Transactions on Information Techology and Biomedicine, 3,* 84–91.

Kruse, W., Koch-Gwinner, P., Nikolaus, T., Oster, P., et al. (1992). Measurement of drug compliance by continuous electronic monitoring: A pilot study in elderly patients discharged from hospital. *Journal of the American Geriatrics Society, 40,* 1151–1155

Leopold, C., Poth, E. & Schandry, R. (1999). Entwicklung und Evaluation eines elektronisch gestützten Asthmaschulungsprogramms. *Verhaltenstherapie, 9 (suppl 1),* 46.

Lloyd, I. (1996). An outline of the European Data Protection Directive. The Journal of Information, Law and Technology (JILT), 1, 1+ (online journal). Retrieved January 8th, 2001, from http://elj.warwick.ac.uk/elj/jilt/dp/intros/

Montani, S., Bellazzi, R., Larizza, C., Riva, A., d´Annunzio, G., Fiocchi, S., Lorini, R. & Stefanelli, M. (1999). Protocol-based reasoning in diabetic patient management. *International Journal of Medical Informatics, 53,* 61–77.

Mucha, R.F., Mutz, G., Stephan, E. & Pauli, P. (1996). Smoking produces a smaller increase in heart rate in the natural smoking environment than in the laboratory. *Drug and Alcohol Dependence, 42,* 209–215.

Navein, J., Arose, D. & Pietermich, A. (1999). A business model for telemedicine. *Journal of Telemedicine and Telecare, 5 (Suppl 1),* S76–78.

Pawlik, K. (1996). Contributions to differential psychology from ambulatory assessment: A researcher´s pladoyer. In J. Fahrenberg & M. Myrtek (Eds.), *Ambulatory assessment: Computer-assisted psychological and psychophysiological methods in monitoring and field studies* (p. 21–28). Göttingen: Hogrefe & Huber.

Pickering, T.G. & James, G.D. (1994). Ambulatory blood pressure and prognosis. *Journal of Hypertension, 12,* S29–33.

Rigby, M. (1999). The management and policy challenges of the globalisation effect of informatics and telemedicine. *Health Policy, 46,* 97–103.

Smeja, M., Foerster, F., Fuchs, G., Emmans, D., Hornig, A. & Fahrenberg, J. (1999). 24-h assessment of tremor activity and posture in Parkinson's disease by multi-channel accelerometry. *Journal of Psychophysiology, 13,* 245–256

Smith, E. & Eloff, J.H.P. (1999). Security in health-care information systems – current trends. *International Journal of Medical Informatics, 54,* 39–54.

Stanberry, B. (1998). The legal and ethical aspects of telemedicine. 3: Telemedicine and malpractice. *Journal of Telemedicine and Telecare, 4,* 72–79.

Stemmler, G. (1996). Strategies and designs in ambulatory assessment. In J. Fahrenberg & M. Myrtek (Eds.), *Ambulatory assessment: Computer-assisted psychological and psychophysiological methods in monitoring and field studies* (p. 257–270). Göttingen: Hogrefe & Huber.

Tattersall, A.B. & Ellis, R. (1989). The use of a hand-held computer to record clinical trial data in general pratice: A pilot study. *Journal of International Medical Research, 17,* 185–189.

The Emerging European Health Telematics Industry. (2000). Market Analysis by Deloitte & Touche on assignment of European Commission-Directorate General Information Society. Health Information Society Technology Based Industry Study. Reference C13.25533.

Theranostics: *The influence of diagnostics on pharmaceutical therapy* (2000). Scrip Clinica reports, May 2000. Richmond: PJB Publications Ltd..

Vogt, M. & Schandry, R. (1995). Symptomwahrnehmung bei Asthmapatienten. *Pneumologie, 49,* 316–321.

Whitten, P.S. & Allen, A. (1995). Analysis of telemedicine from an organizational perspective. *Telemedicine Journal, 1,* 203–213.

Wootton, R., Loane, M., Mair, F., Moutray, M, Harrisson, S., Sivananthan, S., Allen, A., Doolittle, G. & McLernan, A. (1998). The potential for telemedicine in home nursing. *Journal of Telemedicine and Telecare, 4,* 214–218.

Chapter 35
Origins and Developments of Ambulatory Monitoring and Assessment

Jochen Fahrenberg
Forschungsgruppe Psychophysiologie, Department of Psychology, University of Freiburg, Germany

Introduction

Portable data recorders have long been used in the behavioral sciences, but they were not particularly innovative developments of these fields. The recorders' mechanical and electronic components, such as keyboards, sensors, amplifiers, micro-processors and storage components, had already been developed for other applications and purposes. The adoption of this technology in medicine and behavioral sciences, was however followed by the birth of a new methodology notable for its specific design of data acquisition.

The technical progress in recording equipment has of course a longer history: from the mechanical data logger, and the electro-mechanical and electronic recording apparatus to the modern advancements of programmable hand-held PCs. These PCs allow for specific formats and hierarchical branching of the questions and are therefore particularly useful in psychological assessment. The medical instrumentation progressed from the analog (cassette) recorder for physiological measures to digital systems, enabled the signal input to be pre-processed, and which subsequently led to real-time detection of certain parameters of physiological changes. However, many of the computer-assisted methods were yet to be used. These options included the technically available interactive monitoring based on real-time analysis of recordings and contingent feedback, or the communication between portable systems and a control center (via phone or internet). The use of new expert systems has been suggested to assist self-monitoring and self-management in chronic disease and in everyday life. Such systems are desirable in monitoring of man-machine systems and in exceedingly important, but high risk workplaces or in bedside monitoring of the critically ill. A more recent development of this kind has been the use of these applications in telemedicine (see Chapter by Leopold & Schandry, and Stephan et al., this Volume). Further technical progress can be achieved in the miniaturization of sensor devices and in more efficient (intelligent sampling strategy) storage for continuous long-term audio and video (minicam) recordings. This progress will open another door to new assessment strategies in behavior and symptom analysis.

The origins and developments of computer-assisted methodology in ambulatory monitoring could be reviewed from several perspectives. In the present context, however, the discussion seeks to provide a simple outline of the basic developments, and the obvious discrepancies in the acceptance of this new methodology between medicine and psychology. In psychology, there has been an apparent delay in adopting ambulatory monitoring and assessment. Nevertheless, we may anticipate that computer-assisted methodologies will increasingly be used in many fields to attain a higher validity and generalizability of findings in behavior assessment.

Since in most fields of application portable recording devices, that is, hand-held PC and digital recorders which use a small disk or memory card for data storage, are clearly preferred to on-line biotelemetry, the following discussion primarily refers to such recorders. Biotelemetry is useful, for example, in tracking wild-life or in applications which necessarily include real-time communication (telecommand, telestimulation).

Recorder/analyzer for physiological measures

The methodology for monitoring physiological measures in daily life (as an extension of bedside monitoring of the critically ill) was pioneered largely by Holter during the fifties. In the beginning, Holter used radio transmission (biotelemetry) to record animal ECG and EEG, and he subsequently employed a portable cassette recorder for continuous registration of the ECG in heart patients to detect segments of ST-depression (Holter, 1961, 1976). The Holter technique and "holtering" became a synonym for ambulatory monitoring of the ECG and other physiological recordings.

Portable recording systems had been used prior to the Holter technique. For example, motion during walking and running was registered using a pneumatic sensing and recording system (Marey, 1895; cited from Bussmann, 1998). However, the method developed by Holter appears to have been the first project to have generated wide interest. The evident advantages of monitoring heart patients and other subjects like athletes outside the clinic and laboratory met with a positive reaction. The new methodology lends itself to the attainment of more reliable diagnoses and a more valid evaluation of treatment outcome, for example, by testing anti-arrhythmic or anti-hypertensive medication.

The first recordings of intra-arterial blood pressure used tape recorders or biotelemetry (Bachmann, Thebis, Heynen & Graf, 1967; Bevan, Honour & Stott, 1969; cf. Meyer-Sabellek & Gotzen, 1988; O'Brien & Fitzgerald, 1991). At approximately the same time, an automatic device for the non-invasive measurement of blood pressure became available (Schneider, 1968). Pioneering work was also carried out by Sokolow and co-workers in San Francisco who developed a semi-automatic device consisting of an inflatable cuff and a tape recorder for Korotkoff sounds and pressure. In the years to follow, the clinical importance of ambulatory blood pressure monitoring became increasingly evident (Hinman, Engel & Bickford, 1962; Sokolow, Werdegar, Kain & Hinman, 1970; cf. Pickering, 1992).

The ECG and blood pressure enjoy by far the largest number of references in the literature to ambulatory monitoring. These references relate to clinical findings and to methodological issues, for example, technical developments, guidelines for application, and evaluation (quality control) of specific devices. The application is predominantly in the medical field and only to a much smaller extent in the behavioral sciences, for example, in psychophysiology or behavioral medicine (for overviews on ambulatory monitoring and assessment technology/methodology see Amlaner & Macdonald, 1980; Fahrenberg & Myrtek, 1996, 2001; Littler, 1980; Miles & Broughton, 1990; Pawlik & Buse, 1996; Pickering, 1991; Schneiderman, Weiss & Kaufman,1989; Stott, 1982; Suls & Martin, 1993; Turpin, 1985, 1990).

In the first generation, the monitoring systems used tape or cassette analog recorders, for example, the Oxford Medilog™ Series (Oxford Instruments, Oxford). The data analysis was performed off-line. The ISAM Conferences, initiated in 1975 by Stott et al. (Stott, 1976), showed a gradual transition from analog to digital technology and the development of computer-assisted methodologies. The advances in micro-processor technology and storage capacity soon paved the way for multichannel recordings and — another innovative step — led to the on-line analysis of medically important changes, for example, the immediate detection of heart rate changes or ST-depression in the ECG. These applications, of course, had been previously used for bedside monitoring of patients in critical care.

Among the first digital recorders/analyzers was the M2P (Deutsche Versuchsanstalt für Luft- und Raumfahrt, Oberpfaffenhofen, Germany). The innovative concept of the M2P was noteworthy despite its failure to be fully developed following the switching of research programs and termination of research funding: The loss of this and other such promising projects does not appear to be uncommon especially in this field. As an early precursor of digital recorder/analyzer systems a short account of this design provides an appropriate starting point (bearing in mind the own involvement in this project) for the following discussion.

M2P-Project

The M2P Multifactorial Analyzer for Continuous Long-term Assessment of Physiological Data at the Workplace ("Multifaktiorelles Meßsystem zur kontinuierlichen Langzeiterfassung physiologischer Daten am Arbeitsplatz") was developed by

Kunz, Mertens, and Oeste (1980, 1982a, 1982b). It appears to be the first system, besides the Vitalog-System (Miles & Rule, 1982), to be intentionally designed as a digital analyzer consisting of several modules. Its development included the integration of a near sensor pre-processing and semi-conductor storage.

The project was initiated by the Institut für Arbeitsphysiologie, TU München (Prof. Dr. Müller-Limmroth, Dr. Strasser) and a project group (Dipl.-Ing. Mertens) at the Deutsche Versuchsanstalt für Luft- und Raumfahrt DFVLR, Institut für Nachrichtentechnik Oberpfaffenhofen. The funding for this project came from the program "Humanisierung des Arbeitslebens HdA" which was realized by the Bundesminister für Forschung und Technologie.

The project statement for the commissioned work included the following specifications:

(1) A device for long-term monitoring of physiological data at the workplace, suitable for application at various sites.

(2) A recorder and analyzer comprising on-line processing of signal input to obtain meaningful parameters in formats suitable for computer analysis.

(3) An ergonomically designed device that is portable and light-weight, exerts minimal influence on the subject and has control commands that are not accessible to the subject.

(4) Independence of mains and high-frequency transmission (telemetry).

(5) Easy to use and check.

The project statement clearly pointed to the role of the device as a mobile application in order to assess, for example, recovery times, lunch breaks, leisure time, sleep, and working time. Since a generally approved concept of the specific parameters to assess work strain did not exist, the device was to enable the measurement of many parameters thus allowing for empirical correlation and evaluation of data and, thereby preparing the way for effective and economic results. The general design and the selection of parameters was approved at a meeting (Oberpfaffenhofen, 14. 2. 1977) made up of participants from the fields of occupational physiology, medicine and psychophysiology.

A prototype M2P (CPU 6100, 3.145 Hz, 12 KB RAM, 12 KB EPROM, 8 bit AD 100ms, 16 channel multiplexer) with signal modules for ECG, EMG, EOG, was used by the Forschungsgruppe Psychophysiologie, University of Freiburg, between 1978 and 1981. Because a suitable semiconductor storage was not available at that time, the Medilog (Oxford Instruments) analog cassette recorder was used instead. Subsequent to a number of smaller method studies, a larger study was designed for evaluation of the M2P methodology. In 58 students enrolled in physical education, five channels (ECG,2 EMG, EOG and a marker channel) were recorded before, during and after a 1000 m run at the stadium and during sleep as well. The participants were also assessed in a pychophysiology laboratory using conventional technology. The laboratory-field comparison was repeated two months later. The essential findings and suggestions for the further development of the new methodology were published (Fahrenberg, Foerster, Schneider, Müller & Myrtek, 1984; 1986).

A series of subsequent studies was proposed to advance this new methodology. However the DFVLR/HdA project was short-lived, this being due to changes in research policies at that time. Although attempts were made to transfer this innovative technology to manufacturers in the field of medical technology, our efforts were to no avail, and the know-how which had been accumulated, and the financial investment from the large development funds between 1977 and 1982 were lost.

Subsequent developments

The development of the Medilog based on digital technology (Miles & Rule, 1982) has already been mentioned. During the eighties, a number of digital recorders/ analyzers emerged in Germany that used semi-conductor storage: the PHYSIOPORT and PAR-PORT (PAR -Natic, Berlin, see Kiparski & Massmann, 1982; Kiparski & Steffens, 1985).), the BIOPORT and MULTITALENT (Zak, Simbach), the LOGOPORT (Krüger & Vollrath, 1996) and the Cologne System Series VITAPORT (Vitaport GmbH, Cologne, and Temec, Amsterdam, NL, see Stephan, Mutz, Langer, Schmitz & Wemschulte, 1989; Jain, Martens, Mutz, Weiß & Stephan, 1996) and the successor, VARIOPORT (Becker Meditec, Karlsruhe).

Today, more than a dozen recorder/analyzer systems are available from international manufactures – not to mention the even greater number of long-term ECG recorders/analyzers and the long-term-BP recorders. An overview of selected multi-purpose recorder systems is depicted in Table 1. Only a few systems have a multi-channel design, the advantage of which is that they can be applied to a variety of research questions that require different recording channels. Besides the devices suitable for ambulatory recordings and their use in 24-hr or long-term monitoring, a wide range of portable (mobile) equipment designed for in-field measurement does exist. For example, continuous finger arterial pressure (Portapres™, TNO, BioMedical Instrumentation, Amsterdam; see Imholz, Langewouters, van Montfrans, Parati, van Goudoever, Wesseling, Wieling, & Mancia, 1993; Wesseling, Settels & de Wit, 1986), measurement of respiration (Respitrace™), O_2/CO_2 gas exchange and energy expenditure, capnometry and pulse oximetry, polysomnography, cardio-respiratory polygraphic systems, 24 hour pH and motility testing, or fetal monitoring. Furthermore, monitoring systems have been designed for use by patients, for example, for use as blood glucose monitoring systems, respiration and asthma monitoring systems, long-term EEG and EMG monitors.

The pace of these and other developments is so fast that the reader may wish to refer to the *Journal of Medical Engineering & Technology* (Taylor & Francis, Publishers) and related journals or reports like the *International Hospital Equipment* (Elsevier, Publishers). The website of *Medica*, which is the largest medical instrumentation exhibition and trade fair, provides more information (www.medica.de). An overview of neither the device technology in digital recorder/analyzer systems nor the progress in ambulatory assessment of endocrine responses are within the scope of this chapter.

Table 1. Multi-channel digital recorder/analyzer for physiological measurement (modular design).

Name	Manufacturer	Internet
AMI	Ambulatory Monitoring, Inc., Ardsley NY, US	www.ambulatory-monitoring.com
BIOLOG	UFI, Morro Bay CA, US	www.ufiservingscience.com
CARDIOTENS	P.M.S. (Instruments) Ltd., Maidenhead, UK	www.pmsinstruments.co.uk
EMBLA	Flaga, Reykjavik, IS	www.flaga.is
Flexilog	Oakfield Instr., Witney, UK	www.oakfieldinst.com
Mini-Logger VitalSense	Mini-Mitter, Beand OR, US	www.minimitter.com
Medilog	Oxford Instruments, Witney, GB	www.oxinst.com
PAR-PORT	Par Medizintechnik, Berlin, D	www.par-berlin.com
PHYSIO-LOGGER	med-natic, München, D	www.med-natic.de
PHYSIO Modul	Rimkus, Riemerling, D	
VITAPORT, VARIOPORT	Becker Meditec, Karlsruhe, D	
VU-AMS	Free University Amsterdam, NL	www.psy.vu.nl

Custom-made Vests with Easy Access Pockets to House Devices and Connections		
Life Shirt	VivoMetrics, Ventura CA, USA	www.vivometrics.com
MediVest	MediVest, Chicago IL, USA	www.Medivest.com

Note: Technical specifications were omitted here because of the multiplicity of parameters. The reader is referred to the manufacturers' information outlets (e.g., internet homepages). Long-term ECG recorder/analyzer (Holter analysis), ambulatory blood pressure monitors, and polysomnography (sleep or sleep apnea) recorders were not included (cf. Medica: www.medica.de).

A wide selection of physiological variables have been measured in daily life, using mostly non-invasive methods. However, some investigators have made ambulatory recordings of arterial (inter-brachial) blood pressure or gastrointestinal functions. Even more specific sensor techniques and registrations have been used and conducted in medical research. However, the great majority of investigators have employed a few selected measures (for reviews see Fahrenberg & Myrtek, 2001; Fahrenberg & Wientjes, 2000).

The software support which is given by the manufacturers is more or less developed. On the one hand, there is tailor-made software for editing, post-processing (parameterization) of physiological signals, plotting software, data conversion, etc., and on the other hand, there are also standard packages like LabVIEW™ and DASYLab™.

Hand-held PC for data acquisition in field studies

The need for ecological validity in psychological assessment, that is, recording behavior and self-reports under naturalistic conditions (daily life) was urged by Lewin, Brunswik, Barker and other pioneers (for overviews, see Fahrenberg & Myrtek, 2001; Patry, 1982; Pawlik & Buse, 1996; Perrez, 1994). The term ecological validity was introduced by Cicourel (1982) with respect to the agreement between interviews and actual behavior; operational definitions were not proposed by him.

In fact, at this point Cattell (1957) insisted, in his textbook on personality, on recording "life record (or in situ or criterion)" variables: "Indeed, there arises at this point the need for a proper development of measurement techniques particularly as they apply to L-data, both in terms of techniques and units and of frequencies and norms of ordinary everyday behavior ..." (p. 55). However, at that time, his large scale time series studies (P-technique research) extending over weeks and months had to be conducted without the facilitating use of a hand-held PC.

Methods of recording task demands and performance data have a long history in the applied fields (for example, time and motion studies). These and similar assessments have been conducted in differential, developmental, social and clinical psychology. To this end, event recorders for the timed registration of stimuli and responses found their use. Following the growing interest in behavior coding systems in the sixties, the trend toward behavioral assessment became evident in the seventies and eighties. This led to a corresponding increase in demand for new data acquisition technology. Thus, many researchers in psychology, ethnology and social science research developed mechanical, electromechanical and electronic devices (event recorder, data logger). Usually, simple push-button marker or numeric and alphanumeric keyboards were used for data input, rarely an acoustic trigger (voice key). For storage, simple mechanical counters, ticker tapes, punchcards, mark sense cards, and, from the beginning of the seventies magnetic tape recorders (analog cassette recorders) were employed. At the end of that decade semi-conductor storage components, portable PC, and, finally, the smaller hand-held PC were introduced (for overviews, see Farrell, 1991; Heger, 1990a; Mertesdorf, 1980; Pawlik & Buse, 1996; Rugh, Gable & Lemke, 1986; Sidowski, 1977; Totterdell & Folkard, 1992).

Devices consisting of a tailor-made encoder-recorder instrumentation are worth mentioning. These allowed digital data acquisition in field studies ready for computer processing. The Datapack System (Electro/ General Corporation, Minnetouka, MI) was widely applied, initially (1967) using a cassette recorder and later equipped with semi-conductor memory Datamyte 900 (Torgerson, 1977).

In this context, computer-assisted data acquisition is defined according to the following features: (1) The recording equipment is programmable in a basic assembler code or a higher language; (2) The data are stored in a standard format (e.g., ASCII); (3) an interface for data transfer (e.g., RS 232) is available. Portable devices including programmable clock, beeper and other controls were in use already in the late seventies (cf. Mertesdorf, 1980). The development of pocket-sized (hand-held, palm-top) computers then served to ease the acquisition of data considerably. A few years later, Elias (1984) included the Epson HX-20, Hewlett-Packard 75, and Sharp PC 1500 in his list of commercially available hand-held computers for data acquisition in ethnology.

Since 1975, the University of Chicago has been the scene of an alternative development involving Csikszentmihalyi and his collaborators (Csikszentmihalyi & Larson, 1987; de Vries, 1992). Repeated self-reports were elicited by beeper signals. The participants received booklets for the self-protocol, when signaled, of activities, mood, and other variables. Besides a conventional clock (Brandstätter, 1983) or a simple random timer (Hurlburt, 1979), investigators used a programmable wrist watch (e.g., Seiko RC-1000), programmable beeper (Hormuth, 1986) or paging systems ("doctor pagers") to prompt the subject to respond to a questionnaire. The Experience Sampling Method ESM became well-known and has clearly encouraged further developments.

Computer-assisted methodologies, as compared to the ESM, appear to have many advantages, for example, in the flexible adjustment to various tasks, reliability and control of data acquisition, high memory capacity, or easy read-out.

A computer-assisted methodology for data acquisition in field studies was introduced by Pawlik and Buse (1982) in cooperation with the Zak GmbH (Simbach, Germany). The first version of this behavior recorder (8 KB RAM, programmed in assembler code, 16 keys for typing item codes) was further refined as the BIDATA (48 KB RAM, item text display, performance tests, sensors for recording heart rate and finger temperature). The present model, AMBU, is manufactured by PAR company (Berlin) and the features are: 1 MB RAM, 128x64 pixel display, 10 numeric and 5 control keys, 470 g weight, programming in Turbo Pascal or C) This methodology is well suited to ambulatory assessment of settings, mood, and in-field performance testing (Buse & Pawlik, 1996; Buse & Pawlik, this Volume).

Other investigators have preferred to use the commercially available hand-held PCs instead. Noteworthy among these hand-held PCs and software developments were the Sharp PC-1360 employed for the COMRES (Perrez & Reicherts, 1989), and the CASIO PB 1000 which was used for both the protocol on setting, location, activity, and mood (Heger, 1990b; Fahrenberg, Heger, Foerster & Müller, 1991), and the symptom diary for anxiety patients (Taylor, Fried & Kenardy, 1990). The Atari Portfolio was selected for the SONET-CT diary for social network protocols (Perkonigg, Baumann, Reicherts & Perrez, 1993). The software for ambulatory psychological assessment (Heger, 1990b; Käppler, 1994) was refined to the MONITOR methodology for the Psion Series (Brügner, 1998; cf. Fahrenberg, Hüttner & Leonhart, this Volume). Meanwhile, a considerable number of other developments can be noted.

Table 2. Overview on hand-held (palmtop) PCs

Hand-Held PC with Keyboard	
Psion Revo Plus, Psion 5mx Pro	Epoc Release 5
Psion Workabout	Psion OPL
Hewlett Packard Jornada 720	Windows CE
Hand-Held PC with Touchscreen and Pen (Personal Digital Assistant PDA)	
Casio Cassiopeia E-15G (EM-550G)	Windows CE
Compaq Aero 2130, iPAQ	Windows CE
Handspring Visor	Palm OS
Hewlett-Packard Jornada 548	Windows CE
Palm IIIx, V, m100	Palm OS
Special-purpose Hand-held PC	
AMBU Recorder	Turbo Pascal or C

The OBSERVER software (Noldus, 1991) was introduced to ease the recording of behavior observations in field studies in animal and human ethology. This program is available for a number of hand-held PC, for example, Psion and Psion Workabout (cf. Albonetti, 1992; Hile, 1991). This methodology further consists of a Psiwin version and a behavior observation training course available on video casssette (Noldus Information Technology, 1995).

Software to facilitate the use of hand-held PCs in field studies has been developed in many institutions, more or less specific to certain studies. Flexible software systems suited to a variety of applications are still an exception (e. g., Behavior Observation System, Noldus Information Technology, AG Wageningen, NL; MONITOR for various types of self-reports, developed for use with the PSION series, Brügner, 1998; in-field performance testing, cf. Buse & Pawlik, 1996).

There are various sources of data: behavior (performance) measurement, behavior observation, self-reports on experiences, subjective state, etc., and, possibly, environmental aspects, like ambient noise or temperature, which can be recorded in field studies.

The application of a programmable pocket PC in ambulatory assessment has many advantages as compared to conventional paper-and-pencil methods:

- alarm functions for prompting the observer/subject at predefined intervals and a built-in reminder signal;
- reliable timing of input, delay of input, and duration of input;
- flexible layout of questions and response categories;
- branching of questions and tailor-made sequential or hierarchical strategies;
- concealment of previously recorded responses from the observer/subject;
- overcoming the recall-error.

The recall-error or retrospection effect has been a methodological issue in several studies. Even if subjects are told to monitor their stress responses, mood and symptoms several times daily, such questionnaire reports are often done from memory. A specific bias is evident when ratings made in the evening indicate more negative mood and unease than is to be expected from the actual ratings averaged across the day, that is, a *negative* retrospection bias (see Fahrenberg, Hüttner & Leonhart, this Volume).

Many applications for hand-held PCs (electronic diaries) exist, for example, job stress diaries (Rau & Triemer, 1999; Totterdell, Spelten, Smith, Barton & Folkard, 1995) and pain diaries (Lang, Ostermeier, Forster & Handwerker, 1991; Lewis, Lewis & Cumming, 1995; Smith & Safer, 1993); diaries can facilitate the diagnostic assessment of a variety of behavioral disorders (Shiffman, 2000; Shiffman et al, 1994; Suls & Martin, 1993; Wilz & Brähler, 1997; see Chapters in this Volume).

A higher technical reliability and ecological validity of computer-assisted recordings can be generally assumed compared with paper-and-pencil questionnaires and diaries that lack flexibility in data acquisition and exactness when timing responses.

Detection of posture and motion

The recording of posture and motion is another basic issue in the methodology of behavior observation and performance measurement. Calibrated piezoresistive sensors allow the separation of a DC-component indicating degree of inclination, that is, position, and an AC-component representing acceleration, that is, movement. Multi-channel accelerometry can be used for the measurement of posture, specific movements, tremor, gait, and other aspects of motor behavior. Moreover, an automatic detection of posture and motion during ambulatory monitoring can be achieved if an individual's characteristic patterns were obtained with, for example, a standard protocol for walking, standing, and sitting at the beginning of the assessment. Based on such multi-site accelerometry and ambulatory recordings, a continuous record of posture and movement can be achieved rather unobtrusively. In addition to this, accelerometry may be used as a method for the estimation of gross physical activity and energy expenditure. The detection of posture and motion was recently improved and has attained a satisfactory reliability and validity (see Bussmann et. al.; Foerster; Tulen et al., this Volume).

To assist in objective behavior analysis, a range of interesting variables could be measured continuously. However, to date little systematic use has been made of these technically available options. Examples are:

- movement of the head measured by a small accelerometer placed beneath the chin to assess head movement, for example, nodding during a conversation;
- voice signal recorded via a throat sensor (micro);
- ambient conditions recorded via suitable sensors for light, noise, and temperature.

The temporal analysis of speech patterns, that is, speech chronometrics, was used in ambulatory assessment (Krüger & Vollrath, 1996). Behavior channels like nodding and voice (in case an audio recording is not possible) may be used as objective indicants of conversation and social interaction. Pilot studies were encouraging and speak in favor of further developing such methods. Some hand-held PCs allow for audio recordings up to a number of minutes, depending on storage capacity. Digital dictating systems have a capacity up to 240 minutes in long play mode.

In psychological and psychophysiologal research, so far, little use was made of digital mini-cams for recordings of the videostream of behavior. A mini-cam for mobile video transmission (range 300 m) has a housing 18 x 17 x 34 mm, objective lens 1.5 mm diameter. A digital web-cam is available with integrated web-server, that is, transmission via web-site activation or e-mail in JPEG-format.

Psychophysiological monitoring

The scope and the development of ambulatory monitoring was documented in the Proceedings of the International Symposium on Ambulatory Monitoring (Stott, 1976). Most applications were from the medical field, however, psychophysiological research involved in the assessment of behavioral and subjective correlates of physiological changes has since gradually emerged.

A psychological investigation of gradients of arousal in novice and expert parachutists by Fenz and Epstein (1967) was an early example of growing interest in research under naturalistic conditions. (A similar study actually using modern monitoring equipment was conducted by Roth, Breivik, Jørgenson & Hofman, 1996). Noteworthy projects include a field study on blood pressure responses elicited by emotions (Sokolow, Werdegar, Cowan & Brenenstuhl, 1970), changes in heart rate during daily life and self-report on mood changes (Roth, Tinklenberg, Doyle, Horvarth & Kopell, 1976) and the recording of heart rate, physical activity and self-reports (Taylor et al, 1982). Nevertheless, the psychological data were still recorded by paper-and-pencil methods.

Monitoring methodology in psychophysiology requires the concurrent recording of the essential response channels. Because cassette recorders at that time had a substantial wow and flutter, which might cause deviations in the order of several minutes per hour, the necessary post-hoc synchronization required special care using a timer channel, marker, etc. Concurrent recordings of psychological data were made using a small set of keys placed on a watchstrap (Fahrenberg et al., 1984, 1986). The EMOPAD was a specific device for data acquisition and was designed for use with the VITAPORT 1 (Jain, Mutz & Mucha, 1992).

The BIDATA (Buse & Pawlik, 1994, 1996) and the MULTITALENT MT (Zak, Simbach, Germany) were probably the first systems designed as multi-channel recorders for psychological and physiological data. The MT (NSC 800 CPU) had three analog input channels, 20 keys for recording behavioral data, a display for item text, acoustic feedback, and a number of further options. Based on this device, Myrtek et al. (1988) developed the methodology of interactive psychophysiological monitoring (see below).

In 1987, a multimethod strategy for psychophysiological 24-hour monitoring of blood pressure reactivity was developed (see Fahrenberg, 1987, 1990, 1996; Fahrenberg, Heger, Foerster & Müller, 1991; Heger, 1990; Käppler, 1994). This method consisted of recordings of blood pressure, heart rate, physical activity, and respiration rate, and – concurrent to each blood pressure measurement – obtained a computer-assisted self-report on setting, behavior, emotional state, and experience. The equipment in these studies was made up of a four-channel recorder for physiological measures (Physioport, Par-Natic, Berlin), a pocket-sized computer (Casio PB 1000 or Psion 3a), and a dictating system (Walkman recorder, Sony WM 202)

Systolic and diastolic blood pressure were measured intermittently by the auscultatory method, employing a microphone and R-wave gating to detect Korotkoff sounds. During the day, a measurement interval of 30 minutes, with a random component of +5/-5 minutes, and, at night, an interval of 60 minutes (+5/-5) was used. The physical activity index was derived from continuous registration of an three-directional piezoelectric accelerometer. The pocket-computer provided a convenient medium for obtaining a self-report on setting variables and activities, as well as self-ratings of emotional state and level of physical activity. The setting protocol contained four aspects (location, social context, posture, activities). The momentary state was assessed by means of ten seven-point adjective rating scales, and two retrospective ratings related to perceived stress and physical activity in the preceding interval. The pocket-computer was initially programmed to record self-reports at fixed intervals, for example, at intervals of 30 minutes, and subjects were instructed to give additional self-reports when relevant events occurred. In subsequent studies, subjects were instructed to give a self-report immediately after each BP measurement, which in turn was automatically initiated at intervals of 30 (±5) minutes. The dictating system – via a microphone fixed to the subjects' shirt or top – was used to obtain comments on the more specific aspects of behavior settings and events. Such information is also important for estimating the subject's time budget and for the segmentation and evaluation of the 24-hour-record (cf. Fahrenberg, 1996).

Controlled monitoring

The multi-method approach was applied in a number of studies on blood pressure reactivity to obtain 24-hour BP profiles. Although this equipment, in particular its weight and the noisy pump system imposed some restrictions, it was well accepted by nearly all participants and hypertensive patients. Concurrent recordings of physical activity provided means for a segmentation of recordings according to high or low activity. Energy expenditure and posture are essential sources of BP variance and require appropriate controls if BP level and sudden blood pressure surges are to be evaluated adequately. Thus, activity-controlled psychophysiological BP profiles were obtained under conditions of daily life. The methodology allowed for time sampling and for event sampling of blood pressure and subjective state, as well. Furthermore, standardized or semi-standardized measurement periods were included which served as a reference for inter- and intra-individual comparison. As part of the standard protocol in 24-hour monitoring, the subjects performed specific tasks: climbing a stair case, performing a mental test, and participating in a short interview.

Multimethod assessment strategies of this kind, using hand-held PC instead of written diaries, were likewise developed, for example, by Kamarck et al. (1998) and Schmidt and Jain (1996).

Interactive monitoring

The development of recorder equipment suitable for physiological and psychophysiological recordings and on-line (real-time) analysis led to innovative research strategies. Contingent to changes of certain physiological parameters, a patient can be prompted by a beeper signal to record specific events, activities, or symptoms. Myrtek et al. (1988) and Myrtek, Brügner and Müller (1996) developed a new methodology for interactive monitoring of "additional heart rate" and concurrent assessment of subjective state change (cf. Myrtek & Foerster, this Volume). The on-line analysis of ECG changes were used also in detection and early warning of transient myocardial ischemia (Barry, Campbell, Nabel, Mead & Selwyn, 1987; Myrtek, Fichtler, König, Brügner & Müller, 1994; Kinne & Droste, 1996; Kinne, Droste, Fahrenberg & Roskamm, 1999) and in triggering a concurrent blood pressure measurement (Deedwania & Nelson, 1990).

General issues in methodology

Developments in research designs, measurement issues, sampling, and statistical data analysis have been discussed in other chapters of this volume, so that it may suffice here to refer to general issues of the ambulatory assessment approach as a whole.

The interplay between progress in information technology and the development of new research questions is evident. Innovative methodologies were developed to assess physiological and psychological parameters that were previously not accessible or were not accessible in a satisfactory manner, for example, only under the restrictions of the artificial laboratory settings and with highly questionable external validity. Such developments have stimulated new research questions leading to a mutual process of progression and refinement of hardware and software, and, moreover, promoting the development of new strategies in statistical data analysis.

Several issues are noteworthy in discussing the origins and developments of computer-assisted monitoring and assessment. Such issues include the choice between special-purpose or multi-purpose equipment, the acceptance of this methodology by study participants and patients, and the attitude of professionals and potential users regarding these innovations, exchange of know-how, attempts at standardization, and aspects of cost-benefits.

Special- and multi-purpose devices

A prevailing issue concerning the more recent application of monitoring is the question whether equipment which has to be specifically designed for a certain application is to be given preference to a readily available device which does not fulfill all the requirements of that applications. Special-purpose devices are available for certain applications in medicine, especially ECG and BP recorder. Such equipment is produced in a large number and is less expensive than multi-purpose recorders. However, these convenient devices are limited in the sense that the selection of channels, operating characteristics and other features is pre-determined. ECG and BP recorders usually lack channels for concurrent registration of physical activity and psychological data.

Since research evidence has strongly affirmed that blood pressure variability and the effects of energy expenditure and body position (for example, standing upright, body rotation during sleep affecting the distance between cuff and heart level) are confounded, this unwanted (however unknown) variance should be controlled for in a more thorough evaluation of significant blood pressure surges. Ambulatory monitoring studies which have used multi-channel recordings have strongly suggested that the inclusion by manufacturers of at least one channel for a tridimensional accelerometer device would provide the necessary data for an adequate analysis of 24-hour recordings.

Equipment in modular, multi-purpose designs, on the other hand, may be more suitable in many fields of the behavioral sciences for monitoring and assessment because of its flexibility and adaptability to a range of research questions. These devices are probably more expensive and less well supported with application software.

In psychology, computer-assisted data acquisition by hand-held PC may require a choice between a general-purpose hand-held PC and a tailor-made system with, for example, software for recording self-ratings or responses to mental performance tests (cf. Pawlik & Buse, this Volume). A general-purpose hand-held PC will be less costly, but is not provided with the appropriate software. Software development, depending on the range of options required, may amount to a formidable task and most users would prefer to acquire such programs from other institutions or licenses, respectively. Such software developments were referred to in a number of chapters in this Volume.

Acceptance, compliance, and reactivity

From the beginning, there have been concerns raised about the acceptance of monotoring and the validity of monitoring in daily life has been questioned. Ambulatory assessment with a pocket PC or recorder depends on the favorable attitude and motivation of the participating subjects. It is essential that the equipment is readily accepted and that good compliance to instructions is established and sustained. If the ambulatory monitoring is part of a diagnostic process or a treatment program, the patient's consent to the monitoring follows in the course of the interaction with the clinicians. For this reason, the attitude of patients may be different and the acceptance of monitoring may be higher within the health care system than in research projects. The ambulatory assessment should not cause major problems with the social environment. A comprehensive post-monitoring-interview is recommended in order to obtain information on these essential aspects.

The book on "Microcomputers and Clinical Psychology" edited by Ager and Bendall (1991) discussed already many of the essential issues, applications and future developments in this domain. The contributions still referred to the use of stationary PCs, although the pioneer studies employing hand-held PC had been published already. These issues included, for example, computer-assisted assessment of psychological problems, computer-based neuropsychological assessment and cognitive rehabilitation, applications for people with learning disabilities, expert systems and the role of the clinical psychologist. A chapter on psychological aspects of the new technological age referred to client reactions to computerized assessment. In some cases there was a reluctant attitude or even computer-phobia and in others the favorable response of most clients was indicated.

The acceptance of the hand-held computer in field studies and of ambulatory monitoring in general appears to be much higher than initially anticipated by investigators (cf. Fahrenberg & Myrtek, 1996; 2001). The experience of being equipped with a new electronic device can be a motivating condition to participants. Furthermore, motivation can stem from the participation in a diagnostic procedure or research project and the willingness to learn about oneself: "Everybody is his own blood pressure (or stress) researcher." However, it is understandable that at some workplaces and by some subjects this attitude is not shared. Certain environments will be less suited to ambulatory monitoring, however, the registration of the ECG and motion (actometer) are feasible in practically all conditions because these recordings are disguised to the public. Intermittent automatic blood pressure measurements, beeper signals, and the instruction to type a response into a hand-held computer may be a problem in some instances because they distract the participant or elicit positive or negative responses and comments from others. A computer-assisted method for obtaining self-reports and physiological measurements has the specific advantage of being able to register an protocol of the subject's compliance and the exact timing of data acquisition.

Reactivity means that the method of observation and measurement itself is one aspect of the unwanted variance because of specific interactions such as awareness, adaptation, sensitization, and coping tendencies (cf. Haynes & Horn, 1983; Stern, 1986). Such reactivity may include a bias that is common to a class of methods or specific to one method. Non-reactive methods are clearly an exception in psychological assessment and physiological measurement, indeed this an analogy to Heisenberg's uncertainty principle: the attempt to measure a phenomenon may distort this phenomenon.

Three aspects of reactivity, however, appear to be specific to ambulatory assessment. Subjects may: (1) tend to steer clear of certain settings during the recording in order to avoid being monitored there; (2) tend to unintentionally or deliberately manipulate the recording systems, shift settings of the PC and may even try to get access to the program; and (3) try to test their capacities or the equipment by unusual patterns of behavior, exercise or vigorous movements. At present, only a post-monitoring interview can reveal these effects and their actual evaluation is rather difficult. Little is yet known about the advisability of including a few control items and questions in the computer-assisted questionnaire that directly refer to actual (non-)compliance and method-dependent effects; for example, the subject's being irritated by the beeps or having specifically changed the usual routine.

Ethical issues

Ethical issues that are specific to ambulatory monitoring studies have hardly been discussed in the literature. The monitoring could be regarded as a case of "Big brother is watching you", that is, an invasion of privacy. Of course, the guidelines of ethics committees must be adhered to. Appropriate data protection is a concern because ambulatory assessment may violate privacy more easily than alternative methods (Schuler, 1982; Bersoff & Bersoff, 2000). Furthermore, persons not being assessed may become involved in the observation and evaluation of settings when these are being carried out. Obtaining the subject's informed consent before the recording starts is essential, but may be problematic since the exact course of daily activities and events cannot be anticipated. Moreover, it may be more difficult to explain the essential hypothesis of the investigation, variables, and methods of analysis in ambulatory studies than in the laboratory. Especially when psychological data and recordings of behavioral (motor) activities are obtained, the participants should be briefed about the kind of findings and conclusions that can be derived from such protocols. Thus, the post-monitoring interview is well suited to recalling specific events and discussing problematic aspects.

Cost-benefit

Ambulatory assessment methodology has certain advantages compared with stationary equipment. However, the recorder/analyzer will usually be more costly. The expectation is that cheaper devices, suitable for multi-channel physiological recordings, and cheaper pocket-PCs will be developed in future. Thus, a more extensive use of the ambulatory assessment technology is foreseeable as is already the case in single purpose ECG recorders or blood pressure recorders. The higher ecological validity of the ambulatory assessment will encourage such applications.

Exchange of know-how and training

The ISAM Meetings were initiated to provide the first opportunity of its kind for the presentation of new technologies and methodologies of ambulatory monitoring (Stott, 1976; Stott et al., 1978, 1982; Dal Palú & Pessina, 1986). Journals, devoted to this subject, included: *Biotelemetry and Patient Monitoring* (1972–1982, then, *Acute Care* 1983–1989), *Biotelemetry* (1974–1977), *Journal of Ambulatory Monitoring* (1988–1995), *Journal of Medical Engineering & Technology* (1976–), and *Blood Pressure Monitoring* (1996–).

A number of symposia on ambulatory monitoring have taken place at annual meetings of societies, like the Society for Psychophysiological Research, the European Federation of Psychophysiological Societies, and national congresses. On a smaller scale, there were a number of users' meetings over the years regarding, for example, the application of specific systems (like Vitaport-Meetings and Portapres Meetings in Germany, VU-AMS Workshops in Amsterdam, NL). At such workshops, participants from a wide range of institutions and disciplines met who would not normally attend the same annual congresses. The diversity of equipment and research interests, of course, is a severe handicap for in-depth cooperation. There is an obvious need for the exchange of know-how and training, however, this requires more time than is available for conventional workshops at larger congresses. Noteworthy was a training course on "Psychobiological ambulatory monitoring in health psychology", staged by the Research Institute for Psychology and Health (at Utrecht University and Leiden University, NL) in 1997.

Among these meetings were two workshops organized by the Forschungsgruppe Psychophysiologie, Psychology Department, Freiburg University, and funded by the Deutsche Forschungsgemeinschaft. These meetings were encouraging and the resultant manuscripts formed the core of the present volume and the previous book published in 1996.

Physiological measurement and monitoring, as in the laboratory, require specific training, technical assistance, and software development. This can hardly be achieved in a sole person enterprise. It needs team work and adequate funding to foster a continuous development of skills and general competence. One may assume that over the years a large number of multi-purpose recorders were purchased but rarely used because it was realized only to late that the methodology needed is by no means as simple and convenient as in the case of BP or ECG recorders.

Acceptance and impact of computer-assisted monitoring methodology in psychophysiology and psychology

In medicine, the ambulatory monitoring of BP and ECG are now indispensable routine methods. The ever more widespread application of the new methodology can be attributed to its practical usefulness which was evident in the increased validity of diagnosis and in the external validity of therapy outcome evaluation – and in the fact that such applications were paid for by the insurance companies.

In contrast, computer-assisted monitoring and assessment still appear to have had little impact in psychophysiology and psychology. A general scan through journals and congress programs (including symposia, papers, posters) will easily confirm the impression that these applications have largely stagnated. In psychophysiology, for example, over many years a nearly constant percentage of five or less per cent of posters refer to ambulatory monitoring methodology. It fits into this picture that the previous volume "Ambulatory Assessment" had only one review (Turpin, 1999) in international journals.

Standard textbooks on behavioral research methods, for example, Kerlinger and Lee (2000), although acknowledging the specific advantages and disadvantages of both, laboratory and field research, hardly refer to the new methodologies based on computer-assisted data acquisition and monitoring in the natural environment. An exception is Goldstein and Hersen (2000), who at least mention such developments.

This situation may be due to several reasons. In spite of the pioneer work in the late seventies and eighties, this methodology had little influence on present day mainstream research activities. Investigators seemed to be concerned with the possibility that hand-held PC and other monitoring systems might have little acceptance in study participants and patients. This attitude was put into words by van Egeren and Madarasmi (1988): "We initially considered using a small, hand-held programmable microcomputer to log diary information but abandoned the idea because the operation of these devices is too complex and the fear of computers on the part of some people too great to ensure reliable performance. Instead we developed the mark sense diary card ..." (p. 180). However, was this attitude based on empirical evidence ?

The feedback from participants of ambulatory monitoring studies, even in the past, when the equipment was more obtrusive and uncomfortable, was on the whole encouraging. A general acceptance of and, in particular, interest in these new methods was indicated and appeared to motivate the participants. Such compliance was reported by many investigators (see above), although for some populations and some subjects this methodology appears to be less suitable.

The critical attitude seems to be based on theoretical preconceptions or even prejudice and is particularly noteworthy because of the enduring controversy in theoretical psychology about the dichotomy of artificial laboratory setting versus naturalistic observation. This controversy is often misleadingly paralleled with the a dichotomy of internal versus external validity. Both aspects of validity rightly have to be put under scrutiny in laboratory experimentation as well as in ambulatory assessment (for a more extended discussion see Fahrenberg, 1996; Fahrenberg & Myrtek, 2001; Patry, 1982; Pawlik, 1988).

Pawlik (1988, 1996) has pointed out that differential psychology and personality assessment might have taken a basically different course of development had the empirical approach initially been one of data acquisition in daily life instead of mental testing and laboratory experimentation. Of course, ambulatory assessment requires the elaboration of specific designs and strategies (see for example, Stemmler, 1996) and the development of appropriate statistical models for multi-level analyses and rather short time series (for example, Delespaul, 1992; Schwarz & Stone, 1998; Suen & Ary, 1989; Totterdell, Briner, Parkinson & Reynolds, 1996; see also, Ott & Scholz; and Wilhelm, this Volume).

A rather reluctant attitude toward ambulatory monitoring and assessment of individual differences and testing hypotheses under naturalistic conditions may be further due to general assumptions derived from the philosophy of science and the logic of research. The general attitude is one of favoring the testing of theories under highly controlled conditions and not of deliberating to much on inductive approaches, that is, accumulation of empirical facts as raw material for subsequent theory building. This attitude may appear to be adequate in the natural sciences (which has undergone a long and very successful history of data gathering and inductive reasoning), but in the behavioral sciences an inductive-hypothetico-deductive strategy still is a useful approach. For a range of issues, ambulatory monitoring methodology has already shown that findings and conclusions based on laboratory experiments were hardly tenable on empirical grounds, provided that the field studies have been seriously taken into account. Neither the dichotomy internal/external validity nor theory driven/data driven research are adequate descriptions of the basic methodological issues implied here, however, sometimes the discussion and probably the willingness to apply innovative methodology may be hindered by such views.

Following from this, the impression is that the acceptance of this methodology may be greater by study participants and patients than by mainstream psychologists and psychophysiologists. In Germany, for example, where basic research reports on large scale psychological and psychophysiological monitoring studies were published in the early eighties, the impact of these reports was hardly noticeable in spite of the availability of technically advanced equipment in the country. Not even in fields particularly suited to ambulatory assessment methodology, for example, diagnosis and evaluation in behavior therapy, investigation of symptom reports in chronic illness and psychiatric patients, or engineering psychophysiology, was a wide acceptance evident (for reviews, Fahrenberg, 2000; Fahrenberg & Myrtek, 2001; Fahrenberg & Wientjes, 2000).

Two further issues should be mentioned which could explain the hesitant and sceptical attitude of mainstream researchers: costs and necessary training. The price of a hand-held PC, of course, exceeds the cost of paper-and-pencil methods but is not really so high as to hinder its use when the advantages of flexibility of data acquisition, the high technical reliability and exact timing are to be taken into account. Ambulatory assessment methodologies need some training. However, the use of a PC is a common skill today.

Perspectives

During the last two decades, a fast development in microprocessor technology has enabled the design of new instrumentation and, accordingly, new methodologies in medicine and the behavioral sciences. Multi-channel recorders/analyzers and special purpose devices for physiological measures and convenient hand-held PCs for acquisition of psychological data are available. Such systems allow innovative research and practical application in many fields and essential findings have been obtained. In medicine, ambulatory monitoring is an indispensable routine method.

There are two noticeable developments which probably exert an essential influence on the computer-assisted methods in medicine and the behavioral sciences:

— The arrival of the web-based mobile telecommunication (e. g., IMT-2000 and UMTS). The fusion of mobile and fixed networks will stimulate the evolution and progress toward universal mobile telecommunication systems. These new information technologies would allow for personal mobility and for access to, for example, experts and knowledge-based systems.

— The arrival of new patient monitoring equipment appears to revolutionize the way in which patient information is transmitted and used in the healthcare system: "Healthcare institutions are progressively pursuing a reduction in patients lengths of stay as a means of achieving cost containment. Encouraging earlier ambulation while continuing to monitor the patients is just one of the methods applied to attain this goal. This has, in turn, stimulated the development and use of telemetry and telemedicine in both the hospital and home environments." (From a Report on European Patient Monitoring Device Market, 2000, provided by Frost & Sullivan, an international marketing consulting company.). Wireless technology will transform healthcare in many respects (Leopold, this Volume; Walsh, 2000). A bibliography of health care journal articles regarding *Professional and Patient Use of Palm Tops, PDAs, and Hand Helds* was provided by Stoddard, Arizona Health Sciences Library (stoddard@ahsl.arizona.edu).

The benefits of hand-held PC and internet technologies in clinical trials and the care of patients with chronic disease is the subject of an increasing number of publications. At present, we may only speculate about the consequences of such developing information technologies for the health care system and, to some extent, on subsequent developments in applied fields of psychology.

From self-monitoring to self-management

A hand-held PC may be useful in the diagnostic assessment of a variety of behavior disorders, for example, the assessment and self-management of drinking, smoking, and of eating disorders, in facilitating self-management in chronic illness, and moreover in neuropsychological training, in health care of the chronically ill, in patient education, and in behavior therapy:

- relaxation training (Baer & Surman, 1985);
- obesity (Burnett, Taylor & Agras, 1985, 1992);
- hypoglycemia in insulin-dependent diabetes mellitus (Cox et al., 1994; Schvarcz, Palmer, Berne & Bjork, 1991, see Kubiak & Hermanns, this Volume);
- in asthma patients (Osman et al., 1994; Leopold & Schandry, this Volume);
- in ambulatory computer-assisted therapy for anxiety disorder (Newman, Consoli & Taylor, 1999; Newman, Kenardy, Herman & Taylor, 1996).

Computer-programs that are based on a hand-held PC can be used as a component of behavioral therapy: this was the message conveyed by a number of recently published pilot studies. The basic intention of this approach is evident from the following statement by Newman et al. (1999):

"This is the first report of a palmtop computer program developed to increase the efficiency and cost-effectiveness of cognitive behavioral therapy for generalized anxiety disorders (GAD). The computer program offers advantages to researchers, therapists, and clients. These advantages include continuous, unobtrusive collection of data of process data on treatment adherence as well as on the impact of cognitive-behavioral therapy techniques in the client's natural setting. In addition, the computer extends treatment beyond the therapy hour and motivates clients to comply with homework assignments by prompting practice of cognitive behavioral strategies." (p. 597).

The expectation is that the hand-held PCs and the recorder/analyzer for physiological measures will in future become smaller, cheaper and more refined. Further applications can therefore be anticipated. Such developments may include strategies for unrestricted and controlled monitoring, new strategies in interactive monitoring and on-line feedback, monitoring and concurrent recording of audio and video signals (intelligently pre-processed before stored), setting-dependent sampling, new strategies in self-monitoring and self-management in chronic illness. At present, it is hard to conceive to what extent specific expertise systems, and in particular, the wireless application protocol WAP, mobile phone short message systems SMS, and further developments in information technology will direct the course of this methodology.

Acknowledgement
Marcus Cheetham helped to improve the English version of this chapter.

References

Ager, A. & & Bendall, S. (Eds.) (1991). *Microcomputers and clinical psychology: Issues, applications, and future development.* Chichester: John Wiley & Sons.

Albonetti, M.E. et al. (1992). Software multiple review. The Observer: software for behavioral research, version 2.0. *Ethology, Ecology & Evolution, 4,* 401–416.

Amlaner, C.J. & Macdonald, P.W. (Eds.). (1980). *A handbook of biotelemetry and radio tracking.* Oxford: Pergamon Press.

Bachmann, K., Thebis, J., Heynen, H.P. & Graf, N. (1967). Die drahtlose Blutdruckregistrierung unter physiologischen Belastungen. *Verhandlungen der Deutschen Gesellschaft für Kreislauf-Forschung, 33,* 185–188.

Baer, L. & Surman, O.S. (1985). Microcomputer and relaxation. *Perceptual and Motor Skills, 61,* 499–502.

Barry, J., Campbell, S., Nabel, E.G., Mead, K. & Selwyn, A.P. (1987) Ambulatory monitoring of the digitized electrocardiogram for detection and early warning of transient myocardial ischemia in angina pectoris. *American Journal of Cardiology, 60,* 483–488.

Bersoff, D.M. & Bersoff,. D.N. (2000). Ethical issues in the collection of elf-report data. In: A.A. Stonc, J.S. Turkhan, C.A. Bachrach, J.B. Jobe, H.S. Kurtzman and V.S. Cain (Eds.). *The science of self-report. Implications for research and practice (pp. 9–24).* Mahwah N J: Lawrence Erlbaum.

Bevan, A.T., Honour, A.J. & Stott, F.H. (1969). Direct arterial pressure recording in unrestricted man. *Clinical Science, 36,* 329–344.

Brandstätter, H. (1983). Emotional responses for other persons in everyday life situations. *Journal of Personality and Social Psychology, 45,* 871–883.

Brügner, G. (1998). MONITOR: Ein flexibles Programm zur Datenerhebung mittels Pocket-PC. *Zeitschrift für Differentielle und Diagnostische Psychologie, 19,* 145–147.

Burnett, K.F., Taylor, C.B. & Agras, W.S. (1985). Ambulatory computer assisted therapy for obesity: A new frontier for behavior therapy. *Journal of Consulting and Clinical Psychology, 53,* 698–703.

Burnett, K.F., Taylor, C.B. & Agras, W.S. (1992). Ambulatory computer-assisted behavior therapy for obesity: An empirical model for examining behavioral correlates of treatment outcome. *Computers in Human Behavior, 8,* 239–248.

Buse, L. & Pawlik, K. (1994). Differenzierung zwischen Tages-, Setting- und Situationskonsistenz ausgewählter Verhaltensmerkmale, Maßen der Aktivierung, des Befindens und der Stimmung in Alltagssituationen. *Diagnostica, 40,* 2–26.

Buse, L. & Pawlik, K. (1996). Ambulatory behavioral assessment and in-field performances testing. In J. Fahrenberg & M. Myrtek (Eds.). *Ambulatory Assessment: computer-assisted psychological and psychophysiological methods in monitoring and field studies* (pp. 29–50). Seattle, WA: Hogrefe & Huber.

Bussmann, H. (1998). *Ambulatory monitoring of mobility-related activities in rehabilitation medicine.* Delft, The Netherlands: Eburon.

Cattell, R.B. (1957). *Personality and motivation. Structure and measurement.* Yonkers-on-Hudson, NY: World Book Company.

Cicourel, A.V. (1982). Interviews, surveys, and the problem of ecological validity. *American Sociologist,* 17, 11–20.

Cox, D.J., Kovatchev, B.P., Julian, D.M., Gonder-Frederick, L.A., Polonsky, W.H., Schlundt, D.G. & Clarke, W.L. (1994). Frequency of severe hypoglycemia in insulin-dependent diabetes mellitus can be predicted from self-monitoring blood glucose data. *Journal of Clinical Endocrinology and Metabolism, 79,* 1659–1662.

Csikszentmihalyi, M. & Larson, R. (1987). Validity and reliability of the experience-sampling method. *The Journal of Nervous and Mental Disease, 175,* 526–536.

Dal Palù, C. & Pessina, A. (Eds.). (1986). *ISAM 1985.* Padova: Cleup.

Deedwania, P.C. & Nelson, J.R. (1990). Pathophysiology of silent myocardial ischemia during daily life – Hemodynamic evaluation by simultaneous electrocardiographic and blood pressure monitoring. *Circulation, 82,* 1296–1304.

Delespaul, P.A.E.G. (1992). Technical note: devices and time-sampling procedures. In M. de Vries (Ed.), *The experience of psychopathology. Investigating mental disorders in their natural settings* (pp. 363–373). Cambridge: Cambridge University Press.

de Vries, M.W. (Ed.). (1992). *The experience of psychopathology. Investigating mental disorders in their natural settings.* Cambridge: Cambridge University Press.

Elias, M.F. (1984). Handheld computers for recording timed behavior observations. *Ethology and Sociobiology, 5,* 59–60.

Fahrenberg, J. (1987). Extension from the laboratory to the field: On the generalizability of psychophysiological assessments (Abstract). *Psychophysiology, 24,* 569–570.

Fahrenberg, J. (1990). Simultaneous physiological and psychological ambulatory monitoring: Issues in theory and assessment (Abstract). Symposium. Society for Psychophysiological Research. October 1990, Boston. *Psychophysiology, 27,* S10–S11.

Fahrenberg, J. (1996). Concurrent assessment of blood pressure, heart rate, physical activity, and emotional state in natural settings. In J. Fahrenberg & M. Myrtek (Eds.). *Ambulatory Assessment: computer-assisted psychological and psychophysiological methods in monitoring and field studies* (pp. 165–187). Seattle, WA: Hogrefe & Huber.

Fahrenberg, J. (2000). Psychophysiologie und Verhaltenstherapie. In J. Margraf (Ed.), *Lehrbuch der Verhaltenstherapie* (2. Aufl.) (pp. 107–124). Berlin: Springer.

Fahrenberg, J., Foerster, F., Schneider, H.J., Müller, W. & Myrtek, M. (1984). *Aktivierungsforschung im Labor-Feld-Vergleich.* München: Minerva.

Fahrenberg, J., Foerster, F., Schneider, H.J., Müller, W. & Myrtek, M. (1986). Predictability of individual differences in activation processes in a field setting based on laboratory measures. *Psychophysiology, 23,* 323–333.

Fahrenberg, J., Heger, R., Foerster, F. & Müller, W. (1991). Differentielle Psychophysiologie von Befinden, Blutdruck und Herzfrequenz im Labor-Feld-Vergleich. *Zeitschrift für Differentielle und Diagnostische Psychologie, 12,* 1–25.

Fahrenberg, J. & Myrtek, M. (Eds.) (1996). *Ambulatory Assessment: computer-assisted psychological and psychophysiological methods in monitoring and field studies.* Seattle, WA: Hogrefe & Huber.

Fahrenberg, J. & Myrtek, M. (2001). Ambulantes Monitoring und Assessment. In F. Rösler (Ed.), *Enzyklopädie der Psychologie. Serie Biologische Psychologie. Band 4: Grundlagen und Methoden der Psychophysiologie (pp. 657–798).* Göttingen: Hogrefe.

Fahrenberg, J. & Wientjes, C.J.E. (2000). Recording methods in applied environments. In R.W. Backs & W. Boucsein (Eds.), *Engineering psychophysiology: Issues and applications (pp. 111–136).* Mahwah, New Jersey: Lawrence Erlbaum.

Farrell, A.D. (1991). Computers and behavioral assessment: Current applications, future possibilities, and obstacles to routine use. *Behavioral Assessment, 13,* 159–179.

Fenz, W.D. & Epstein, S. (1967).Gradients of physiological arousal in parachutists as a function of an approaching jump. *Psychosomatic Medicine, 29,* 33–51.

Goldstein, G. & Hersen, M. (2000). *Handbook of psychological assessment. (3rd ed.).* Amsterdam: Pergamon-Elsevier

Haynes, S.N. & Horn, W.F. (1983). Reactivity in behavioral observation: A review. *Behavioral Assessment, 4,* 369–385.

Heger, R. (1990a). Apparative Datenerfassung in Feldstudien. *Diagnostica, 36,* 60–80.

Heger, R. (1990b). *Psychophysiologisches 24-Stunden-Monitoring. Methodenentwicklung und erste Ergebnisse eines multimodalen Untersuchungsansatzes bei 62 normotonen und blutdrucklabilen Studenten.* Frankfurt: Lang.

Hile, M.G. (1991). Hand-held behavioral observations: The Observer. *Behavioral Assessment, 13,* 187–196.

Hinman, A.T., Engel, B.T. & Bickford, A.F. (1962). Portable blood pressure recorder: accuracy and preliminary use in evaluating intra-daily variations in pressure. *American Heart Journal, 63,* 663–668.

Holter, N.J. (1961). New methods for heart studies. *Science, 134,* 1214–1220.

Holter, N.J. (1976). Historical background and development of ambulatory monitoring. In N.K. Jacobsen & S.R. Yarnall (Eds.), *Ambulatory ECG Monitoring* (pp. 1–9). Seattle, Washington: MCSA

Hormuth, S.E. (1986). The sampling of experiences in situ. *Journal of Personality, 54,* 262–293.

Hurlburt, R.T. (1979). Random sampling of cognitions and behavior. *Journal of Research in Personality, 13,* 103–111.

Imholz, B.P.M., Langewouters, G.J., van Montfrans, G.A., Parati, G., van Goudoever, J., Wesseling, K.H., Wieling, W. & Mancia, G.(1993). Feasibility of ambulatory, continuous 24-hour finger arterial pressure recording. *Hypertension, 21,* 65–73.

Jain, A., Martens, W.L.J., Mutz, G., Weiß, R.K. & Stephan, E. (1996). Towards a comprehensive technology for recording and analysis of multiple physiological parameters within their behavioral and environmental context. In J. Fahrenberg & M. Myrtek (Eds.). *Ambulatory Assessment: computer-assisted psychological and psychophysiological methods in monitoring and field studies* (pp. 215–235). Seattle, WA: Hogrefe & Huber.

Jain, A., Mutz, G. & Mucha, R.F. (1992). Emopad: A device to collect useful background data for psychophysiological recordings in the field (Abstract). *Journal of Psychophysiology, 6,* 358.

Käppler, C. (1994). *Psychophysiologische Bedingungsanalyse von Blutdruckveränderungen im alltäglichen Lebenskontext.* Frankfurt a.M.: Lang.

Kamarck, T.W., Shiffman, S.M, Smithline, L., Goodie, J.L, Thompson, H.S, Ituarte, P.H.G, Jong, J., Yi-Kuan, Pro, V., Paty, J.A, Kassel, J. D, Gnys, M. and Perz, W. (1998). The diary of ambulatory behavioral states: A new approach to the assessment of psychosocial influences on ambulatory cardiovascular activity. In S. Krantz & A. Baum (Eds.), *Technology and methods in behavioral medicine* (pp. 163–193). Mahwah, NJ: Lawrence Erlbaum.

Kerlinger, F.N. & Lee, H.B. (2000). *Foundations of behavioral reseach*: Forth Worth TX: Harcourt.

Kinne, G. & Droste, C. (1996).Psychophysiological monitoring of transient ischaemic states in patients with coronary heart disease. In J. Fahrenberg & M. Myrtek (Eds.). *Ambulatory Assessment: computer-assisted psychological and psychophysiological methods in monitoring and field studies* (pp. 347–363). Seattle, WA: Hogrefe & Huber.

Kinne, G., Droste, C., Fahrenberg, J. & Roskamm, H. (1999). Symptomatic myocardial ischaemia (heart pain) is linked to the psychological context in daily life. Implications for a clinical use of interactive monitoring. *Journal of Psychosomatic Research*, 46, 369–377.

Kiparski, R. v. & Massmann, W. (1982). Die digitale Speicherung als neues Verfahren zur Aufzeichnung von Beanspruchungsprofilen am Arbeitsplatz. *Zeitschrift für Arbeitswissenschaft, 36,* 77–82.

Kiparski, R. v. & Steffens, H. P. (1985). Möglichkeiten der drahtlosen Biosignalerfassung mittels digitaler Speicherung. *Biomedizinische Technik, 30,* 76–84.

Krüger, H.-P. & Vollrath, M. (1996). Temporal analysis of speech patterns in the real world using the LOGOPORT. In J. Fahrenberg & M. Myrtek (Eds.). *Ambulatory Assessment: computer-assisted psychological and psychophysiological methods in monitoring and field studies* (pp. 101–113). Seattle, WA: Hogrefe & Huber.

Kunz, B., Mertens, K. & Oeste, B. (1980). A portable microprocessor based system for long-term simultaneous registration of several physiological data. In F.D. Stott, E.B. Raftery & L. Goulding (Eds.), *ISAM 1979* (pp. 487–491). London: Academic Press.

Kunz, B., Mertens, K. & Oeste, B. (1982a). Near sensor reduction of physiological data by use of a portable microprocessor-system. In F.D. Stott, E.B. Raftery, D.L. Clement & S.L. Wright (Eds.), *ISAM-Gent-1981. Proceedings of the Fourth International Symposium on Ambulatory Monitoring* (pp. 464–468). London: Academic Press.

Kunz, B., Mertens, K. & Oeste, B. (1982b). *Multifaktorielles Meßsystem zur kontinuierlichen Langzeiterfassung physiologischer Daten am Arbeitsplatz. Arbeitsbericht.* Oberpfaffenhofen: Deutsche Forschungs- und Versuchsanstalt für Luft- und Raumfahrt e.V. (DFVLR), Institut für Nachrichtentechnik.

Lang, E., Ostermeier, M., Forster, C. & Handwerker, H.O. (1991). Die Rating-Box – ein neues Gerät zur ambulanten Erfassung von subjektiven Variablen. *Biomedizinische Technik, 36,* 210–212.

Lewis, B., Lewis, D. & Cumming, G. (1995). Frequent measurement of chronic pain: An electronic diary and empirical findings. *Pain, 60,* 341–347.

Littler, W.A. (Ed.). (1980). *Clinical and ambulatory monitoring.* London: Chapman & Hall.

Mertesdorf, F. (1980). Mobile Datenerfassungsgeräte als Registrierungshilfen bei der Beobachtung von (nonverbalem) Verhalten. *Gruppendynamik, 11,* 328–343.

Meyer-Sabellek, W. & Gotzen, R. (Eds.). (1988). *Indirekte 24-Stunden-Blutdruckmessung* (S. 71–87). Darmstadt: Steinkopff.

Miles, L.E. & Broughton, R.J. (Eds.). (1990). Medical monitoring in the home and work environment. New York: Raven Press.

Miles, L.E. & Rule, R.B. (1982). Long term monitoring of multiple physiological parameters using a programmable portable microcomputer. In F.D. Stott, E.B. Raftery, D.L. Clement & S.L. Wright (Eds.), *ISAM-Gent 1981* (pp. 249–257). London: Academic Press.

Myrtek, M., Brügner, G., Fichtler, A., König, K., Müller, W., Foerster, F. & Höppner, V. (1988). Detection of emotionally induced ECG changes and their behavioral correlates: A new method for ambulatory monitoring. *European Heart Journal, 9* (Supplement N), 55–60.

Myrtek, M., Brügner, G. & Müller, W. (1996). Interactive monitoring and contingency analysis of emotionally induced ECG changes: Methodology and applications. In J. Fahrenberg & M. Myrtek (Eds.). *Ambulatory Assessment: computer-assisted psychological and psychophysiological methods in monitoring and field studies* (pp. 115–127). Seattle, WA: Hogrefe & Huber.

Myrtek, M., Fichtler, A., König, K., Brügner, G. & Müller, W. (1994). Differences between patients with asymptomatic and symptomatic myocardial infarction: The relevance of psychological factors. *European Heart Journal, 15,* 311–317.

Newman, M.G., Consoli, A. & Taylor, C.B. (1999). A palmtop computer program for the treatment of generalized anxiety disorder. *Behavior Modification, 23*, 597–619.

Newman, M.G., Kenardy, J., Herman, S. & Taylor, C.B. (1996). The use of hand-held computers as an adjunct to cognitive-behavior therapy. *Computers in Human Behavior, 12,* 135–143.

Noldus, L.P.J.J. (1991). The Observer: A software system for collection and analysis of observational data. *Behavior, Research Methods, Instruments & Computers, 23,* 415–429.

Noldus Information Technology (Ed.). (1995). *Base Package for Windows. Reference Manual.* Groningen: Author.

O'Brien, E. & Fitzgerald, D. (1991). The history of indirect blood pressure measurement. In E.O'Brien & K.O. Malley (Eds.). *Blood pressure measurement. Handbook of hypertension. Vol. 14.* Amsterdam: Elsevier.

Osman, L.M., Abdalla, M.I., Beattie, J.A.G., Ross, S.J., Russell, I.T., Friend, J.A., Legge, J.S. and Douglas, J.G. (1994). Reducing hospital admission through computer supported education for asthma patients. *British Medical Journal,* 308, 568–571.

Patry, J.L. (Ed.) (1982). *Feldforschung. Methoden und Probleme sozialwissenschaftlicher Forschung unter natürlichen Bedingungen.* Bern: Huber.

Pawlik, K. (1996). Contributions to differential psychology from ambulatory assessment: A researcher's plaidoyer. In J. Fahrenberg & M. Myrtek (Eds.). *Ambulatory Assessment: computer-assisted psychological and psychophysiological methods in monitoring and field studies* (pp. 21–25). Seattle, WA: Hogrefe & Huber.

Pawlik, K. (1988). "Naturalistische" Daten für Psychodiagnostik: Zur Methodik psychodiagnostischer Felderhebungen. *Zeitschrift für Differentielle und Diagnostische Psychologie, 9,* 169–181.

Pawlik, K. & Buse, L. (1982). Rechnergestützte Verhaltensregistrierung im Feld: Beschreibung und erste psychometrische Überprüfung einer neuen Erhebungsmethode. *Zeitschrift für Differentielle und Diagnostische Psychologie, 3,* 101–118.

Pawlik, K. & Buse, L. (1996). Verhaltensbeobachtung in Labor und Feld. In K. Pawlik (Ed.), *Enzyklopädie der Psychologie. Differentielle Psychologie und Persönlichkeitsforschung. Band 1. Grundlagen und Methoden der Differentiellen Psychologie* (S. 359–394). Göttingen: Hogrefe.

Perkonigg, A., Baumann, U., Reicherts, M. & Perrez, M.(1993). Soziale Unterstützung und Belastungsverarbeitung: Eine Untersuchung mit computergestützter Selbstbeobachtung. In A. Laireiter (Ed.). *Soziales Netzwerk und soziale Unterstützung* (S. 128–153). Bern: Huber.

Perrez, M. (1994). Felddiagnostik mit besonderer Berücksichtigung der computerunterstützten Diagnostik. In R.D. Stieglitz & U. Baumann (Eds.), *Psychodiagnostik bei psychischen Störungen* (pp. 149–161). Stuttgart: Enke.

Perrez, M. & Reicherts, M. (1989). Belastungsverarbeitung: Computerunterstützte Selbstbeobachtung im Feld. *Zeitschrift für Differentielle und Diagnostische Psychologie, 10,* 129–139.

Pickering, T.G. (1991). *Ambulatory monitoring and blood pressure variability.* London: Science Press.

Pickering, T. (1992). Ambulatory blood pressure monitoring: An historical perspective. *Clinical Cardiology, 15 (Suppl I),* II–3–II–5.

Rau, R. & Triemer, A. (1999). Instrumente der Arbeits- und Organisationspsychologie. *Zeitschrift für Arbeits- und Organisationspsychologie, 43,* 226–231.
Roth, W.T., Breivik, G., Jørgensen, P.E. & Hofmann, S. (1996). Activation in novice and expert parachutists while jumping. *Psychophysiology, 33,* 63–72.
Roth, W.T., Tinklenberg, J.R., Doyle, C.M., Horvath, T.B. & Kopell, B.S. (1976). Mood states and 24-hour cardiac monitoring. *Journal of Psychosomatic Research, 20,* 179–186.
Rugh, J.D., Gable, R.S. & Lemke, R.R. (1986). Instrumentation for behavioral assessment. In A.R. Ciminero, K.S. Calhoun & H.E. Adams (Eds.), *Handbook of behavioral assessment* (2nd ed.) (pp. 79–108). New York: Wiley.
Schmidt, T.H. & Jain, A. (1996). Continuous assessment of finger blood pressure and other haemodynamic and behavioral variables in everyday life. In J. Fahrenberg & M. Myrtek (Eds.). *Ambulatory Assessment: computer-assisted psychological and psychophysiological methods in monitoring and field studies* (pp. 189–213). Seattle, WA: Hogrefe & Huber.
Schneider, R.A. (1968). A fully automated portable blood pressure recorder. *Journal of Applied Physiology, 24,* 115–119.
Schneiderman, N., Weiss, S.M. & Kaufmann, P.G. (Eds.). (1989). *Handbook of research methods in cardiovascular medicine.* New York: Plenum.
Schvarcz, E., Palmer, M., Berne, C. & Bjork, E. (1991). Incidence of symptomatic mild hypoglycaemic events: a prospective study in adult patients with insulin-treated diabetes mellitus using a portable microcomputer-based data-logger. *Diabetes-Research, 16,* 25–28.
Schuler, H. (1982). Ethische Probleme. In J.L. Patry (Ed.), Feldforschung (pp 341–364). Bern: Huber.
Schwarz, J.E. & Stone, A.A. (1998). Strategies for analyzing ecological momentary assessment data. *Health Psychology, 17,* 6–16.
Shiffman, S. (2000). Real-time self-report of momentary states in the natural environment: Computerized ecological momentary assessment. In: A.A. Stone, J.S. Turkhan, C.A. Bachrach, J.B. Jobe, H.S. Kurtzman and V.S. Cain (Eds.). *The science of self-report. Implications for research and practice (pp. 277–296).* Mahwah N J: Lawrence Erlbaum.
Shiffman, S., Fischer, L.A., Paty, J.A., Gnys, M., Hickcox, M. & Kassel, J. D. (1994). Drinking and smoking: A field study of their association. *Annals of Behavioral Medicine, 16,* 203–209.
Sidowski, J.B. (Ed.). (1977). Special report section observational research methods: Portable event recording systems. *Behavior Research Methods & Instrumentation, 9,* 403–455.
Smith, W.B. & Safer, M.A. (1993). Effects of present pain level on recall of chronic pain and medication use. *Pain, 55,* 355–361.
Sokolow, M., Werdegar, D., Perloff, D.B., Cowan, R.M. & Brenenstuhl, H. (1970). Preliminary studies relating portably recorded blood pressure to daily life events in patients with essential hypertension. In M. Koster, H. Musaph & P. Visser (Eds.), *Psychosomatics in essential hypertension* (pp. 164–189). Basel: Karger.
Stemmler, G. (1996). Strategies and designs in ambulatory assessment. In J. Fahrenberg & M. Myrtek (Eds.), *Ambulatory Assessment: computer-assisted psychological and psychophysiological methods in monitoring and field studies* (pp. 257–268). Seattle, WA: Hogrefe & Huber.
Stephan, E., Mutz, G., Langer, S., Schmitz, D. & Wemschulte, B. (1989). A portable microprocesssor-controlled psychophysiological data-acquisition-system. *Journal of Psychophysiology, 3,* 338.
Stern, E. (1986). *Reaktivitätseffekte in Untersuchungen zur Selbstprotokollierung des Verhaltens im Feld.* Frankfurt: Lang.
Stott, F.D. (1976). Proceedings of the International Symposium on Ambulatory Monitoring ISAM 1975. *Postgraduate Medical Journal, 52* (Suppl. 7)
Stott, F.D. (1982). Ambulatory monitoring. *Journal of Physics. E: Scientific Instruments, 15,* 619–626.
Stott, F.D., Raftery, E.B., Clement, D.L. & Wright, S. L. (1982). *ISAM – Gent – 1981.* London: Academic Press.
Stott, F.D., Raftery, E.B., Sleight, P. & Goulding, L. (1978). *ISAM 1977.* London: Academic Press.
Suen, H.K. & Ary, D. (1989). *Analyzing quantitative behavioral observational data.* Hillsdale, N.J.: Lawrence Erlbaum.

Suls, J. & Martin, R.E. (1993). Daily recording and ambulatory monitoring methodologies in behavioral medicine. *Annals of Behavioral Medicine, 15*, 3–7.

Taylor, C.B., Fried, L. & Kenardy, J. (1990). The use of a real-time computer diary for data acquisition and processing. *Behaviour Research and Therapy, 28,* 93–97.

Taylor, C.B., Kraemer, H.C., Bragg, D.A., Miles, L.E., Rule, B., Savin, W.M. & DeBusk, R.F. (1982). A new system for long-term recording and processing of heart rate and physical activity in outpatients. *Computers and Biomedical Research, 15,* 7–17.

Torgerson, L. (1977). Datamyte 900. *Behavior Research Methods and Instrumentation, 9,* 405–406.

Totterdell, P., Briner, R.B., Parkinson, B. & Reynolds, S. (1996). Fingerprinting time series: Dynamic patterns in self-report and performance measures uncovered by a graphical non-linear method. *British Journal of Psychology, 87,* 43–60.

Totterdell, P. & Folkard, S. (1992). In situ repeated measures of affect and cognitive performance facilitated by use of a hand-held computer. *Behavior Research Methods, Instruments & Computers, 24,* 545–553.

Totterdell, P., Spelten, E., Smith, L., Barton, J. and Folkard, S. (1995). Recovery from work shifts: how long does it take?. *Journal of Applied Psychology. 80,*43–57.

Turpin, G. (1985). Ambulatory psychophysiological monitoring: techniques and applications. In: D. Papakostopoulos, S. Butler & I. Martin (Eds.), *Clinical and experimental neuropsychophysiology* (pp. 695–728). London: Croom Helm.

Turpin, G. (1999). Book review: "Ambulatory Assessment: Computer-assisted psychological and psychophysiological measures in monitoring and field studies". *Journal of Psychophysiology, 13,* 58–60.

Turpin, G. (1990). Ambulatory clinical psychophysiology: an introduction to techniques and methodological issues. *Journal of Psychophysiology, 4,* 299–304.

Van Egeren, L..F. & Madarasmi, S. (1988). A computer-assisted diary (CAD) for ambulatory blood pressure monitoring. *American Journal of Hypertension, 1,* 179S–185S.

Walsh, P.J. (2000). Wireless technology transforms healthcare delivery and tracking. *MD computing: computers in medical practice. 17*, 45–48.

Wesseling, K.H., Settels, J.J. & de Wit, B. (1986). The measurement of continuous finger arterial pressure noninvasively in stationary subjects. In T.H. Schmidt, T.M. Dembroski & G. Blümchen (Eds.). *Biological and psychological factors in cardiovascular disease* (pp. 355–376). Berlin. Springer.

Wilz, G. & Bröhler, E. (Ed.) (1997). *Tagebücher in Therapie und Forschung. Ein anwendungsorientierter Leitfaden.* Göttingen: Hogrefe.

Subject Index

List of Contributors

Alfer, Dirk, Dipl. Psych.
Psychologisches Institut, Universität Köln, Herbert-Lewin-Str. 2, D-50931 Köln, Germany

Alpers, Georg W., Dipl. Psych.
Department of Psychiatry and Behavioral Sciences, Stanford University, PAVAHCS (116F-PAD), 3801 Miranda Avenue, Palo Alto, CA 94304-1207, USA
alpers@stanford.edu

Aschenbrenner, Eveline, Dipl. Psych.
Forschungsgruppe Psychophysiologie, University of Freiburg, Belfortstrasse 20, D-79085 Freiburg, Germany

Bazański, Jan, Dr.
National Aerospace Laboratory, NLR Man-Machine Integration & Human Factors Research P.O. Box 90502, 1006 BM Amsterdam, The Netherlands

Baumann, Urs, Prof. Dr.
Institut für Psychologie, Universität Salzburg, Hellbrunnerstrasse 34, A-5020 Salzburg, Austria
urs.baumann@sbg.ac.at

Berndt, Andre
Institut und Poliklinik für Arbeits- u. Sozialmedizin, Med. Fakultät TU Dresden, Fetscherstr. 74,
D-01307 Dresden, Germany

Bohus, Martin, Dr.
Department of Psychiatry, University of Freiburg, Hauptstrasse5, D-79085 Freiburg, Germany

Boucsein, Wolfram, Prof. Dr.
Physiologische Psychologie, University of Wuppertal, D-42119 Wuppertal, Germany
boucsein@uni-wuppertal.de

Buse, Lothar, Prof. Dr.
Psychologisches Institut I, Universität Hamburg, Von-Melle-Park 11, D-20146 Hamburg, Germany
buse@uni-hamburg.de

Bussmann, J.B.J., Ph.D.
Department of Rehabilitation, University Hospital Rotterdam, PO Box 2040, NL-3000 CA Rotterdam, The Netherlands
bussmann@revd.azr.nl

Cavelaars, Marinel
Erasmus Medical Center Rotterdam, Department of Internal Medicine, room L253, Dr. Molewaterplein 40, NL-3015 GD Rotterdam, The Netherlands
marinel@mediaport.org

de Geus, Eco, Ph.D.
Department of Biological Psychology, Vrije Universiteit, Van der Boechorststraat 1, NL-1081 BT, Amsterdam, The Netherlands
Eco@psy.vu.nl

Dekkers, Caroline
Department of Health Psychology, Utrecht University, PO Box 80 140, NL-3508 TC Utrecht, The Netherlands
C.Dekkers@FSS.UU.NL

Fahrenberg, Jochen, Prof. Dr.
Forschungsgruppe Psychophysiologie, University of Freiburg, Belfortstrasse 20, D-79085 Freiburg, Germany
fahrenbe@psychologie.uni-freiburg.de

Feichtinger, Ludwig, Dr.
Institut für Psychologie, Universität Salzburg, Hellbrunnerstrasse 34, A-5020 Salzburg, Austria
ludwig.feichtinger@sbg.ac.at

Feist, Ansgar, Dr.
Psychologisches Institut, Universität Köln, Herbert-Lewin-Str. 2, D-50931 Köln, Germany
Ansgar.eist@uni-koeln.de

Fischer, Joachim
Swiss Federal Institute of Technology, Department of Behavioral Sciences, Turnerstrasse 1, CH-8092, Zurich, Switzerland

Foerster, Friedrich, Dipl. Math.
Forschungsgruppe Psychophysiologie, University of Freiburg, Belfortstrasse 20, D-79085 Freiburg, Germany
foerster@uni-freiburg.de

Freedman, Robert R., Prof. Ph.D.
Wayne State University School of Medicine, Behavioral Medical Lab, C.S. Mott Ctr, 275 E. Hancock Ave, Detroit, MI 48201, USA
aa2613@wayne.edu

Fricke, Leonie, Dipl. Psych.
Psychologisches Institut, Universität Köln, Herbert-Lewin-Str. 2, D-50931 Köln, Germany

Geenen, Rinie
Department of Health Psychology, Utrecht University, PO Box 80 140, NL-3508 TC Utrecht, The Netherlands
R.Geenen@FSS.UU.NL

Godaert, Guido L.R., Dr.
Department of Health Psychology, Utrecht University, PO Box 80 140, NL-3508 TC Utrecht, The Netherlands
G.Godaert@FSS.UU.NL

Grathwol, Tanja, Dipl. Psych.
Michael-Balint-Klinik, D-78126 Königsfeld, Germany

Groeneveld, Wim
Erasmus Medical Center Rotterdam, Department of Biomedical Physics and Technology, P.O.Box 1738, NL-300 DR Rotterdam, The Netherlands

Fischer, Joachim, Dr.
Swiss Federal Institute of Technology, Department of Behavioral Sciences, Turnerstrasse 1, CH-8092, Zurich, Switzerland

Häseli, Alexandra, Dipl. Natw. ETH
Swiss Federal Institute of Technology, Department of Behavioral Sciences, Turnerstrasse 1, CH-8092, Zurich, Switzerland

Hank, Petra, Dr.
Fachbereich Psychologie, Universität Trier, D-54286 Trier, Germany
hank@uni-trier.de

Hanson, Eamonn, Dr.
National Aerospace Laboratory, NLR Man-Machine Integration & Human Factors Research P.O. Box 90502, 1006 BM Amsterdam, The Netherlands
hanson@nlr.nl

Hermanns, Norbert, Dr.
Forschungsinstitut der Diabetes-Akademie Mergentheim, Diabetes Zentrum Mergentheim, Th.-Klotzbücher-Strasse 12, D-97980 Bad Mergentheim, Germany
hermanns@diabetes-zentrum.de

Hinkel, Michael, Dipl. Psych.
Vogelsangstr. 12, D-53498 Goennersdorf, Germany
Michael.Hinkel@web.de

Horner, Monique
Psychologisches Institut, Universität Fribourg, Rue de Faucigny 2 CH-1701, Switzerland
Monique.Horner@unifr.ch

Hufford, Michael R., Dr.
invivodata, inc., 2100 Wharton St., Ste. 505, Pittsburgh, PA 15203, USA
mhufford@invivodata.com

Hüttner, Paul, Dipl. Phys.
Forschungsgruppe Psychophysiologie, University of Freiburg, Belfortstrasse 20, D-79085 Freiburg, Germany
huettner@psychologie.uni-freiburg.de

Käppler, Christoph, Dr.
Departemento de Psicologia, Universidade Federal de Minas Gerais, Belo Horizonte, Brazil, and Department of Psychology, University of Freiburg, Belfortstrasse18, D-79085 Freiburg, Germany
kaeppler@hotmail.com

Kastner, Michael, Prof. Dr. Dr.
Universität Dortmund, FB 14, Organisationspsychologie, Emil-Figge-Straße 50, D-44227 Dortmund, Germany
iapam@t-online.de

Knöpfel, Dieter, Dipl. Ing.
Institut und Poliklinik für Arbeits- u. Sozialmedizin, Med. Fakultät TU Dresden, Fetscherstr. 74,
D-01307 Dresden, Germany

Kubiak, Thomas, Dipl. Psych.
Forschungsinstitut der Diabetes-Akademie Mergentheim, Diabetes Zentrum Mergentheim, Th.-Klotzbücher-Strasse 12, D-97980 Bad Mergentheim, Germany
kubiak@diabetes-zentrum.de

Leonhart, Rainer
Forschungsgruppe Psychophysiologie, University of Freiburg, Belfortstrasse 20, D-79085 Freiburg, Germany
leonhart@psychologie.uni-freiburg.de

Leopold, Christian, Dr.
Nets Healthcare GmbH, Bayerstrasse 89, D-80335 Munich, Germany
christian.leopold@nets-ag.de

Meuret, Alicia E., Dipl. Psych.
Department of Psychiatry and Behavioral Sciences, Stanford University, PAVAHCS (116F-PAD), 3801 Miranda Avenue, Palo Alto, CA 94304-1207, USA
alpers@stanford.edu

Mühlensiep, Markus, Dipl. Psych.
Psychologisches Institut, Universität Köln, Herbert-Lewin-Str. 2, D-50931 Köln, Germany

Mussgay, Lutz, Dr.
Psychosomatische Fachklinik St.-Franziska-Stift, Franziska-Puricelli-Straße 3, D-55543 Bad Kreuznach, Germany
mussgay@t-online.de

Mutz, Gerhard, Dipl. Psych.,
Psychologisches Institut, Universität Köln, Herbert-Lewin-Str. 2, D-50931 Köln, Germany
gerhard.mutz@uni-koeln.de

Myrtek, Michael. Prof. Dr.
Forschungsgruppe Psychophysiologie, University of Freiburg, Belfortstrasse 20, D-79085 Freiburg, Germany
myrtek@psychologie.uni-freiburg.de

Niegot, Frithjof, Dipl. Psych.
Psychosomatische Fachklinik St.-Franziska-Stift, Franziska-Puricelli-Straße 3, D-55543 Bad Kreuznach, Germany
St-Franziska-Stift@t-online.de

Ott, Ralf, Dipl. Psych.,
100world Institute, Nuremberg, Germany,
ralf.ott@100world.com.de

Paty, Jean, Dr.
invivodata, inc., 2100 Wharton St., Ste. 505, Pittsburgh, PA 15203, USA
jean@ invivodata.com

Pawlik, Kurt, Prof. Dr.
Psychologisches Institut I, Universität Hamburg, Von-Melle-Park 11, D-20146 Hamburg, Germany
pawlik@uni-hamburg.de,

Perrez Meinrad, Prof. Dr.
Psychologisches Institut, Universität Fribourg, Rue de Faucigny 2 CH-1701, Switzerland
Meinrad.Perrez@unifr.ch

Peters, Madelon, Dr.
Department of Medical, Clinical and Experimental Psychology, Maastricht University, The Netherlands
Madelon.Peters@Dep.Unimaas.NL

Rau, Renate, Dr.
Institut für Arbeits-, Organisations- u. Sozialpsychologie, TU Dresden, Mommsenstr. 13, D-01069 Dresden, Germany
rau@psy1.psych.tu-dresden.de

Rieder, Stephan, Dipl. Psych.
Department of Psychology, University of Freiburg, Belfortstrasse18, D-79085 Freiburg, Germany
Rieder.as@t-online.de

Riese, Harriëtte, Ph.D.
Department of Biological Psychology Vrije Universiteit, Van der Boechorststraat 1, NL-1081 BT Amsterdam, The Netherlands
h.riese@psy.vu.nl

Roth, Walton T., Prof.
Veterans Administration Palo Alto Health Care System (116F-PAD),
3801 Miranda Avenue, Palo Alto, CA 94304-1207, USA
wtroth@stanford.edu

Rüddel, Heinz, Prof. Dr.
Psychosomatische Fachklinik St.-Franziska-Stift, Franziska-Puricelli-Straße 3, D-55543 Bad Kreuznach, Germany
St-Franziska-Stift@t-online.de

Schaefer, Florian, Dr.
Physiologische Psychologie, University of Wuppertal, D-42119 Wuppertal, Germany
schaefe2@uni-wuppertal.de

Schandry, Rainer, Prof. Dr.
Institut für Psychologie, Klinische Psychologie, Universität München, Leopoldstr. 13, D-80802 München, Germany
schandry@psy.uni-muenchen.de

Scheuch, Klaus, Prof. Dr.
Institut und Poliklinik für Arbeits- u. Sozialmedizin, Med. Fakultät TU Dresden, Fetscherstr. 74,
D-01307 Dresden, Germany
Klaus.Scheuch@mailbox.tu-dresden.de

Schoebi, Dominik
Psychologisches Institut, Universität Fribourg, Rue de Faucigny 2 CH-1701, Switzerland
Dominik.Schoebi@unifr.ch

Scholz, O. Berndt, Prof. Dr.
Klin. und Angew. Psychologie, Psychologisches Institut der Universität Bonn,Römersstraße 164, D-53117 Bonn, Germany
o.berndt.scholz@uni-bonn.de

Schuman, Jens
Fachbereich Psychologie, Universität Trier, D-54286 Trier

Schwenkmezger, Peter, Prof. Dr.
Fachbereich Psychologie, Universität Trier, D-54286 Trier
schwenkm@uni-trier.de

Seibt, Reingard, Dr.
Institut und Poliklinik für Arbeits- u. Sozialmedizin, Med. Fakultät TU Dresden, Fetscherstr. 74,
D-01307 Dresden, Germany
Reingard.Seibt@mailbox.tu-dresden.de

Shiffman, Saul, Ph.D.
University of Pittsburgh, Department of Psychology, Pittsburgh PA 15260, USA, invivodata, inc., Scientific Affairs, 2100 Wharton St., Ste. 505, Pittsburgh, PA 15203, USA
shiffman@pitt.edu

Sieb, Jörn P., Dr.
Max-Planck-Institut für Psychiatrie, Kraepelinstrasse 10, D-80804 München, Germany
sieb@mpipsykl.mpg.de

Sommer, Thorsten, Dipl. Psych.
Physiologische Psychologie, University of Wuppertal, D-42119 Wuppertal, Germany

Sorbi, Marjolijn, Dr.
Department of Health Psychology, Utrecht University, PO Box 80 140, NL-3508 TC Utrecht, The Netherlands
m.sorbi@fss.uu.nl

Stam, Henk J., Dr.
Department of Rehabilitation, PO Box 2040, NL-3000 CA Rotterdam, The Netherlands

Stephan, Egon, Prof. Dr.
Psychologisches Institut, Universität Köln, Herbert-Lewin-Str. 2, D-50931 Köln, Germany
Egon.stephan@uni-koeln.de

Steptoe, Andrew, Prof. Dr.
Department of Epidemiology and Public Health, 1-19 Torrington Place, University College London, London WC1E 6BT, UK
a.steptoe@ucl.ac.uk

Stiglmayr, Christian, Dipl. Psych.
Institut für Klinische Psychologie, Freie Universität, Habelschwerdter Allee 45, D-14195 Berlin, Germany
Christian_Stiglmayr@web.de

Stone, Arthur, Prof. Dr.
Department of Psychiatry, Putnam Hall, State University of New York, Stony Brook New York,
NY 11794-8790, USA
Arthur.Stone@sunysb.edu

Stronks, Dirk
Erasmus Medical Center Rotterdam, Departments of Psychiatry and Medical Psychology and Psychotherapy, Dr. Molewaterplein 40, NL-3015 GD Rotterdam, The Netherlands

Thiele, Claudia, Dr.
Institut für Eriehungswissenschaften, Universität Salzburg, Akademiestrasse 26, A-5020 Salzburg, Austria
claudia.thiele@sbg.ac.at

Tulen, Joke H. M., Ph.D.
Erasmus Medical Center Rotterdam, Departments of Psychiatry and Medical Psychology and Psychotherapy, Dr. Molewaterplein 40, NL-3015 GD Rotterdam, The Netherlands
tulen@psy.fgg.eur.nl

van den Berg-Emons, Hendrika J. G., Dr.
Department of Rehabilitation, PO Box 2040, NL-3000 CA Rotterdam, The Netherlands

Vogt, Joachim, Dr.
Universität Dortmund, FB 14, Organisationspsychologie, Emil-Figge-Strasse 50, D-44227 Dortmund, Germany
vogt@orgapsy.uni-dortmund.de

Volkers, Anita
Erasmus Medical Center Rotterdam, Departments of Psychiatry and Medical Psychology and Psychotherapy, Dr. Molewaterplein 40, NL-3015 GD Rotterdam, The Netherlands

Vrijkotte, Tanja G. M., MS
Department of Biological Psychology Vrije Universiteit, Van der Boechorststraat 1, NL-1081 BT Amsterdam, The Netherlands
tgm.vrijkotte@psy.vu.nl

Weiss, Rolf K., Dr.
Psychologisches Institut, Universität Köln, Herbert-Lewin-Str. 2, D-50931 Köln, Germany

Wilhelm, Frank H., Dr.
Department of Psychiatry and Behavioral Sciences, Stanford University, PAVAHCS (116F-PAD), 3801 Miranda Avenue, Palo Alto, CA 94304-1207, USA
fwilhelm@stanford.edu
Wilhelm, Peter, Dipl. Psych.
Psychologisches Institut, Universität Fribourg, Rue de Faucigny 2 CH-1701, Switzerland
Peter.Wilhelm@unifr.ch

Wilson, Glenn F., Ph.D.
Air Force Research Laboratory, AFRL/HECP, 2255 H Street, Wright-Patterson Air Force Base, OH 45433-7022, USA
Glenn.Wilson@wpafb.af.mil

Zanda, Denis, Dipl. Psych.
Forschungsgruppe Psychophysiologie, University of Freiburg, Belfortstrasse 20, D-79085 Freiburg, Germany

Zeier, Hans, Prof. Dr.
Swiss Federal Institute of Technology, Department of Behavioral Sciences, Turnerstrasse 1, CH-8092, Zurich, Switzerland
Zeier@ifv.gess.ethz.ch